DATE DUE

Demco, Inc. 38-293

Surgical Pathology of the Female Reproductive System and Peritoneum

Surgical Pathology of the Female Reproductive System and Peritoneum

Editors

Stephen S. Sternberg
Attending Pathologist, Memorial Hospital
Memorial Sloan-Kettering Cancer Center
New York, New York

Stacey E. Mills
Associate Professor of Pathology
Division of Surgical Pathology
University of Virginia Medical Center
Charlottesville, Virginia

Contributors

Geoffrey Altshuler
Philip B. Clement
Christopher P. Crum
Henry F. Frierson, Jr.
Michael R. Hendrickson

Richard L. Kempson
Robert J. Kurman
Michael T. Mazur
Gerard Nuovo
Robert E. Scully

Robert H. Young

Raven Press New York

Raven Press, 1185 Avenue of the Americas, New York, New York 10036

Printed in Hong Kong

Library of Congress Cataloging-in-Publication Data

Surgical pathology of the female reproductive system and peritoneum/
    editors, Stephen S. Sternberg, Stacy E. Mills; contributors,
    Geoffrey Altshuler . . . [et al.].
        p.   cm.
    "Reprinted from the much larger Raven Press book. Diagnostic
surgical pathology, edited by Stephen S. Sternberg . . . [et al.]"—
Pref.
    Includes bibliographical references.
    Includes index.
    ISBN 0-88167-726-4
    1. Generative organs, Female—Diseases—Histopathology.
2. Peritoneum—Diseases—Histopathology.   3. Pathology, Surgical.
4. Pathology, Gynecological.   I. Sternberg, Stephen S.   II. Mills,
Stacey E.   III. Altshuler, Geoffrey.   IV. Diagnostic surgical
pathology.
    [DNLM: 1. Genital Diseases, Female—diagnosis.   2. Genital
Diseases, Female—pathology.   3. Peritoneum—pathology.   WP 141
S961]
RG77.S87   1991
618.1'07—dc20
DNLM/DLC
for Library of Congress   90-8902
                                                              CIP

9 8 7 6 5 4 3 2 1

Preface

Surgical Pathology of the Female Reproductive System and Peritoneum is reprinted from the much larger Raven Press book, *Diagnostic Surgical Pathology,* edited by Stephen S. Sternberg, Donald A. Antonioli, Darryl Carter, the late Joseph C. Eggleston, Stacy E. Mills, and Harold A. Oberman. It focuses on practical diagnostic decisions in gynecologic pathology and emphasizes problems having important clinical implications. We believe that this book will be of value to pathologists in training and practice who want a comprehensive review of gynecologic pathology but have elected not to purchase *Diagnostic Surgical Pathology.* We especially believe that gynecologists and other clinicians involved in the care of the female patient will find this text of value. Gynecologists have, by tradition and, perhaps, necessity, been interested and well versed in the varied pathology of the female genital tract. Their typically frequent interactions with pathologists result in optimal patient management and should serve as a model to other, less "pathologically inclined" surgical specialists.

This book serves two useful functions for gynecologists and other nonpathologist clinicians. First, it will aid in the more conventional function of reviewing the myriad pathologic abnormalities encountered in the female genital tract. Second, we believe that it provides considerable insight into the diagnostic pitfalls faced by surgical pathologists who examine gynecologic specimens. The diagnostic pitfalls are often lacking in many "textbook" presentations that ignore the problematic variations in favor of the prototypical appearance of a lesion.

The chapter authors were chosen not only for their widely recognized knowledge of a specific area but also for their demonstrated ability to communicate effectively using the written word. Moreover, we asked the authors to give their chapters the flavor of a personal consultation. Because surgical pathologic diagnosis is a visual exercise, the book is generously illustrated with color and black-and-white photographs. Finally, the authors have liberally cited pertinent and up-to-date references, thereby easing the reader's return to the primary literature.

Stephen S. Sternberg
Stacey E. Mills

Contents

Contributors

Geoffrey Altshuler, M.D.   *Professor of Pathology and Clinical Professor of Pediatrics, University of Oklahoma Health Sciences Center, and Oklahoma Children's Memorial Hospital, Oklahoma City, Oklahoma 73126*

Philip B. Clement, M.D.   *Department of Pathology, Vancouver General Hospital, and Associate Professor of Pathology, University of British Columbia, Vancouver, British Columbia, Canada V5Z1M9*

Christopher P. Crum, M.D.   *Associate Professor of Pathology, Microbiology, and Obstetrics and Gynecology, University of Virginia Medical Center, Charlottesville, Virginia 22908*

Henry F. Frierson, Jr., M.D.   *Assistant Professor of Pathology, University of Virginia Medical Center, Charlottesville, Virginia 22908*

Michael R. Hendrickson, M.D.   *Associate Professor of Pathology, Stanford University Medical Center, Stanford, California 94305*

Richard L. Kempson, M.D.   *Professor of Pathology, and Co-Director, Division of Surgical Pathology, Stanford University Medical Center, Stanford, California 94305*

Robert J. Kurman, M.D.   *Professor of Pathology, Obstetrics and Gynecology, Georgetown University School of Medicine, Washington, D.C. 20007*

Michael T. Mazur, M.D.   *Professor of Pathology, State University of New York Health Science Center, Syracuse, New York 13210*

Stacey E. Mills, M.D.   *Associate Professor of Pathology, Division of Surgical Pathology, University of Virginia Medical Center, Charlottesville, Virginia 22908*

Gerard Nuovo, M.D.   *Research Fellow in Pathology and Microbiology, Columbia University College of Physicians and Surgeons, New York, New York 10032*

Robert E. Scully, M.D.   *Professor of Pathology, Massachusetts General Hospital, Harvard Medical School, Boston, Massachusetts 02115*

Robert H. Young, M.D.   *Associate Professor of Pathology, Massachusetts General Hospital, Harvard Medical School, Boston, Massachusetts 02115*

Surgical Pathology of the Female Reproductive System and Peritoneum

*Surgical Pathology of the Female
Reproductive System and Peritoneum,*
edited by Stephen S. Sternberg
and Stacey E. Mills. Raven Press, Ltd,
New York © 1991.

CHAPTER 1

Gestational Trophoblastic Disease

Michael T. Mazur and Robert J. Kurman

Gestational trophoblastic disease (GTD) describes a spectrum of lesions that includes disorders of the placenta characterized by abnormal proliferation and maturation of trophoblast, as well as neoplasms derived from trophoblast. The diversity of the entities subsumed under the rubric of GTD has been underscored by recent morphologic, epidemiologic, immunohistochemical, and cytogenetic studies. For example, partial mole is now recognized as a distinct form of hydatidiform mole, and the placental-site trophoblastic tumor (PSTT) has been clearly identified as a distinct form of solid trophoblastic tumor. The recognition and separation of these various forms of GTD remains essential, since each disease entity has distinctive clinical ramifications. Furthermore, these disorders mimic growth patterns encountered in normal placental development and in nonmolar abortions, so an understanding of the morphologic forms of GTD remains important in order to avoid confusing these lesions with normal physiologic changes of pregnancy. Fortunately, most cases of GTD have characteristic presentations and pathologic features and present little difficulty in diagnosis.

Recent scientific committees of the World Health Organization (1) and the International Society of Gynecological Pathologists have proposed standardized nomenclature for the different morphologic forms of GTD (Table 1). This classification will be used in this chapter.

HYDATIDIFORM MOLE

Hydatidiform mole, complete or partial, represents a placenta characterized by marked villous enlargement due to central edema of the stroma. Variable hyperplasia of the villous trophoblast also is present, and this hyperplasia may be marked. Complete mole is separated from partial mole by the amount of villous involvement. The edema is generalized in complete mole, whereas in partial mole the edematous change affects only a portion of the villi. Most molar pregnancies are complete, and 25% to 43% are partial (2–4). Recent literature indicates clinical, pathologic, and cytogenetic differences between these two forms, yet all molar pregnancies have the potential for persistent GTD.

Considerable amounts of data have accrued concerning the epidemiology of hydatidiform mole. For instance, molar pregnancy has a marked variation in incidence between countries and parts of the world (5–8). It occurs more frequently in parts of Asia, Latin America, and the Middle East than it does in North America or Europe. In Europe and the United States, hydatidiform mole occurs in 1 in 1,000 to 2,000 pregnancies, whereas in Singapore, Japan, or Malaysia the incidence is 1 in 500 to 800 pregnancies (5,6,9).

Many studies have shown that increased maternal age correlates with an increased incidence of hydatidiform mole. The relative risk clearly becomes greater after age 40 and much greater after age 45 (5,6,10,11). Conversely, there appears to be a somewhat greater risk for molar pregnancy in women under age 20 in some studies.

Most epidemiologic studies concerning molar gestation have not separated complete mole from partial mole. Since complete moles predominate in most series, the data gathered so far probably are most correct for this subtype. Few studies have examined epidemiologic profiles of partial mole. One study from Hawaii found that the frequency of partial mole was one in 346 naturally terminating pregnancies, whereas complete mole occurred in one in 762 pregnancies (12). Molar pregnancy can even be found incidentally in elective abortion specimens (13), and one study from the United States found hydatidiform mole with a frequency of 1 in 600 elective abortions (14). Maternal age and race appear to have no effect on the incidence of partial mole (10). Recent data also indicate that some molar gestations, especially partial moles, may abort early and

1

TABLE 1. *Classification of gestational trophoblastic disease*

Hydatidiform mole
  Complete
  Partial
Invasive mole
Choriocarcinoma
Placental-site trophoblastic tumor
Trophoblastic lesion, miscellaneous
  Exaggerated placental site
  Trophoblastic lesion, unclassified

escape detection. Failure to include these "silent moles" may further skew results.

Substantial problems with methodology in early studies cast doubt on conclusions regarding the epidemiology of hydatidiform mole and GTD in general. Specifically, the population at risk is often not clearly defined. Many studies used denominators such as number of deliveries or number of live births in determining incidence rates, but the preferred denominator is the number of pregnancies. Use of an inappropriate denominator leads to over-reporting of the true incidence of any form of GTD. Confounding factors in epidemiologic studies include lack of consistent terminology, use of data only from referral medical centers, and lack of separation of complete from partial mole. Recent advances in the cytogenetic analysis of molar gestations appear to offer important clues in the evolution of hydatidiform mole that may have relevance to other epidemiologic considerations.

Cytogenetic analysis of moles has suggested different mechanisms of origin for complete and partial moles. The 46,XX complete mole is androgenetic, usually formed from duplication of a haploid paternal genome (23,X) and lacking functional maternal DNA (15). Over 90% of complete moles contain this paternal chromosomal composition (16–19). The remaining group of complete moles also are androgenetic but are 46,XY and formed by dyspermy, i.e., fertilization of an ovum lacking functional maternal chromosomes by two spermatozoa (16,20,21).

Partial moles are different (21), being triploid with two sets of chromosomes of paternal origin (diandric) and a haploid maternal set (17,21,22). This triploid chromosomal composition is known as *diandric*. Usually the triploid set is XXY (58%). Less commonly it is XXX (40%) or XYY (2%) (21). Thus a predominance of paternal chromosomes characterizes the cytogenetics of molar pregnancy. The ratio of paternal to maternal chromosomes is 2:0 in complete mole and 2:1 in partial mole.

Further chromosomal analysis and flow cytometry studies of ploidy in molar gestations have indicated that the cytogenetic distinctions between complete and partial moles may not be as clear as earlier studies have suggested (23–26).

Morphologic Features

Complete Mole

Complete mole often is voluminous, consisting of 300 to over 500 cc of bloody tissue. Prior spontaneous passage of a portion of the tissue may decrease this volume substantially, however. The hallmark of the complete mole is gross, generalized villous edema. Enlarged villi form grape-like, transparent vesicles measuring 1 to 2 cm across. When the complete mole is encountered in a hysterectomy specimen, the uterus is enlarged and molar vesicles protrude on opening. Only rarely is an embryo or fetus associated with complete mole. In most of these cases this represents a twin gestation.

The primary histologic feature of complete mole is generalized hydropic villous change (Fig. 1). Most villi show edematous stroma (Fig. 2), and many have cisterns. The latter are central, acellular fluid-filled spaces devoid of mesenchymal cells (Fig. 3). A small rim of mesenchyme separates the cistern from the surrounding layer of trophoblast. Often the border of the mesenchyme with the acellular cistern is abrupt and well defined. Necrosis and patchy calcification of villous stroma may be seen.

The other hallmark of complete mole is proliferation of villous trophoblast (Fig. 2). This proliferation is irregular, affecting villi unevenly; some, including smaller villi, show a marked overgrowth of trophoblast, whereas

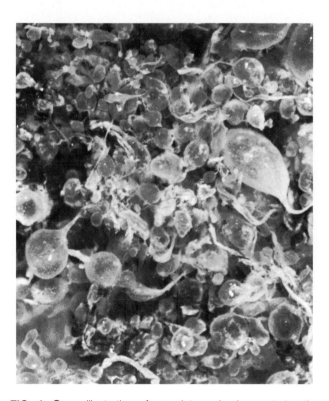

FIG. 1. Gross illustration of complete mole demonstrates the marked, generalized villous hydrops characteristic of molar gestation.

others, including some huge villi, show little trophoblastic hyperplasia. The proliferating trophoblast, composed of syncytiotrophoblast, cytotrophoblast, and intermediate trophoblast shows a random, circumferential growth from the villous surface, in marked contrast to the orderly, polar growth of trophoblast emanating from the surface of anchoring villi in early nonmolar placentas. The trophoblast of a mole, in addition to being hyperplastic, often shows considerable cytologic atypia (Fig. 4) with nuclear and cytoplasmic enlargement, irregularity of nuclear outlines, and hyperchromasia. The amount of trophoblastic growth is highly variable in molar gestations; it may be exuberant or it may be focal and minimal. Consequently, while this feature is an integral component of hydatidiform mole, it does not have to be prominent to establish the diagnosis.

In addition to the marked villous swelling and trophoblastic hyperplasia, complete mole is typically characterized by an absence of development of the embryo/fetus. Neither fetal parts nor amnion is found, and the villous stroma lacks blood vessels that would normally form if embryogenesis had occurred. Rare, small degenerating vascular spaces may be found in complete mole, and their presence does not exclude the diagnosis.

Partial Mole

Several features separate partial mole from complete mole (Table 2). First, the amount of tissue is generally

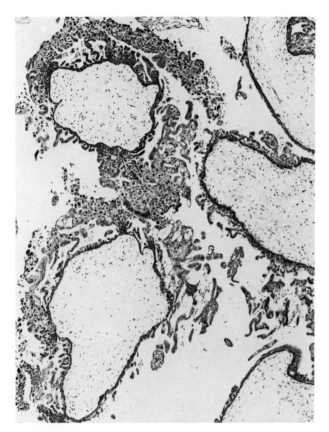

FIG. 2. Low-magnification view of complete mole demonstrates generalized villous swelling with circumferential hyperplasia of trophoblast.

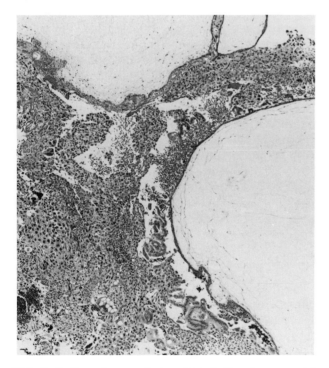

FIG. 3. Portion of a massively enlarged villus from complete hydatidiform mole demonstrates central cistern formation with an acellular central core. Note the circumferential hyperplasia of proliferative trophoblast growing from the villous surface.

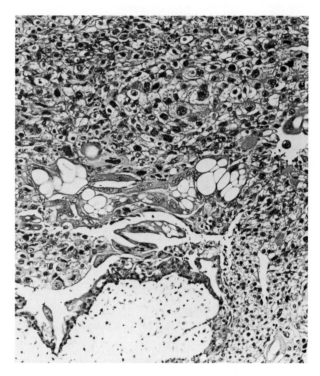

FIG. 4. High magnification of trophoblast growing from the surface of villi in complete hydatidiform mole. A mixture of syncytiotrophoblast, cytotrophoblast, and intermediate trophoblast is present. Cytologic atypia accompanies the proliferation.

TABLE 2. *Morphology of complete mole versus that of partial mole*

	Complete mole	Partial mole
Villous swelling:	Generalized	Partial
Trophoblastic proliferation:	Variable, may be marked	Focal, minimal
Trophoblastic atypia:	Often present	Rare

less than that found in complete mole, and the total volume is often no greater than 200 cc. The gross specimen shows large, hydropic villi like those seen in complete mole mixed with nonmolar placental tissue (27), an important distinguishing point. In some cases of partial mole a fetus is present and, when seen, may show gross developmental abnormalities (27).

Microscopically, the hallmark of partial mole is a mixture of large, edematous villi and small, normal-sized villi (2,27) (Fig. 5). At least some of the hydropic villi show the central, acellular cistern like that seen in complete mole. The small villi often show fibrosis. Trophoblastic hyperplasia is limited and focal. As in complete mole, the trophoblastic overgrowth, where present, is circumferential rather than polar.

Other histologic features commonly are found in partial mole. One typical feature is an irregular, scalloped outline to the villi (27) (Fig. 6). These irregular outlines

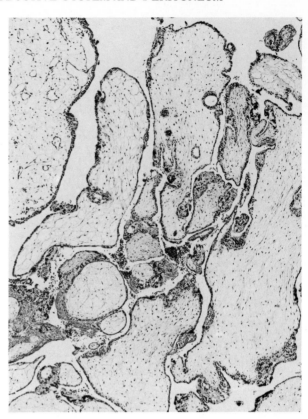

FIG. 6. Hydropic villi of partial mole show scalloped outlines, trophoblastic inclusions, and haphazard proliferation of trophoblast.

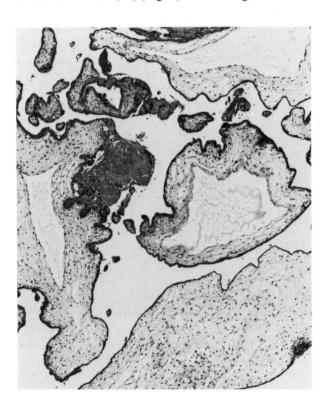

FIG. 5. Partial hydatidiform mole demonstrating mixture of small villi and large hydropic villi with an irregular, scalloped outline. Note cisterns in large villi, along with minimal proliferation of trophoblast.

produce infoldings of the trophoblast into the villous stroma which, when prominent and sectioned tangentially, appear to be stromal inclusions (Fig. 7). Evidence of a fetus with fetal parts or an amnion is seen in many cases. With fetal development, stromal vasculature often persists, and these vessels may contain nucleated erythrocytes.

Immunohistochemistry for human chorionic gonadotropin (hCG) and placental alkaline phosphatase (PlAP) can help in the distinction of complete and partial mole. The distribution of hCG is much greater than that of PlAP in complete mole. The opposite is found in partial mole with greater staining of PlAP (28).

Differential Diagnosis

The differential diagnosis of hydatidiform mole, complete or partial, usually includes early, nonmolar pregnancy (29,30). The nonmolar abortus can have several morphologic features that may mimic changes found in molar pregnancy. First, early nonmolar gestations are associated with marked growth of trophoblast that must be distinguished from the trophoblastic hyperplasia of mole (Fig. 8). Second, immature villi have loose, edematous stroma. Finally, the hydropic villi of

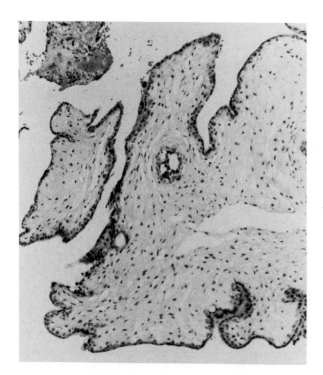

FIG. 7. Partial mole demonstrating minimal trophoblastic proliferation, inclusions, and a cistern.

the so-called "blighted ovum," in which there was no development of an embryo, demonstrate a moderate amount of edema (Fig. 9).

The edema of the nonmolar abortus including the blighted ovum is separated from the molar pregnancy by degree. Most importantly, in the nonmolar gestations, central cistern formation is not a significant component. Edema may be present but is usually only a microscopic finding, and trophoblastic proliferation from chorionic villi shows polarity characterized by column-like growth emanating from only one pole of the villi (Fig. 8). In addition, the trophoblast in the nonmolar gestation does not show cytologic atypia like that seen in many moles, especially complete moles. When the abortion must be separated from partial mole where hydropic change is less generalized, the secondary features of the partial mole such as irregular, scalloped borders, although not completely specific, can be helpful in making the distinction. Furthermore, immunohistochemical staining for PlAP is only focal in abortions with hydropic change, whereas it is more diffuse in partial moles (28).

Although molar pregnancies usually present with a moderate volume of tissue, occasionally the amount of material obtained is very scant, and helpful gross features are absent. This problem may be encountered in cases in which suction curettage has been performed, with the device causing collapse of villi on the gauze used to collect the specimen. Only histologic examina-

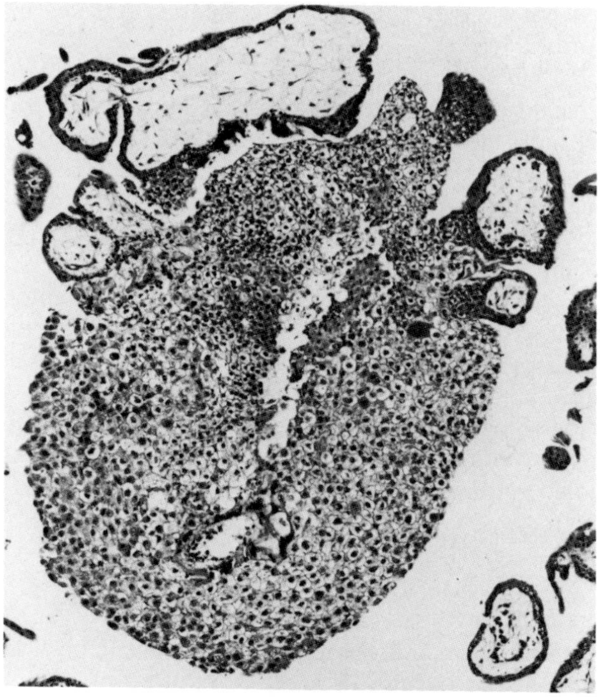

FIG. 8. Nonmolar first-trimester abortion demonstrates small villi with loose, edematous-appearing stroma. Trophoblast projects from the villous surface but maintains polarity, growing from only one end of the villi. Despite the proliferative activity, significant atypia is absent in the trophoblastic cells.

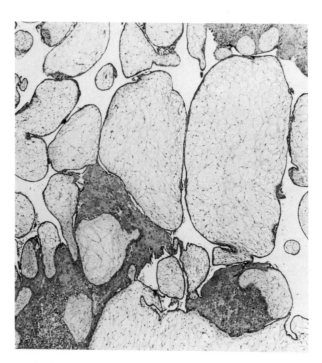

FIG. 9. Hydropic villi of a blighted ovum. There is villous edema, but this is a microscopic finding. No cisterns are present, and there is no proliferation of trophoblast from the villous surface.

tion of the tissue attached to the gauze establishes the diagnosis.

Repeat curettage after initial evacuation of a hydatidiform mole may contain proliferating trophoblast, raising the possibility of choriocarcinoma following mole. If villi are present, however, choriocarcinoma cannot be diagnosed, and the lesion represents retained intracavitary mole. Conversely, neither invasive mole nor choriocarcinoma are excluded, and meticulous follow-up with serum hCG titers is needed. Importantly, nonvillous trophoblast after evacuation of a mole does not necessarily indicate the presence of choriocarcinoma (29).

Clinicopathologic Correlation

Complete mole typically presents between the 11th and 25th week of pregnancy, with an average gestational age of about 16 weeks (31–33). Excessive uterine enlargement is common and is often accompanied by other symptoms such as severe vomiting (hyperemesis gravidarum) and pregnancy-induced hypertension (PIH) (31,34). The PIH associated with molar pregnancy may be a clinical clue to the diagnosis since PIH generally occurs in later gestation (third trimester) in nonmolar pregnancies. Often, patients with complete mole spontaneously abort, presenting with vaginal bleeding or passage of molar vesicles. Ovarian enlargement due to multiple theca-lutein cysts (hyperreactio luteinalis) occurs in some patients with complete mole. The hCG level is markedly elevated. Ultrasonography often discloses a classic "snowstorm" appearance.

With partial mole, the duration of pregnancy tends to be greater than with complete mole, with an average gestational age of about 19 weeks (2,35,36) (Table 3). Often the gestational age is greater than 20 weeks.

Usually the patient presents with abnormal uterine bleeding and is clinically thought to have a spontaneous or missed abortion (2,35,36). This contrasts with complete mole where the patient with abnormal bleeding is diagnosed as having molar pregnancy before curettage. With partial mole, the uterus is typically normal or small in size for the gestational age, and serum hCG levels generally do not show the marked elevation seen in complete mole (37). PIH also may occur in partial mole.

Finally, the clinical outcome of complete mole differs considerably from that of partial mole. Complete mole has a greater risk for persistent GTD (38). It has long been recognized that hydatidiform mole, once evacuated, may be followed by persistent molar disease in the uterine cavity, invasive hydatidiform mole, or choriocarcinoma. Most of the studies that have examined the long-term follow-up of hydatidiform mole were completed before the partial mole was recognized as a distinctive variant, so comprehensive comparison of the two forms is not always feasible. Nonetheless, available data indicate that 10% to 30% of patients with complete moles will require therapy for persistent GTD, as evidenced by a plateau or rise in hCG titers or the presence of metastases (31,39,40). The overt malignancy, choriocarcinoma, is the most serious form of persistent GTD, and it occurs in about 2% to 3% of patients with complete moles (39,41). Other sequelae are (a) persistent uterine cavity disease and (b) invasive mole that either penetrates the myometrium or embolizes to the vagina and/or lungs.

Partial mole has less risk for persistent GTD, and the percentage of patients requiring therapy following partial mole has ranged from 4% to 11% (2–4,35,36,42). Importantly, there are no well-documented reports of choriocarcinoma following partial mole; the sequelae have been persistent intrauterine disease and, rarely, documented examples of invasive mole (43,44).

Because of the risk of continued GTD, close monitoring of serum beta-hCG levels is necessary following the diagnosis of any form of hydatidiform mole until levels fall to, and remain in, the normal range (34,39,40). A chest radiograph after diagnosis also is useful for detecting early metastases as well as serving as a baseline should pulmonary disease ensue.

INVASIVE MOLE

Invasive hydatidiform mole is almost invariably a sequela to hydatidiform mole, complete or partial (33,38,45,46). The pathologic diagnosis of invasive mole is made when molar villi grow into the myometrium and broad ligament or are associated with trophoblast at distant sites, almost always the vagina, vulva, or lung. Rare examples of deportation to other sites (such as

TABLE 3. *Comparison of complete and partial mole*[a]

	Complete mole	Partial mole
Preoperative diagnosis		
Mole:	+++	+/−
Spontaneous abortion:	++	++
Missed abortion:	+/−	+++
Heavy bleeding:	+++	+
Toxemia:	++	+/−
Uterus large for dates:	++	+/−
Uterus small for dates:	+/−	++
Fetus present:	−	+
Serum hCG level:	+++	+/++
Cytogenetics:	XX (all paternal)	XXY or XXX (2:1, paternal: maternal)
Behavior:	10–30% persistent GTD	4–11% persistent GTD

[a] hCG, human chorionic gonadotropin; GTD, gestational trophoblastic disease.

paraspinal soft tissues) have been reported (47). This clinical diagnosis is made when hCG titers plateau or rise following evacuation of a mole. A pathologic diagnosis is rarely made, since persistent uterine disease and metastatic lesions that may represent invasive mole often are treated with chemotherapy without the need to perform a hysterectomy (46). The exact frequency of invasive mole is thus difficult to determine because of the lack of pathologic confirmation for most cases (33). Overall, invasive mole is a clinically significant sequela in about 15% of cases.

Morphologic Features

Grossly, invasive mole in the uterus results in an irregular, often hemorrhagic, lesion that penetrates into the myometrium. It may grow through the myometrium, perforating the serosa or expanding the broad ligament and involving the adnexa.

Microscopically, invasive mole is diagnosed when molar villi with associated trophoblast are found either within the myometrium (Fig. 10), within myometrial blood vessels, or at distant sites. The villi present in invasive mole are enlarged but are often not as enlarged

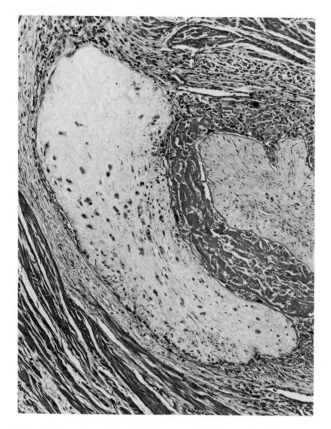

FIG. 10. Invasive mole within the myometrium demonstrates enlarged chorionic villi away from the endometrial surface. In this area, there is minimal proliferation of trophoblast. Other examples of invasive mole often show more proliferative trophoblast in association with the villi.

as the villi of a typical complete intrauterine mole. The amount of trophoblast proliferating around the molar villi is highly variable; it may be marked and obscure the presence of the molar villus. In such cases, careful scrutiny for villi is necessary to avoid misclassification of the lesion as choriocarcinoma. Likewise, trophoblastic lesions at distant sites following evacuation of a hydatidiform mole may also show invasive mole with a marked proliferation of trophoblast, underscoring the need for careful sectioning and scrutiny to ensure the correct diagnosis.

Clinicopathologic Correlation

Invasive hydatidiform mole may cause severe and life-threatening hemorrhage if it perforates the uterus and involves the parametrial tissues (48,49). Currently, this is an unusual event; the greater significance of invasive mole is the difficulty in separating this entity from choriocarcinoma when the patient is managed medically. Persistently elevated or rising serum hCG titers following evacuation of a mole may represent either invasive mole or choriocarcinoma. Since tissue is generally not available to make the distinction, elevated serum hCG titers are usually attributed to "persistent GTD" without further classification. The risk of invasive mole progressing to choriocarcinoma appears to be no greater than that of progression from intracavitary hydatidiform mole, and presumably many lesions of invasive mole would regress spontaneously if given appropriate opportunity. Nonetheless, persistent or elevated hCG titers are generally treated with chemotherapy in the absence of a histologic diagnosis, and the lesions usually respond.

Differential Diagnosis

Invasive mole must be distinguished from noninvasive hydatidiform mole, choriocarcinoma, and placenta increta/percreta (30). Invasive mole should only be diagnosed when there is clear-cut evidence of extension of molar tissue into the myometrium and its vessels or deportation to distant sites. Marked trophoblastic proliferation associated with an intracavitary hydatidiform mole does not necessarily indicate the presence of invasive mole. Invasive mole may be difficult to distinguish from choriocarcinoma, since both entities can show a proliferation of trophoblast in the myometrium, vagina, or lungs, but invasive mole is only diagnosed when chorionic villi are present.

Placenta increta and percreta represent growth of nonmolar placental tissue into the myometrium. These disorders lack the villous hydrops and abnormal trophoblastic proliferation found in invasive mole. Furthermore, invasive mole usually is a sequela to intracavitary hydatidiform mole.

CHORIOCARCINOMA

Gestational choriocarcinoma is a malignant tumor derived from the trophoblast of the placenta. It is a tumor allograft in the host mother and is thus almost unique among human malignancies. Choriocarcinoma theoretically could arise from the trophoblastic lining of the primitive blastocyst before implantation, yet most cases of choriocarcinoma seem to follow a recognizable pregnancy event. The more abnormal the pregnancy, the more likely that it will be followed by choriocarcinoma. Complete hydatidiform mole is the most common preceding gestational event, accounting for about 50% of all choriocarcinomas (41,50). About one-quarter of all choriocarcinomas follow abortions, and the remaining cases occur following normal pregnancy or, rarely, following ectopic gestation.

The epidemiology of choriocarcinoma tends to parallel that of hydatidiform mole, and the geographic variations are similar (5,6,8). Choriocarcinoma occurs with a frequency of one in 20,000 to 40,000 pregnancies in the United States and Europe. Maternal age influence is similar to that seen with hydatidiform mole, with an increased frequency for women who become pregnant after age 45 and a smaller, but still increased, frequency for women aged 40 to 44 (6). The relative risk for choriocarcinoma in the older age groups is greater than that for hydatidiform mole, although the trends are similar.

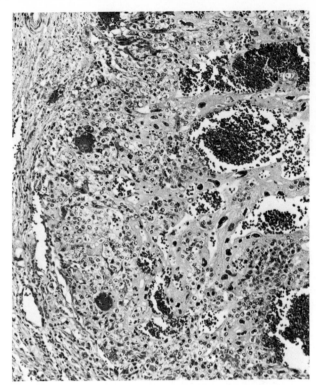

FIG. 12. Choriocarcinoma within the uterus. There is a biphasic mixture of syncytiotrophoblastic and cytotrophoblastic cells with intermediate trophoblastic cells intermixed. Note the red-cell lakes within the syncytiotrophoblast on the right side.

Again, these epidemiologic evaluations suffer from methodologic problems similar to those found in studies of hydatidiform mole. Failure to separate other forms of persistent GTD from choriocarcinoma confounds data in many studies.

Morphologic Features

The gross appearance of choriocarcinoma typically is that of a circumscribed, hemorrhagic mass (48,49,51, 52). This is due to its rapid proliferation, combined with its propensity to invade blood vessels. The tumors vary from small, pinpoint-sized lesions to large destructive masses (Fig. 11). The central portion of the tumor is typically hemorrhagic and necrotic with only a thin rim of recognizable tumor at the periphery of the nodule.

The classic histologic pattern of choriocarcinoma has been described as bilaminar, dimorphic, or biphasic, these terms referring to the alternating arrangement of cytotrophoblast and syncytiotrophoblast that characterize choriocarcinoma (53) (Figs. 12 and 13). A third form of trophoblastic cell, the intermediate trophoblast, is another important component of trophoblastic lesions including choriocarcinoma (54,54a) (Table 4). The intermediate cell, described in greater detail in the PSTT,

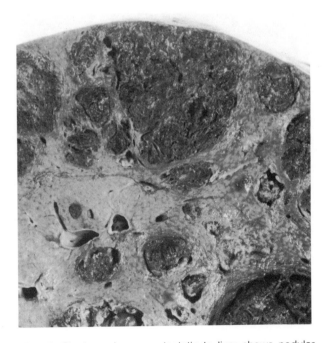

FIG. 11. Choriocarcinoma metastatic to liver shows nodular, hemorrhagic growth.

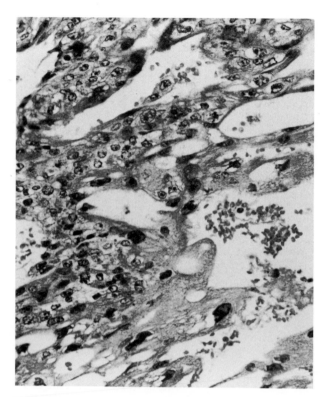

FIG. 13. High magnification of choriocarcinoma demonstrates the alternating arrangement of syncytiotrophoblast and cytotrophoblast.

pearing chorionic villi (56). These villi do not show molar change. Chorionic villi in association with trophoblastic proliferations under any other circumstance rule out the diagnosis of choriocarcinoma.

The component cells of choriocarcinoma each have their own set of cytologic characteristics that facilitate recognition of the growth patterns (Table 4) (33). The cytotrophoblastic cells are the primitive, germinative component that show mitotic activity. Typically, they are small to moderately sized mononucleate cells that contain a small amount of pale granular to clear cytoplasm (Fig. 13). Cell borders are prominent. The syncytiotrophoblastic cells, in contrast, are highly developed multinucleate cells that are terminally differentiated and therefore do not show mitotic activity. The cytoplasm is dense and stains deeply eosinophilic to basophilic (Fig. 15). The cytoplasm often contains multiple vacuoles, due to (a) dilated cytoplasmic endoplasmic reticulum and (b) lacunae formed by complex infoldings of the syncytiotrophoblastic surface. Erythrocytes may be seen in the lacunae. Sometimes a distinct brush border is identified along the membrane surfaces of syncytiotrophoblast. The intermediate trophoblastic cells, as their name implies, have features in between those of cytotrophoblast and syncytiotrophoblast. Typically, these cells are large and polyhedral with one or several nuclei and abundant cytoplasm (Fig. 14). The cytoplasm is densely eosinophilic to amphophilic and lacks the vacuolation seen in syncytiotrophoblast. Cell membranes tend to be less distinct in intermediate trophoblast than they are in cytotrophoblast. When the intermediate trophoblasts become dispersed, cell borders are prominent, however. All of the cell types found in choriocarcinoma may show cytologic aberrations (Fig. 14). There can be marked variations in the amount of cytologic atypia encountered. Nuclear pleomorphism and hyperchromasia is often marked, and nucleoli can be prominent.

Most choriocarcinomas have the typical biphasic pattern, but variations may exist. Portions of tumors can show a predominance of cytotrophoblastic, interme-

has features that bridge the cytologic aspects of cytotrophoblast and syncytiotrophoblast (55) (Fig. 14).

Because of the extensive necrosis associated with choriocarcinoma, trophoblastic tissue may be scant, and extensive sectioning may be necessary to find the diagnostic biphasic pattern. Vascular invasion often is prominent in choriocarcinoma. Chorionic villi are not a component, except for the rare cases of choriocarcinoma arising in the normally developing placenta. In these few cases that have been described, the choriocarcinoma clearly arises from the surface of normal-ap-

TABLE 4. Morphologic features of trophoblastic cells[a]

	Cytotrophoblast	Intermediate trophoblast	Syncytiotrophoblast
Nucleus:	Single	One to several	Multiple
Mitotic activity:	High	Low	Absent
Shape:	Round	Variable; polyhedral to spindle	Irregular; highly variable
Cytoplasm:	Scant; clear to granular-cell borders	Abundant; amphophilic; occasional vacuoles	Abundant; dense; multiple vacuoles; lacunae; red cell lakes
Immunostaining			
hCG:	−	+	++++
hPL:	−	++++	++

[a] ++++ denotes semiquantitative scoring of proportion of cells showing a positive reaction; hCG, human chorionic gonadotropin; hPL, human placental lactogen.

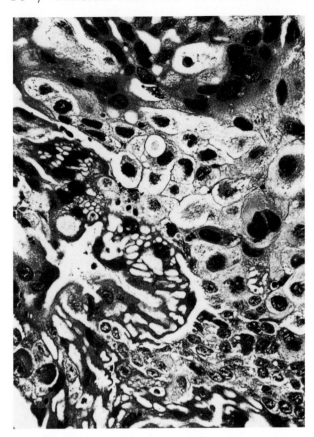

FIG. 14. Gestational choriocarcinoma with prominent syncytio-trophoblast in the upper and left lower portions of the micrograph. Both cytotrophoblastic and intermediate trophoblastic cells are interspersed.

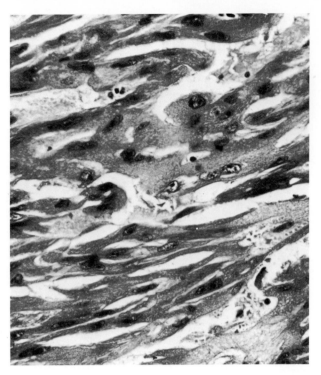

FIG. 15. An area of choriocarcinoma showing a predominance of the syncytiotrophoblastic cells. Note the dense cytoplasm that is finely vacuolated. Large, slit-like spaces separate the cytoplasm of the syncytiotrophoblastic cells.

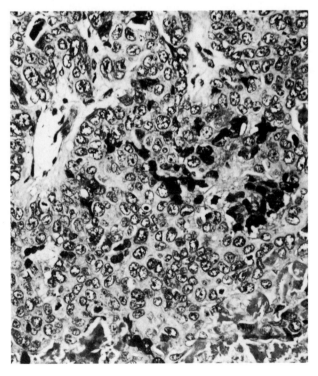

FIG. 16. Metastatic gestational choriocarcinoma following chemotherapy. The syncytiotrophoblastic cells have become less distinct, with reduced cytoplasm. The syncytiotrophoblast at right center show dark, clustered nuclei.

diate trophoblastic, or syncytiotrophoblastic cells (48,49,53). Usually, further sampling will reveal the more typical alternating arrangement of cytotrophoblastic and syncytiotrophoblastic cells. The syncytiotrophoblast is the most distinctive cell in choriocarcinoma, so it is the most important diagnostic cell. We have found examples of choriocarcinoma in which syncytiotrophoblastic cells were particularly difficult to identify, even with extensive sectioning. In such cases, the predominant cell is somewhat larger than cytotrophoblast, has one or several nuclei, and has indistinct cell membranes, features suggesting intermediate trophoblastic cell differentiation (54b). The syncytiotrophoblastic cells may be less conspicuous following chemotherapy (Fig. 16) (53).

Syncytiotrophoblast and intermediate trophoblast are hormonally active cells, so immunohistochemical studies using antibodies to hCG or human placental lactogen (hPL) can be extremely helpful in evaluating cases of suspected choriocarcinoma (54). In typical choriocarcinoma, the syncytiotrophoblastic cells stain intensely with beta-hCG and to a variable but lesser extent with hPL. Furthermore, the staining pattern can help define the regular alternating network of syncytiotrophoblast and cytotrophoblast. Intermediate cells also stain to some extent with hCG and hPL. Ultrastructurally, trophoblastic cells show marked epithelial differentiation including desmosomes and tonofilaments. Consequently, choriocarcinoma is broadly reactive to antibodies for cytokeratin that recognize both low- and high-molecular-weight species. All trophoblastic cells, including cytotrophoblast, are positive.

Differential Diagnosis

Choriocarcinoma is often considered in the differential diagnosis of normal trophoblast from early gestations and in the proliferation of trophoblast associated with hydatidiform mole (29,30). Rarely, choriocarcinoma arises from trophoblast covering villi in a normally developing placenta, but other than this exception, chorionic villi associated with trophoblastic proliferations represent hydatidiform mole or a nonmolar abortion specimen. When trophoblastic proliferations are encountered in uterine tissues and no chorionic villi are found, the differential includes choriocarcinoma and an abortion specimen in which no villi have persisted. The distinction between the trophoblast of abortions and that of choriocarcinoma is based on the quality of the trophoblast. In a normal abortion without villi, there is usually only a small amount of trophoblastic tissue present. In choriocarcinoma, the tissue tends to be more abundant and the trophoblast predominates in the sections. Choriocarcinoma can be established when there are sheets of trophoblast without villi that show the characteristic bilaminar pattern. In addition, choriocarcinoma shows tumor necrosis and cytologic atypia. Often, trophoblast without villi in curettings may be suspicious for choriocarcinoma but may be difficult to categorize with certainty (29). A careful obstetric history in such cases may be extremely helpful. Atypical trophoblast without villi is more likely to represent choriocarcinoma if the preceding pregnancy was nonmolar, whereas similar trophoblast after evacuation of mole may only represent persistent intrauterine mole (29,30). In questionable cases, careful monitoring of serum beta-hCG levels, accompanied by chest radiographs, may help establish the diagnosis.

At metastatic sites, the differential diagnosis includes deported invasive mole, ordinary epithelial malignancies with areas of choriocarcinomatous differentiation, and pleomorphic epithelial malignancies with tumor giant cells. Choriocarcinoma is distinguished from invasive mole by the absence of chorionic villi, especially when evaluating lesions of the lung, vagina, or vulva following molar gestation. In nongestational tumors with choriocarcinomatous differentiation or with areas that mimic choriocarcinoma, the differential diagnosis

may be difficult, especially in young women in whom gestational trophoblastic disease would be highly suspected. Choriocarcinoma occurs as a form of differentiation in some primary visceral neoplasms such as carcinomas of the gastrointestinal tract or the bladder (57–59). In such cases, the sections also usually reveal areas of typical adenocarcinoma or transitional-cell carcinoma that clarify the diagnosis. Rarely, trophoblastic tissue may be the only cytologic component of a neoplasm where it is not possible to determine whether the tumor represents gestational choriocarcinoma, a germ-cell malignancy with choriocarcinoma predominance, or choriocarcinomatous differentiation of a more typical epithelial tumor.

Germ-cell tumors often are associated with a large adnexal mass, a helpful differential feature. In addition, germ-cell tumors often contain a mixture of other histologic types such as dysgerminoma, teratoma, or yolk sac tumor. Alpha fetoprotein (AFP) is typically produced by yolk sac tumor and less commonly by teratoma, so immunostaining tissue and serum AFP levels can be useful in diagnosing these mixed germ-cell tumors. When the differential diagnosis includes epithelial malignancy with giant-cell change, immunohistochemistry may be useful in establishing the correct diagnosis. In choriocarcinoma, the syncytiotrophoblast and the intermediate trophoblast stain with hCG and hPL, while the giant cells in nontrophoblastic proliferations do not. Occasionally, an epithelial malignancy arising at an extrauterine site may focally produce hCG or hPL (60), and immunostaining must be correlated with the histologic pattern to arrive at the diagnosis. In questionable cases the serum evaluations for beta-hCG can be helpful. The differential diagnosis of the PSTT with choriocarcinoma is considered in the discussion of the PSTT.

Clinicopathologic Correlation

Generally, choriocarcinoma follows an identifiable gestational event (hydatidiform mole, abortion, or term gestation) by a few months, but choriocarcinomas not associated with hydatidiform mole are often not suspected clinically (52,61). Patients most frequently present with abnormal uterine bleeding. Choriocarcinoma may regress in the uterus without causing symptoms, and metastases may be the first sign of the tumor (53,61–63). Rare examples of extended latent periods for choriocarcinoma have been reported (64).

Metastatic lesions most commonly occur in the lung, since choriocarcinoma is disseminated hematogenously (33,48,49,52). Other common metastatic sites include the brain, liver, and gastrointestinal tract (48). Vaginal nodules are often found in choriocarcinoma and may bleed profusely if biopsied. Kidney, skin, and other unusual locations may also be sites of spread.

Prior to modern cytotoxic chemotherapy, hysterectomy was the only treatment and survival was only 41% if no metastases were present and 19% with metastases (65). Chemotherapy has dramatically improved the prognosis. The survival rate is 81% for all patients, although it is only 71% for those with metastatic disease (50). In contrast, the overall survival rate for all cases of persistent and metastatic GTD is now over 90% (32,50).

Death from choriocarcinoma is usually due to hemorrhagic tumor at metastatic sites, pulmonary insufficiency caused by a large tumor burden, or the effects of irradiation and cytotoxic chemotherapy (53,66).

Several prognostic factors help predict the response to treatment. Poor prognostic factors include advanced disease at diagnosis, cerebral or hepatic metastases, symptoms of disease for greater than 4 months, failure of prior chemotherapy, and a pretreatment serum beta-hCG titer of greater than 40,000 mIU/ml (67–69). Metastases limited to the lung or vagina are not, by themselves, poor prognostic signs. Choriocarcinoma following a term gestation has a somewhat worse prognosis that is attributed to delays in treatment and the presence of metastases beyond the lungs and vagina (62,70). No histologic features thus far have been found to have prognostic importance. Chemotherapy may alter the histologic appearance in isolated cases (53, 54b), but the influence of these microscopic changes on clinical outcome has not been established. Some investigators have suggested that all forms of gestational trophoblastic disease showing minimal differentiation toward syncytiotrophoblast have a worse prognosis (71). Further study is needed to determine whether or not such histologic patterns do, in fact, have clinical significance.

PLACENTAL-SITE TROPHOBLASTIC TUMOR

The placental-site trophoblastic tumor (PSTT) is the rarest form of GTD. Terminology for this distinctive form of neoplasm has only recently been clearly defined. The tumor has been described intermittently for many years under terms such as *atypical chorioepithelioma, atypical choriocarcinoma, syncytioma, chorioepitheliosis,* and *trophoblastic pseudotumor,* but none of these terms is now appropriate (33,72). In addition, these tumors also have been mistakenly classified as sarcomas. The epidemiologic and risk factors for the PSTT are not well known, since the entity has only recently been recognized as a distinct form of trophoblastic disease. So far there are only approximately 80 reported and unreported cases of PSTT known to us (72). As expected, this is a disorder of the reproductive years, although several patients have been over 50 years of age when the tumors have been diagnosed (73,74). Most patients have been parous; several have had a preceding hydatidiform mole (74–76). Both term pregnancies and spontaneous abortions have preceded the diagnosis of

PSTT. Usually the relation to the previous gestations is uncertain, since the tumors are diagnosed long after the last known pregnancy.

Morphologic Features

The gross appearance of PSTT is highly varied. The lesions range from microscopic to diffuse tumors that enlarge and distort the fundus. Usually the tumors are well defined, yet some are poorly demarcated. Tumor may project into the uterine cavity or may have predominant growth into the myometrium. Often the neoplasm is soft and tan and may have areas of hemorrhage or necrosis. Many cases have been associated with invasion through the entire thickness of the myometrium, extending to the serosa. Perforation or extension into the broad ligament or adnexa may occur.

Microscopically, PSTT is composed predominantly of intermediate trophoblast (Table 4) (54,54a,55). There is a secondary component of syncytiotrophoblast. The typical growth pattern is that of infiltration of the myometrium by large, polygonal, intermediate trophoblastic cells that insinuate themselves between the smooth-muscle fibers, causing little apparent tissue destruction (Fig. 17). The cells may be present singly or in large nests or masses. Usually the cells have a polyhedral outline, yet portions of the tumor may have a spindle-cell shape. Extensive deposition of fibrinoid material is characteristic. This neoplasm also tends to invade the walls of blood vessels from the lumen to the periphery, eventually replacing the entire wall. Fibrinoid material is also deposited in the vessel wall (Fig. 18). Typically, a central lumen containing erythrocytes is maintained that identifies the structure as a vessel. These tumors also have a secondary component of larger syncytiotrophoblastic cells (Fig. 19) sometimes containing vacuolated cytoplasm. Cytotrophoblastic cells are not a conspicuous component. PSTT is generally not associated with the presence of chorionic villi. Decidua may also be present in the uninvolved endometrium.

Malignant PSTT have some cytologic features that may help predict their aggressive course. Often they are composed of larger masses and sheets of cells, and the component cells tend to have clear, instead of amphophilic, cytoplasm (Fig. 20). Necrosis is more extensive in the malignant tumors and the mitotic rate is higher. In benign PSTT, the mean mitotic rate has been two mitotic figures per 10 high-power fields, with the highest reported rate being five mitotic figures per 10 high-power fields. In contrast, malignant lesions generally have more than five mitotic figures per 10 high-power fields. In one fatal case, however, the mean mitotic rate was only two per 10 high-power fields. Furthermore, the malignant cases tend to stain more diffusely for hCG than hPL, more closely resembling the distribution of

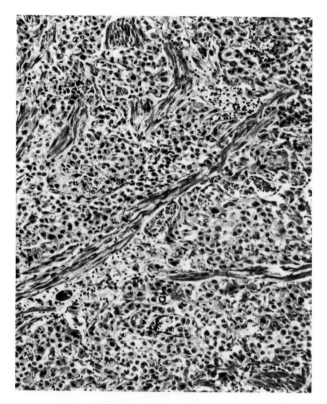

FIG. 17. Placental-site trophoblastic tumor with sheets of intermediate trophoblastic cells separating smooth muscle of the myometrium.

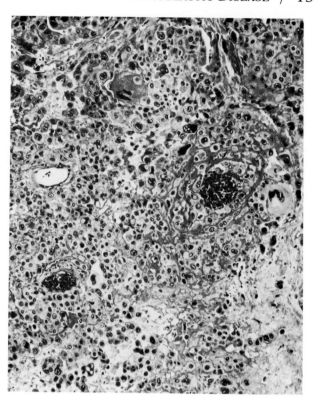

FIG. 19. An area of placental-site trophoblastic tumor demonstrating some pleomorphism of cells. Scattered syncytiotrophoblastic cells are admixed with the intermediate trophoblastic cells. To the right center, a vessel wall has been replaced by intermediate trophoblastic cells and fibrin.

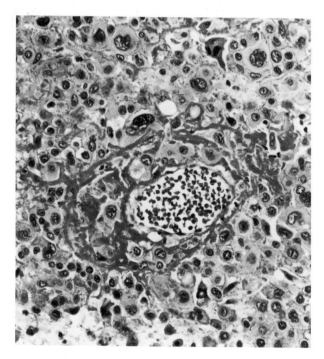

FIG. 18. High magnification of placental-site trophoblastic tumor demonstrates replacement of a vascular wall by intermediate trophoblastic cells in fibrinoid material. Characteristically, the lumen is preserved and contains erythrocytes. Note scattered multinucleate syncytiotrophoblast.

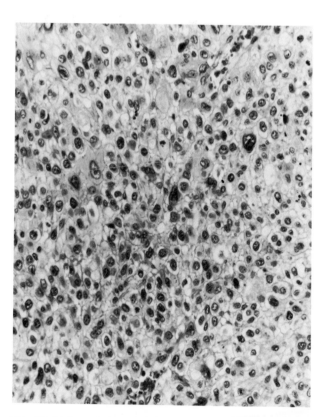

FIG. 20. Malignant placental-site trophoblastic tumor composed of intermediate trophoblastic cells with clear cytoplasm.

these hormones in choriocarcinoma. Abnormal mitotic figures may be found in either benign or malignant tumors.

Differential Diagnosis

PSTT must be differentiated from choriocarcinoma, other forms of neoplasia, and an exaggerated implantation site. Usually the distinction of PSTT from choriocarcinoma is not difficult. PSTT is composed predominantly of intermediate trophoblastic cells. Syncytiotrophoblast may be present, but these cells are widely scattered in PSTT, in contrast to their alternating biphasic arrangement in choriocarcinoma. We have seen cases of choriocarcinoma in which more intermediate trophoblast than cytotrophoblast alternated with the syncytiotrophoblast, but the biphasic pattern persists in contrast to the monomorphic growth of PSTT.

PSTT has a different immunohistochemical staining pattern than does choriocarcinoma. Since the tumor is composed primarily of intermediate trophoblast, staining for hPL is diffusely distributed throughout the neoplasm. In contrast, hCG immunostaining is usually focal because syncytiotrophoblastic cells are less prominent (54). Typically, in choriocarcinoma the beta-hCG levels are high, ranging from 1,000 mIU/ml to over 100,000 mIU/ml, whereas in PSTT the levels are generally low.

PSTT can be confused with a wide variety of other malignancies, especially epithelioid leiomyosarcoma. This can be a difficult problem in the differential diagnosis, since PSTT often has a highly infiltrative pattern within the myometrium, dissecting among the smooth-muscle fibers and simulating origin from the latter cells. Helpful clues in the differential diagnosis include the distinctive pattern of vessel invasion and the deposition of fibrinoid material in PSTT that are not found in leiomyosarcomas or most other malignancies. Immunostaining for hPL and hCG can also help distinguish PSTT from other malignancies. In addition, PSTT shows a diffuse distribution for cytokeratin, whereas sarcomas do not. Other tumors may, on occasion, stain focally for hCG and/or hPL, but the combination of histologic features and the more diffuse and intense immunostaining for hPL and hCG in PSTT should resolve difficult cases.

The normal implantation site is composed of intermediate trophoblastic cells much like those seen in PSTT. Consequently, curettage or hysterectomy specimens that include an implantation site without accompanying villi and villous trophoblast can mimic the PSTT. This can be particularly problematic when there is a prominent proliferation of intermediate trophoblast, the so-called "exaggerated placental site." In the past this was termed "syncytial endometritis." The exagger-

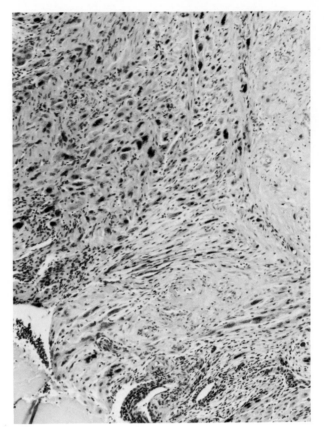

FIG. 21. Exaggerated placental site showing nests of internal trophoblast infiltrating the superficial myometrium. The pattern of invasion closely simulates placental-site trophoblastic tumor but is focal and not confluent.

ated placental site is composed of large nests of intermediate cells infiltrating the decidua and the superficial myometrium (Fig. 21). An exaggerated placental site is only a focal phenomenon, in contrast to the larger tumor formed by PSTT. Furthermore, PSTT usually forms a mass or nodular lesion, whereas the exaggerated placental site is merely an infiltrative process of intermediate cells that does not distort normal architecture to such a significant degree. At times it may be extremely difficult to determine in curettings whether or not the process represents an exaggerated implantation site or a PSTT. In such cases, close clinical follow-up with monitoring of hCG levels is prudent. In normal gestations the hCG levels should return to normal and menstruation should resume. In contrast, with PSTT the elevated serum hCG levels often persist following curettage. In view of the low propensity for spread beyond the uterus, careful clinical follow-up with monitoring of serum hCG levels is a safe procedure in the questionable case. Plateauing or rising hCG titers, however, signal the need for hysterectomy in view of the apparent lack of response to chemotherapy of these neoplasms.

Clinicopathologic Correlation

Patients with PSTT can present either with amenorrhea or with abnormal bleeding (74–76). Often the uterus is enlarged, so the patient may be thought to be pregnant. The results of pregnancy tests are variable but are almost always positive when a sensitive immunologic assay is used. When progressive uterine enlargement ceases, a diagnosis of missed abortion may be made. One case of PSTT has been associated with virilization (77). A few PSTT have been associated with an apparently unique form of renal disease in which the nephrotic syndrome is a major component (78).

PSTT tends to have an indolent behavior. In most cases the tumor remains confined to the uterus. Because of the deep myometrial penetration, perforation may occur during curettage. Approximately 10% to 15% of the cases known to us have resulted in death of the patient (72,79–81). In the few overtly malignant cases, lungs, liver, abdominal cavity, and brain have been involved by metastases, and the metastases retain the same histologic pattern as that of the uterine primary. Usually, metastases develop rapidly after the initial diagnosis, but one reported case recurred 5 years after hysterectomy (80). The malignant cases have not responded to the multiagent chemotherapy used to treat choriocarcinoma.

REFERENCES

1. World Health Organization Scientific Group on Gestational Trophoblastic Disease. *Gestational trophoblastic diseases.* Technical Report Series, No. 692. Geneva, 1983.
2. Czernobilsky B, Barash A, Lancet M. Partial moles: a clinicopathologic study of 25 cases. *Obstet Gynecol* 1982;59:75–77.
3. Szulman AE, Surti U. The clinicopathologic profile of the partial hydatidiform mole. *Obstet Gynecol* 1982;59:597–602.
4. Wong LC, Ma HK. The syndrome of partial mole. *Arch Gynecol* 1984;234:161–166.
5. Bracken MB, Brinton LA, Hayashi K. Epidemiology of hydatidiform mole and choriocarcinoma. *Epidemiol Rev* 1984;6:52–75.
6. Buckley J. Epidemiology of gestational trophoblastic diseases. In: Szulman AE, Buchsbaum HJ, eds. *Gestational trophoblastic disease.* New York: Springer-Verlag, 1987:8–26.
7. Craighill MC, Cramer DW. Epidemiology of complete molar pregnancy. *J Reprod Med* 1984;29:784–787.
8. Grimes DA. Epidemiology of gestational trophoblastic disease. *Am J Obstet Gynecol* 1984;150:309–318.
9. Womack C, Elston CW. Hydatidiform mole in Nottingham: a 12-year retrospective epidemiological and morphological study. *Placenta* 1985;6:93–106.
10. Matsuura J, Chin D, Jacobs PA, Szulman AE. Complete hydatidiform mole in Hawaii: an epidemiologic study. *Genet Epidemiol* 1984;1:271–284.
11. Stone M, Bagshawe KD. An analysis of the influences of maternal age, gestational age, contraceptive method, and the mode of primary treatment of patients with hydatidiform moles on the incidence of subsequent chemotherapy. *Br J Obstet Gynaecol* 1979;86:782–792.
12. Jacobs PA, Hunt PA, Matsuura JS, Wilson CC, Szulman AE. Complete and partial hydatidiform mole in Hawaii: cytogenetics, morphology and epidemiology. *Br J Obstet Gynaecol* 1982;89:258–266.
13. Yuen BH, Callegari PB. Occurrence of molar pregnancy in patients undergoing elective abortion: comparison with other clinical presentations. *Am J Obstet Gynecol* 1986;154:273–276.
14. Cohen BA, Burkman RT, Rosenshein NB, Antienza MF, King TM, Parmley TH. Gestational trophoblastic disease within an elective abortion population. *Am J Obstet Gynecol* 1979;135:452–455.
15. Kajii T, Ohama K. Androgenetic origin of hydatidiform mole. *Nature* 1977;268:633–634.
16. Kajii T, Kurashige H, Ohama K, Uchino F. XY and XX complete moles: clinical and morphologic correlations. *Am J Obstet Gynecol* 1984;150:57–64.
17. Szulman AE, Surti U. The syndromes of hydatidiform mole. I. Cytogenetic and morphologic correlations. *Am J Obstet Gynecol* 1978;131:665–671.
18. Vassilakos P, Riotton G, Kajii T. Hydatidiform mole: two entities. A morphologic and cytogenetic study with some clinical considerations. *Am J Obstet Gynecol* 1977;127:167–170.
19. Wake N, Takagi N, Sasaki M. Androgenesis as a cause of hydatidiform mole. *J Natl Cancer Inst* 1978;60:51–57.
20. Surti U, Szulman AE, O'Brien S. Dispermic origin and clinical outcome of three complete hydatidiform moles with 46,XY karyotype. *Am J Obstet Gynecol* 1982;144:84–87.
21. Surti U. Genetic concepts and techniques. In: Szulman AE, Buchsbaum HJ, eds. *Gestational trophoblastic disease.* New York: Springer-Verlag, 1987:111–121.
22. Jacobs PA, Szulman AE, Funkhouser J, Matsuura JS, Wilson CC. Human triploidy: relationship between parental origin of the additional haploid complement and development of partial hydatidiform mole. *Ann Hum Genet* 1982;46:223–231.
23. Davis JR, Kerrigan DP, Way DL, Weiner SA. Partial hydatidiform moles: deoxyribonucleic acid content and course. *Am J Obstet Gynecol* 1987;157:969–973.
24. Hemming JD, Wuirke P, Womack C, et al. Diagnosis of molar pregnancy and persistent trophoblastic disease by flow cytometry. *J Clin Pathol* 1987;40:615–620.
25. Ohama K, Ueda K, Oka B, Moto E, Takenaka M, Fujiwara A. Cytogenetic and clinicopathologic studies of partial moles. *Obstet Gynecol* 1986;68:259–262.
26. Vejerslev LO, Fisher RA, Surti U, Walke N. Hydatidiform mole: cytogenetically unusual cases and their implications for the present classification. *Am J Obstet Gynecol* 1987;157:180–184.
27. Szulman AE, Surti U. The syndromes of hydatidiform mole. II. Morphologic evolution of the complete and partial mole. *Am J Obstet Gynecol* 1978;132:20–27.
28. Brescia RJ, Kurman RJ, Main C, Surti U, Szulman AE. Immunocytochemical localization of chorionic gonadotropin, placental lactogen, and placental alkaline phosphatase in the diagnosis of complete and partial hydatidiform moles. *Int J Gynecol Pathol* 1987;6:213–229.
29. Elston CW, Bagshawe KD. The diagnosis of trophoblastic tumours from uterine curettings. *J Clin Pathol* 1972;25:111–118.
30. Elston CW. The histopathology of trophoblastic tumors. *J Clin Pathol* 1976;10:111–131.
31. Curry SL, Hammond CB, Tyrey L, Creasman WT, Parker RT. Hydatidiform mole: diagnosis, management, and long-term followup of 347 patients. *Obstet Gynecol* 1975;45:1–8.
32. Hertig AT, Sheldon WH. Hydatidiform mole. A pathologico-clinical correlation of 200 cases. *Am J Obstet Gynecol* 1947;53:1–36.
33. Mazur MT, Kurman RJ. Gestational trophoblastic disease. In: Kurman RJ, ed. *Blaustein's pathology of the female genital tract.* New York: Springer-Verlag, 1987:835–875.
34. Goldstein DP, Berkowitz RS. *Gestational trophoblastic neoplasms. Clinical principles of diagnosis and management.* Philadelphia: WB Saunders, 1982.
35. Szulman AE. Partial hydatidiform mole. In Szulman AE, Buchsbaum HJ, eds. *Gestational trophoblastic disease.* New York: Springer-Verlag, 1987:37–44.
36. Berkowitz RS, Goldstein DP, Bernstein MR. Natural history of partial molar pregnancy. *Obstet Gynecol* 1985;66:677–681.
37. Smith EB, Szulman AE, Hinsaw W, Tyrey L, Surti U, Hammond CB. Human chorionic gonadotropin levels in complete and partial hydatidiform moles and in nonmolar abortuses. *Am J Obstet Gynecol* 1984;149:129–132.

38. Szulman AE. Complete hydatidiform mole: clinico-pathologic features. In: Szulman AE, Buchsbaum HJ, eds. *Gestational trophoblastic disease.* New York: Springer-Verlag, 1987:27–36.

39. Lurain JR, Brewer JI, Torok EE, Halpern B. Natural history of hydatidiform mole after primary evacuation. *Am J Obstet Gynecol* 1983;145:591–595.

40. Bagshawe KD, Wilson H, Dublon P, Smith A, Baldwin M, Kardana A. Follow-up after hydatidiform mole: studies using radioimmunoassay for urinary human chorionic gonadotrophin (HCG). *J Obstet Gynaecol Br Commonw* 1973;80:461–468.

41. Hertig AT, Mansell H. Tumors of the female sex organs. Part 1. Hydatidiform mole and choriocarcinoma. In: *Atlas of tumor pathology,* section 9, fascicle 33. Washington, DC: Armed Forces Institute of Pathology, 1956.

42. Mostoufi-Zadeh M, Berkowitz RS, Driscoll SG. Persistence of partial mole. *Am J Clin Pathol* 1987;87:377–380.

43. Gaber LW, Redline RW, Mostoufi-Zadeh M, Driscoll SG. Invasive partial mole. *Am J Clin Pathol* 1986;85:722–724.

44. Szulman AE, Ma HK, Wong LC, Hsu C. Residual trophoblastic disease in association with partial hydatidiform moles. *Obstet Gynecol* 1981;57:392–394.

45. Takeuchi S. Nature of invasive mole and its rational treatment. *Semin Oncol* 1982;9:181–186.

46. Dehner LP. Gestational and nongestational trophoblastic neoplasia. A historic and pathobiologic surgery. *Am J Surg Pathol* 1980;4:43–58.

47. Delfs E. Quantitative chorionic gonadotrophin: prognostic value in hydatidiform mole and chorionepithelioma. *Obstet Gynecol* 1957;9:1–24.

48. Elston CW. Trophoblastic tumors of the placenta. In: Fox H, ed. *Pathology of the placenta.* Philadelphia: WB Saunders, 1978:368–425.

49. Elston CW. Development and structure of trophoblastic neoplasms. In: Luke YW, Whyte A, eds. *Biology of trophoblast.* New York: Elsevier, 1983:188–232.

50. Lurain JR, Brewer JI, Torok EE, Halpern B. Gestational trophoblastic disease: treatment results at the Brewer Trophoblastic Disease Center. *Obstet Gynecol* 1982;60:354–360.

51. Novak E, Seah CS. Choriocarcinoma of the uterus. A study of 74 cases from the Mathieu Memorial Chorionepithelioma Registry. *Am J Obstet Gynecol* 1954;67:933–961.

52. Ober WB, Edgcomb JH, Price EB. The pathology of choriocarcinoma. *Ann NY Acad Sci* 1971;179:299–321.

53. Mazur MT, Lurain JR, Brewer JI. Fatal gestational choriocarcinoma. Clinicopathologic study of patients treated at a trophoblastic disease center. *Cancer* 1982;50:1833–1846.

54. Kurman RJ, Young RH, Norris HJ, Main CS, Lawrence WD, Scully RE. Immunocytochemical localization of placental lactogen and chorionic gonadotropin in the normal placenta and trophoblastic tumors, with emphasis on intermediate trophoblast and the placental site trophoblastic tumor. *Int J Gynecol Pathol* 1984;3:101–121.

54a. Duncan DA, Mazur MT. Trophoblastic tumors. Ultrastructural comparison of choriocarcinoma and placental–site trophoblastic tumor. *Hum Pathol* 1989;20:370–381.

54b. Mazur MT. Metastatic gestational choriocarcinoma. Unusual pathologic variant following therapy. *Cancer* 1989;63:1370–1377.

55. Kurman RJ, Main CS, Chen HC. Intermediate trophoblast: a distinctive form of trophoblast with specific morphological, biochemical and functional features. *Placenta* 1984;5:349–370.

56. Brewer JI, Mazur MT. Gestational choriocarcinoma: its origin in the placenta during seemingly normal pregnancy. *Am J Surg Pathol* 1981;5:267–277.

57. Kubosawa H, Nagao K, Kondo Y, et al. Coexistence of adenocarcinoma and choriocarcinoma in the sigmoid colon. *Cancer* 1984;54:866–868.

58. Obe JA, Rosen N, Koss LG. Primary choriocarcinoma of the urinary bladder. Report of a case with probable epithelial origin. *Cancer* 1983;52:1405–1409.

59. Savage J, Subby W, Okagaki T. Adenocarcinoma of the endometrium with trophoblastic differentiation and metastases as choriocarcinoma: a case report. *Gynecol Oncol* 1987;26:257–262.

60. Heyderman E, Chapman DV, Richardson TC, Calvert I, Rosen SW. Human chorionic gonadotropin and human placental lactogen in extragonadal tumors: an immunoperoxidase study of ten non-germ cell neoplasms. *Cancer* 1985;56:2674–2682.

61. Hammond CB, Hertz R, Ross GT, Lipsett MB, Odell WD. Diagnostic problems of choriocarcinoma and related trophoblastic neoplasms. *Obstet Gynecol* 1967;29:224–229.

62. Olive DL, Lurain JR, Brewer JI. Choriocarcinoma associated with term gestation. *Am J Obstet Gynecol* 1984;148:711–716.

63. Hou PC, Pang SC. Chorionepithelioma: An analytical study of 28 necropsied cases with special reference to the possibility of spontaneous retrogression. *J Pathol Bacteriol* 1956;72:95–104.

64. Dougherty CM, Cunningham C, Mickal A. Choriocarcinoma with metastases in a postmenopausal woman. *Am J Obstet Gynecol* 1978;132:700–701.

65. Brewer JI, Smith RT, Pratt GB. Choriocarcinoma. Absolute 5 year survival rates of 122 patients treated by hysterectomy. *Am J Obstet Gynecol* 1963;85:841–843.

66. Lurain JR, Brewer JI, Mazur MT, Torok EE. Fatal gestational trophoblastic disease: an analysis of treatment failures. *Am J Obstet Gynecol* 1982;144:391–395.

67. Bagshawe KD. Risk and prognostic factors in trophoblastic neoplasia. *Cancer* 1976;38:1373–1385.

68. Hammond CB, Borchert LG, Tyrey L, Creasman WT, Parker RT. Treatment of metastatic trophoblastic disease. Good and poor prognosis. *Am J Obstet Gynecol* 1973;115:451–457.

69. Surwit EA, Alberts DS, Christian CD, Graham VE. Poor-prognosis gestational trophoblastic disease: an update. *Obstet Gynecol* 1984;64:21–26.

70. Berkowitz RS, Goldstein DP, Bernstein MR. Choriocarcinoma following term gestation. *Gynecol Oncol* 1984;17:52–57.

71. Deligdisch L, Driscoll SG, Goldstein DP. Gestational trophoblastic neoplasms: morphologic correlates of therapeutic response. *Am J Obstet Gynecol* 1978;130:801–806.

72. Young RE, Kurman RT, Scully RE. Proliferations and tumors of intermediate trophoblast of the placental site. *Semin Diagn Pathol* 1988;5:223–237.

73. Nickels J, Risberg B, Melander S. Trophoblastic pseudotumor of the uterus. *Acta Pathol Microbiol Scand [A]* 1978;86:14–16.

74. Eckstein RP, Paradinas FJ, Bagshawe KD. Placental site trophoblastic tumour (trophoblastic pseudotumour): a study of four cases requiring hysterectomy including one fatal case. *Histopathology* 1982;6:211–226.

75. Kurman RJ, Scully RE, Norris HJ. Trophoblastic pseudotumor of the uterus. *Cancer* 1976;38:1214–1226.

76. Gloor E, Hurlimann J. Trophoblastic pseudotumor of the uterus. Clinicopathologic report with immunohistochemical and ultrastructural studies. *Am J Surg Pathol* 1981;5:5–13.

77. Nagelberg SB, Rosen SW. Clinical and laboratory investigation of a virilized woman with placental site trophoblastic tumor. *Obstet Gynecol* 1985;65:527–534.

78. Young RE, Scully RE, McCluskey RT. A distinctive glomerular lesion complicating placental site trophoblastic tumor: report of two cases. *Hum Pathol* 1985;16:35–42.

79. Eckstein RP, Russell P, Friedlander ML, Tattersall MHN, Bradfield A. Metastasizing placental site trophoblastic tumor: a case study. *Hum Pathol* 1983;16:632–636.

80. Gloor E, Dialdas J, Hurlimann J, Ribolzi J, Barrelet L. Placental site trophoblastic tumor (trophoblastic pseudotumor) of the uterus with metastases and fatal outcome. *Am J Surg Pathol* 1983;7:483–486.

81. Hopkins M, Nunez C, Murphy JR, Wentz WB. Malignant placental site trophoblastic tumor. *Obstet Gynecol* 1985;66:95S–100S.

Surgical Pathology of the Female Reproductive System and Peritoneum, edited by Stephen S. Sternberg and Stacey E. Mills. Raven Press, Ltd, New York © 1991.

CHAPTER 2

The Placenta

Geoffrey Altshuler

Many descriptions and discussions of placental pathology are available in textbooks, articles, and reviews. In 1984, Perrin edited an excellent volume on the pathology of the placenta (1). For 20 years, Benirschke and Driscoll's book has been the outstanding tome (2). Fox also has written a succinct textbook in this area (3). Nonetheless, some discussions of placental pathology contain controversial, conflicting, and even substantially incorrect statements. For example, one textbook states that "Histological examination of the placenta of a macerated fetus is of no value whatsoever." This chapter emphasizes a practical, morphologic approach to placental pathology. Where the author's procedures differ from prior publications, these differences and their rationale are discussed in detail.

MEDICOLEGAL INDICATIONS FOR PLACENTAL EXAMINATIONS

Because of huge litigations, many obstetricians have quit practice. Placental findings can prove that clinical management is usually not the primary cause of adverse neonatal outcome. The placenta is a diary of gestational life; as is the case for all other surgical biopsies, it can often reveal the pathogenesis of disease (4). In some states, litigations of perinatal cases can be filed for 18 years after alleged medical negligence. Hospitals are thus now well advised to save representative parts of all placentas. A nurse practitioner and pathology technician can complete a checklist (Table 1) and prepare paraffin blocks for storage. If needed, the gross placental information can be obtained, and the paraffin blocks processed, for light-microscopic examination. The cost would be defrayed by successful use of placental findings as opposed to making incorrect judgments.

The role of placentas in medicolegal medicine has been discussed in a recent review (5). Several of the statements in this prior study (5) differ from the current author's approach. Because of the increasing medicolegal implications of proper placental examination, the following differences with the prior review should be emphasized:

1. "A microscopic examination is needed . . . if a placenta is grossly abnormal." Many placentas are grossly abnormal, but there are often no associated clinical problems. Fox exaggerates this point: "Very few gross lesions of the placenta are therefore of any clinical or functional significance . . . and they have been discussed at some length . . . only in an attempt to emphasize their banality (3)."

2. "Troublesome (placental) artifacts can appear within 48 hours during refrigeration." I have examined thousands of placentas within a week of delivery and have not encountered troublesome refrigeration artifacts. For microbiologic study, one can sterilize the placental amniotic surface and obtain a noncontaminated chorionic specimen even 4 days after delivery.

3. "The only bacterium that is widely recognized to cause villitis is *Listeria monocytogenes*." Campylobacter, mycobacteria, and viruses may not be widely known causes of villitis, but there are many reports and descriptions of villitis caused by *Escherichia coli* and syphilis.

4. Meconium-induced epithelial changes, notably pseudostratification of the amniotic epithelial cells, is said to occur within an hour of the time that meconium first appears in the amniotic fluid. The methods of the cited study, however, were performed *in vitro* (6). Sequential *in vivo* changes are not necessarily identical.

CLINICAL INDICATIONS FOR GROSS AND LIGHT-MICROSCOPIC PLACENTAL EXAMINATION

Clinical indications for a prompt placental examination include recurrent reproductive failure (a maternal

TABLE 1. *Gross placental report*

General:

Trimmed weight: _____ g

Size: _____ × _____ × _____ cm

Complete placenta (yes/no):

Cord:

Site of cord insertion:

Number of cord vessels:

Membranes:

Placental sac rupture: _____ cm from margin

Membrane insertion: _____ % marginal

_____ % circummarginate

_____ % circumvallate

Placenta:

Color of fetal surface:

Infarcts (yes/no):

Acute infarcts or ischemia <50% (yes/no):

Chronic infarcts or ischemia <50% (yes/no):

Abruption (%):

Maternal floor:

Comment:

_____ , M.D.

---

history of stillbirth, spontaneous abortion, and/or prematurity in one or more pregnancy), diabetes, dysmorphism, dysmaturity, erythroblastosis, multiple births, and meconium staining.

ACCESSION, STORAGE, PROCESSING, AND ARTIFACTS

Placentas should never be frozen. Freezing distorts the villi, obscures meconium, and compromises diagnoses. Placentas of normal pregnancies and deliveries should be temporarily stored. Our personnel refrigerate them for 1 week, at 4°C. If a clinician requests a placental examination, we obtain the specimen that would otherwise be incinerated. Methods of examination have been provided in detail (7–9). We document the gross features that are listed in Table 1.

When a placenta is refrigerated, it progressively loses blood and fluid. The associated weight loss does not detract from appreciation of clinically meaningful pathological size.

Artifacts occur when placentas are fixed prior to examination. Fixation in buffered formalin causes more than a 12% increase in weight. It prevents the success of many microbiological tests, produces distention of blood vessels, and causes congested thrombotic and villitis lesions to appear hemorrhagic. Distention of blood vessels simulates effects of cord obstruction and fetal cardiac failure.

Bouin's fixative masks fusobacteria (Fig. 1). In my experience, the Brown and Hopps method of staining bacteria is convenient and reliable (10). Other stains often fail to show organisms.

Light-microscopic items that should be evaluated are listed in Table 2.

Details of placental processing include the following:

1. Umbilical cord vascular anastomoses are present near the placenta. To avoid an incorrect diagnosis of single umbilical artery, the cord should be sampled 4 cm or more from its insertion into the placenta.

2. The membrane roll should be sampled by making a roll in which the rupture site is at the center of the roll.

3. Placental blocks for fixation ideally should be approximately 2.5 cm depth by 2 cm width by 1.5 cm thickness.

4. Care should be taken to compensate for placental congestion. The volume of buffered 10% formalin used for fixation should be at least 10 times greater than the total volume of tissue segments.

5. The use of new blades enables optimal sampling of amniotic epithelium. Blunt blades disrupt the amnion from the underlying tissue.

6. Representative sections should include a block with a segment of umbilical cord and membrane roll, a block with a segment of superficial placenta near the umbilical cord insertion site, two blocks of tissue from nonmarginal superficial placental sites, and two blocks of nonmarginal placenta with maternal floor. Samples of lesions should also be processed.

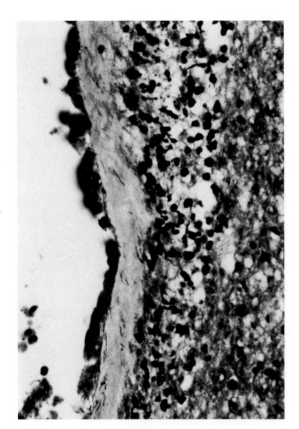

FIG. 1. Placental surface. Fusobacteria are present beneath the necrotic epithelial surface. Beneath the bacteria there is a band of necrotic inflammatory cells. (Brown and Hopps.)

MULTIPLE PREGNANCY

Benirschke has provided methods for the placental examination of specimens from multiple births (11). Reviews of clinicopathologic, teratologic, and other aspects of twins are also available (12,13). The examination of placentas from twins is similar to that for a singleton. Tissue pieces are trimmed into five blocks from each placenta, plus blocks of each umbilical cord, pla-

TABLE 2. *Features examined by light microscopy*

1. Meconium staining	15. Amnion nodosum
2. Membranitis	16. Chorioamnionitis
3. Cord vasculitis	17. Funisitis
4. Perivillositis	18. Tissue ischemia
5. Infarction	19. Intervillous fibrin
6. Thrombi	20. Endovasculitis
7. Avascular villi	21. Intravillous hemosiderin
8. Chorangiosis	22. Dysmaturity
9. Intravillous hemorrhage	23. Hydrops
10. Fetal nucleated red blood cells	24. Intervillous thrombi
11. Specific villitis	25. Villitis of unknown etiology
12. Proliferative villitis	26. Necrotizing villitis
13. Granulomatous villitis	27. Lymphohistiocytic villitis
14. Lymphoplasmacytic villitis	28. Basal villitis

cental sac, and interplacental partition. Placentas from triplets and quadruplets also can be similarly examined. Because monochorionic twin placentas have only one disk, their interplacental partition does not include chorionic or decidual tissue (Fig. 2). It is transparent and has only two layers of amnion. Diamnionic, dichorionic placental partitions have two separate chorionic layers or fused (originally bilayered) chorions (Fig. 3). They therefore tend to be opaque. Amniotic tissue does not have blood vessels. The presence of any vessel within an interplacental partition means that the placentation is dichorionic.

Twin Transfusion Syndrome

Monochorionic twin placentas share artery-to-artery, vein-to-vein, and artery-to-vein anastomoses. Injection of easily seen liquid or roentgenographic dye can demonstrate these anastomoses. Identification of superficial anastomoses is facilitated by the fact that, where a vessel overlies another, the more superficial vessel is arterial. When blood transfused from a donor is insufficiently returned, the twin transfusion syndrome occurs (11–13). The donor twin is then small and pale, and the recipient twin is large and plethoric. The donor twin suffers anemia, and the recipient twin suffers high output cardiac failure. In fatal cases, there is typically discordancy of

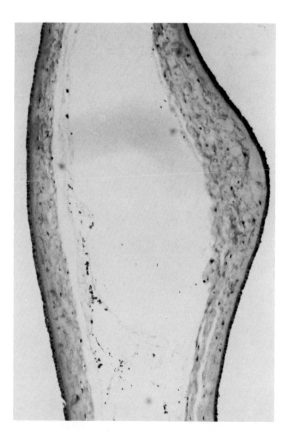

FIG. 2. Monochorionic interplacental partition.

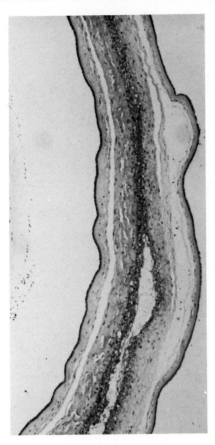

FIG. 3. Dichorionic interplacental partition.

organ size. The heart is the first organ thus affected. The donor has small organs, and the recipient twin has large organs. This syndrome is the major cause of midtrimester, twin pregnancy mortality. In symptomatic liveborns, the diagnosis is made by a combination of clinical and placental findings; typically, there is a lack of large, superficial placental anastomoses. One side of the monochorionic disk may be congested, and the other side may be pale. Because human dichorionic twins never have interplacental anastomoses, they never have the twin transfusion syndrome.

NORMAL PLACENTAL DEVELOPMENT

Gross Features

The placenta should consist of a single disk without any kind of accessory lobe. At midtrimester, the umbilical cord insertion is central and, as gestation proceeds, the cord insertion becomes eccentric. The cord should have two arteries and one vein. Severe eccentricity of cord insertion is abnormal, as is irregular insertion of the membranes (Fig. 4). Often, gross placental abnormalities are not associated with symptomatic disease or malformation.

Light-Microscopic Features

Changes of placental maturation include diminution in the size of villi, condensation of trophoblast, and development of syncytiotrophoblast knots (Figs. 5A–C).

MAJOR GROSS ABNORMALITIES

Size and Shape

Although some authors believe that routinely weighing the placenta should be discontinued because of difficulty in quantifying or controlling the amount of fetal

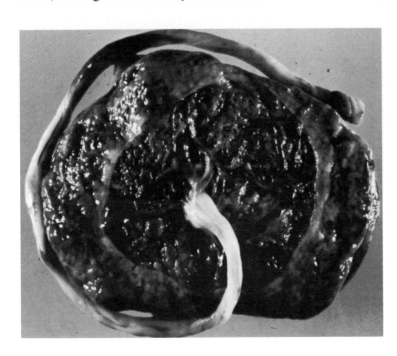

FIG. 4. Circumvallate placenta. There is a peripheral cup-like insertion of the membranes at the placental surface.

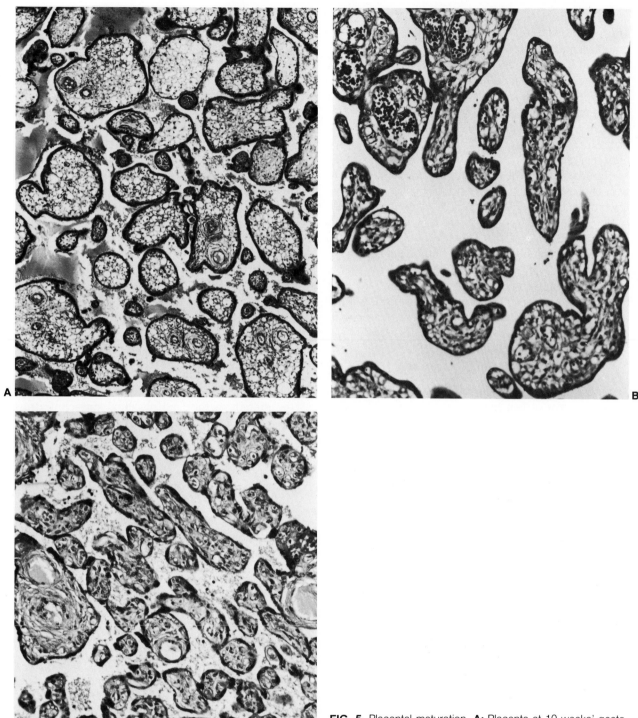

FIG. 5. Placental maturation. **A:** Placenta at 10 weeks' gestation. The villi have a hydropic appearance. **B:** Placenta at 30 weeks' gestation. Severe congestion distends these villi, but they are not hydropic. **C:** Placenta at 40 weeks' gestation. The villi are much smaller than those of the first and second trimester. Also, they are bordered by condensed syncytiotrophoblast and syncytiotrophoblastic knots.

blood remaining (14), I disagree. Despite the aforementioned consideration, the following pertains with normal placentas. At 20 weeks' gestation, the trimmed unfixed and fresh placenta should not exceed 150 g; at 30 weeks' gestation, it should not be more than 375 g; and at term gestation, it should not weigh more than 600 g. The cause of placentomegaly is usually inapparent. Frequently recognized causes include diabetes, chronic intrauterine infection, immunohemolytic anemia, and maternal anemia.

Abnormal placental shapes usually are not associated with clinical problems. Accessory placental lobes or bidiscoid placentas with anastomoses between the disks can predispose a newborn to blood loss. The mechanism of this is the same as that which occurs with vascular rupture of velamentously inserted umbilical cords (Fig. 6). When pieces of placenta are retained in the uterus, the mother may suffer postpartum hemorrhage. The placental shape is usually normal, but inspection of the maternal floor readily reveals the incomplete cotyledons.

Fetal Placental Surface Color

A normal fetal placental surface has a light blue or blue-pink color. When acute meconium staining occurs and the meconium has been on the placenta for only a few minutes, the placental surface and membranes have a green discoloration. They have viscid surfaces. The longer a placenta has been exposed to meconium, the more its appearance changes from a slimy green color to mud-brown discoloration. Chorioamnionitis, in its early phase, does not have any grossly visible change. Severe or chronic chorioamnionitis has a dull, yellow-gray color. Fusobacteria can cause the fetal placental surface to appear light green. When we have seen the characteristic color, we have taken a chorionic specimen for culture and have isolated fusobacteria. Abruptio placentae is typically accompanied by blood clots. Remote episodes of placental abruption often cause red-brown placental discoloration. The cause of that color is hemosiderin or blood pigment.

Not uncommonly, the fetal placental surface has tan-pink or tan-gray discolorations that result from plaques of chorionic fibrin. The size and extent of these changes should be noted within the gross description.

Membrane Insertion

Normal placentas have membranes that insert directly into their edge. There is no villous tissue beyond the margin of the fetal placental surface. Extrachorial

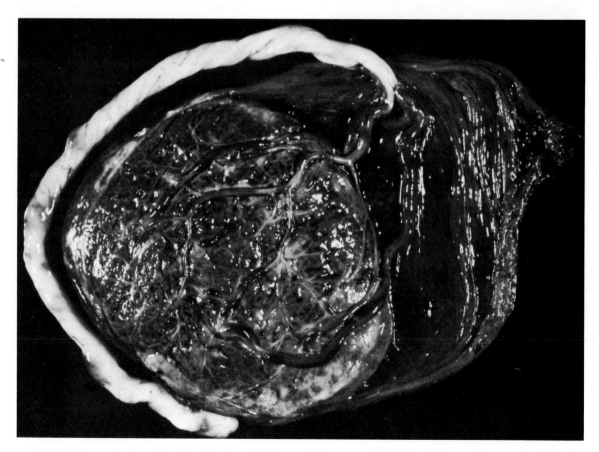

FIG. 6. Velamentous insertion of umbilical cord. At the top right aspect of the illustration, the umbilical cord is seen to insert into the placental membranes.

placentas are either circummarginate or circumvallate. Circummarginate placentas have a margin with thin, fibrous, flat tissue. Circumvallate placentas have a peripheral protuberance of villous tissue (Fig. 4). In large population studies, extrachorial placentas with cysts or other aberrations correlate with maternal and fetal abnormalities. The mother may have an abnormal uterus. The newborn may have an overt or inapparent malformation. Circummarginate placentas usually do not have any accompanying clinical problem. Severe circumvallate placentation results from repeated marginal hemorrhages. Associated clinical manifestations include a maternal history of uterine bleeding, cramping, and hydrorrhea (15).

Fetal Placental Surface Lesions

Acute hemorrhages are often present near the umbilical cord insertion. They are caused by cord traction and usually do not have clinical significance. If 0.2- to 0.4-cm amniotic lesions are present, a sample should be taken for light-microscopic examination. Very small amniotic granules or nodules indicate amnion nodosum. Crateriform amniotic lesions of similar size are usually caused by stratified squamous metaplasia. These abnormalities are discussed in the section on major light-microscopic abnormalities.

Cysts

With or without a content of blood, cysts can be present at the surface of a placenta or anywhere

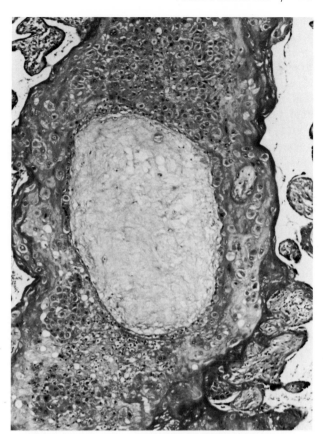

FIG. 8. X-cell cyst. There are many X-cells about the microcyst. They have vesicular nuclei and basophilic cytoplasm.

throughout its cotyledons (Fig. 7). The cysts are lined by cells that are called "X-cells" (Fig. 8). They have a fetal origin and are most abundant in degenerate and ischemic placentas of growth-retarded fetuses (16,17). Their secretory function is poorly understood, but they appear to be involved with the metabolism of prostaglandins and with suppression of labor (17,18).

Infarcts and Intervillous Thrombi

Acute infarcts may have a red-purple color but often they are grossly unrecognizable. Chronic infarcts are tan-gray. Thrombi of intervillous laminated fibrin have a pink-red color. The volume of that tissue should be documented as accurately as possible. This includes record of focal and diffuse changes and one light-microscopic slide for each affected area. Even if less than half of the placenta has these lesions, there may be untoward outcome of the associated newborn. This is particularly true if the rest of the placenta has villous shrinkage, inflammation, and other pathological features. Only when the entire features of the placenta are known can one adduce the extent to which placental pathology is significant. Severe gross lesions can be free of ill outcome, and subtle abnormalities may be associated with perinatal morbidity and mortality.

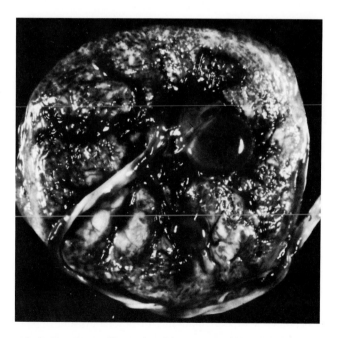

FIG. 7. X-cell cyst. Hemorrhage is present within and about the central X-cell cyst.

Maternal Floor Infarction

A layer of degenerative maternal floor tissue has been called "maternal floor infarction" (19). It consists of a gross gray-white or gray-tan decidual 0.2- to 0.4-cm thickening. This abnormality does not result from ischemic necrosis but is comprised of a fibrinoid replacement of decidua (Fig. 9). Cut surfaces of these placentas are more firm than usual. Although it has been suggested that maternal floor infarction is only a postmortem change, seen when several days or weeks have elapsed between fetal death and abortion (20), this has not been my experience. Many of these placentas that I have seen have been associated with neonates who have suffered from a variety of diseases. From specimens and data of the Collaborative Perinatal Study, Naeye has found that 50% of gravidas with maternal floor infarction have had prior abortions and stillbirths (21).

Calcification

Placentas with numerous foci of calcification are pathologic but are not necessarily associated with a poor outcome of the associated newborn. Often, however, these placentas have fibrinoid entrapment of villi, X-cell proliferation, and diffuse chronic infarction. Because of

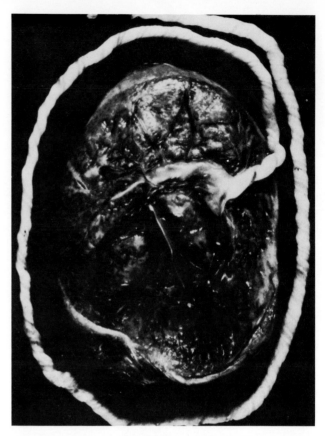

FIG. 10. Placenta with long umbilical cord. Also note the diagonal structure near the cord insertion. It is a fetal vessel with an intravascular luminal cushion of fibrin thrombus.

reduced uteroplacental circulation that causes the latter abnormalities, fetal growth retardation and neonatal morbidity and mortality may result.

Umbilical Cord Abnormalities

The mean length of an umbilical cord at term is between 50 cm and 60 cm (22). Obstruction and thrombi may occur when an umbilical cord is very long (Fig. 10). Short cords have been associated with conditions of impaired fetal mobility. Examples include oligohydramnios, maternal uterine malformation, the amniotic band syndrome, and congenital neuromuscular diseases (22). Experimental studies of Moessinger et al. support the opinion that longitudinal cord growth is influenced by tensile forces and depends on fetal motor activity and space available for movement (23). Rupture of a cord that inserts into the placental membranes may occur during labor (Fig. 6). This can cause anemia of fetal blood loss. Usually, velamentously inserted umbilical cords are not associated with increased morbidity or mortality. A higher incidence of deformational defects has been suggested to result from intrauterine mechanical factors that cause the fetus and placenta to compete for space at the implantation site (24).

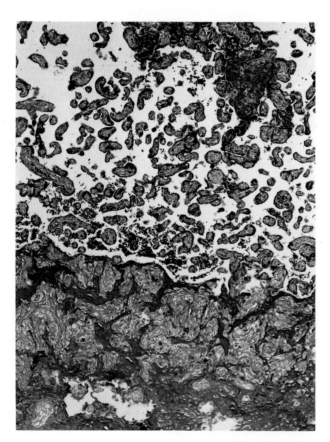

FIG. 9. Maternal floor infarction. Fibrinoid degeneration of the maternal floor is herein complicated by shrinkage of the adjacent villi.

THE PLACENTA / 25

Single umbilical artery (SUA) occurs in approximately 1% of term deliveries. It is found in about 2% of perinatal autopsies. There is a sevenfold incidence of associated anomalies, but no particular organ system is therein affected. Twins have an increased incidence of SUA; acardiac twins usually have the anomaly. When newborns with SUA survive the neonatal period, they are at no greater risk of mortality than non-SUA neonates. Heifetz has provided a major review of SUA (25).

Rare omphalomesenteric duct cysts and tumors of the umbilical cord have been reviewed relatively recently (26,27).

Miscellaneous Considerations

The gross examination should include documentation of blood clots and the rupture site of the extraplacental membranes. In the absence of cesarean section, marginally ruptured membranes indicate that the placenta had implanted near the cervix.

MAJOR LIGHT-MICROSCOPIC ABNORMALITIES

Chorioamnionitis

Definition and Significance

The term "chorioamnionitis" designates inflammation of the extraplacental membranes and the placental amnion and chorion (Figs. 1 and 11). Beyond 30 weeks' gestation, umbilical cord vasculitis and funisitis are often additionally present. The fundamental importance of chorioamnionitis is that it causes prematurity.

Historical Considerations

Almost 40 years ago, Knox et al. postulated the pathogenesis of chorioamnionitis: "It seemed logical that an infectious process in the cervical canal might extend itself to the membranes overlying the internal os" (28). Within the next 10 years, Benirschke and Blanc separately described pathways by which a fetus can become infected (29,30). Those pathologists regarded chorioamnionitis as being synonymous with ascending intrauterine infection. Not everyone agreed. Dominguez claimed that hypoxia could cause chorioamnionitis (31). Both before and after the development of sophisticated microbiologic techniques, several investigators were unable to demonstrate a causal relationship between infection and chorioamnionitis (32–34).

Inferential Considerations

Inferences from basic pathology indicate that infection causes chorioamnionitis:

a. Organisms are often demonstrable.
b. Microabscesses are often part of the inflammatory process.

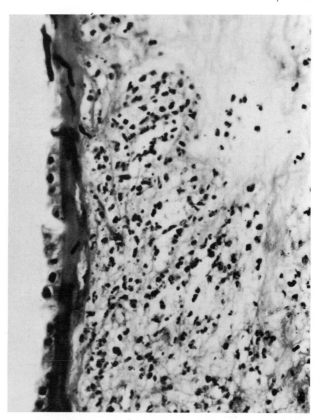

FIG. 11. Amnionitis with *Candida albicans*. Hyphae are present at the top left aspect of the illustration. (Gomori methenamine silver.)

c. Light-microscopic examination of chorioamnionitis frequently shows apparent chemotaxis between organisms at the amniotic surface and fetal leukocytes that transgress vessels of the chorionic plate and umbilical cord (Fig. 12).
d. Within an inflamed membrane roll, whose center has the membrane rupture site, maximal inflammation at the center of the roll indicates ascent of an infectious agent from the cervix.

With twins, one never sees chorioamnionitis in the placenta of the second born in the absence of similar inflammation of the placenta of the first born (35). This provides evidence that in chorioamnionitis, organisms have ascended from the vagina and cervix to the placenta.

Microbiologic Methods

Because of cost, there has never been a totally comprehensive investigation of aerobic and anaerobic bacteria, mycoplasma, chlamydia, and viruses. A successful method of obtaining a specimen begins with sterilizing the amniotic surface with a hot spatula. Sterile scissors and forceps are then used to obtain underlying chorionic tissue (36). Some investigators have used a swab to obtain specimens (37). Both methods have led to the dem-

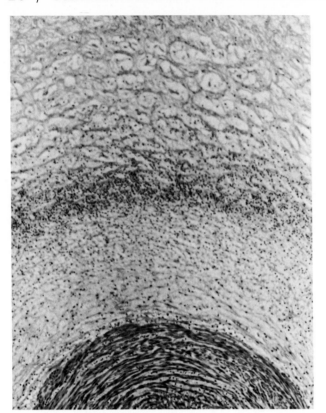

FIG. 12. Amniotropism. In this illustration, a band of polymorphonuclear leukocytes is present within the Wharton jelly of an umbilical cord.

onstration of a relationship between infection and chorioamnionitis (36,37). This is particularly noteworthy because neither of these studies included tests for viruses. There is no *a priori* reason to assume that viruses cannot cause chorioamnionitis.

Obstetrical Significance of Chorioamnionitis

Major contributions have been published in the obstetrical literature regarding this point (38,39). Obstetricians diagnose chorioamnionitis in clinical terms of maternal fever, tachycardia, uterine tenderness, leukocytosis, and a foul odor during labor. Gibbs and colleagues have studied chorioamnionitis at term (38,39). Prolonged rupture of membranes increases the incidence of chorioamnionitis, but placental inflammation is more often a cause of ruptured membranes than a consequence. Minkoff has comprehensively reviewed the infectious etiology of chorioamnionitis (40).

Relationship of Chorioamnionitis to Neonatal Disease

In a clinicopathologic study, my colleagues and I showed a relationship between chorionic microabscesses and infection of the associated newborn (41). The investigation was performed in a predominantly intensive

care population (41). Russell came to the same conclusion in an investigation of 7,505 placentas associated with consecutive singleton infants delivered after 20 weeks' gestation (42).

Specific Causes of Chorioamnionitis

Mycoplasma infection

Twenty years ago, Kundsin and Driscoll drew attention to the role of mycoplasma as a cause of chorioamnionitis and reproductive failure (43). In a later study of 572 placentas, these investigators found that perinatal morbidity and mortality are associated with colonization of the chorionic surface by *Ureaplasma urealyticum* or *Mycoplasma hominis,* or both (44). Although the investigation included 125 perinatal deaths and 293 placentas from neonatal intensive care patients, *Chlamydia trachomatis* was not isolated from any placenta (44). This absence raises some question regarding the methods of the study (see below). There have been many investigations of genital mycoplasmas. They substantiate a causal relationship between *Ureaplasma urealyticum* (T-mycoplasmas), chorioamnionitis, and perinatal morbidity and mortality (45–48). *Mycoplasma hominis* is a common inhabitant of the female genital tract but is less prone to produce chorioamnionitis and reproductive failure (45,48).

Chlamydia trachomatis infection

Schachter's review of chlamydial infections is an important reference (49). He has provided extensive details of microbiology, pathogenesis, and resultant diseases (49). In 1981, Heggie et al. reported chlamydial infection in 28% of 95 infants born vaginally to infected mothers; conjunctivitis occurred in 20 of 21 infants with chlamydial infection of the conjunctivae, but the chlamydial pneumonia syndrome occurred in only 3 of 18 infants with nasopharyngeal infection (50). Several investigators have shown associations between *Chlamydia trachomatis* infection and perinatal morbidity and mortality in humans (51–53). Their findings indicate that this infection can produce chorioamnionitis or ascending intrauterine infection. At the International Academy of Pathology Congress in 1982, Rettig and I described a rat model of *Chlamydia trachomatis* amniotic infection syndrome. Chorioamnionitis was found in all placentas of *Chlamydia trachomatis* fetal sac inoculations and, by immunofluorescent light-microscopic study, *Chlamydia trachomatis* was demonstrable within the amniotic and yolk sac tissue (Fig. 13). Inflammation was rarely present in controls. By immunohistochemical methods, chlamydial antigens have been demonstrated in 4 of 19 cases with severe endometritis (54). It is of

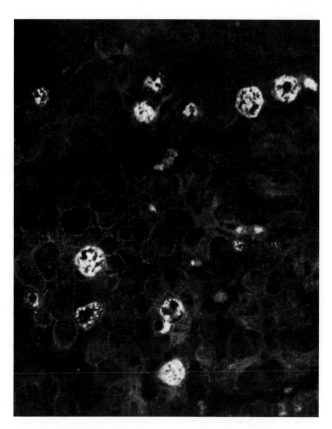

FIG. 13. *Chlamydia trachomatis*. Monoclonal antibody enables easy visualization of organisms in rat placental membrane.

interest that although chlamydial antibodies are commercially available, reports of chlamydial chorioamnionitis are noticeably lacking.

Infection with group B, beta-hemolytic streptococcus

Innumerable reports of perinatal group B, beta-hemolytic streptococcal (GBS) infection are available in many journals. Reports of associated chorioamnionitis are greatly lacking (55,56). On many occasions, I have found minimal chorioamnionitis in the placentas of GBS-infected newborns who have died within the first postnatal day.

Infection with nontypable Haemophilus influenzae

Since 1965, there have been numerous reports of neonatal infection with nontypable *Haemophilus influenzae*. Recent publications include review of 107 cases (57,58). These neonates have suffered pneumonia, meningitis, and sepsis similar to that which occurs with early onset group B, beta-hemolytic streptococcus sepsis (57–60). There has been a strong association with prematurity; more than 80% of the cases have been born at less than 37 weeks' gestation (57). The associated chorioamnionitis has varied in severity (58) and has occurred

with intact amniotic membranes (61). The organisms are fastidious in culture. With the Brown and Hopps stain (9), these short gram-negative bacilli are recognizable within the placental inflammatory process.

Fusobacteria chorioamnionitis

Fusobacteria in infancy was described 30 years ago (62), and neonatal fusobacterium bacteremia was reported more than 20 years ago (63). In contrast, the first detailed description of fusobacteria chorioamnionitis is relatively recent (64,65). We discovered the entity during a study of placental villitis (64). The organisms are pleomorphic and filamentous (Fig. 1). They have occurred in as many as 18% of our chorioamnionitis cases (65). We initially found them with the Warthin-Starry stain. For convenience, we now recommend the Brown and Hopps method of bacterial staining (10). We have often confirmed the diagnosis by culture or by immunofluorescent light-microscopic examination. Fusobacteria are very difficult to see with hematoxylin and eosin. Bouin's fixation severely masks them. Reports of fusobacterium amnionitis are receiving increasing attention in clinical literature (66). We have found that if fusobacteria are unaccompanied by other organisms, they rarely cause neonatal pneumonia, meningitis, or sepsis. The organisms produce phospholipase A_2 and may thereby induce premature onset of labor (67).

Bacteroides fragilis

In European literature, there are reports of infection with *Bacteroides fragilis* (68,69). *Bacteroides fragilis* are very small organisms with a safety-pin-type configuration. On the uncommon occasion that they cause chorioamnionitis, they may be recognizable on hematoxylin and eosin or standard bacterial stains. The role of diagnosis by immunofluorescent light-microscopic examination has been emphasized (69).

Miscellaneous causes of chorioamnionitis

Additional causes of chorioamnionitis include *Staphylococcus aureus, Escherichia coli, Listeria monocytogenes, Candida albicans,* and *Herpes simplex* virus (70–77). Further information is obtainable from recent reviews (70,71).

Conclusion with regard to chorioamnionitis. Infection causes chorioamnionitis and, thereby, prematurity. Chorioamnionitis is also a significant finding in cases of stillbirth (78).

Villitis

Inflammation of the placental villi results from the passage of an infectious agent from the mother's intervillous vascular sinusoids to the villi of the fetus. Intervillositis may also be present (Fig. 14). Organisms reported to cause placental infection are listed in Table 2. These agents are potentially capable of producing villitis. Congenital rubella, toxoplasmosis, and tuberculosis are now rare. Today, the most common specific villitides are caused by cytomegalovirus, herpesvirus, syphilis, *Escherichia coli, Listeria monocytogenes,* and probably enteroviruses, hepatitis viruses, and chlamydia. Campylobacters, which previously were classified in the genus *Vibrio,* rarely cause fetoplacental infection in humans within North America.

Patterns of Villitis

Cytomegalovirus, syphilis, and rubella virus produce lymphoplasmacytic villitis (Fig. 15) and vasculopathy of fetal placental blood vessels. Proliferative endovasculitis (Fig. 16), acute and chronic thrombotic lesions, avascular villi, and intravillous hemosiderin deposits are characteristic of those infections. Cytomegalovirus inclusions are seen in less than one-third of cytomegalovirus

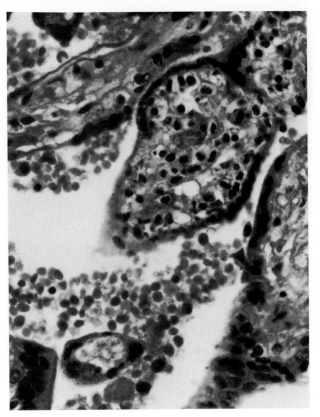

FIG. 15. Lymphoplasmacytic villitis.

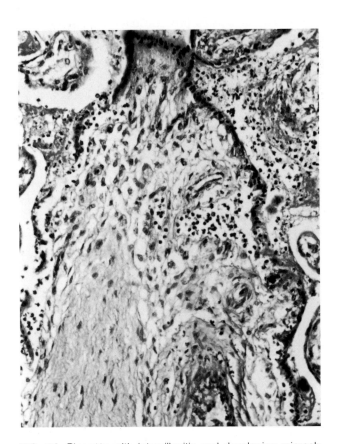

FIG. 14. Placenta with intervillositis and developing microabscess of villus.

placentitis. If any penicillin has been given to a syphilitic mother, spirochetes will not be demonstrable. Alternately, the Warthin-Starry method is an effective means of identifying syphilis (65).

Exudative villitis, with or without demonstrable bacteria, is typical of *Escherichia coli, Listeria monocytogenes,* and campylobacters (Fig. 14). Also, these organisms may cause proliferative and necrotizing perivillositis.

With cytomegalovirus and *Herpes simplex* virus, one usually finds bland, necrotizing lesions in the decidua of the membranes and placenta. The latter infection is additionally characterized by amniotic microvesicles, lymphoplasmacytic or mononuclear chorioamnionitis, and necrotizing villitis.

Villitis of Unknown Etiology

Many years ago, several pathologists briefly mentioned obscure inflammatory lesions of placental villi. A review in 1973 emphasized the importance of these lesions and adopted the term, "villitis of unknown etiology" (79,80). Numerous confirmatory reports have been forthcoming from various investigators in this country and abroad (81–90). The acronym "VUE" is now used to diagnose inflammatory placental lesions that have no morphologically or clinically apparent, specific infectious cause (Fig. 17).

There are many histologic patterns of VUE that may be present within the one placenta. Typical descriptive terms include: proliferative (Fig. 17), necrotizing, granulomatous (Fig. 18), evanescent (Fig. 19), lymphohistiocytic, lymphocytic, and histiocytic. Plasmacytic and lymphoplasmacytic inflammatory-cell infiltrates usually are associated with specific villitides. Reports of VUE include mention of associated chorangiosis and endovasculitis and thrombosis of fetal placental blood vessels (79,80,89).

Sander has claimed that hemorrhagic endovasculitis and hemorrhagic villitis is a "unique (placental) vascular lesion" that occurs in 20% of the placentas referred to his Michigan Placental Registry (83,84). Dr. Susan Shen-Schwarz has found hemorrhagic endovasculitis (HEV) in only 0.67% of placentas at the Magee Women's Hospital (89). Her experience is similar to mine in Cincinnati and Oklahoma City (Figs. 20 and 21). I rarely see HEV in the absence of VUE or thrombotic fetal vasculopathy.

Because lesions of "HEV" feature fragmented red blood cells rather than inflammatory cells, I designate them as "endovasculopathy" rather than as "endovasculitis." I reserve the term "endovasculitis" for lesions like those of Fig. 16.

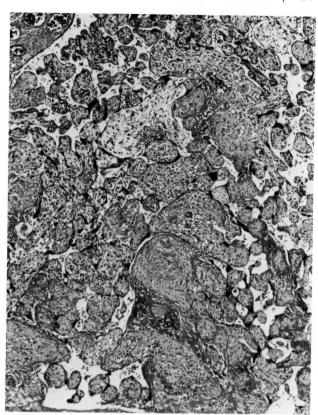

FIG. 17. Villitis of unknown etiology. Toward the center, pepper-like granules of inflammatory cells characterize proliferative villitis.

Twenty-four of Sander's 32 originally reported HEV cases had chronic villitis (83). Sander acknowledges that "intravascular coagulation (DIC) may be basic to the entire process" (84).

Placental hemorrhagic endovasculopathy is very common. It is identified by fetal vascular microhemorrhages and by fragmented red cells with thrombotic and obliterative fetal vascular lesions (Figs. 20–24). Affected placentas often do not have chorioamnionitis, villitis, or accompanying clinical signs of maternofetal infection (90–92). Associated placental changes include fetal vascular occlusion by fibrosis (Fig. 20), organized thrombi (Fig. 22), recanalized thrombi (Fig. 23), and fibrin with endovasculitis (Fig. 24). Associated clinical features frequently include acidosis, hypoxia, diabetic ketoacidosis, intravascular coagulation, spontaneous abortion, and stillbirth.

The more that VUE is investigated with new microbiologic techniques, the more likely it is that many cases will be rediagnosed as a specific infection. Because of the inflammatory diversity within many cases of VUE, it is probable that dual or multiple infections are etiologic.

VUE is associated with fetal growth retardation, stillbirth, and perinatal morbidity and mortality (79–90). Cases of recurrent VUE also have been reported (87,88,90,93). In my experience, one cannot reliably estimate the severity of fetal growth retardation by looking

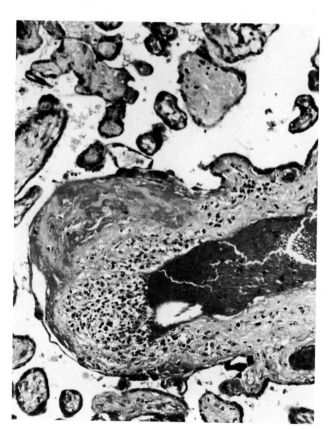

FIG. 16. Proliferative endovasculitis. Also note the avascular, sclerotic villi at the top.

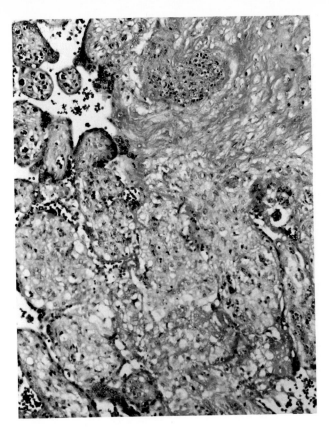

FIG. 18. Granulomatous villitis. Histiocytic cells are extensively present. Also, at top there is a vessel with hemorrhagic endovasculopathy.

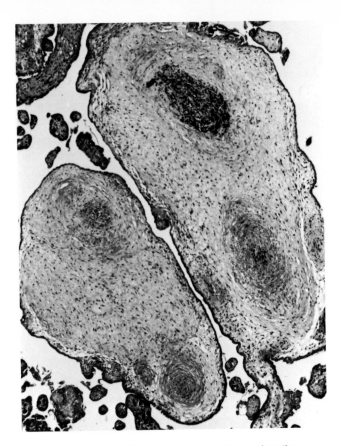

FIG. 20. Villus with hemorrhagic endovasculopathy.

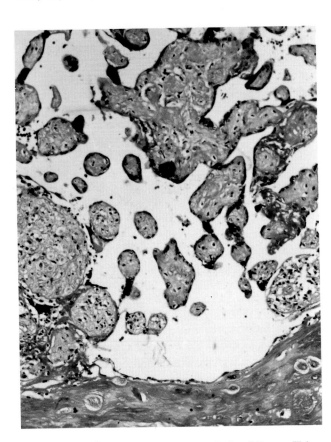

FIG. 19. Evanescent villitis. The avascularity of these villi is a result of remote endovasculitis.

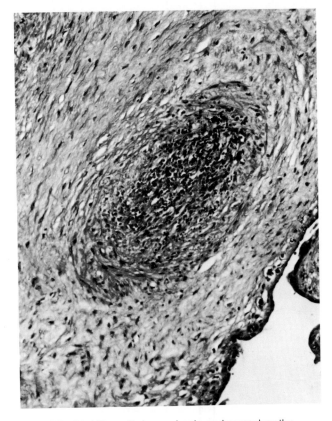

FIG. 21. Villus with hemorrhagic endovasculopathy.

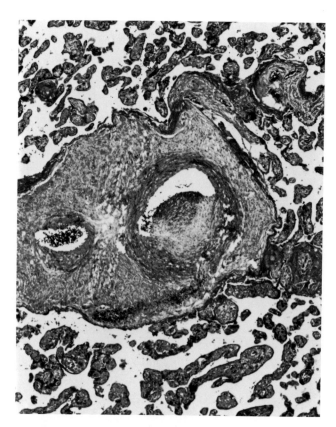

FIG. 22. Villus with intimal fibrin cushion lesion. This appearance is typical of the lesion grossly apparent in Fig. 10.

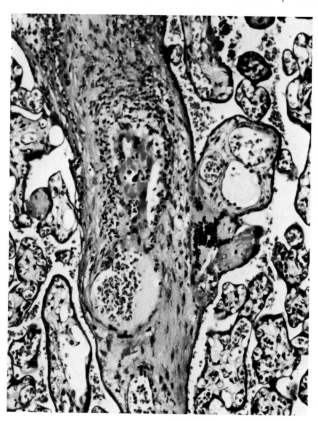

FIG. 24. Placental villus with endovasculitis about intravascular fibrin.

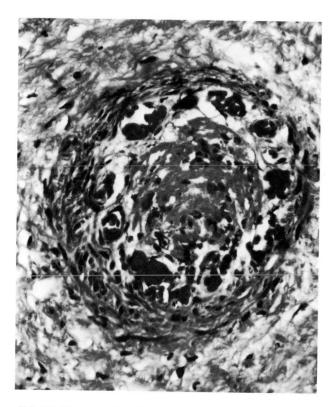

FIG. 23. Placental villus. Fibrin within a recanalized thrombus.

at the numerical severity of villitis lesions. Coexistent placental infarcts and ischemic changes are confounding variables that must additionally be considered.

NONINFECTIOUS LESIONS OF THE AMNION

Meconium Staining

Amniotic epithelium becomes necrotic when the fetus defecates meconium. Epithelial changes ensue within a time frame that has medicolegal significance. Meconium discharge is a sign of fetal distress. If the amnion is necrotic, the meconium discharge very likely occurred within 3 hours of delivery. Beyond that time, the changes are expected to consist of vacuolated large amniotic epithelium and meconium-laden macrophages progressively deep within the subamniotic connective tissue (Fig. 25).

Meconium discharge in baboons has been investigated (94) and *in vitro* meconium-induced changes have been described (6). There are no reported *in vivo* studies of sequential meconium-induced amniotic changes.

Stratified Squamous Metaplasia of the Amnion

The gross appearances of this histologically defined entity consist of crateriform lesions that are each less

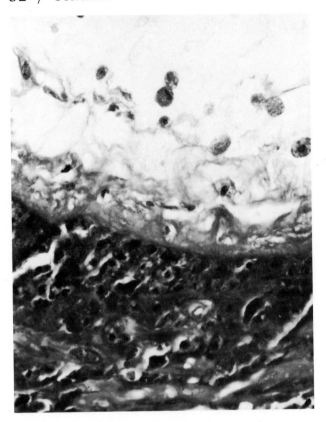

FIG. 25. Placental surface. Chronic meconium staining is evidenced by meconium-laden macrophages deeply located near the chorion.

than 0.4 cm in diameter. The lesions do not have any clinical significance.

Amnion Nodosum and Amniotic Squamous Balls

Chronic leakage of amniotic fluid, as well as dysplastic, nonfunctioning, or absent kidneys, causes oligohy-

dramnios. Amnion nodosum results from these events (Fig. 26). At light-microscopic examination, one sees nodular conglutination of squames and vernix in continuity with a unicellular layer of amniotic epithelium. Lesions of amnion nodosum are often not seen grossly. In my experience, there is no correlation between the severity of the lesions and the extent of symptomatic or fatal disease.

Oligohydramnios may simultaneously be accompanied by amnion nodosum and amniotic squamous balls (Fig. 27). Rarely, I have seen placental amniotic squamous balls unaccompanied by amnion nodosum (95). Whenever a newborn requires high-pressure ventilation, the clinician and pathologist should determine if there are oligohydramnios, lung hypoplasia, and amniotic lesions.

Conclusion With Regard to Amniotic Lesions

For certainty of interpretation, I recommend light-microscopic examination. Amniotic lesions are very difficult to diagnose with the naked eye.

FOCAL AND DIFFUSE VILLOUS DYSMATURITY

The sequence of placental maturation throughout gestation was described earlier in this chapter. In many placentas, rare foci of dysmaturity are randomly present (Fig. 28). There is no associated clinical significance. Alternately, generalized villous dysmaturity is frequently a sign of growth retardation or anomaly in the associated fetus. It is characterized by persistence of cytotrophoblast, deficient development of syncytiotrophoblast knots, persistent abundance of stromal or Hofbauer cells, and delayed diminution in the size of villi (Fig. 29).

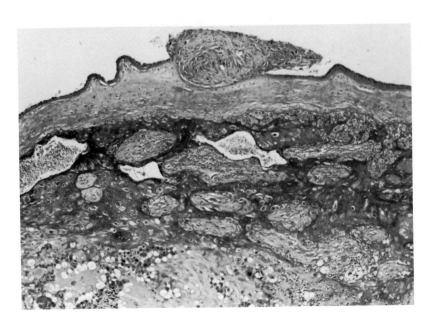

FIG. 26. Placental amnion nodosum.

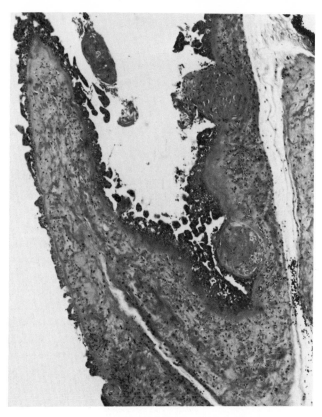

FIG. 27. Placental amniotic squamous balls. Numerous balls of amniotic epithelium are present across the epithelial surface. At the top there is an oval-shaped fragment of conglutinated squames; this resembles sloughed amnion nodosum.

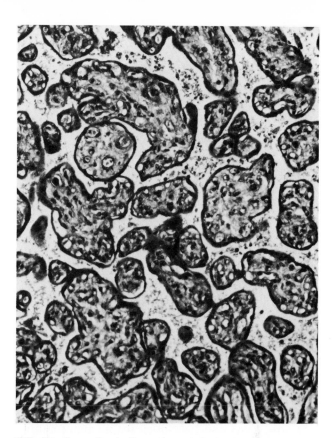

FIG. 29. Generalized villous dysmaturity in the term gestation placenta of a diabetic mother. The villi are enlarged and have increased numbers of Hofbauer cells and reduced syncytiotrophoblastic knots.

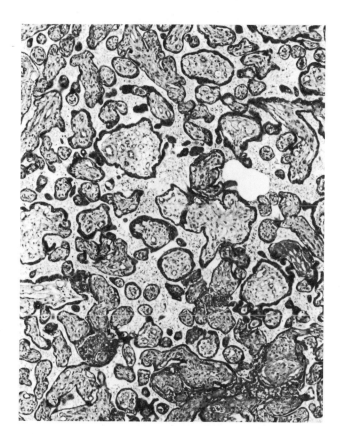

FIG. 28. Focal placental immaturity. Noteworthy features include hydropic villi with syncytiotrophoblastic knots in the sinusoids between them.

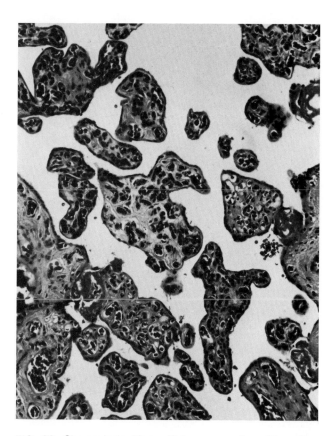

FIG. 30. Chorangiosis. Many villi have more than 10 capillary lumens.

CHORANGIOSIS

The following are criteria for a light-microscopic diagnosis of chorangiosis: There should be at least 10 different fields in 10 different placental areas, with 10 villi that have 10 capillary lumens in each villus (Fig. 30). The vessels may be present in more than one plane of section. Chorangiosis is different from congestion in which vasculature is numerically normal. The excessive vascularity may be masked by edema of high-output fetal cardiac failure (Fig. 31). Chorangiosis never occurs in normal placentas of normal pregnancies and deliveries; it occurs in 5% of placentas from newborns hospitalized in intensive care units (96). I continue to find mortality and congenital anomalies in approximately 30% of associated neonates. Chorangiosis is more often present with diabetes and maternal hypertension syndrome than with other conditions. Thus, it probably results from low-grade tissue hypoxia caused by decidual vasculopathy.

DIABETES

Diverse gross and light-microscopic abnormalities occur with diabetes. These include placentomegaly, in-farcts, hydrops, dysmaturity, chorangiosis, and basement membrane abnormalities of trophoblast and capillaries (97,98). From ultrastructural findings of the placenta in diabetes, Asmussen has suggested that diabetic metabolism induces a proliferative small-vessel disease in combination with accelerated aging (99).

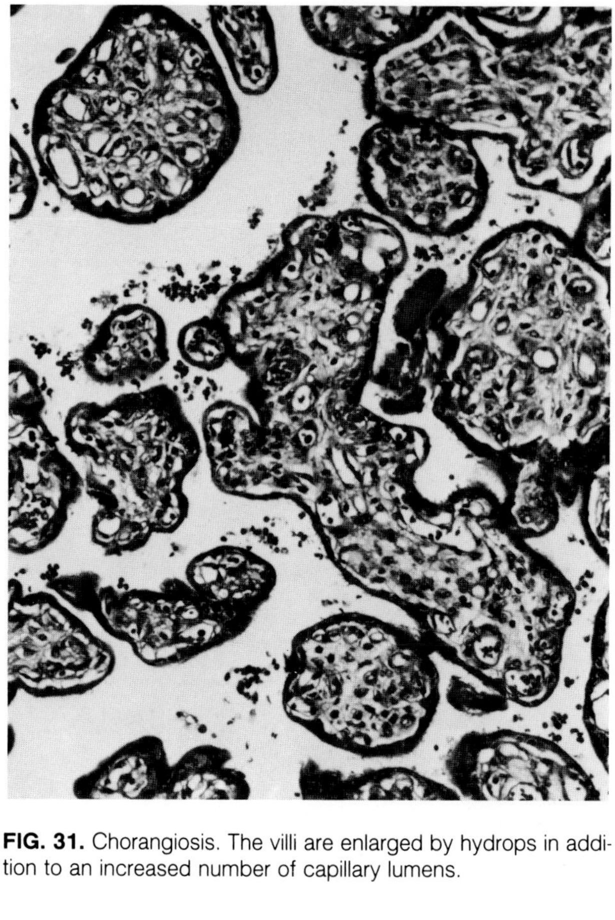

CLOSING COMMENTS

Many gross and light-microscopic abnormalities indicate risk of neonatal disease or compromise. Signs of potential prepartum fetal jeopardy include diffuse villous dysmaturity, chorangiosis, severe villitis, fetal thrombotic lesions, meconium staining, and nucleated red blood cells within fetal placental vessels. I have often seen numerous fetal placental nucleated red blood cells associated with a high level of similar cells per 100 white blood cells in a postnatal blood specimen. Either at those times or subsequently, there have been clinical signs of hypoxic brain disease or cerebral palsy.

The placenta, like all other tissues, is a specimen that the surgical pathologist can meaningfully report. By that action, there will be clarification of many disease processes and absolution of many an ill-accused obstetrician.

FIG. 31. Chorangiosis. The villi are enlarged by hydrops in addition to an increased number of capillary lumens.

REFERENCES

1. Perrin Eugene VDK. *Pathology of the placenta.* Contemporary issues in surgical pathology, vol. 5. Churchill Livingstone, New York: 1984.
2. Benirschke K, Driscoll SG. *The pathology of the human placenta.* New York: Springer-Verlag, 1967.
3. Fox H. *Pathology of the placenta.* Major problems in pathology, vol. 7. Philadelphia: WB Saunders, 1978.
4. Altshuler G. *Diseases of the placenta and their effect on transport.* Placental transport. Mead Johnson symposium on perinatal and developmental medicine, no. 18, 1981:35–43.
5. Naeye RL. Functionally important disorders of the placenta, umbilical cord, and fetal membranes. *Hum Pathol* 1987;18:680–691.
6. Miller PW, Coen RW, Benirschke K. Dating the time interval from meconium passage to birth. *Obstet Gynecol* 1985;66:459–462.
7. Benirschke K. Examination of the placenta. *Obstet Gynecol* 1961;18:309–333.
8. Altshuler G. The placenta, how to examine it, its normal growth and development. In: Naeye RL, Kissane JM, Kaufman N, eds. *Perinatal disease.* IAP monograph. Baltimore: Williams & Wilkins, 1981:5–22.
9. Altshuler G. Placental infection and inflammation. In: Perrin Eugene VDK, ed. *Pathology of the placenta,* New York: Churchill Livingstone, 1984:141–163.
10. Brown and Hopps method for gram-positive and gram-negative bacteria. In: Luna L, ed. *Manual of histologic staining methods of the Armed Forces Institute of Pathology,* 3rd edition. New York: McGraw–Hill, 1968:224–225.
11. Benirschke K. Accurate recording of twin placentation. A plea to the obstetrician. *Obstet Gynecol* 1961;18:334–347.
12. Benirschke K, Kim CK. Multiple pregnancy. *N Engl J Med* 1973;288:1276–1329.
13. Altshuler G. Developmental aspects of twins, twinning, and chimerism. In: Rosenberg HS, Bernstein J, eds. *Perspectives in pediatric pathology.* New York: Masson, 1982:121–136.
14. Fox H. *Pathology of the placenta.* Major problems in pathology, vol. 7. Philadelphia: WB Saunders, 1978:478.

15. Naftolin F, Khudr G, Benirschke K, Hutchinson DL. The syndrome of chronic abruptio placentae, hydrorrhea, and circumvallate placenta. *Am J Obstet Gynecol* 1973;116:347–350.

16. Ermocilla R, Altshuler G. An enigma: the origin of "X-cells" of the human placenta and their possible relationship to intra-uterine growth retardation. *Am J Obstet Gynecol* 1973;117:1137–1140.

17. Altshuler G, Ermocilla R, Russell P. The placental pathology of the small for gestational age infant. *Am J Obstet Gynecol* 1975;121:351–359.

18. Alan NA, Clary P, Russell PT. *Prostaglandins* 1973;4:363.

19. Benirschke K, Driscoll SG. *The pathology of the human placenta.* New York: Springer-Verlag, 1967:232.

20. Fox H. *Pathology of the placenta.* Philadelphia: WB Saunders, 1978:265.

21. Naeye RL. Maternal floor infarction. *Hum Pathol* 1985;16:823–828.

22. Mills JL, Harley EE, Moessinger AC. Standards for measuring umbilical cord length. *Placenta* 1983;4:423–426.

23. Moessinger AC, Blanc WA, Marone PA, Polsen DC. Umbilical cord length as an index of fetal activity: experimental study and clinical implications. *Pediatr Res* 1982;16:109–112.

24. Robinson LK, Jones KL, Benirschke K. The nature of structural defects associated with velamentous and marginal insertion of the umbilical cord. *Am J Obstet Gynecol* 1983;146:191–193.

25. Heifetz SA. Single umbilical artery. A statistical analysis of 237 autopsy cases and review of the literature. *Perspect Pediatr Pathol* 1984;8:345–378.

26. Heifetz SA, Rueda-Pedraza ME. Omphalomesenteric duct cysts of the umbilical cord. *Pediatr Pathol* 1983;1:325–335.

27. Heifetz SA, Rueda-Pedraza ME. Hemangiomas of the umbilical cord. *Pediatr Pathol* 1983;1:385–398.

28. Knox IC, Hoerner JK. The role of infection in premature rupture of the membranes. *Am J Obstet Gynecol* 1950;59:190–194.

29. Benirschke K. Routes and types of infection in the fetus and the newborn. *AMA J Dis Child* 1960;99:714.

30. Blanc WA. Amniotic infection syndrome. *Clin Obstet Gynecol* 1959;2:715–734.

31. Dominguez R, Segal AJ, O'Sullivan JA. Leucocytic infiltration of the umbilical cord: manifestation of fetal hypoxia due to reduction in blood flow in the cord. *J Amer Med Assoc* 1960;173:346–349.

32. Olding L. Value of placentitis as a sign of intrauterine infection in human subjects. *Acta Pathol Microbiol Scand [A]* 1970;78:256–264.

33. Chellam VG, Rushton DI. Chorioamnionitis and funiculitis in the placentas of 200 births weighing less than 2.5 kg. *Br J Obstet Gynaecol* 1985;92:808–814.

34. Svensson L, Ingemarsson I, Mardh PE. Chorioamnionitis and the isolation of microorganisms from the placenta. *Obstet Gynecol* 1986;67:403–409.

35. Benirschke K. Twin placenta and perinatal mortality. *NY State J Med* 1961;61:1499.

36. Pankuch GA, Appelbaum PC, Lorenz RP, et al. Placental microbiology and histology and the pathogenesis of chorioamnionitis. *Obstet Gynecol* 1984;64:802–806.

37. Aquino TI, Zhang J, Kraus FT, et al. Subchorionic fibrin cultures for bacteriologic study of the placenta. *Am J Clin Pathol* 1984;81:482–486.

38. Gibbs RS, Blanco JD, St Clair PJ, et al. Quantitative bacteriology of amniotic fluid from women with clinical intraamniotic infection at term. *J Infect Dis* 1982;145:1–8.

39. Dong Y, St. Clair PJ, Ramzy I, et al. A microbiologic and clinical study of placental inflammation at term. *Obstet Gynecol* 1987;70:175–182.

40. Minkoff H. Prematurity: infection as an etiologic factor. *Obstet Gynecol* 1983;62:137–144.

41. Keenan WJ, Steichen JJ, Mahmood K, Altshuler G. Placental pathology compared with clinical outcome. *Am J Dis Child* 1977;131:1224–1227.

42. Russell P. Inflammatory lesions of the human placenta. *Am J Diagn Gynecol Obstet* 1979;1:127–137.

43. Kundsin RB, Driscoll SG, Ming PL. Strain of mycoplasma associated with human reproductive failure. *Science* 1967;157:1573–1574.

44. Kundsin RB, Driscoll SG, Pelletier PA. Ureaplasma urealyticum

45. Shurin PA, Alpert S, Rosner B, et al. Chorioamnionitis and colonization of the newborn infant with genital mycoplasmas. *N Engl J Med* 1975;293:5–8.

46. Tafari N, Ross S, Naeye RL, et al. Mycoplasma T strains and perinatal death. *Lancet* 1976;108–109.

47. Dische MR, Quinn PA, Czegledy-Nagy E, et al. Genital mycoplasma infection. *Am J Clin Pathol* 1979;72:167–174.

48. Embree JE, Krause VW, Embil JA, et al. Placental infection with mycoplasma hominis and ureaplasma urealyticum: clinical correlation. *Obstet Gynecol* 1980;56:475–481.

49. Schachter J. Chlamydial infections, Part 1. *N Engl J Med* 1978;298:428–435. Part II. *N Engl J Med* 1978;298:490–495. Part III. *N Engl J Med* 1978;298:540–549.

50. Heggie AD, Lumicao GG, Stuart LA, et al. *Chlamydia trachomatis* infection in mothers and infants. *Am J Dis Child* 1981;135:507–511.

51. Martin DH, Koutsky L, Eschenbach DA, et al. Prematurity and perinatal mortality in pregnancies complicated by maternal chlamydia trachomatis infections. *JAMA* 1982;247:1585–1607.

52. Thompson SE, Dretler RH. Epidemiology and treatment of chlamydial infections in pregnant women and infants. *Rev Infect Dis* 1982;4(suppl):S747–S757.

53. Alexander ER, Harrison HR. Role of chlamydia trachomatis in perinatal infection. *Rev Infect Dis* 1983;5:713–719.

54. Winkler B, Reumann W, Mitao M, et al. Chlamydial endometritis. *Am J Surg Pathol* 1984;8:771–778.

55. Becroft DMO, Farmer K, Mason GH, et al. Perinatal infections by group B beta-haemolytic streptococci. *Br J Obstet Gynaecol* 1976;83:960–966.

56. Desa DJ, Trevenen CL. Intrauterine infections with group B beta-haemolytic streptococci. *Br J Obstet Gynaecol* 1984;91:237–239.

57. Friesen CA, Cho CT. Characteristic features of neonatal sepsis due to *Haemophilus influenzae. Rev Infect Dis* 1986;8:777–780.

58. Campognone P, Singer DB. Neonatal sepsis due to nontypable Haemophilus influenzae. *Am J Dis Child* 1986;140:117–121.

59. Lilien LD, Yeh TF, Novak GM, Jacobs NM. Early-onset *Haemophilus sepsis* in newborn infants: clinical, roentgenographic, and pathologic features. *Pediatr* 1978;62:299–303.

60. Wallace RJ, Baker CJ, Quinones FJ, et al. Nontypable *Haemophilus influenzae* (biotype 4) as a neonatal, maternal, and genital pathogen. *Rev Infect Dis* 1983;5:123–136.

61. Winn HN, Egley CC. Acute *Haemophilus influenzae* chorioamnionitis associated with intact amniotic membranes. *Am J Obstet Gynec* 1987;156:458–459.

62. Hurst V. Fusiforms in the infant mouth. *J D Res* 1957;36(4):513–515.

63. Robinow M, Simonelli FA. Fusobacterium bacteremia in the newborn. *Am J Dis Child* 1965;110:92–94.

64. Altshuler G, Hyde S. Fusobacteria chorioamnionitis: human and murine evidence of an important cause of prematurity. *Lab Invest* 1985;52:2A.

65. Altshuler G, Hyde S. Fusobacteria. An important cause of chorioamnionitis. *Arch Pathol Lab Med* 1985;109:739–743.

66. Easterling TR, Garite TJ. Fusobacterium: anaerobic occult amnionitis and premature labor. *Obstet Gynecol* 1985;66:825–828.

67. Bejar R, Curbelo V, Davis C, Gluck L. Premature labor. II. Bacterial sources of phospholipase. *Obstet Gynecol* 1981;57:479–482.

68. Larroche J CL, Paul G, Helffer L, Beaudoin M. *Bacteroides fragilis.* Contamination materno-placento-foetale. *Arch Fr Pediatr* 1981;38:41–45.

69. Evaldson GR, Malmborg AS, Nord CE. Premature rupture of the membranes and ascending infection. *Br J Obstet Gynecol* 1982;89:793–801.

70. Blanc WA. Pathology of the placenta, membranes, and umbilical cord in bacterial, fungal, and viral infections in man. In: Kaufman N, ed. *Perinatal diseases.* Baltimore: Williams & Wilkins, 1981:67–132, Chapter 6.

71. Altshuler G. Placental infection and inflammation. In: Perrin Eugene VDK, ed. *Pathology of the placenta.* New York: Churchill Livingstone, 1984;141–163, Chapter 6.

72. Delprado WJ, Baird PJ, Russell P. Placental candidiasis: report of

three cases with a review of the literature. *Pathology* 1982;14:191–195.

73. Hood IC, Desa DJ, Whyte RK. The inflammatory response in candidal chorioamnionitis. *Hum Pathol* 1983;14:984–990.

74. Altshuler G. Pathogenesis of congenital herpesvirus infection. *Am J Dis Child* 1974;127:427–429.

75. Robb JA, Benirschke K, Mannino F, Voland J. Intrauterine latent herpes simplex virus infection. II. Latent neonatal infection. *Hum Pathol* 1986;17:1210–1217.

76. Witzleben CL, Driscoll SF. Possible transplacental transmission of herpes simplex infection. *Pediatrics* 1965;36:192–199.

77. Von Herzen JL, Benirschke K. Unexpected disseminated herpes simplex infection in a newborn. *Obstet Gynecol* 1977;50:728–730.

78. Quinn PA, Butany J, Taylor J, Hannah W. Chorioamnionitis: its association with pregnancy outcome and microbial infection. *Am J Obstet Gynecol* 1987;156:379–387.

79. Altshuler G. Placental villitis of unknown etiology: harbinger of serious disease? *J Reprod Med* 1973;11:215–222.

80. Altshuler G, Russell P. The human placental villitides. A review of chronic intrauterine infection. In: *Current topics in pathology, vol. 60.* New York: Springer-Verlag, 1975:63–112.

81. Russell P. Inflammatory lesions of the human placenta. II. *Am J Diagn Gynecol Obstet* 1979;1:229–346.

82. Russell P. Inflammatory lesions of the human placenta. III. The histopathology of villitis of unknown aetiology. *Placenta* 1980;1:227–244.

83. Sander CH. Hemorrhagic endovasculitis and hemorrhagic villitis of the placenta. *Arch Pathol Lab Med* 1980;104:371–373.

84. Sander CH, Kinnane L, Stevens NG, Echt R. Haemorrhagic endovasculitis of the placenta: a review with clinical correlation. *Placenta* 1986;7:551–574.

85. Knox WF, Fox H. Villitis of unknown aetiology: its incidence and significance in placentae from a British population. *Placenta* 1984;5:395–402.

86. Kaplan CG, Bienstock J, Baker DA. Villitis of unknown etiology: incidence and implications in an unselected population. *Lab Invest* 1985;1:33A.

87. Althabe O, Labarrere C. Chronic villitis of unknown aetiology and intrauterine growth-retarded infants of normal and low ponderal index. *Placenta* 1985;6:369–373.

88. Redline RW, Abramowsky CR. Clinical and pathologic aspects of recurrent placental villitis. *Hum Pathol* 1985;16:727–731.

89. Shen-Schwarz S. Hemorrhagic endovasculitis of the placenta: relationship with villitis and fetal thrombosis. *Lab Invest* 1986;1:49.

90. Altshuler G. Human placental villitis of unknown etiology. In: Schenker JG, Rippman ET, Weinstein D, eds. *Recent advances in pathophysiological conditions in pregnancy.* Amsterdam/New York: Elsevier, 1984:314.

91. Fujikura T, Benson RC. Placentitis and fibrous occlusion of fetal vessels in the placentas of stillborn infants. *Am J Obstet Gynecol* 1964;89:225–229.

92. Ornoy A, Crone K, Altshuler G. Pathological features of the placenta in fetal death. *Arch Pathol Lab Med* 1976;100:367–371.

93. Russell P, Atkinson K, Krishnan L. Inflammatory lesions of the human placenta. III. The histopathology of villitis of unknown etiology. *J Reprod Med* 1980;24:93–98.

94. Block MF, Kallenberger DA, Kern JD, Nepveux RD. *In utero* meconium aspiration by the baboon fetus. *Obstet Gynecol* 1981;57:37–40.

95. Altshuler G, Jordan J. A stillbirth with aspirated squamous pearls and fetoplacental thromboembolism: a new finding and reminder of the importance of placental and fetal pathologic conditions. *Am J Obstet Gynecol* 1986;155:106–107.

96. Altshuler G. Chorangiosis. An important placental sign of neonatal morbidity and mortality. *Arch Pathol Lab Med* 1984;108:71–74.

97. Haust MD. In: Naeye RL, Kissane JM, Kaufman N, eds. *Perinatal diseases international academy of pathology monograph.* Maternal diabetes mellitus—effects on the fetus and placenta. Baltimore: Williams & Wilkins, 1981:201–284.

98. Singer DB. The placenta in pregnancies complicated by diabetes mellitus. *Perspect Pediatr Pathol* 1984;8:199–212.

99. Asmussen I. Ultrastructure of the villi and fetal capillaries of the placentas delivered by non-smoking diabetic women (white group D). *Acta Pathol Microbiol Immunol Scand [A]* 1982;90:95–101.

Surgical Pathology of the Female Reproductive System and Peritoneum, edited by Stephen S. Sternberg and Stacey E. Mills. Raven Press, Ltd, New York © 1991.

CHAPTER 3

The Vulva and Vagina

Henry F. Frierson, Jr. and Stacey E. Mills

VULVA

Normal Anatomy and Histology

The vulva is covered by both skin and mucous membrane. It consists of the mons pubis, labia majora and minora, clitoris (with prepuce and frenulum), vulvovaginal glands, Skene's (paraurethral) glands, vestibule, vestibular bulbs, urethral meatus, and hymen. Keratinized squamous epithelium covers most of the vulvar surface, but it becomes nonkeratinized at the introitus. The labia majora have sebaceous, eccrine, and apocrine glands, and much of their thickness is due to abundant adipose tissue. The labia minora are rich in blood vessels, elastic fibers, and sebaceous glands and have few, if any, sweat glands and little or no adipose tissue. Bartholin's glands, which are homologous to Cowper's glands in the male, are composed of lobules of mucus-secreting acini located bilaterally in the stroma of the vestibule, inferior to the hymen. They are palpable sometimes in thin women and are more easily detected when enlarged by inflammation or neoplasm (1). The major excretory duct of each Bartholin's gland empties posterolaterally at the junction of the hymenal ring and labium minus. Each major duct, as well as each of the ductules, is lined by stratified transitional-type epithelium that changes to stratified squamous epithelium at its orifice. The lesser vestibular glands (Littre's glands in the male) are lined by a single layer of tall columnar mucinous cells. Robboy et al. (2) found from one to several hundred (usually two to 10) of these glands in nine of 19 autopsied fetuses and young women whose vulvae were serially blocked for microscopic examination. Skene's paraurethral glands, homologues to the prostatic glands, form a network that surrounds the urethra, primarily posteriorly and laterally (3). Most of the ducts open into the distal one-third of the urethral canal. Skene's glands are lined by low columnar to tall cylindrical cells with occasional mucus-secreting cells. The paraurethral ducts are lined by columnar epithelium that changes to stratified squamous epithelium or transitional epithelium near their urethral openings.

The lymphatic channels of the anterior portion of the labia majora and minora and the prepuce of the clitoris drain into the superficial and deep femoral lymph nodes via the dense lymphatic network at the symphysis pubis (the presymphyseal plexus), or else they drain into the superficial inguinal lymph nodes (4). The superficial inguinal nodes form a horizontal chain between the skin and deep fascia, just inferior to the inguinal ligament. Lymph drainage ultimately proceeds to the external iliac system. Unilateral vulvar injection studies show lymph flow to contralateral pelvic nodes via anastomotic channels between both sides of the vulva or the pelvis (5). The obturator lymph node, located in the obturator fossa of the pelvis near the obturator nerve, is often large and is found inferior and lateral to the other external iliac nodes. Cloquet's (or Rosenmüller's) lymph node is either the most superior lymph node of the deep femoral chain or the most inferior external iliac node that projects below the inguinal ligament. Way noted that only about 8% of individuals have nodal tissue at this location (6). Iversen and Aas (5), however, using radioactive injections, found that the medial lacunar node of the external iliac chain (which perhaps is Cloquet's node) had nearly half of the total activity detected in removed pelvic nodes. In his vital dye studies, Eichner (7) noted that Cloquet's node was always involved initially; he also noted that if the node was not stained, then dye was absent in the superficial and deep femoral nodes and in the iliac nodes. The lymphatic channels of the posterior vulva reach the femoral lymph nodes, bypassing the presymphyseal plexus.

Conflicting data exist concerning the lymphatic drainage of the clitoris. Most of the drainage is into the superficial femoral lymph nodes via the presymphyseal plexus. Plentl and Friedman emphasized direct lymphatic communications from the clitoris to pelvic nodes (4). Way, however, has stated that there is no evidence for spread of cancer from the clitoris to the pelvic lymph nodes without initial involvement of the inguinal lymph nodes (6). Moreover, Iversen and Aas (5) failed to find a direct lymphatic pathway from the clitoris to the pelvic lymph nodes.

Lymph drainage from midline vulvar structures, such as the clitoris and perineum, is often bilateral. Most unilateral vulvar squamous-cell carcinomas that metastasize do so to the ipsilateral groin lymph nodes. Approximately 5% of carcinomas located on one side of the vulva metastasize to the contralateral lymph nodes only, and 15% of unilateral cancers metastasize bilaterally (6).

Approach to Specimens

Several types of vulvar biopsy and excision specimens may be submitted to the surgical pathology laboratory. For excisions of carcinoma, it is important to identify the primary tumor, search for multifocal lesions, document the depth of tumor penetration, check the margins of resection, and examine all lymph nodes. A labeled picture protocol is often useful to indicate the sites selected for microscopic study. Alternatively, the specimen may be placed upside down on clear plastic and photocopied. Wide excision vulvar specimens contain underlying adipose tissue and fascia. A partial vulvectomy specimen retains as much normal vulva as possible. The tissue from the "skinning" vulvectomy consists of only epidermis and dermis. The total (simple) vulvectomy specimen contains the entire vulva, including subcutaneous tissue down to the deep fascia. The traditional radical vulvectomy with lymphadenectomy is an *en bloc* resection of the entire vulva, inguinal skin and subcutaneous tissue, femoral and inguinal lymph nodes, and portions of the saphenous vein. At present, some surgeons have abandoned the *en bloc* resection, utilizing separate incisions for the inguinal-node dissections. The radical hemivulvectomy is a unilateral radical vulvectomy with separate incisions for the groin dissections.

Congenital Anomalies

There are a variety of congenital abnormalities of the vulva. Most are rare. They may be categorized as genital manifestations of specific genetic anomalies, developmental defects affecting the external genitalia only, and congenital abnormalities associated with anomalies of other anatomic regions, especially the urinary and gastrointestinal tracts. A newborn with ambiguous genitalia may be a virilized female, an imperfectly masculinized male, or a true hermaphrodite. The external genitalia of a true hermaphrodite also may have primarily male or female features (8). *Female pseudohermaphroditism* results from prenatal virilization and manifests as clitoral hypertrophy and, often, labial fusion. There may be a persistent urogenital sinus or penis with a penile urethra. Most frequently, female pseudohermaphroditism is caused by *congenital adrenal hyperplasia.* Virilization results from an excess in adrenal androgens caused by deficiencies in converting enzymes (9). Masculinization also develops from exposure to exogenous or maternal androgens. Although virilization is sometimes induced by exogenous *testosterone* or the synthetic androgen *danazol* (10,11), most instances have resulted from exposure to *progestational* compounds that were used for the treatment of threatened abortion (12,13). Female pseudohermaphroditism has resulted from maternal androgen-producing neoplasms such as *luteoma* of pregnancy (14–16) as well as from *Krukenberg tumor* with stromal luteinization (17–20). A purported maternal Sertoli-Leydig cell tumor causing congenital virilization more likely represents a luteoma (21). Congenital virilization also may be secondary to maternal adrenal adenoma (22–24), adrenal hyperplasia (25), or undetermined causes.

Malformations of the external genitalia are sometimes an isolated finding but are often associated with gastrointestinal or urinary tract defects (26,27). Complete *absence* or *duplication* of the external genitalia occurs virtually always in association with multiple anomalies, many of which are not compatible with life. Severe cases of *labial fusion* (chiefly due to the exposure to androgens *in utero*) result in the covering of the vaginal and urethral orifices and the formation of a urogenital sinus. Midline *labial adhesions,* which are congenital or acquired, usually obliterate the urethral and vaginal orifices. Unilateral or bilateral *hypertrophy* of the *labium minus* is a common finding that, in actuality, may be a normal variant (28). A single case of an *ectopic labium majus* has been described (29). The clitoris may be absent, hypoplastic, hypertrophic, or bifid. *Clitoral hypertrophy* is most often associated with exposure to androgens *in utero,* but it is also found in rare conditions such as the Beckwith-Wiedemann syndrome (9). A *bifid* clitoris may be a solitary abnormality or may be found with epispadias or exstrophy of the bladder (26). The hymen may be *imperforate, microperforate,* or *rigid.* An imperforate hymen is often not recognized until after puberty. A microperforate hymen is usually detected before menarche, because it results in recurring vulvovaginitis and urinary tract infections (30). A *persistent urogenital membrane sinus* develops from fusion of the membrane with the inner labia minora obliterating the introitus (31). The shallow sinus is covered by a thick membrane that contains a small aperture; the vagina and urethra open separately into the sinus.

Anomalies of the urinary tract that occur with malformations of the female external genitalia include *epi-

spadias, exstrophy of the bladder, and *ectopic ureteral orifices.* Ectopic ureters, which usually are accessory, open into the vagina or the vestibule. An ectopic ureterocele is sometimes seen as a cystic mass at the introitus (32). An *ectopic anus* opens more anteriorly in the perineum than normal or is found in the inferior portion of the vagina. In the *persistence of the cloaca,* the fused labial folds cover only a single narrow channel that empties onto the perineum via a small orifice; the bladder, genital tract, and bowel each open into this common cavity (26).

Cysts

The most common vulvar cyst, the *epidermoid cyst* (33), occurs as a round or oval, painless nodule primarily on the anterior half of the labia majora. Frequently, multiple cysts are present. The cyst is found chiefly in adults, but one report described an epidermoid cyst of the labium majus in a newborn, who also had a bifid clitoris and skeletal anomalies (34). So-called traumatic inclusion cysts, also lined by squamous epithelium, are found at sites of previous surgery. They are seen most often in episiotomy scars. Some have occurred in Nigerian women and children who have undergone ritual circumcision (35).

A *pilonidal cyst* (or sinus) uncommonly occurs in the vulva (36) and consists of an abscess cavity filled with hair shafts that elicit a foreign-body granulomatous reaction. A squamous lining may cover the superficial portion of the sinus tract, but most of the sinus tract is surrounded by granulation tissue.

Skene's duct cyst (paraurethral cyst) is usually less than 2 cm in diameter but may cause urethral obstruction (33). The cyst is lined by transitional epithelium, sometimes with squamous or ciliated cells (2,37–39). Although inflammation has been considered causal, most women lack a history of infection. When found in the newborn, Skene's duct cyst must be distinguished clinically from ectopic ureterocele, urethrocele, and urethral diverticulum (37). Spontaneous drainage of the cyst in the newborn occurs within a few weeks or months (39).

Hymenal cyst is the most common cyst of the female newborn (39). It is 0.5 to 1 cm in diameter and is lined by squamous epithelium. Spontaneous drainage of a milky fluid is characteristic.

The *cyst of the canal of Nuck,* similar to the hydrocele of the spermatic cord, results from incomplete obliteration of the processus vaginalis (40). This hydrocele is located along the course of the round ligament and is bordered by its occluded ends at the inguinal ring and labium majus. The nontender, elongated cyst varies in size, is occasionally multiple, and transilluminates. Unlike a hernia, it is typically irreducible. An inguinal hernia is present in one-third of the cases, however (40,41). The cyst contains clear fluid and is lined by a single layer of cuboid or flattened mesothelial cells. The cyst must be excised, because recurrence follows aspiration (41).

The *mucous* or *mucinous cyst* of the vestibule (2,42–44) virtually never occurs before puberty and is probably related to hormonal stimulation. Twenty percent of the cysts are multiple, and the mean size is approximately 1 cm (43). The cyst is usually unilocular and contains abundant mucoid material. It is lined by a single layer of tall columnar, mucus-secreting cells that have basal nuclei (Fig. 1). Papillary groups of cells, reserve-cell hyperplasia, ciliated cells, and squamous metaplasia may also be present. The lining is surrounded by a fibrovascular stroma without smooth-muscle cells. A müllerian origin was postulated formerly (42), but the mucous cyst is now considered to derive from urogenital sinus (minor vestibular gland) epithelium (2,43). Inflammation usually does not cause cystic dilatation of minor vestibular glands but may cause pain or dyspareunia (45).

Bartholin's duct cyst results from occlusion of the major duct with persistent secretion of the glands. The cyst occurs chiefly during the reproductive years and is usually unilocular, unilateral, and nontender (33). Large cysts may block the entrance to the vestibule. Unless infected, the cyst fluid is mucoid and clear. Transitional-type epithelium is the most common lining, but cuboid, columnar, ciliated, and squamous cells may be observed in varying proportions (Fig. 2) (1). The cyst wall contains chronic inflammatory cells and normal acini. *Mucocele-like* changes of Bartholin's gland are observed after rupture of obstructed, dilated ducts with leakage of mucin (46). Vacuolated histiocytes are conspicuous in the stroma.

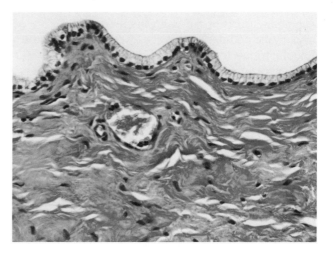

FIG. 1. Mucous cyst. The cyst is lined by a single layer of columnar, mucus-producing cells surrounded by a fibrovascular stroma.

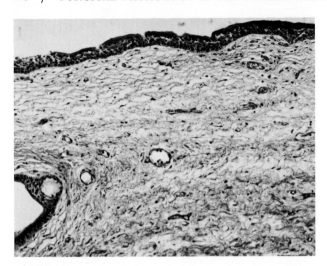

FIG. 2. Bartholin's duct cyst. The cyst is lined most often by multilayered transitional-type epithelium.

Gartner's duct cyst (mesonephric or Wolffian cyst) occurs less often in the vulva than in the vagina. A lining of nonmucinous, cuboid or low columnar cells is sometimes accompanied by focal squamous metaplasia (Fig. 3). Smooth-muscle fibers may be found in the cyst wall.

Fox-Fordyce disease is a chronic pruritic eruption of multiple, 1- to 3-mm papules or microcysts (47). The condition manifests wherever there are apocrine glands. It predilects the axilla and vulva, is very rare before puberty, and is uncommon after menopause. Microscopically, the superior portion of the hair follicle is obstructed by a keratin plug that also occludes the ostium of the apocrine duct. A vesicle then forms in the wall of the follicle after ductal rupture. Acanthosis and spongiosis of the follicle, dilatation of apocrine gland acini, and chronic inflammation of the dermis are also present. Multiple histologic sections are often necessary to identify the diagnostic microcysts (retention vesicles) (47).

Endometriosis of the vulva manifests as blue or red, firm, cystic nodules that enlarge cyclically with menses. Endometriotic foci are found at sites of previous surgery, especially episiotomy, but have also been noted after incision and drainage of Bartholin's gland abscess and radical vulvectomy (48).

Infectious Diseases

Bacteria

The chancre of primary *syphilis* (*Treponema pallidum*) occurs as a painless, eroded papule or indurated ulcer with round, raised edges and a smooth, erythematous base. Microscopically, the central surface epithelium is attenuated or ulcerated. There is an intense infiltrate of lymphocytes and plasma cells in the edematous

ulcer bed and prominent proliferation of capillaries with swollen endothelial cells. The characteristic spiral organisms in smears of the exudate may be visualized using dark-field examination or fluorescent antitreponemal antibodies (49). In paraffin sections, the organisms may be seen with the Warthin-Starry or Levaditi stains, or with antisera using the immunoperoxidase technique (50). Secondary syphilis of the vulva, condyloma latum, manifests as moist, gray-white patches or flat-topped papules that usually appear 3 to 6 weeks after the chancre. They are highly contagious, containing many spirochetes. Pseudoepitheliomatous hyperplasia is conspicuous, and neutrophils may migrate into the epithelium. The inflammatory and endothelial cell changes are similar to those of the chancre. Tertiary syphilis is rarely observed in the vulva.

Vulvar infection by *Neisseria gonorrhoeae* is essentially limited to Skene's glands and Bartholin's glands and is usually accompanied by gonococcal cervicitis, urethritis, or proctitis. The vulvar glands are swollen and painful with abscess formation. Culture of the organism is essential for diagnosis. Although gonococci were believed responsible for most abscesses of Bartholin's gland, in one study they were cultured from only 17% of the abscesses that contained bacteria (51).

Granuloma inguinale (*Calymmatobacterium granulomatis*) is rare in the United States and is largely confined to the southern states (52). It manifests as solitary or multiple, painless papules that ulcerate and have serpiginous, rolled borders. Marked tissue destruction may ensue with extensive scarring and elephantiasis (49,52). Inguinal lymphadenopathy is generally not marked. Microscopically, there is exuberant pseudoepitheliomatous hyperplasia (53), granulation tissue, and an inflammatory infiltrate with plasma cells, scattered polymor-

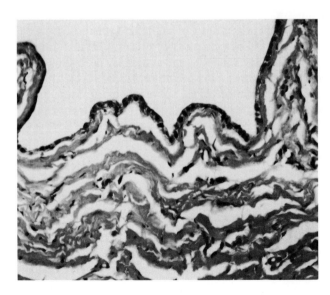

FIG. 3. Gartner's duct cyst. A single layer of cuboid, nonmucus-producing cells lines the cyst.

phonuclear leukocytes, and characteristic vacuolated histiocytes. The histiocytes contain 0.6- to 2.0-μm encapsulated rods with bipolar granules (Donovan bodies). The gram-negative bacteria are difficult to identify in hematoxylin-and-eosin-stained paraffin sections but are better visualized with Wright, Giemsa, toluidine blue, or Warthin-Starry stains. They are readily apparent in Papanicolaou-stained smears (54) and in appropriately stained, thin plastic sections. The florid pseudoepitheliomatous hyperplasia must not be confused with squamous-cell carcinoma. There are, however, well-documented reports of vulvar squamous-cell carcinoma arising in areas of chronic granuloma inguinale infection (55,56).

Chancroid (Hemophilus ducreyi) is a rare venereal disease in the United States. It begins as a small papule or pustule, usually on the vestibule. Later, painful, soft, single or multiple ulcers have ragged edges with erythematous borders. Enlarged inguinal lymph nodes with suppuration (buboes) are present in approximately 25% of cases (57). Beneath the surface ulceration and necrotic debris, endothelial proliferation is prominent and there may be lumenal compromise and thrombosis. Lymphocytes and plasma cells densely populate the deep dermis. Culture isolation of the organism is necessary for diagnosis (58).

The vulva is the least common site for tuberculosis of the female genital tract (59). Vulvar tuberculosis results from hematogenous dissemination or spread from the upper genital tract. It also may be transmitted sexually from a male partner harboring tuberculous epididymitis. Grossly, the infected vulva is ulcerated or hypertrophic, mimicking squamous-cell carcinoma. Culture is usually necessary for diagnosis, given the low sensitivity of acid-fast stains (60).

Erythrasma (Corynebacterium minutissium) forms symmetrical, erythematous inguinal macules that may simulate infection with tinea or candida. The condition is asymptomatic and is almost never biopsied. The organisms are located in the horny layer of the epidermis. Diagnosis is confirmed by orange-red fluorescence with a Wood's lamp (61).

Folliculitis and erysipelas of the vulva are typically caused by staphlococci and streptococci, respectively. These microorganisms, as well as a variety of other aerobic and anaerobic bacteria (almost always in combination), are also involved in necrotizing fasciitis of the vulva (62). This toxic, systemic illness follows surgery or minor trauma. The disease is rapidly progressive and frequently fatal, especially in diabetics. Grossly, the vulva is erythematous and swollen. The superficial fascia and subcutaneous tissue are necrotic, but the underlying muscular layer is spared. Microscopically, the subcutaneous tissue shows necrosis, acute inflammation, and thrombosis of small vessels. Aggressive surgical resection is the most important therapeutic modality.

Hidradenitis suppurativa is a chronic inflammation commencing in anatomic areas replete with apocrine glands. The disease is virtually never seen prior to puberty and has a peak incidence in the third decade of life (63). Follicular occlusion by keratin with perifolliculitis leads to the formation of abscesses. Chronic inflammatory cells, foreign-body giant cells, granulation tissue, fibrosis, and deep sinus tracts follow destruction of cutaneous appendages. Cultures usually reveal a spectrum of bacterial pathogens (63). Surgery is the mainstay of therapy (64).

Chlamydia

Chlamydia trachomatis serotypes L1 through L3 cause lymphogranuloma venereum, and serotypes D through K are associated with sexually transmitted oculogenital disease (65). The most important technique for the identification of oculogenital chlamydia is culture isolation. In the vulva, C. trachomatis has been isolated from duct exudate of Bartholin's gland (66).

The initial manifestation of lymphogranuloma venereum is a small, asymptomatic vesicle or ulcer, frequently on the posterior vulva (49). Swollen inguinal lymph nodes with suppuration may occur after a few weeks. The histopathologic features of the ulcer are nonspecific. The lymph nodes show follicular hyperplasia and characteristic, but nonspecific, stellate microabscesses. In long-standing infection, there is extensive scarring, with strictures and fistulas of the vulva, urethra, vagina, and rectum. Chronic lymphedema and obstruction may result in elephantiasis. Squamous-cell carcinoma of the vulva has been reported in women with previous infection (56).

Viruses

Herpes simplex is the most common cause of vulvar ulcers. Approximately 90% of infections are caused by the type 2 virus, whereas 10% are caused by type 1 (67). An intraepithelial herpetic vesicle forms from acantholysis of the squamous epithelium as a result of ballooning and reticular degeneration. Subsequent rupture forms a superficial ulcer. The inflammatory infiltrate in the dermis varies; polymorphonuclear leukocytes and vasculitis may be present. At the periphery of the ulcers, multinucleated epithelial cells contain "ground-glass" nuclei or eosinophilic intranuclear inclusions. The inclusions are seen in both hematoxylin-and-eosin-stained histologic sections as well as in Papanicolaou- or Giemsa-stained cytologic preparations.

Herpes zoster (68), vaccinia (69), and Epstein-Barr virus (70) rarely affect the vulva.

Human papillomaviruses comprise a heterogeneous group that causes squamous proliferations of the skin and mucous membranes. A review of papillomavirus infection of the female genital tract has been provided by Syrjanen (71). Papillomavirus infection occurs anywhere on the external genitalia and is most commonly observed in women of childbearing age. Vulvar warts (condylomata acuminata) appear as pink or gray-white, soft, sessile or verrucous growths that may become confluent. Vulvar squamous papillomatosis (small pruritic growths on the vestibule) is also due to papillomavirus (72). Recurrence of genital warts is due to reinfection or latent viral activation (73). Microscopically, condyloma acuminatum is characterized by delicate, branching fibrovascular cores lined by squamous epithelium showing acanthosis, papillomatosis, hyperkeratosis, and parakeratosis (Fig. 4). The parabasal layer is thickened, and there is minimal nuclear enlargement and pleomorphism. Orderly maturation and normal cellular polarity are retained. Mitotic figures are identifiable, but atypical mitoses are absent. Koilocytosis is the characteristic cytopathic effect of papillomavirus infection. Koilocytes are superficial squamous cells with single or occasionally multiple, enlarged, hyperchromatic, and wrinkled nuclei. Surrounding the nucleus is a prominent clear space or "halo" that abuts a thickened zone of peripheral cytoplasm. Electron-microscopic, immunocytochemical, and in situ hybridization studies have shown that the viral particles are concentrated in the nuclei of koilocytes and parakeratotic cells (74).

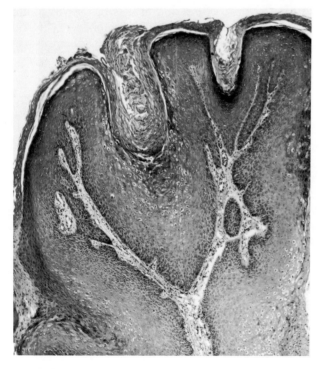

FIG. 4. Condyloma acuminatum. Acanthotic squamous epithelium is supported by branching fibrovascular cores. Hyperkeratosis, parakeratosis, orderly maturation of cells, and koilocytes are characteristic.

Podophyllin therapy for condyloma acuminatum may produce cytologic changes mimicking intraepithelial neoplasia. Microscopically, the effects are most pronounced within 48 hours after treatment and are absent after 1 week (75). Typically, there is intercellular edema, necrosis of the basal half of the epidermis, and an edematous, inflamed papillary dermis. Mitotic figures (with a few bizarre forms) are markedly increased. Unlike intraepithelial neoplasia, orderly squamous-cell maturation is present; marked nuclear atypia and dyskeratotic cells are absent.

Condyloma acuminatum is usually easy to distinguish from vulvar intraepithelial neoplasia. For the latter, the following features are conspicuous: pleomorphic, enlarged, and hyperchromatic parabasal nuclei; disorderly maturation; and abnormal mitotic figures (76). The nuclei of condyloma acuminatum are diploid or polyploid, whereas those of intraepithelial neoplasia are typically aneuploid (74,77). Focal koilocytotic atypia and cellular maturation may be observed in, or adjacent to, intraepithelial neoplasia. In addition, some squamous proliferations of the vulva have microscopic features intermediate between condyloma and intraepithelial neoplasia. There is increasing evidence at clinical, light-microscopic, ultrastructural, immunocytochemical, and molecular levels that human papillomavirus infection is associated with premalignant and malignant squamous proliferations of the vulva (71,74,78–87). Human papillomavirus DNA has been noted in 80% to 100% of genital intraepithelial neoplasia and bowenoid papulosis (80,86,87). Viral DNA has also been demonstrated in verrucous carcinoma (82,83) and squamous-cell carcinoma of the vulva (80,84). Viral types 6 and 11 are frequently observed in vulvar condylomata acuminata (73,80,82,85), whereas type 16 has been found more often in precancer and cancer (80,84).

Molluscum contagiosum is a DNA poxvirus that has a predilection for the vulva. This mildly contagious infection appears as multiple, 1- to 4-mm papules with central umbilication. The papules often disappear spontaneously after approximately 6 months, but others may remain for several years (88). Microscopically, the follicular epithelium expands to produce rounded lobules containing cells and keratinized debris (89). Eosinophilic intracytoplasmic inclusion bodies enlarge and become basophilic as they migrate from the deeper layers of the epidermis. The diagnostic viral inclusions may also be observed in cytologic material obtained from scrapings of the papules.

Fungi and Parasites

Tinea cruris causes erythematous, scaly patches in the perineal, inguinal, and vulvar areas. The diagnosis is determined by culture or identification of hyphae in potassium hydroxide-treated skin scrapings.

Vulvar *candidiasis* commonly accompanies vaginal infection. The erythematous, pruritic lesions may involve large areas of the vulva and perineum. Severe infection is associated with obesity, pregnancy, and diabetes mellitus. Microscopically, the epidermis is mildly thickened and spongiotic; a chronic inflammatory infiltrate is present in the dermis. The surface exudate contains degenerated squamous cells, polymorphonuclear leukocytes, yeast, and pseudohyphae (90).

Deep fungal infections of the vulva are very rare. Clinically, they may simulate necrotizing fasciitis. *Phycomycosis* of the vulva has been reported in a diabetic woman (91).

Invasive parasitic infestation of the vulva is rare in North America. Vulvar elephantiasis sometimes results from lymphatic obstruction by *filariform* worms. *Schistosomiasis* may cause ulcers or papillary nodules that simulate condylomata acuminata (92).

Miscellaneous Benign Lesions

Seborrheic keratosis and *fibroepithelial polyp* occur on the labia majora of middle-aged or elderly women. Two cases of *verruciform xanthoma* of the vulva have been described (93). The lesion is characterized by uniform acanthosis, hyperkeratosis, and parakeratosis with deep extension into the rete pegs and an associated neutrophilic infiltrate. There is also hyalinization of dermal collagen and infiltration of xanthoma cells into the papillary dermis between the rete pegs. *Sebaceous-gland hyperplasia* forms smooth, soft dermal nodules up to 1.5 cm in diameter on the labia minora or majora (94). Minor vestibular gland *adenoma* occurs as a firm nodule less than 2 cm in size (95). *Pilar tumor,* usually found on the scalp, has been documented on the vulva (96). Benign pigmented lesions of the vulva include *melanotic macule (lentigo)* (97) and *nevi* (congenital or acquired). Junctional or compound vulvar nevi in premenopausal women may be atypical and have some architectural features of melanoma, including (a) wide lateral extent, confluence, and variation in size and shape of junctional nests and (b) involvement of adnexal structures (98). Unlike melanoma, atypical vulvar nevi have a well-demarcated epidermal melanocytic component, lack melanocytes at all levels of the epidermis, and show maturation of melanocytes from the epidermis to the dermis (98).

A variety of dermatologic conditions may involve the vulva, either as a localized process or as part of generalized disease (Table 1). *Radiation damage* to the vulva, although uncommon, results in loss of pubic hair and sclerosis of the connective tissue and blood vessels. The shallow, circinate erosions of *Reiter's syndrome* are exceedingly rare; histologically, there is focal ulceration with acute inflammation of the superficial dermis (99).

TABLE 1. *Dermatologic conditions that may occur on the vulva*

Allergic contact dermatitis	Pemphigus vulgaris
Irritant dermatitis	Familial benign pemphigus
Seborrheic dermatitis	Bullous pemphigoid
Psoriasis	Benign mucosal pemphigoid
Lichen planus	Darier's disease
Vitiligo	Acantholytic dermatosis
Erythema multiforme	Herpes gestationis
Acanthosis nigricans	Subcorneal pustular dermatosis
	Dermatitis herpetiformis

Behcet's syndrome, a chronic, relapsing disease, manifests as small vesicles or pustules that may develop into deep ulcers. Microscopically, there are (a) a necrotizing vasculitis with swollen endothelial cells, (b) a fibrinoid necrosis of vascular walls, and (c) a lymphocytic perivascular infiltrate (100). Persistent red-brown glistening papules and erosions are characteristic of *vulvitis circumscripta plasmacellularis* (101). The microscopic features include an inflamed epidermis, parakeratosis, and a dense dermal infiltrate of plasma cells and hemosiderin-laden macrophages.

Lipoma and *fibrolipoma* occur on the labium majus as solitary subcutaneous nodules and pedunculated masses (102). *Sclerosing lipogranuloma,* caused by trauma or injection of foreign oils, is characterized by vacuolated cysts lined by adipocytes or giant cells with adjacent bands of hyalinized tissue. The lesion may be locally infiltrative and should be distinguished from liposarcoma (103). Vulvar *leiomyomas* may have cytologic atypia, increased cellularity, and bizarre tumor giant cells. Tavassoli and Norris developed criteria for benign and malignant smooth-muscle tumors of the vulva (104). In contrast to leiomyomas, leiomyosarcomas are often 5 cm or more in diameter, have infiltrating margins, and have five or more mitotic figures per 10 high-power fields. Tumors lacking one or all of these features may recur, however. Epithelioid leiomyoma (104,105) appears to have a greater proclivity to recur than the usual spindle-cell type. Leiomyomas excised during pregnancy may have extensive myxoid change, hemorrhage, or foci of necrosis (104). Vulvar *neurofibroma* occurs as an isolated lesion or as part of von Recklinghausen's disease (106,107). Other neural tumors such as *schwannoma* (108), *plexiform schwannoma* (109), and *traumatic neuroma* may arise in the vulva. *Granular-cell tumor* occurs as a single (or multiple) superficial nodule on the labium majus or clitoris and has a strong predilection for black women (110,111). The overlying pseudoepitheliomatous hyperplasia may mimic well-differentiated squamous-cell carcinoma. *Nodular fasciitis* (112), *desmoid tumor* (113), and genital *rhabdomyoma* (114) only rarely involve the vulva.

Benign vascular lesions of the vulva include *capillary* (*strawberry*) *hemangioma, senile hemangioma, cavernous hemangioma, angiokeratoma, lobular capillary hemangioma* (*pyogenic granuloma*) (102), and *varicosities.* Lobular capillary hemangioma and varicosities are seen most often during pregnancy. Cavernous hemangioma may involve the clitoris, simulating pseudohermaphroditism (115). Angiokeratomas are often multiple 2- to 10-mm papillary, warty, or globular lesions of the labia majora (116). They are associated with pregnancy and increased venous pressure. Microscopically, dilated, often thrombosed, capillaries are found in the upper dermis, surrounded by acanthosis and hyperkeratosis of the overlying squamous epithelium. *Glomus tumor,* arising on the labium minus or clitoris, causes persistent pain and dyspareunia (117,118). *Lymphangiomas* are rarely observed on the vulva. *Lymphangiectasis* (acquired lymphangioma) arises as multiple vesicles or warty papules on the labia majora, developing in chronic lymphedematous states after radiation therapy or lymphatic surgery for cervical carcinoma (119,120). Microscopically, thin-walled, ectatic lymphatic channels are located superiorly in the papillary dermis.

Accessory breast tissue is found on the labium majus and is bilateral in 25% of cases (121). Rarely, a nipple is present. Because of hormone-induced swelling, about half of the cases are diagnosed during pregnancy or lactation. Fibrocystic changes, lactating adenoma (122), fibroadenoma (123), and intraductal papilloma (124) have all developed in vulvar breast tissue. Adenocarcinoma may arise in vulval breast tissue (125,126) and must be distinguished from invasive Paget's disease, adenocarcinoma of adnexal origin, and metastatic mammary carcinoma.

Crohn's disease involves the vulva by direct extension from the anus or as a discontinuous "metastatic" ulcer. The latter shows granulomatous inflammation, acute and chronic inflammation, fibrosis, and, sometimes, ex-

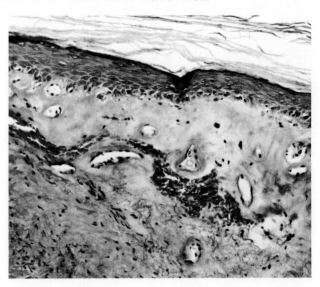

FIG. 5. Lichen sclerosus. The thin, hyperkeratotic epidermis with a vacuolated basal layer overlies a hyalinized dermis containing telangiectatic vessels.

tensive pseudoepitheliomatous hyperplasia (127). *Sarcoidosis* (128), *malacoplakia* (129,130), *amyloidosis* (131), *tumoral calcinosis* (132), *lymphoid hamartoma* (133), and *choristoma* (134) of the vulva also have been described.

Dystrophy and Squamous Intraepithelial Neoplasia

Standardized terminology for vulvar dystrophy and squamous intraepithelial neoplasia has evolved over the last two decades (Table 2) (135,136). Biopsy of one or more vulval lesions in a particular patient is essential because of the variable and overlapping clinical appearances for dystrophic and dysplastic conditions.

Lichen sclerosus, a persistent and recurring condition found in all ages, is seen predominantly in postmenopausal women. Two-thirds of affected children have spontaneous involution before or at puberty (137). All or any part of the vulva may be involved, with occasional extension to the perianal region and inner thighs. Initially, pale pink or white maculopapules coalesce to form dry, rough, scaly plaques. Advanced lesions appear wrinkled and "parchment-like," with telangiectasia and ecchymoses frequently being observed (138). Extensive vulvar contracture may lead to agglutination of the labia minora and stenosis of the introitus. Microscopically, there is epithelial thinning, loss of rete pegs, hyperkeratosis, and plugging of follicles (Fig. 5). The basal cells are vacuolated and, occasionally, subepidermal bullae are present. Melanin pigment and melanocytes are lost from the epithelium. The atrophic dermis is edematous, hyalinized, and sparsely cellular. Sweat glands and pilosebaceous apparatuses are absent. Dermal vessels are

TABLE 2. *Classification of vulvar dystrophy and squamous intraepithelial neoplasia (VIN)*

A. Dystrophic conditions
  1. Lichen sclerosus
  2. Squamous hyperplasia (hyperplastic dystrophy)
  3. Mixed lichen sclerosus and squamous hyperplasia
B. Squamous intraepithelial neoplasia[a]
  1. VIN I (mild dysplasia)
  2. VIN II (moderate dysplasia)
  3. VIN III (severe dysplasia/carcinoma *in situ*)
C. Dystrophy with squamous intraepithelial neoplasia[a]
  1. Squamous hyperplasia with VIN
  2. Lichen sclerosus with VIN
  3. Mixed dystrophy (squamous hyperplasia and lichen sclerosus) with VIN

[a] The presence of changes suggestive of human papillomavirus infection should be noted.

telangiectatic, and there is loss of elastic fibers. A variable number of lymphocytes and plasma cells lie just below the atrophic dermis. Lichen sclerosus is commonly observed in association with intraepithelial neoplasia and invasive squamous-cell carcinoma (139), but there is no evidence that the lichen sclerosus component is a premalignant process. Hart et al. followed 92 patients with lichen sclerosus for a median follow-up interval of 9 years (140). The single patient who subsequently developed an invasive squamous-cell carcinoma initially had coexistent mild intraepithelial neoplasia. In the same series, each of five patients with simultaneous lichen sclerosus and invasive carcinoma had neoplasms that tended to arise in areas of minimal dystrophy or in areas of normal vulvar skin. Melanoma (141) and basal-cell carcinoma (142) also have occurred coincidentally with lichen sclerosus.

Squamous hyperplasia (hyperplastic dystrophy) is related to chronic irritation. Many cases probably represent neurodermatitis (lichen simplex chronicus) (138). Two-thirds of the patients are premenopausal (143). The lesions occur on the labia majora or mons and have a highly variable appearance but are usually discrete red or white plaques that may be multiple and lichenified (138). Scales and excoriations are often present. Microscopically, the acanthotic epidermis contains cells with orderly maturation and uniform nuclei. Hyperkeratosis is frequent, sometimes with parakeratosis and hypergranulosis. Thickened rete pegs are club-shaped or pointed and may become confluent. The dermis contains a variable number of chronic inflammatory cells and minimal edema. Squamous hyperplasia is sometimes observed adjacent to invasive squamous-cell carcinoma. The risk of development of invasive carcinoma for women treated for squamous hyperplasia without intraepithelial neoplasia is minimal (143).

Approximately 45% to 50% of patients with vulvar dystrophy have squamous hyperplasia, and 40% have lichen sclerosus (143,144); 10% to 15% of the patients have mixed dystrophies. Squamous hyperplasia may be present adjacent to, or remote from, lichen sclerosus. Sometimes, squamous hyperplasia overlies an atrophic dermis (Fig. 6). Approximately 10% of biopsies of squamous hyperplasia have foci of intraepithelial neoplasia (143,144). Although studies of untreated women with long follow-up intervals are not available, there is probably only a small risk of invasive squamous-cell carcinoma for women with squamous hyperplasia and mild intraepithelial neoplasia.

Vulvar intraepithelial neoplasia (VIN) is a designation promulgated to replace other terms for *in situ* squamous proliferations of the vulva such as: atypia; dysplasia; Bowen's disease; bowenoid atypia; bowenoid papulosis; erythroplasia of Queyrat; and carcinoma *in situ*, simplex type (136). It is controversial whether bowenoid papulosis should be retained as a specific clinicopathologic

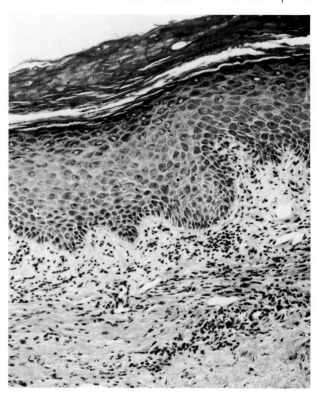

FIG. 6. Squamous hyperplasia and lichen sclerosus. The thickened epidermis shows hyperkeratosis, hypergranulosis, and orderly maturation of cells without nuclear atypia. The dermis contains chronic inflammatory cells and shows areas of hyalinization superficially.

entity or whether it should be abandoned in favor of VIN. Prior to 1970, VIN was found most often in women in the fifth or sixth decade of life (145); currently, however, about half of the patients are less than 40 years old. VIN in young women is frequently multiple and is associated with human papillomavirus infection. Progression to carcinoma appears to be uncommon in this age group (146). Older women with VIN more often have solitary lesions with a higher risk for progression to cancer (146). The clinical appearance of VIN is variable. Discrete or coalescent papules or macules are gray, white, red, or darkly pigmented. They may be scaly or eczematoid. Some lesions mimic condyloma grossly. Microscopically, VIN consists of crowded cells that have the following: high nuclear-to-cytoplasmic ratios; hyperchromatic, pleomorphic nuclei; and increased numbers of mitotic figures (with abnormal forms) (76,136). Hyperkeratosis, parakeratosis, and dyskeratotic cells are often observed (147). The cells of VIN I (mild dysplasia) are confined to the lower one-third of the epithelium. Mitotic figures (with occasional abnormal forms) are also confined to the basal layers. Orderly, mature squamous epithelium is found overlying the dysplastic cells. VIN II (moderate dysplasia) contains cells with enlarged, crowded nuclei in the lower two-thirds of the epithelium. Cellular maturation is present at the uppermost one-third of the epithelial surface. Mitotic figures (including abnormal forms) and dyskeratotic cells are found in the dysplastic cell layers. VIN III (severe dysplasia/carcinoma *in situ*) contains immature, dysplastic cells that extend up more than two-thirds of the thickness of the epidermis (Fig. 7). The dysplastic cells often extend into the outer portions of hair follicles. Some examples of VIN III have cells with copious mature cytoplasm that retain dysplastic nuclei. The rete pegs may be thickened and branched, and intraepithelial squamous pearls may be located at their tips (77). Multinucleated, giant dysplastic cells (bowenoid cells) are frequently seen in VIN III. Koilocytotic atypia and evidence of human papillomavirus are often associated with intraepithelial neoplasia (76,81). Condyloma may be seen adjacent to VIN, or there may be a gradual transition from condyloma to VIN. Sometimes, atypical lesions have features of both VIN and condyloma (76). Human papillomavirus type 16 has been found in VIN of young women (87).

Approximately 25% of women with VIN III have persistent or recurrent disease after local excision (81,146,148), whereas 2% to 10% of women treated for VIN III develop invasive squamous-cell carcinoma (77,145,146,148). The presence of invasive cancer is due to progression of intraepithelial neoplasia or to the development of carcinoma away from the area of VIN.

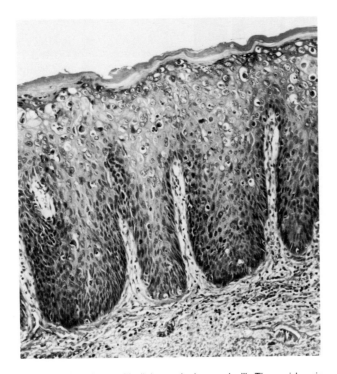

FIG. 7. Vulvar intraepithelial neoplasia, grade III. The epidermis has thickened rete ridges and is filled with crowded cells having high nuclear-to-cytoplasmic ratios and hyperchromatic, pleomorphic nuclei. Mitotic figures and dyskeratotic cells are numerous.

One-fifth to one-third of invasive squamous-cell carcinomas have adjacent foci of VIN III (139,149). Patients with VIN are at high risk for the development of dysplasia or invasive squamous-cell carcinoma of the vagina and cervix. Between 20% and 30% of patients with VIN III have vaginal or cervical dysplasia or carcinoma (77,145,148).

Bowenoid papulosis (87,150) and *Bowenoid dysplasia* (151) represent a subset of VIN in which multiple, small, red-brown papules occur chiefly in young women from 20 to 40 years of age. The lesions are sometimes found during pregnancy. If untreated, bowenoid papulosis may regress spontaneously (150,151). Human papillomavirus DNA has been documented in bowenoid papulosis (87). Some authors have reported that the cells of bowenoid papulosis show a lesser degree of dysplasia and more maturation than those of VIN III (150,151). It has also been noted that bowenoid papulosis tends to (a) involve the acrosyringium and (b) spare the acrotrichium (150,151). Although the natural history of bowenoid papulosis is not completely known, the risk of progression to invasive carcinoma appears to be small.

Malignant Neoplasms

Squamous-cell carcinoma accounts for approximately 90% of all primary invasive vulvar neoplasms. Three-fourths arise on the labia (usually the labia majora), and most of the remainder are located on the clitoris or fourchette (152–155). The age range is broad, but most neoplasms develop in women in the seventh or eighth decade of life (152,155,156). Very rarely are patients less than 20 years of age. Prior conditions associated with vulvar squamous-cell carcinoma include lymphogranuloma venereum (56), granuloma inguinale (55,56), human papillomavirus infection (78,79,81), immunosuppression (157), and Fanconi's anemia (158). Women with vulvar cancer have an increased risk for dysplasia and invasive carcinoma of the cervix and vagina.

Grossly, the tumors appear as erythematous or white plaques, as ulcers, as nodules, or as fungating, papillomatous growths (156). The important factors in clinical staging include tumor size, extension, and the clinical status of the inguinal and femoral lymph nodes (Table 3). The clinical evaluation of groin lymph nodes is often unreliable. Up to 43% of clinically negative groin lymph nodes contain carcinoma, microscopically (159). Conversely, up to 45% of clinically positive inguinal-femoral lymph nodes lack tumor upon microscopic examination (156). Stage Ia, a proposed modification of the FIGO classification (Table 3), defines a subset of squamous-cell carcinomas that are 2 cm or less in diameter and have 1 mm or less of stromal invasion (measured from the epithelial-stromal junction of the adjacent, most superficial dermal papilla to the deepest point of invasion) (160).

TABLE 3. *International Federation of Obstetrics and Gynecology (FIGO) staging system for invasive squamous-cell carcinoma of the vulva*[a]

Stage	Definition
I	Lesion confined to the vulva with a maximum diameter of 2 cm or less and without suspicious groin nodes
Ia[b]	Lesion confined to the vulva with a maximum diameter of 2 cm or less and with 1 mm or less of stromal invasion
II	Lesion confined to the vulva with a diameter greater than 2 cm and without suspicious groin nodes
III	Lesion of any size extending beyond the vulva (to urethra, vagina, perineum, or anus) without suspicious inguinal nodes or lesion of any size with suspicious groin nodes
IV	Lesion of any size with grossly positive groin nodes; lesion involving mucosa of rectum, bladder, or urethra or involving bone; palpable deep pelvic nodes or distant metastasis

[a] Criteria set forth were approved at the VIth Congress of FIGO in 1970.
[b] Proposed by the International Society for the Study of Vulvar Disease in 1984.

Important pathologic factors for vulvar squamous-cell carcinoma include tumor size, thickness or depth of stromal invasion, grade, pattern of infiltration, capillary invasion, multifocality, margins of excision, and status of groin lymph nodes. Although strict criteria for grading these neoplasms have not been well delineated in most studies, the criteria set forth by Broders [originally for lip cancer (161)] or Jakobsson [for carcinoma of the larynx (162)] generally have been applied. Most squamous-cell carcinomas of the vulva are keratinizing tumors. Approximately 5% to 15% are poorly differentiated or anaplastic with marked nuclear pleomorphism, high nuclear-to-cytoplasmic ratios, and minimal or no keratinization. Although the data are conflicting concerning the relationship of tumor grade to groin lymph-node status and overall prognosis (155,156,159,163–174), many studies have shown that high-grade tumors more often metastasize to inguinal and femoral nodes, resulting in a poorer outlook (155,156,159,165–168,173,174). Infiltration by tumor may manifest as papillary fronds, discrete nests, small strands or cords, and dispersed single cells. Vulvar squamous cancers generally have either a broad, pushing, circumscribed front or an irregular, infiltrating margin. Tumors with an infiltrating margin may contain dissociated cells, or they may contain cells forming small, angulated nests or cords that incite a prominent desmoplastic response (diffuse, stellate, or spray pattern) (Fig. 8) (165,169, 172,175). Such neoplasms, even those that are small and superficially invasive, have a proclivity for lymph-node metastasis. *Confluent growth* is a poorly defined term that often refers to an amount of tumor filling at least 1

mm of a microscopic field (166,169,170). It primarily correlates with tumor thickness and depth of stromal invasion. The use of the term "confluent" should be discouraged. Patients with squamous cancers having a marked lymphocytic stromal response may have a better prognosis than patients with tumors that incite a minimal lymphoplasmacytic reaction (156,164,172). The presence of vascular permeation clearly increases the risk for nodal metastasis (166,167,169,172,173, 176,177). Using multiple-step sections, Donaldson et al. (177) found capillary permeation in 34% of tumors that had less than 5 mm of stromal invasion and in 71% of neoplasms that had more than 5 mm of stromal infiltration. Seventy-nine percent of their patients with vascular invasion had inguinal lymph-node metastases, as compared with only 6% of patients whose tumors lacked invasion. Permeation of vascular channels is observed more often in tumors that are poorly differentiated than in those that are well differentiated. For stage I carcinomas, Iverson et al. (176) found that 6 of 15 tumors with vascular invasion metastasized to lymph nodes, whereas only 2 of 61 that lacked vascular permeation metastasized. The 5-year survival rate for their patients whose tumors lacked vascular invasion was 85%, compared with 52% survival for patients having neoplasms with vessel invasion (176). The relationship of perineural invasion to recurrence, lymph-node metastasis, prognosis, and other histologic parameters has not been examined.

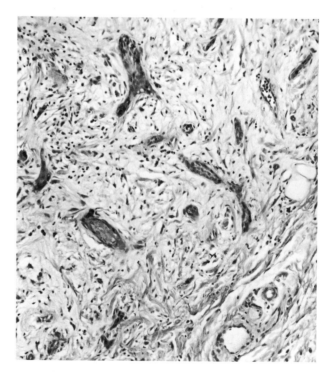

FIG. 8. Squamous-cell carcinoma. Small nests, strands, and angulated cords of cells embedded in a loose fibrous stroma characterize the "spray" pattern of invasion.

Microinvasive, superficially invasive, and *early invasive* are descriptions for squamous-cell carcinomas that are thin and have small amounts of stromal penetration. Unfortunately, these terms have not been applied uniformly, resulting in considerable confusion. Franklin and Rutledge (174) initially defined *microinvasive squamous-cell carcinoma of the vulva* as a tumor 2 cm or less in diameter with 5 mm or less of stromal invasion. More recently, 3 mm (164,166,171) and 1 mm (160) have been used as upper limits for stromal invasion. Neoplasms that are 2 cm or less in diameter and have 1 mm or less of stromal invasion have been classified as stage Ia tumors in the FIGO staging system (160). In a literature review, Wilkinson found that 15% of tumors with stromal invasion of 5 mm or less metastasized to groin lymph nodes, whereas 12% of tumors that invaded to a depth of 3 mm or less resulted in nodal metastases (178). There are no reports of metastasis for tumors having 1 mm or less of stromal invasion or that are less than 2 mm thick (179).

A variety of measuring points have been used to determine the depth of stromal invasion. The most frequently used methods for assessing tumor depth (or thickness) include: (A) measurements from the surface of the tumor to the deepest point of invasion (thickness) (163,171,172,176) (B) measurements from the epithelial-stromal junction of the adjacent most superficial dermal papilla to the deepest point of infiltration (165,166), and (C) measurements from the tip of the adjacent non-neoplastic rete ridge to the deepest point of invasion (171). Currently, there is debate as to whether the optimal technique of measurement should be the depth of stromal invasion (method B) (178) or tumor thickness (method A) (179). Only a large study comparing the ease and reproducibility of the two methods will resolve this issue. We believe that tumor thickness is a simpler and more reproducible measurement than depth of stromal invasion. The form of measurement, whichever is preferred, should be mentioned in the pathology report. A calibrated ocular micrometer is essential for accuracy.

At times, the separation of minimally invasive squamous-cell carcinoma from intraepithelial neoplasia is difficult. Sections that are completely perpendicular to the tumor surface are essential for evaluation. The diagnosis of invasion is readily made when small nests or buds of cells are separate from the overlying surface or when a desmoplastic stromal response is present. Clearly, difficulties arise in individual cases, especially for lesions that are predominantly papillary and have broad, pushing rete pegs.

Historically, the standard treatment for vulvar squamous-cell carcinoma has been radical vulvectomy with *en bloc* bilateral inguinal-femoral lymph-node dissection. Currently, more conservative operative procedures are used for small, unilateral tumors. For patients without groin node metastasis, the 5-year survival rate is 81% to 96%; for those with positive groin lymph nodes, it is 43% to 66% (152–154,159,168,172). The mortality increases with the number of nodes involved by tumor (154,168), bilateral involvement of groin nodes (168,172), and metastasis to pelvic lymph nodes (154,168,172,173).

Adenoid squamous-cell carcinoma consists of a single layer of squamous cells lining pseudoacini that contain dyskeratotic, acantholytic cells. Adenoid changes in squamous-cell carcinoma may be focal or predominant (180,181). Neoplasms with a predominantly adenoid pattern are poorly differentiated and have a poor prognosis. Underwood et al. (181) noted only a 6% 5-year survival for such patients, as compared with a 77% survival for patients with conventional squamous-cell carcinoma. Ultrastructurally, some adenoid squamous cancers may have features suggesting glandular differentiation (181). For these cases, *adenosquamous carcinoma* (of possible skin appendage origin) seems a better designation (181). *Spindle-cell carcinoma* is a rare, aggressive variant of squamous-cell carcinoma that may involve the vulva (182,183). Grossly, the tumor is often polypoid. It is composed of spindle-shaped cells and, sometimes, highly pleomorphic, sarcomatoid cells (Fig. 9). Ulceration, hemorrhage, necrosis, and numerous mitotic figures are typical. Spindle-cell carcinoma must be distinguished from melanoma and sarcoma. The diagnosis of spindle-cell carcinoma is secure when foci of

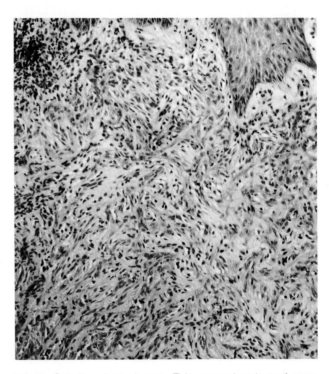

FIG. 9. Spindle-cell carcinoma. This unusual variant of squamous-cell carcinoma consists of dispersed spindle-shaped cells that mimic the cells of sarcoma and melanoma.

conventional squamous-cell carcinoma or overlying intraepithelial neoplasia are observed. In histologically difficult cases, the identification of tonofilaments and desmosomes ultrastructurally finalizes the diagnosis of squamous cancer. Immunohistochemical positivity for keratin or epithelial membrane antigen may also be helpful but does exclude certain sarcomas, such as epithelioid and synovial types.

Verrucous carcinoma, a distinctive clinicopathologic subtype of squamous-cell carcinoma, was initially documented on the vulva by Kraus and Perez-Mesa (184). This exquisitely well-differentiated tumor occurs in patients with a broad age range, but it occurs chiefly in those in the sixth or seventh decade of life (185). Grossly, it is bulky, exophytic, and cauliflower-like. Ulceration is present in one-third of the cases. Microscopically, there is prominent acanthosis, hyperkeratosis, and parakeratosis (Fig. 10). The broad and elongated papillary processes lack prominent fibrovascular cores. The bulbous rete pegs are well circumscribed and push deeply into the dermis. Keratin microcysts are sometimes present centrally in the acanthotic pegs. Minimally pleomorphic cells are confined to the lower layers, and the overlying stratified squamous epithelium is mature. Mitotic figures are few and are confined primarily to the basal layer.

The microscopic diagnosis of verrucous carcinoma is usually difficult, and appropriate clinical information is

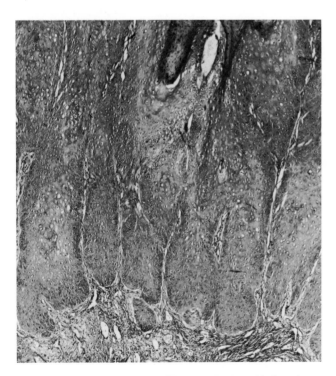

FIG. 10. Verrucous carcinoma. The acanthotic epithelium forms prominent bulbous rete pegs and contains mature cells with minimal pleomorphism. Unlike condyloma acuminatum, large branching fibrovascular cores are not conspicuous.

imperative. Indeed, diagnosis may be impossible with small, superficial specimens. Deep biopsies that include underlying stroma are usually necessary. The distinction from condyloma and squamous-cell carcinoma is often a challenge. Although verrucous carcinoma may have vacuolated cells at the surface, the papillae lack the characteristic central fibrovascular cores seen in condyloma. The papillary fronds of verrucous carcinoma also penetrate deeper into the dermal tissues than do the papillae of condyloma. It is our opinion that the so-called giant condyloma of Buschke-Loewenstein represents verrucous carcinoma and that this former designation has historical interest only.

In spite of its distinction from condyloma, verrucous carcinoma also has been associated with human papillomavirus infection. In one study, half of the patients with verrucous carcinoma had vulvar condylomas 3 to 10 years previously (185). Human papillomavirus DNA also has been identified in verrucous carcinoma (82,83). Papillary (warty) squamous-cell carcinoma with a well-differentiated surface and small nests and cords of cells irregularly penetrating the dermis should be separated from verrucous carcinoma because the former is a more aggressive, metastasizing lesion. Unlike verrucous carcinoma, papillary squamous-cell carcinoma has (a) squamous pearls at the invasive front and (b) more nuclear pleomorphism. Verrucous carcinoma, especially if it is massive, tends to recur and may prove fatal as a result of direct extension into vital structures. Inguinal-femoral lymph nodes may be enlarged, but metastases have not been described (185). In one study (185), the 5-year survival rate for patients treated with complete excision alone was 94%.

Basal-cell carcinoma of the vulva occurs in middle-aged or elderly Caucasian women (186,187). Histologically and biologically, the tumor is identical to basal-cell carcinoma elsewhere on the skin. Basal-cell carcinoma with an adenoid pattern (188) must be distinguished from adenoid cystic carcinoma. The former neoplasm originates from the basal layer of the epidermis, grows in a serpiginous fashion, focally shows cribriform and gland-like patterns, and has a palisading arrangement of cells at the periphery of nests. Squamous differentiation and solid foci are also observed in adenoid basal-cell carcinoma. Basal-cell carcinoma of the vulva may recur following excision, or new tumors may arise; metastases, however, are very rare (189).

Primary *adenocarcinoma* of the vulva may have origin from the epidermal appendages, accessory breast tissue, minor vestibular glands, periurethral glands, or Bartholin's gland. Approximately 275 carcinomas of Bartholin's gland have been documented. The histologic features of many of these neoplasms have not been described in detail. Approximately 40% are adenocarcinomas, and a similar number are *squamous-cell carcinomas* (190,191). Most of the remaining cases include *adenoid cystic carcinomas, undifferentiated carcinomas,* or carcinomas having both squamous and glandular features. Tumors reported as transitional-cell carcinoma are poorly described microscopically; it is likely that most, if not all, represent nonkeratinizing squamous-cell carcinomas.

To be considered as a primary tumor of Bartholin's gland, a neoplasm must be located in the correct anatomic location, and the patient must not have a histologically similar neoplasm elsewhere (191). Intact overlying squamous epithelium and residual normal acini adjacent to the tumor are helpful for determining origin in Bartholin's gland. *In situ* squamous carcinoma or adenocarcinoma in ducts or acini is also helpful but is not essential for the diagnosis (191). A large ulcerated tumor in the proper anatomic position might represent a Bartholin's gland carcinoma, especially if intraepithelial neoplastic changes of the skin, vagina, and anus are absent. It may be impossible, however, to determine the exact origin of extensive, deeply invasive lesions.

Clinically, carcinoma of Bartholin's gland is often unsuspected, but it should be considered in a women 40 years of age or older who has any clinical abnormality of the gland. Microscopically, most of the adenocarcinomas produce mucus and are well or moderately differentiated. Approximately 10% are adenoid cystic carcinomas (192); the tumors are histologically identical to their counterparts in salivary glands and elsewhere (193). They have a propensity for perineural invasion, recurrence, and distant metastasis, but metastases to inguinal femoral lymph nodes have occurred in only one instance (194).

The standard treatment for a carcinoma of Bartholin's gland is radical vulvectomy with bilateral inguinal lymphadenectomy (190). Recently, some authors advocated wide local excision, ipsilateral inguinal lymphadenectomy, and radiation therapy (191). Leuchter et al. (190) noted (a) a 52% survival for patients with negative inguinal nodes and (b) a 36% survival for those with positive inguinal-femoral lymph nodes. In a more recent study, Copeland et al. (191) found an overall 5-year survival rate of 84%. For 18 patients with adenoid cystic carcinoma and follow-up, five died with disease, five are living with tumor, and eight are alive without evidence of carcinoma (follow-up of less than 5 years for six of the patients).

Endodermal sinus tumor of the vulva has been described in four patients ranging in age from 22 months to 26 years; three of the four died of disease within 2 years. Each of three elderly women reported with *Merkel-cell carcinoma* of the vulva died of disease within 2.5 years (196–198). One tumor was associated with vulvar intraepithelial neoplasia (197), and another had an invasive squamous-cell carcinoma component (196).

Approximately 60% of vulvar *melanomas* arise on the labium minus or clitoris, and 40% occur on the labium

majus (Fig. 11) (199–202). Melanoma is found primarily in Caucasian women, and 70% of these patients are postmenopausal (199). The vulvar lesions can be classified as superficial spreading, nodular, or acral lentiginous types (200). One case of neurotropic melanoma has been documented (202). Most vulvar melanomas are grossly pigmented. The prognosis depends chiefly on the thickness of the neoplasm. Unfortunately, about 80% of the tumors are greater than 1.5 mm thick (201). Clark's levels of invasion are not applicable because the papillary dermis is absent or poorly defined in the vulva (199). Tumor thickness ranged from 0.6 to 28.0 mm, with a median thickness of 9.0 mm in one study (200). The minimum thickness for nonsurvivors was 2.6 mm (200). The overall survival, which is approximately 30% to 40% (199–201), correlates with the status of groin lymph nodes (201).

A variety of *sarcomas* have arisen on the vulva (203–217) (Table 4); *leiomyosarcoma* is the most common (203,204). Criteria for the distinction of benign and malignant smooth-muscle tumors have been described in the discussion concerning leiomyoma. Two-thirds of vulvar sarcomas develop in the labium majus; most of the remainder are found in the fourchette as well as in the deep tissues near Bartholin's gland (204). *Epithelioid sarcoma* sometimes arises in the lower dermis and subcutaneous fat of the vulva. The prognosis is poorer than that for patients with extragenital epithelioid sarcoma (209).

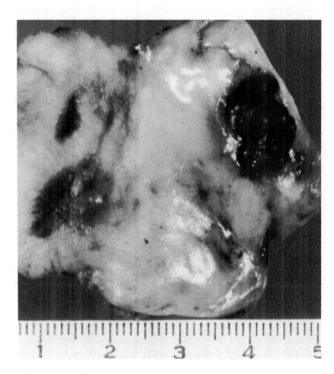

FIG. 11. A 1.5-cm polypoid melanoma and two foci of precancerous melanosis are present in this excision specimen of the vulva.

TABLE 4. *Primary sarcomas of the vulva*

Sarcoma	Reference
Leiomyosarcoma	104, 203, 204
Malignant fibrous histiocytoma	204–206
Rhabdomyosarcoma (embryonal, alveolar)	203, 207, 208
Malignant schwannoma	203, 204
Epithelioid sarcoma	204, 209
Fibrosarcoma	203, 204, 210
Dermatofibrosarcoma protuberans	204, 211
Angiosarcoma	204
Kaposi's sarcoma	212
Hemangiopericytoma	204, 213, 214
Alveolar soft part sarcoma	215
Malignant granular-cell tumor	216
Liposarcoma	217

Aggressive angiomyxoma occurs in the vulva, vagina, perineum, or soft tissues of the pelvis (218,219). It presents as a large, slowly growing, polypoid mass or swelling in women in their third or fourth decade of life. Grossly, the tumor is rubbery and white or is soft and gelatinous. Microscopically, stellate and spindle-shaped mesenchymal cells are embedded in a loose myxoid stroma with a few collagen fibers (Fig. 12). The cells are small and bland, and they lack nuclear atypia. Small or medium-sized veins and arteries within the tumor often are grouped together and may show medial hypertrophy. Blood vessels of various caliber are typically widely dilated, and extravasation of red blood cells is usual. Aggressive angiomyxoma is characteristically hypocellular and lacks necrosis and mitotic figures. Invasion of skeletal muscle and fat is usual. Small nerves are often trapped within the neoplasm. The tumor cells have fibroblastic or myofibroblastic properties ultrastructurally. The microscopic differential diagnosis includes neurofibroma, intramuscular myxoma, spindle-cell lipoma, myxoid malignant fibrous histiocytoma, myxoid liposarcoma, and embryonal rhabdomyosarcoma. The therapy for aggressive angiomyxoma is complete excision. Local recurrence is common, but metastases have not been described.

Non-Hodgkin's lymphoma (220) and *Hodgkin's disease* (221) of the vulva are primarily manifestations of systemic disease. There are rare reports of primary *plasmacytoma* (222) and diffuse large-cell lymphoma, immunoblastic type (223), of the labium majus.

Rose et al. (224) reported a case of vulvar *eosinophilic granuloma* and summarized 24 cases from the literature. Except for one example that was localized to the vulva, all lesions were a manifestation of systemic disease. Most of the patients were adults. Vulvar eosinophilic granuloma may regress spontaneously, but low-dose radiation therapy is indicated for large destructive tumors.

In one series of 22 *metastatic carcinomas* to the vulva, 10 originated from the cervix, whereas eight arose in the endometrium, urethra, vagina, or ovary (225). Three of the four women with primary neoplasms of the breast, kidney, or lymph nodes presented with metastases to the vulva as the initial manifestation of recurrent disease. Squamous-cell carcinoma metastatic to the vulva usually appears as a circumscribed subepithelial mass, whereas metastatic adenocarcinoma tends to invade the surface epithelium. Most patients with vulvar metastases have disseminated disease and a very poor prognosis (225).

Extramammary Paget's Disease and Sweat-Gland Neoplasms

Vulvar *Paget's disease,* often controversial and misunderstood, occurs in three forms: (i) Most commonly, by far, it is an intraepithelial adenocarcinoma that is probably derived from a multipotential cell in the basal layer of the epidermis or adnexa; (ii) it may be an invasive adenocarcinoma arising from intraepithelial adenocarcinoma (invasive Paget's disease); and (iii) it may represent (a) Pagetoid extension or metastasis to the skin by a primary adenocarcinoma of the cervix (226,227) or Bartholin's gland (228) or (b) a transitional-cell carcinoma of the bladder or urethra (229). It is incorrect to assume that intraepithelial Paget's disease with dermal invasion represents epidermotropic spread or metastasis

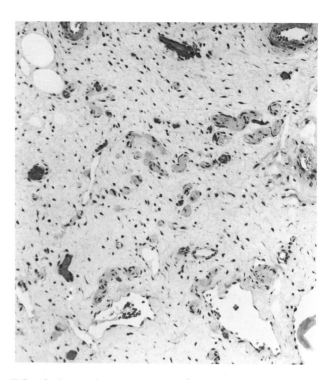

FIG. 12. Aggressive angiomyxoma. Spindle-shaped and stellate cells without nuclear atypia are loosely arranged in a myxoid stroma. Dilated blood vessels and vessels with thickened walls are frequently observed. Entrapped nerves and adipocytes are also present.

from an underlying invasive sweat-gland carcinoma. Approximately 29% of patients with Paget's disease have an additional, unrelated synchronous or metachronous carcinoma, most commonly arising from the genitourinary tract, gastrointestinal tract, or breast (230).

Intraepithelial Paget's disease is a slowly growing neoplasm of long duration which is sometimes mistaken clinically for a chronic, intractable dermatitis. Most cases are seen in postmenopausal Caucasian women, chiefly in the seventh decade of life (226,231). Vulvar Paget's disease is extremely rare in Negro women. Grossly, intraepithelial Paget's disease appears as a flat or slightly raised, granular, moist, erythematous patch. It primarily occurs on the labia majora; however, it is often extensive, involving the labia minora, perineum, perianal skin, thighs, mons, and lower abdomen. Occasionally, there is extension along the mucosa of the vagina, cervix, urethra, bladder, or ureter (229,231,232). Extension into the ducts of the periurethral glands, the mucus-secreting glands of the vestibule, and the endocervical mucous glands also occurs (226,229). Clinically, Paget's disease is sharply demarcated and may be multifocal (233). Typically, however, there is microscopic extension into grossly normal skin.

Microscopically, intraepithelial Paget's disease consists of large pale cells, predominantly in the basal layer of the epidermis (Fig. 13). Single cells, nests, and well-formed glands are present and sometimes extend into the upper layers of the epithelium. The squamous epithelium is acanthotic, often with hyperkeratosis and parakeratosis. Paget's cells frequently involve (a) the basal layers of pilosebaceous structures and (b) the ducts and acini of sweat glands (226,234,235). Paget's cells have abundant clear or eosinophilic, granular cyto-

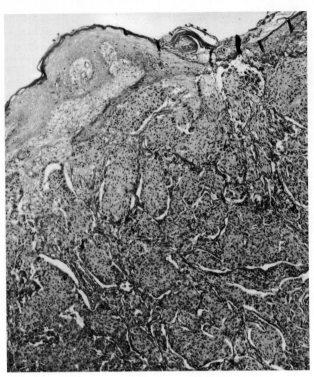

FIG. 14. Invasive Paget's disease. The dermis is infiltrated by nests of adenocarcinoma. The intraepithelial component from this case is illustrated in Fig. 13.

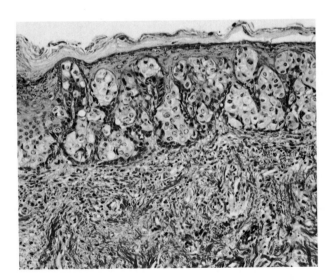

FIG. 13. Intraepithelial Paget's disease. The epidermis contains nests of cells with abundant clear cytoplasm as well as with large pleomorphic nuclei exhibiting vesicular chromatin and conspicuous nucleoli.

plasm. Their large nuclei have vesicular chromatin and often have prominent nucleoli. Mitotic figures are easily identified. Signet-ring cells may be observed (226). Some Paget's cells are invariably positive with (a) mucicarmine, (b) PAS after diastase pretreatment, (c) colloidal iron after hyaluronidase pretreatment, (d) aldehyde Fuchsin, or (e) alcian blue stains (226,235). The dermis contains a variable number of inflammatory cells, and dermal vessels may be increased in number and size. Infrequently, patients with intraepithelial Paget's disease have areas of dermal invasion. It is important not to mistake intraepithelial involvement of sweat glands or ducts for invasive tumor. The cells of invasive Paget's disease infiltrate the dermis from the intraepidermal (or adnexal) component. They invade as cords, nests, and sheets of cells (Fig. 14). The cells may also form trabeculae, tubules, and glands with intraluminal secretions.

Immunocytochemically, Paget's cells are reactive for carcinoembryonic antigen (236,237), cytokeratin (237), and epithelial membrane antigen (237). Normal eccrine and apocrine glands and ducts are immunoreactive for carcinoembryonic antigen, but squamous epithelium, hair follicles, and sebaceous glands lack positivity (236). In addition, Paget's cells are immunoreactive for gross cystic-disease fluid protein, which is found in normal eccrine and apocrine cells (237). Ultrastructurally, Paget's cells have some features of apocrine or eccrine cells (238,239).

The differential diagnosis for Paget's disease includes melanoma and squamous intraepithelial neoplasia. The presence of intracytoplasmic melanin does not exclude a diagnosis of Paget's disease, because 60% of cases contain cells with a few, coarse melanin granules (235). Unlike Paget's disease, melanoma contains the following: theques of cells at the dermal-epidermal junction; fine, diffuse granules of melanin; and immunoreactivity for S-100 protein and more specific melanoma-associated antigens. Melanoma also lacks mucin and immunoreactivity for carcinoembryonic antigen.

Patients with intraepithelial Paget's disease are treated with wide excision or simple vulvectomy (231,234). Because the sharply demarcated clinical lesion belies microscopic extension into grossly normal epithelium, adequate margins should be obtained by frozen sections or, prior to excision, by numerous perilesional biopsies. Local recurrence of intraepithelial tumor develops in approximately one-third of the cases after surgical excision (226). The therapy for invasive Paget's disease is radical vulvectomy and bilateral inguinal-femoral lymph-node dissection (231,234,240). Lymph-node metastases occur in about 85% of patients with invasive anogenital Paget's disease (235). Long-term survival for patients with groin lymph-node metastasis is unusual (226,234,235). The prognosis appears to be better for patients with invasion and negative inguinal-femoral lymph nodes (226,235). No studies have correlated the

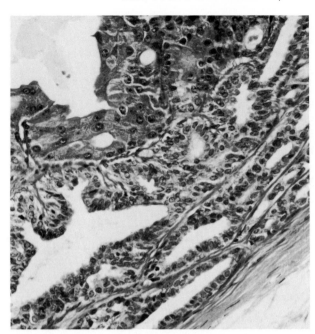

FIG. 16. Hidradenoma papilliferum. Acini are lined by a single or double layer of cuboid or low columnar cells. Apocrine differentiation is present in this example.

thickness or depth of invasion with the status of groin lymph nodes and survival.

Hidradenoma papilliferum (papillary hidradenoma) is the most frequent benign sweat-gland tumor of the vulva. In two series totaling 120 patients, no cases were found in Negro women (241,242). The tumor is virtually nonexistent in prepubertal females. It is usually single and less than 1 cm in diameter. Eighty percent are on the labia majora or labia minora (241,242). Grossly, the lesion appears as a round or oval, firm nodule that sometimes ulcerates and bleeds. On cut section, the tumor is a well-circumscribed, soft, gray-white to red, solid or cystic dermal nodule. Microscopically, hidradenoma papilliferum has papillary and complex glandular patterns (Fig. 15). Acini contain eosinophilic material and are lined by a single or double layer of cuboid cells. Papillary foci usually contain two layers of cells supported by fibrovascular stroma. The superficial cells are columnar and have basal nuclei. The smaller cells adjacent to the basement membrane are cuboid with clear cytoplasm and myoepithelial features. Mild, focal nuclear atypia and occasional mitotic figures may be observed. Some cells have brightly eosinophilic cytoplasm, and others exhibit overt apocrine differentiation (Fig. 16). Apocrine differentiation is also evident histochemically and ultrastructurally (243). Hidradenoma papilliferum sometimes resembles intraductal papilloma or nipple adenoma of the breast. Complete excision of the neoplasm is curative. There are no convincing cases of transformation to carcinoma (244).

A few *mixed tumors* and *syringomas* of the vulva

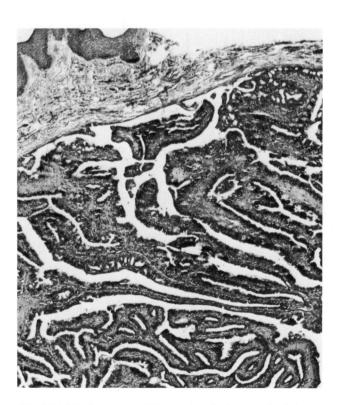

FIG. 15. Hidradenoma papilliferum. A well-circumscribed dermal nodule is composed of papillae having prominent fibrovascular cores.

have been documented. Mixed tumors occur on the labia majora, and most are of long duration (245). Microscopically, they are identical to salivary-gland mixed tumors, and they probably arise from labial sweat glands. There are no convincing cases of mixed tumor arising in Bartholin's gland or malignant mixed tumor of the vulva. Vulvar syringoma, histologically identical to syringoma of the face, manifests as small papules less than 5 mm in diameter. They are found in girls and young adults (246). Syringomas are usually found on both labia majora, but they may be unilateral or may arise on the labium minus. Vulvar lesions may be accompanied by extragenital syringomas.

Vulvar sweat-gland neoplasms reported as isolated examples include *clear-cell hidradenoma (eccrine acrospiroma)* (247), *ductal eccrine adenocarcinoma* (248), *eccrine porocarcinoma* (248), *clear-cell hidradenocarcinoma* (248), and *apocrine carcinoma* (249).

VAGINA

The vagina is that segment of the female genital tract between the hymenal ring and the uterine cervix. It is lined by stratified squamous epithelium overlying a lamina propria, a muscular coat, and an adventitial layer. Keratinized epithelium, normally absent, may be found after mucosal prolapse. The squamous mucosa undergoes cyclic hormonal changes. Cytoplasmic glycogen is most abundant at the time of ovulation. Atrophy of the epithelium occurs at menopause. The lamina propria contains collagen, elastic fibers, fibroblasts, blood vessels, and lymphatic channels. A few lymphocytes are typically present. The muscular coat has an inner layer of circular smooth-muscle fibers and an outer longitudinal layer. The adventitia contains loose connective tissue, a well-developed venous plexus, and a few nerve branches.

The vaginal lymphatic drainage is complex, and pathways from specific regions are not always predictable (4). In general, the channels that flow from the superior posterior vagina drain into the rectal lymph nodes, whereas those from the superior anterior vagina lead to the interiliac nodes. Lymphatics from the middle region of the posterior wall terminate in the deep pelvic nodes. From the middle portion of the anterior wall, lymphatics lead to the lymph nodes of the lateral pelvic wall (especially the interiliac lymph nodes) or to the vesical nodes. Lymphatic channels from the distal vagina communicate with pelvic lymph nodes or with anastomoses from the vestibule that drain into lymph nodes of the femoral triangle. All portions of the vagina have lymphatic channels that (a) drain into lateral collecting vessels around the vaginal artery and (b) lead to the superior gluteal nodes and, sometimes, to the common iliac nodes.

Congenital Anomalies, Including Those Resulting from Intrauterine Exposure to Diethylstilbestrol

Vaginal *agenesis* results from defective formation of the distal portions of the müllerian ducts. Agenesis is typically associated with abnormal development of the uterus and, often, renal and skeletal anomalies (Meyer-Rokitansky-Kuster-Hauser syndrome) (250–252). *Longitudinal* or *transverse vaginal septa* are either complete or partial. Transverse septa are most often observed at the junction of the middle and upper one-third of the vagina and have central or eccentric openings. Microscopically, a core of fibrovascular tissue and smooth muscle is lined on both sides by squamous epithelium (253). Mucinous glandular epithelium is generally absent. Vaginal *duplication* is commonly associated with duplication of the uterus. Other congenital vaginal malformations include *oblique septa* and *distal vaginal atresia* (252).

Congenital abnormalities of the vagina that result from *in utero* exposure to diethylstilbestrol (DES) include *mucosal membrane, corolla-like mucosal elevation, fibrous band, apical narrowing, forniceal obliteration, transverse* or *longitudinal vaginal septa,* and *adenosis* (254). Excluding adenosis, structural malformations of the vagina or cervix occur in about 25% of DES-exposed women (255). Adenosis is the presence of müllerian glands in the vagina after birth. This condition was described in women exposed *in utero* to DES in 1971, when clear-cell adenocarcinoma of the vagina also was linked to DES (256). The drug had been used for over 20 years for women with high-risk pregnancies. Robboy et al. (257), using intact reproductive tracts from human embryos and fetuses grown in athymic (nude) mice, showed that *in vivo* exposure to DES resulted in developmental anomalies of the female reproductive tract, including vaginal adenosis. Adenosis, however, is not limited to women with *in utero* exposure to DES, having been identified in 2.3% of unexposed women (258). When caused by DES, the frequency of adenosis is related to the total drug dose, the duration of pregnancy at the onset of its administration, and the duration of exposure (258,259). Almost all women exposed to DES *in utero* at or before the eighth week of pregnancy have developed adenosis, compared with only 6% exposed at or after the 15 week of gestation (258). Thirty-four percent of women with DES exposure, examined after review of their prenatal records, had vaginal epithelial changes in the form of adenosis or squamous metaplasia (259).

Adenosis occurs chiefly in the upper one-third of the vagina but may extend to the lower two-thirds. There may be only a few glands having extensive involvement. The epithelial changes are characteristically located at the mucosal surface and in the superficial lamina propria. Microscopically, endocervical-type mucous glands predominate, but endometrial and tubal-type glands are frequently present (Figs. 17 and 18). The glands may be simple, complex, cystic, or papillary (260). Cysts resembling cervical nabothian cysts are lined by a single layer of columnar mucinous cells or are occasionally lined by papillary fronds. Tuboendometrial glands, when present, are found in the upper vagina in approximately 20% of cases and in the lower vagina in almost 100% of cases (261). Occasionally, small embryonic-type glands composed of low columnar or cuboid cells are found in patients exposed to DES (262). They are also found in women without a history of exposure to DES.

The microscopic appearance of adenosis in women without exposure to DES is similar to that for women with *in utero* exposure (262). With age, vaginal adenosis is replaced by small nests or pegs of squamous metaplasia that reside in the superficial lamina propria. Sparse intraluminal or intracytoplasmic droplets of mucus that may be present can be detected with the mucicarmine stain (263). Squamous metaplasia is ultimately replaced by fully glycogenated squamous epithelium (264). The incidence of squamous dysplasia of the vagina or cervix is twice as high in women exposed to DES than in non-exposed cohorts (265).

Adenosis must be distinguished from endometriosis, clear-cell adenocarcinoma, and *mesonephric remnants.* Mesonephric (wolffian) tubules are located deep in the lateral vaginal wall, are lined by nonciliated, nonmucinous cuboid cells, and have dense, eosinophilic luminal secretions (Fig. 19) (266). The remnants are surrounded by a loose fibrovascular stroma that may

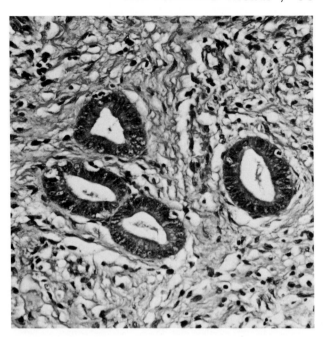

FIG. 18. Vaginal adenosis. Endometrial-type glands are sometimes present in adenosis. Unlike endometriosis, endometrial stroma is absent.

contain smooth-muscle fibers. Clear-cell adenocarcinoma might be confused with the glands of adenosis that undergo *microglandular hyperplasia* (267). Unlike clear-cell adenocarcinoma, microglandular hyperplasia consists of small, uniform, crowded glands without prominent intervening stroma. The cells contain mucin but lack glycogen. Nuclear pleomorphism and prominent nucleoli are absent.

Although adenosis comprised of a variety of cell types may be found adjacent to clear-cell adenocarcinoma, tuboendometrial glands are most common, being found in up to 94% of cases (268). It is hypothesized that carcinoma develops from adenosis through an intermediate form of atypical adenosis (atypical tuboendometrial glands) (268). The latter glands are seen adjacent to about 75% of vaginal clear-cell adenocarcinomas (268). The glands of atypical adenosis have smooth borders, are lined by a single layer of cells, and occasionally show intraglandular bridging. Their enlarged, hyperchromatic, and pleomorphic nuclei have prominent nucleoli. Glands with severely atypical nuclei may represent *in situ* clear-cell adenocarcinoma.

Infectious Diseases

At least 90% of infectious vaginitis is caused by *Candida* species, *Gardnerella vaginalis,* and *Trichomonas vaginalis.* The diagnosis in each instance is readily made by examination of an isotonic saline wet-mount preparation, a Papanicolaou stain of a cervicovaginal smear, or culture isolation.

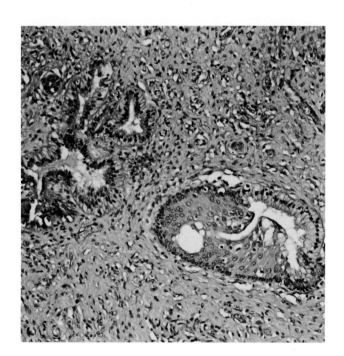

FIG. 17. Vaginal adenosis. Columnar, mucus-producing epithelium (endocervical type) is most often observed in adenosis. The glands are eventually replaced by squamous metaplasia.

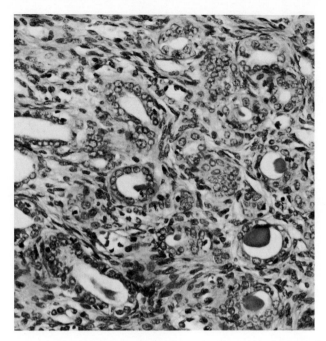

FIG. 19. Mesonephric remnants. Cuboid cells are not ciliated and do not produce mucus. Dense, eosinophilic secretions are present in the lumens.

Bacteria

Gardnerella vaginalis is responsible for the majority of cases of "nonspecific vaginitis" (bacterial vaginosis) (269) as a result of synergism with anaerobic bacteria (270); it is sexually transmitted. The organism does not invade the vaginal epithelium and does not stimulate a local inflammatory response (269). Hence, the vaginal epithelium has a normal microscopic appearance. In a Papanicolaou-stained cervicovaginal smear, the coccobacilli reside on the surface of the superficial squamous cells (clue cells), causing the disappearance of distinct cytoplasmic borders. Polymorphonuclear leukocytes are not a conspicuous component of the cervicovaginal smear.

Neisseria gonorrhoeae rarely causes vaginitis in adults but may infect children who have less resistant vaginal squamous epithelium. The chancre of primary syphilis occasionally occurs in the vagina. *Granuloma inguinale* and *chancroid infection* may involve the vagina, most often in instances of long-standing, destructive vulvar disease. Other organisms that are unusual agents in bacterial vaginitis include *staphylococci, streptococci,* and *M. tuberculosis.* Some strains of *S. aureus* produce an exoprotein ("toxic shock syndrome toxin 1") that is responsible for toxic shock syndrome (271). The association of menstruation and tampon use with toxic shock syndrome results from a complex interaction that includes exposure to a strain of toxin-producing *S. aureus,* lack of immunity, and optimal growth conditions in the vagina for the production of toxin (272). Microscopic

examination of the vagina in women who die of toxic shock syndrome reveals mucosal ulceration, separation of the epithelium beneath the basal layer, vascular congestion, thrombosis, acute inflammation, bacteria within the epithelium, and surface fibrin (273).

A polypoid *xanthogranulomatous pseudotumor* of the vagina was found to be composed of sheets of large histiocytes with abundant eosinophilic, granular cytoplasm that mimicked granular-cell tumor (274). Infection by a mucoid form of *Escherichia coli* was causative (274). Although similar to malacoplakia, the lesion lacked Michaelis-Gutmann bodies. The vagina is the most frequent site of malacoplakia when it occurs in the female genital tract (275). *Escherichia coli* is often cultured from the urine or the specific lesion of genital malacoplakia (275).

Viruses, Chlamydia, and Mycoplasma

Herpesvirus and *human papillomavirus* usually involve the vagina as a part of multicentric infection. Vaginal condylomata may be flat, inverted, or warty. Using Southern blot DNA hybridization techniques, human papillomavirus DNA has been identified in vaginal condylomata (80), vaginal intraepithelial neoplasia (276), and verrucous carcinoma (277). Human papillomavirus types 6 and 11 have been reported in vaginal condyloma (80), and types 1–3,5,6, and 16 have been described in vaginal intraepithelial neoplasia (80,276).

The vagina may be affected by *lymphogranuloma venereum* (*C. trachomatis*) as a part of severe local infection. *Mycoplasma* species and *Ureaplasma urealyticum* normally inhabit the vagina, but, rarely, each may be the predominant isolate in cases of vaginitis (278).

Fungi and Parasites

Candida (usually *C. albicans*), is probably the single most common agent in vaginitis. It is chiefly observed in women during the childbearing years, and it manifests as mucosal erythema or a thick, white exudate (thrush). Histologically, there is mild acanthosis and spongiosis, with congestion and edema of the lamina propria. Lymphocytes, plasma cells, and a few neutrophils are observed in the stroma (90). The organism resides on the epithelial surface and does not penetrate the mucosa. Necrotic debris, neutrophils, and yeast form a surface exudate. About 10% of fungal vaginitis is caused by *Candida* (formerly *Torulopsis*) *glabrata* (279).

Trichomonas vaginalis is a 15- to 20-μm unicellular, flagellate protozoan that is sexually transmitted, primarily during the reproductive years. Some infections are asymptomatic, but in most instances the protozoan causes acute or chronic vaginitis. Microscopic changes include mild acanthosis, spongiosis, congestion, edematous papillae, and small stromal hemorrhages (280). Lymphocytes, plasma cells, and a few neutrophils are observed in the lamina propria. Minute pseudoabscesses may form beneath the epithelium. Necrotic debris and neutrophils sometimes lie on the mucosal surface. The changes are less severe in chronic infection, and no microscopic abnormalities are observed in the asymptomatic patient.

Pinworms, schistosomiasis, and *Entamoeba histolytica* (281) are rare causes of parasitic vaginal infection.

Miscellaneous Benign Conditions

Atrophic vaginitis results from withdrawal of estrogen. The vaginal mucosa appears pale and lacks prominent rugae. Microscopically, the attenuated epithelium is reduced to the basal layer and a few overlying parabasal and intermediate-type squamous cells. The prominent basal and parabasal cells should not be mistaken for dysplastic epithelium. Lymphocytes, plasma cells, and a few neutrophils are present in the lamina propria. *Desquamative inflammatory vaginitis,* histologically similar to atrophic vaginitis, occurs characteristically in the vaginal vault of women with normal estrogen levels (282). The mucosa may be ulcerated superficially with acute and chronic inflammation as well as stromal hemorrhages. The cause is unknown, but in some instances the persistent condition responds to intravaginal application of corticosteroids (282). *Emphysematous vaginitis,* also known as *vaginitis emphysematosa,* occurs in postpubertal women as asymptomatic, gas-filled cysts in the superficial lamina propria. The cysts are usually multiple and measure up to 2 cm in diameter. They are surrounded by multinucleate giant cells, histiocytes, fibroblasts, or collagen (Fig. 20). Occasionally, there is a partial lining of squamous epithelium. Scattered inflammatory cells, including multinucleate giant cells and mononuclear histiocytes, are found in the surrounding fibrotic stroma. The condition has been associated with *Trichomonas* or *Gardnerella* infection and usually disappears after eradication of these organisms (283).

Noninfectious causes of vaginitis include irradiation and a variety of physical and chemical agents. Tampons, especially those of the superabsorbent variety, sometimes cause epithelial drying, layering, and ulceration (284). Granulation tissue, acute and chronic inflammation, and monofilament foreign-body material (synthetic cellulose acetate) have been observed in tampon-related ulcers (285). *Crohn's disease* rarely involves the vagina, manifesting as enterovaginal fistulas (286), sinuses, and abscesses.

Epidermal inclusion cyst occurs as a small asymptomatic cyst in the anterior or posterior vaginal wall. In most instances it is related to previous trauma (287,288). *Mucous cyst,* variously located in the vagina

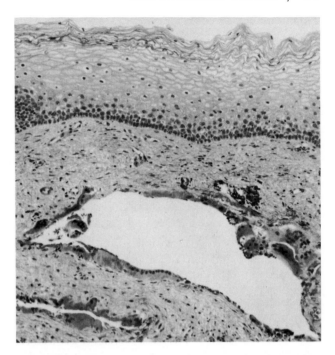

FIG. 20. Emphysematous vaginitis. The lamina propria contains cysts surrounded by multinucleate giant cells, histiocytes, fibroblasts, and collagen.

(287,288), is unilocular and typically measures between 0.5 and 7.0 cm in diameter. It is lined by a single layer of columnar mucous cells, but ciliated cells and squamous metaplasia may be observed focally (287). This cyst, of course, may appear identical to a cystically dilated gland of adenosis. *Gartner's duct (mesonephric) cyst* is a rare vaginal cyst. It is small, single, and characteristically found along the lateral or anterolateral wall. The cyst is lined by a single layer of cuboid, nonmucinous cells. A basement membrane and smooth-muscle fibers in the surrounding stroma are not always present (287). An ectopic ureter may drain into Gartner's duct cyst (289). Vaginal *endometriosis* arises from implantation of shed endometrial fragments into areas of trauma or, more commonly, from pelvic implants along the posterior vaginal fornix (290). The *hymenal cyst* (39) of the newborn is discussed in the section on cystic vulvar lesions. Rare cases of vaginal *dermoid cyst* have been reviewed (291).

The stromal cells of the lamina propria may undergo *decidual metaplasia,* giving rise to a polypoid mass or indurated ulcer that clinically suggests vaginal cancer (292). Spontaneous resolution occurs in the postpartum interval. *Trophoblastic tissue* in the vaginal wall, found rarely in association with normal pregnancy but in up to 10% of patients with hydatidiform mole (293,294), appears as one or more red or purple nodules that readily bleed on palpation. Trophoblastic cells and villi present in the nodules presumably result from hematogenous dissemination and should not be mistaken for choriocarcinoma. A case of vulvar *ectopic pregnancy* has been reported (295).

Granulation tissue, found in the vaginal vault after hysterectomy, occurs chiefly within a few weeks or months after surgery but has appeared after 14 years (296). Granulation tissue is biopsied because it simulates carcinoma clinically, and it is of utmost concern in women who have had a prior hysterectomy for neoplasia. This clinical appearance also may be recapitulated by a *prolapsed fallopian tube* (297,298). Tubal prolapse develops most often after vaginal hysterectomy. The symptoms (abdominal pain, vaginal bleeding, discharge, or dyspareunia) usually occur within 6 months postoperatively but may develop as late as 28 years after surgery (298). Grossly, the prolapsed tube appears as an erythematous, granular, and polypoid mass. It can be diagnosed clinically, when a probe is passed through its lumen or when its traction causes pain (297,298). Microscopically, it easily is overdiagnosed as adenocarcinoma. Marked inflammation, distortion, atypia, and a pseudoinvasive pattern are common (Fig. 21) (297,298). The diagnosis is made upon recognition of hyperplastic tubal epithelium surrounded by smooth-muscle bundles. The therapy is complete excision through the vaginal cuff. Cautery, usually therapeutic for granulation tissue, is not effective (297).

Ectopic *thyroid* and *parathyroid* glands in the wall of the vagina have been described (291).

Benign melanocytic lesions of the vagina include *melanotic macule (lentigo)* (299), *atypical melanocytic hyperplasia* (300), *blue nevus* (301), and *cellular blue nevus*

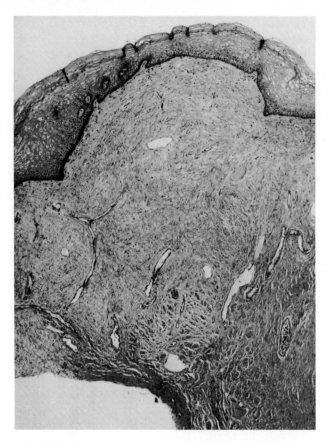

FIG. 22. Vaginal stromal polyp. In this example, dense fibrovascular stroma lies beneath an intact squamous epithelium.

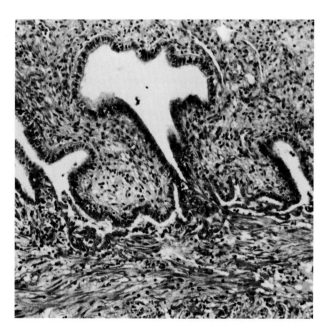

FIG. 21. Fallopian tube prolapsed into vaginal vault. Disorganized, inflamed tubal glands are associated with smooth-muscle bundles.

(302). Three percent of vaginas from women at necropsy have melanocytes in the epithelium (303).

Vaginal *stromal polyps* are generally found in adults but may occur in newborns (304). The designation "pseudosarcoma botryoides" as a synonym for stromal polyp is confusing, and its use should be abandoned (305). The polypoid or pedunculated stromal polyp is found along the lateral walls of the lower one-third of the vagina. It ranges in size from 0.5 to 4 cm and is soft or rubbery, gray-white, and covered by an intact squamous epithelium. The underlying fibrovascular stroma is loose or dense and contains abundant blood vessels (Fig. 22). Approximately half of the cases have atypical stromal cells with large nuclei and abundant cytoplasm. Pleomorphic, hyperchromatic, and occasionally multiple nuclei sometimes have prominent nucleoli. Mitotic figures are rare, but abnormal mitotic forms have been described (304). Stromal polyp may arise from expansion of the subepithelial myxoid stromal zone that extends from the cervix to the vulva. One-quarter of normal women have stromal cells with bizarre nuclear features within this subepithelial myxoid stroma (306). Stromal polyp is cured by simple local excision. Unlike rhabdomyosarcoma it lacks rapid growth, invasion of adjacent tissues, hypercellularity, a cambium layer, and cells with cytoplasmic cross-striations.

"Mesonephric" papilloma is a very rare polypoid or papillary growth in the vagina or cervix of young girls generally less than 6 years of age (307–309). The lesion has a central loose or dense fibrovascular stroma that is lined by nonmucinous cuboid cells. Tall columnar cells and squamous epithelium may be present focally. The papillae vary in size and shape, and the fibrovascular stroma may be infiltrated by neutrophils and lymphocytes. Despite its designation, there is no evidence for mesonephric derivation (309).

The vaginal *mixed* tumor is situated most often just above the hymenal ring in adults (310). It presents as a nonencapsulated, well-circumscribed subepithelial nodule that in most instances is not connected to the surface epithelium. Microscopically, the tumor is dissimilar to the usual mixed tumor of salivary gland, skin, or vulva. Vaginal mixed tumor is composed of small stromal-type cells that surround nests of mature squamous cells and glands lined by mucinous epithelium (Fig. 23). A pseudopapillary arrangement, spindle-shaped stromal cells arranged in fascicles, and hyaline stromal cores may be present. Although the histogenesis is uncertain, the

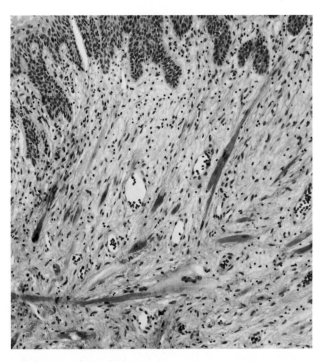

FIG. 24. Vaginal rhabdomyoma. The dermis contains abundant long, spindle-shaped cells with dense, eosinophilic cytoplasm. Nuclei have vesicular chromatin and small nucleoli and lack pleomorphism.

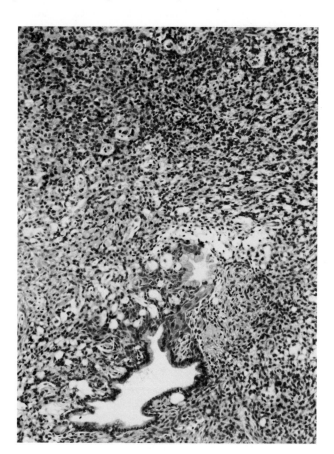

FIG. 23. Mixed tumor of vagina. The neoplasm consists of small stromal-type cells with occasional hyaline stromal cores, mature squamous cells, and glands lined by endocervical-type epithelium.

tumor does not arise from minor vestibular glands. Reported cases of *intramural papilloma* (331) and *Brenner tumor* (312) of the vagina have microscopic features quite similar to vaginal mixed tumor and might be examples of this neoplasm. Local excision for vaginal mixed tumor appears to be curative (310).

Single cases of vaginal *glomus* tumor (313) and *paraganglioma* (314) have been documented. Other benign soft-tissue tumors of the vagina include *leiomyoma* (102,315), *rhabdomyoma* (114,316,317), *nodular fasciitis* (318), *hemangioma* (102), *granular-cell tumor* (319), *neurofibroma* (320), and *neurofibroma* with *rhabdomyomatous differentiation* (benign "Triton" tumor) (321). Leiomyoma is the most common vaginal mesodermal neoplasm. The authors of one study of 60 vaginal smooth-muscle tumors developed criteria for malignancy (leiomyosarcoma) that included moderate to marked cytologic atypia and at least five mitotic figures per 10 high-power fields (315). Vaginal leiomyomas with epithelioid features are very uncommon.

Vaginal *rhabdomyoma* occurs as an asymptomatic polypoid mass in middle-aged women (317). The nonencapsulated, poorly circumscribed lesion generally measures less than 3 cm in diameter. Microscopically, it is distinct from both adult and fetal types of rhabdomyoma. Vaginal rhabdomyoma is composed of interlacing oval or spindle-shaped cells which have large vesicular nuclei with nucleoli but which lack overt atypia (Fig. 24). Large striated-muscle cells may be conspicuous. The cells lie in a collagenous or myxoid stroma that contains thin-walled blood vessels. Cytoplasmic cross-striations may be abundant focally, but they form only a small proportion of the total cell population. Mitotic figures are generally absent. Skeletal-muscle differentiation is evident ultrastructurally (316). The differential diagnosis of rhabdomyoma includes stromal polyp and sarcoma botryoides.

Reactive postoperative sarcoma-like lesions of the vagina include *spindle-cell nodule* (322) and *fibrohistiocytic proliferation* (323). Postoperative spindle-cell nodule, also found in the urinary tract, measures up to 4 cm in diameter and is usually located at a surgical incision site. Resembling spindle-cell sarcoma light microscopically, it is composed of interlacing fascicles of plump spindle cells replacing collagenous stroma and smooth muscle. Nuclei have vesicular chromatin and prominent nucleoli. Mitotic figures are numerous. Unlike sarcoma, marked nuclear pleomorphism, hyperchromatism, and bizarre mitotic figures are absent. There is a single report of a reactive fibrohistiocytic proliferation that developed postoperatively at the vaginal apex in a woman 5 months after hysterectomy. Microscopically, it consisted of foamy histiocytes, foreign-body-type giant cells, polarizable material, and bundles of spindle-shaped cells in a storiform pattern, simulating fibrous histiocytoma.

Malignant Neoplasms

Vaginal intraepithelial neoplasia (VAIN) and *squamous-cell carcinoma* are often associated with intraepithelial and invasive squamous neoplasms of the cervix and vulva (324,325). This multicentricity represents a "field effect" involving the epithelium of the lower female genital tract. Squamous neoplasms that involve both the cervix and vagina are arbitrarily classified as cervical in origin, and those that involve the vagina and vulva are categorized as vulvar tumors. Criteria are not standardized with regard to the classification of *in situ* and invasive squamous lesions of the vagina that manifest as new primary vaginal neoplasms following cervical *in situ* or invasive squamous tumors. For a subsequent lesion confined to the vagina to be classified as a new, separate vaginal neoplasm (325), some authors have required more than a 5-year disease-free interval after treatment for cervical squamous-cell carcinoma and more than a 2-year disease-free interval after therapy for cervical intraepithelial neoplasia. Hence, *in situ* and invasive squamous-cell carcinomas involving the vagina are undoubtedly underclassified as primary vaginal lesions.

VAIN is found typically in the upper one-third of the vagina. Although the age range is broad, most patients are postmenopausal. Approximately one-third have had prior hysterectomy for benign conditions (324). VAIN is

multifocal or diffuse in about one-half of the cases (324,326). The criteria for grading VAIN (I, mild dysplasia; II, moderate dysplasia; III, severe dysplasia/CIS) are similar to those for grading intraepithelial neoplasia of the cervix (327). Morphologic changes of human papillomavirus infection may also be identified in, or adjacent to, VAIN. In one study of VAIN III, subsequent disease was noted in 12% of patients who had complete excision and in 34% of patients who had equivocal or incomplete surgical margins (324). Three of 136 women treated for VAIN III developed invasive squamous-cell carcinoma after 10 to 48 months (324).

Squamous-cell carcinoma accounts for over 90% of all primary invasive neoplasms of the vagina (328–330). Occasionally, squamous-cell carcinoma develops in young adult women, and, rarely, they arise in direct association with vaginal condylomata (331) or in split-thickness skin grafts created as neovaginas for women with vaginal agenesis (332). The clinical staging system for squamous-cell carcinoma of the vagina is based on that set forth by the International Federation of Obstetrics and Gynecology (Table 5) (333). Size and specific location of the tumor in the vagina are not considered in clinical staging.

Grossly, squamous-cell carcinoma is nodular, ulcerative, indurative, or exophytic. Approximately one-third are keratinizing and over one-half are nonkeratinizing, moderately differentiated tumors (328). Adequate data that compare grade with prognosis are not available. The concept of microinvasive squamous-cell carcinoma of the vagina recently has been formulated as a means to identify patients who appear to have a good prognosis and who might be treated more conservatively (334). Peters et al. (334) found that each of six patients who had partial or complete vaginectomy for squamous cancers less than 2.5 mm thick and lacking vascular invasion were alive without disease (follow-up 51–172 months). A large study is necessary to determine whether thickness correlates with prognosis for women with vaginal carcinoma. Treatment of squamous-cell carcinoma is individualized; external beam or implant radiation is often preferred, with surgery reserved for

TABLE 5. *International Federation of Obstetrics and Gynecology (FIGO) staging system for invasive squamous-cell carcinoma of the vagina*[a]

Stage	Definition
I	Neoplasm limited to vaginal wall
II	Neoplasm extending to subvaginal tissue but not to pelvic wall
III	Neoplasm extending to pelvic wall
IV	Neoplasm extending to the mucosa of the bladder or rectum or beyond true pelvis

[a] Criteria accepted by the General Assembly of FIGO in 1970.

selected cases (327–330). The 5-year survival is largely determined by the clinical stage; typically it is 70% to 75% for stage I tumors and 45% overall (329,330).

Verrucous carcinoma of the vagina invades on a broad front with a pushing border. There may be extensive local spread, with invasion of the rectum and coccyx (335). Human papillomavirus DNA has been identified in vaginal verrucous cancer (277). *Spindle-cell carcinoma* (squamous-cell carcinoma with sarcoma-like stroma) of the vagina has gross and light-microscopic features similar to those neoplasms that arise in the upper respiratory and digestive tracts (183).

The association of vaginal and cervical *clear-cell adenocarcinoma* with *in utero* exposure to diethylstilbestrol is well known (256,336,337); however, up to one-third of patients lack exposure (337). Over 500 cases of vaginal and cervical clear-cell adenocarcinoma have been accessioned in the Registry for Research on Hormonal Transplacental Carcinogenesis (336,337). The patients range in age from 7 to 37 years, and the median age is 19 years (336,337). The tumor is distinctly uncommon before age 12 and after age 30. Grossly, the neoplasm appears as a polypoid, nodular, flat, or ulcerated mass, usually in the anterior or lateral wall of the upper vagina (338). Rarely, it is confined to the lamina propria with overlying normal squamous epithelium. Clear-cell adenocarcinoma varies in size from microscopic to more than 10 cm in diameter (338).

Microscopically, about 60% of cervical and vaginal tumors show a predominantly tubulocystic growth pattern (337). Twenty percent have a predominantly solid pattern of growth, and 12% are papillary (337). A mixture of growth patterns is usual (Fig. 25). Solid sheets of tumor are composed of cells with abundant clear cytoplasm. Tubules, cysts, and papillae are lined chiefly by hobnail cells or flat cells. Cords of cells having eosinophilic cytoplasm may also be observed. Nuclear pleomorphism is variable. Flat cells that line dilated cysts often have a bland cytologic appearance (338). Approximately 75% of all neoplasms have no more than one mitotic figure per 10 high-power fields (337). Foci of atypical adenosis are usually observed adjacent to the tumor (268). Clear-cell adenocarcinoma must not be confused with microglandular hyperplasia (arising in adenosis) and the Arias-Stella phenomenon (267,338). The neoplasm must also be distinguished from endodermal sinus tumor and metastatic renal-cell carcinoma. Cells of clear-cell adenocarcinoma contain abundant glycogen, but mucin, which may be present in the lumina of tubules, is absent in the cytoplasm. Ultrastructurally, vaginal and cervical clear-cell adenocarcinomas are identical to clear-cell adenocarcinoma that arises in the ovary or endometrium (339). Intracytoplasmic glycogen and short, blunt surface microvilli are conspicuous features.

The prognosis for cervical or vaginal clear-cell adeno-

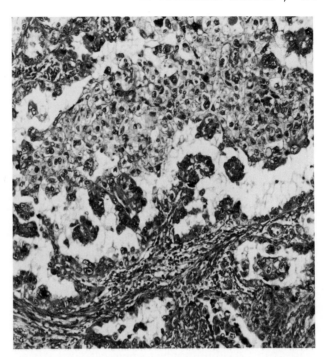

FIG. 25. Clear-cell adenocarcinoma. The neoplasm consists of sheets of cells with pleomorphic nuclei and clear cytoplasm. Tubules and papillae often contain cells with dense, eosinophilic cytoplasm.

carcinoma is related primarily to the clinical stage. The overall actuarial 10-year survival rate is 79% (337). Patients with stage I vaginal tumors have a 90% 10-year actuarial survival rate after therapy (340). In one study, recurrences developed in almost 25% of the patients overall, most of whom died (338). When it metastasizes, clear-cell adenocarcinoma has a propensity for the pelvis, lungs, and supraclavicular lymph nodes.

Some adenocarcinomas of the vagina are *papillary* or *mucinous,* and a few have a squamous component (*adenosquamous*) (325). *Mucin-producing adenocarcinoma* originating in vaginal adenosis has been documented in women without prior *in utero* exposure to DES (341). *Intestinal-type adenocarcinoma* rarely develops in ileal or colorectal grafts, used to create neovaginas (332). One case of *paravaginal wolffian duct (mesonephric) adenocarcinoma* has been described (342). *Small-cell undifferentiated carcinoma* of the vagina portends a very poor prognosis (325). One of the reported tumors also contained areas of intestinal-type adenocarcinoma (343). Two cases of so-called *malignant mixed tumor* were composed of (a) epithelial cells arranged in tubules and acini and (b) spindle-shaped cells (334,345). Light microscopically, some areas in the two cases resembled stromal sarcoma with epithelial-like elements ("uterine-sex-cord-like tumor").

Vaginal or paravaginal carcinoma or sarcoma sometimes arises in endometriosis. The rectovaginal septum is the most common extraovarian site for a malignant tumor occurring in endometriosis (346). Neoplasms that have originated in endometriosis of the vagina or rectovaginal septum include *endometrioid adenocarcinoma, clear-cell adenocarcinoma, carcinosarcoma,* and *stromal sarcoma* (346–349). Criteria promulgated for malignancy arising in endometriosis include the presence of endometriosis near the neoplasm, histology consistent with origin from endometrial glands or stroma, and absence of a primary tumor elsewhere (346). Atypical endometrial glands, when present, provide further support for origin of carcinoma in endometriosis.

Endodermal sinus tumor of the vagina invariably occurs in infants 3 years of age or younger (350). Grossly, the neoplasm is sessile or polypoid with areas of ulceration. On cut section, it is soft, friable, and tan-white, with areas of hemorrhage and necrosis (351). Clinically, it may simulate sarcoma botryoides (309). Vaginal endodermal sinus tumor is microscopically identical to pure yolk sac tumors of the ovary and testis (Fig. 26) (351). Immunohistochemical positivity for alpha-fetoprotein may be of value for distinguishing this neoplasm from clear-cell adenocarcinoma. The prognosis has improved greatly since the addition of chemotherapy (350–352). Local excision plus chemotherapy appears to be the optimal treatment (352). Since 1970, 26 of 38 patients are alive (median follow-up 46 months) (352).

Vaginal *melanoma* presents as an ulcerated, blue or black polypoid nodule most frequently in the lower

TABLE 6. *Primary sarcomas of the vagina*

Sarcoma	Reference
Rhabdomyosarcoma	360, 362
Leiomyosarcoma	315, 361–363
Malignant fibrous histiocytoma	364
Hemangiopericytoma	365, 366
Malignant schwannoma	362, 363
Endometrial stromal sarcoma	362, 363, 367
Malignant mixed müllerian tumor	363
Alveolar soft part sarcoma	368, 369

one-third of the vagina (353). Postmenopausal Caucasian women are chiefly affected. The neoplasm tends to be large: the median diameter in one series was 3 cm (299). Junctional activity may be extensive. Sometimes the neoplasm consists of pleomorphic cells, spindle-shaped cells, or small cells (299,353). In such instances, the differential diagnosis includes a variety of other highly malignant neoplasms. The 5-year survival rate for women with vaginal melanoma, based on a literature summary, is a dismal 7% (354).

Non-Hodgkin's lymphoma and *granulocytic sarcoma* (355) may involve the vagina as a part of widespread disease. Rarely, primary *plasmacytoma* (222,356) and non-Hodgkin's lymphoma (357,358) arise in the vagina. Diffuse, large-cell lymphoma appears to be the predominant subtype of vaginal lymphoma, although nodular lymphoma has also been described. The vagina is rarely the site of *eosinophilic granuloma* (359).

A variety of sarcomas have arisen in the vagina or paravaginally (Table 6) (315,360–369). *Leiomyosarcoma* is by far the most frequent; criteria for its separation from leiomyoma are discussed under benign smooth-muscle tumors of the vagina (315). In one study, 35% of patients with vaginal sarcoma had prior pelvic radiation for cervical carcinoma, and each of the four patients with *malignant mixed müllerian tumor* had received radiation therapy (363). *Aggressive angiomyxoma* (218,219) of the pelvis is discussed in the section on malignant neoplasms of the vulva.

Vaginal *embryonal rhabdomyosarcoma* is found in infants and children up to 6 years of age (median age 1.8 years) (360). The neoplasm presents as soft botryoid nodules that fill, and often protrude out of, the vagina. On cut section, the smooth-surfaced nodules appear gray-white or hemorrhagic. Microscopically, small, round or spindle-shaped cells with scanty cytoplasm are embedded in a myxoid stroma (Fig. 27). A subepithelial condensation of malignant cells ("cambium" layer) and rhabdomyoblasts are observed. Cross-striations may be identified, sometimes after prolonged examination. Immunohistochemical stains for muscle in general (actin, desmin) or skeletal muscle (myoglobin) may be a valuable diagnostic adjunct. The prognosis for patients with vaginal rhabdomyosarcoma has improved as a result of

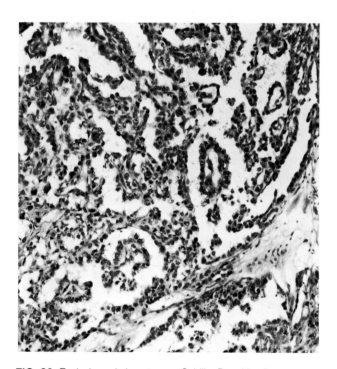

FIG. 26. Endodermal sinus tumor. Schiller-Duval bodies are conspicuous in this neoplasm from a 13-month-old female infant.

a multimodal therapeutic approach. Because of the effectiveness of chemotherapeutic agents, primary pelvic exenteration can be avoided. Only one tumor-related death was found among 24 evaluable children who were admitted to the Intergroup Rhabdomyosarcoma Study (360).

Malignant neoplasms that involve the vagina by local extension or recurrence include carcinomas of the *cervix, vulva, bladder, urethra,* and *rectum.* Other tumors that have metastasized to the vagina include carcinomas of the *endometrium* (370), *ovary* (371), *kidney* (372), and *breast* (373). Following primary therapy, approximately 9% of patients with endometrial adenocarcinoma develop vaginal recurrences, two-thirds of which are solitary (370). The recurrences may be small clinically and resemble granulation tissue. In an autopsy study of 86 women with advanced ovarian cancer, 12% had vaginal involvement (371). Gestational *choriocarcinoma* metastasizes to the vagina in about 25% of cases (294,374,375). Over 90% of choriocarcinomas metastatic to the vagina are found in the lower portion, most often in the anterior wall beneath the urethra or at the urethral orifice (374). The majority of renal-cell carcinomas metastatic to the vagina arise from the left kidney, suggesting a retrograde venous route via the ovarian vein and vaginal venous plexuses. The initial presentation may be as a nodule in the vagina (372). Light microscopically and ultrastructurally, renal-cell carcinoma is distinguishable from primary vaginal clear-cell adenocarcinoma.

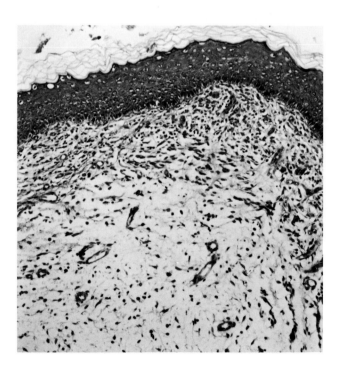

FIG. 27. Embryonal rhabdomyosarcoma. Small, round or spindle-shaped cells in a myxoid stroma and a "cambium" layer are characteristic.

REFERENCES

1. Rorat E, Ferenczy A, Richart RM. Human Bartholin gland, duct, and duct cyst. Histochemical and ultrastructural study. *Arch Pathol Lab Med* 1975;99:367–374.
2. Robboy SJ, Ross JS, Prat J, Keh PC, Welch WR. Urogenital sinus origin of mucinous and ciliated cysts of the vulva. *Obstet Gynecol* 1978;51:347–351.
3. Huffman JW. The detailed anatomy of the paraurethral ducts in the adult human female. *Am J Obstet Gynecol* 1948;55:86–101.
4. Plentl AA, Friedman EA. *Lymphatic system of the female genitalia. The morphologic basis of oncologic diagnosis and therapy.* Philadelphia: WB Saunders, 1971:15–26,51–56.
5. Iversen T, Aas M. Lymph drainage from the vulva. *Gynecol Oncol* 1983;16:179–189.
6. Way S. *Malignant disease of the vulva.* Edinburgh: Churchill Livingstone, 1982:13–19.
7. Eichner E. Vulvar carcinoma. *Am J Obstet Gynecol* 1961;81:1280.
8. Jones HW Jr, Ferguson-Smith MA, Heller RH. Pathologic and cytogenetic findings in true hermaphroditism. Report of 6 cases and review of 23 cases from the literature. *Obstet Gynecol* 1965;25:435–447.
9. Simpson JL. Genetic aspects of gynecologic disorders occurring in 46,XX individuals. *Clin Obstet Gynecol* 1972;15:157–182.
10. Shaw RW, Farquhar JW. Female pseudohermaphroditism associated with danazol exposure *in utero.* Case report. *Br J Obstet Gynaecol* 1984;91:386–389.
11. Kingsbury AC. Danazol and fetal masculinization: a warning. *Med J Aust* 1985;143:410–411.
12. Wilkins L, Jones HW Jr, Holman GH, Stempfel RS Jr. Masculinization of the female fetus associated with administration of oral and intramuscular progestins during gestation: non-adrenal female pseudohermaphrodism. *J Clin Endocrinol Metab* 1958;18:559–585.
13. Wilkins L. Masculinization of female fetus due to use of orally given progestins. *JAMA* 1960;172:1028–1032.
14. Malinak LR, Miller GV. Bilateral multicentric ovarian luteomas of pregnancy associated with masculinization of a female infant. *Am J Obstet Gynecol* 1965;91:251–259.
15. Jenkins ME, Surana RB, Russell-Cutts CM. Ambiguous genitals in a female infant associated with luteoma of pregnancy. Report of a case. *Am J Obstet Gynecol* 1968;101:923–928.
16. Verkauf BS, Reiter EO, Hernandez L, Burns SA. Virilization of mother and fetus associated with luteoma of pregnancy: a case report with endocrinologic studies. *Am J Obstet Gynecol* 1977;129:274–280.
17. Fox LP, Stamm WJ. Krukenberg tumor complicating pregnancy. Report of a case with androgenic activity. *Am J Obstet Gynecol* 1965;92:702–710.
18. Spadoni LR, Lindberg MC, Mottet NK, Herrmann WL. Virilization coexisting with Krukenberg tumor during pregnancy. *Am J Obstet Gynecol* 1965;92:981–991.
19. Connor TB, Ganis FM, Levin HS, Migeon CJ, Martin LG. Gonadotropin-dependent Krukenberg tumor causing virilization during pregnancy. *J Clin Endocrinol Metab* 1968;28:198–214.
20. Bell RJM. Fetal virilisation due to maternal Krukenberg tumour. *Lancet* 1977;1:1162–1163.
21. Brentnall CP. A case of arrhenoblastoma complicating pregnancy. *J Obstet Gynaecol Br Emp* 1945;52:235–240.
22. Murset G, Zachmann M, Prader A, Fischer J, Labhart A. Male external genitalia of a girl caused by a virilizing adrenal tumour in the mother. Case report and steroid studies. *Acta Endocrinol* 1970;65:627–638.
23. Fuller PJ, Pettigrew IG, Pike JW, Stockigt JR. An adrenal adenoma causing virilization of mother and infant. *Clin Endocrinol* 1983;18:143–153.
24. van de Kamp JJP, van Seters AP, Moolenaar AJ, van Gelderen HH. Female pseudo-hermaphroditism due to an adrenal tumour in the mother. *Eur J Pediatr* 1984;142:140–142.
25. Kai H, Nose O, Iida Y, Ono J, Harada T, Yabuuchi H. Female pseudohermaphroditism caused by maternal congenital adrenal hyperplasia. *J Pediatr* 1979;95:418–420.
26. Dewhurst CJ. Congenital malformations of the genital tract in

childhood. *J Obstet Gynaecol Br Commonwealth* 1968;75:377–391.

27. Lubinsky MS. Female pseudohermaphroditism and associated anomalies. *Am J Med Genet* 1980;6:123–136.
28. Radman HM. Hypertrophy of the labia minora. *Obstet Gynecol* 1976;48:78s–80s.
29. So EP, Brock W, Kaplan GW. Ectopic labium and VATER association in a newborn. *J Urol* 1980;124:156–157.
30. Capraro VJ, Dillon WP, Gallego MB. Microperforate hymen. A distinct clinical entity. *Obstet Gynecol* 1974;44:903–905.
31. Nesbitt REL Jr, Abdul-Karim RW. Persistent urogenital membrane sinus as a clinical entity. *JAMA* 1968;205:91–94.
32. Rocereto TF, Campbell WA III. Ureterocele presenting as a perineal cyst. *Obstet Gynecol* 1980;55:54s–56s.
33. Kaufman RH. Cystic tumors. In: Gardner HL, Kaufman RH, eds. *Benign diseases of the vulva and vagina*, 2nd edition. Boston: GK Hall, 1981;95–130.
34. Zivkovic SM. Epidermoid cyst of anterior commissure of labia majora and separated pubic bones. *Urology* 1981;17:467–468.
35. Onuigbo WIB. Vulval epidermoid cysts in the Igbos of Nigeria. *Arch Dermatol* 1976;112:1405–1406.
36. Betson JR Jr, Chiffelle TL, George RP. Pilonidal sinus involving the clitoris. A case report. *Am J Obstet Gynecol* 1962;84:543–545.
37. Kimbrough HM Jr, Vaughan ED Jr. Skene's duct cyst in a newborn: case report and review of the literature. *J Urol* 1977;117:387–388.
38. Blaivas JG, Pais VM, Retik AB. Paraurethral cysts in female neonate. *Urology* 1976;7:504–507.
39. Merlob P, Bahari C, Liban E, Reisner SH. Cysts of the female external genitalia in the newborn infant. *Am J Obstet Gynecol* 1978;132:607–610.
40. Kucera PR, Glazer J. Hydrocele of the canal of Nuck. A report of four cases. *J Reprod Med* 1985;30:439–442.
41. Block RE. Hydrocele of the canal of Nuck. A report of five cases. *Obstet Gynecol* 1975;45:464–466.
42. Hart WR. Paramesonephric mucinous cysts of the vulva. *Am J Obstet Gynecol* 1970;107:1079–1084.
43. Friedrich EG Jr, Wilkinson EJ. Mucous cysts of the vulvar vestibule. *Obstet Gynecol* 1973;42:407–414.
44. Oi RH, Munn R. Mucous cysts of the vulvar vestibule. *Hum Pathol* 1982;13:584–586.
45. Woodruff JD, Parmley TH. Infection of the minor vestibular gland. *Obstet Gynecol* 1983;62:609–612.
46. Freedman SR, Goldman RL. Mucocele-like changes in Bartholin's glands. *Hum Pathol* 1978;9:111–114.
47. Shelley WB, Levy EJ. Apocrine sweat retention in man. II. Fox-Fordyce disease (apocrine miliaria). *Arch Dermatol* 1956;73:38–49.
48. Binder SS. Endometriosis of the vulva and perineum. Report of a case. *Pacific Med Surg* 1965;73:294–296.
49. Lynch PJ. Sexually transmitted diseases: Granuloma inguinale, lymphogranuloma venereum, chancroid, and infectious syphilis. *Clin Obstet Gynecol* 1978;21:1041–1052.
50. Beckett JH, Bigbee JW. Immunoperoxidase localization of *Treponema pallidum*. *Arch Pathol Lab Med* 1979;103:135–138.
51. Lee YH, Rankin JS, Alpert S, Daly AK, McCormack WM. Microbiological investigation of Bartholin's gland abscesses and cysts. *Am J Obstet Gynecol* 1977;129:150–153.
52. Kuberski T. Granuloma inguinale (Donovanosis). *Sex Transm Dis* 1980;7:29–36.
53. Davis CM. Granuloma inguinale. A clinical, histological, and ultrastructural study. *JAMA* 1970;211:632–636.
54. de Boer AI, de Boer F, Van der Merwe JV. Cytologic identification of Donovan bodies in granuloma inguinale. *Acta Cytol* 1984;28:126–128.
55. Alexander LJ, Shields TL. Squamous cell carcinoma of the vulva secondary to granuloma inguinale. *Arch Dermatol* 1953;67:395–402.
56. Saltzstein SL, Woodruff JD, Novak, ER. Postgranulomatous carcinoma of the vulva. *Obstet Gynecol* 1956;7:80–90.
57. Margolis RJ, Hood AF. Chancroid: diagnosis and treatment. *J Am Acad Dermatol* 1982;6:493–499.
58. Werman BS, Herskowitz LJ, Olansky S, Kleris G, Sottnek FO. A clinical variant of chancroid resembling granuloma inguinale. *Arch Dermatol* 1983;119:890–894.
59. Brenner BN. Tuberculosis of the vulva. Case reports. *S Afr Med J* 1976;50:1798–1800.
60. Millar JW, Holt S, Gilmour HM, Robertson DHH. Vulval tuberculosis. *Tubercle* 1979;60:173–176.
61. Friedrich EG Jr. *Vulvar disease*, 2nd edition. Philadelphia: WB Saunders, 1983:126.
62. Addison WA, Livengood CH III, Hill GB, Sutton GP, Fortier KJ. Necrotizing fasciitis of vulvar origin in diabetic patients. *Obstet Gynecol* 1984;63:473–479.
63. Thomas R, Barnhill D, Bibro M, Hoskins W. Hidradenitis suppurativa: a case presentation and review of the literature. *Obstet Gynecol* 1985;66:592–595.
64. Bhatia NN, Bergman A, Broen EM. Advanced hidradenitis suppurativa of the vulva. A report of three cases. *J Reprod Med* 1984;29:436–440.
65. Winkler B, Crum CP. *Chlamydia trachomatis* infection of the female genital tract. Pathogenetic and clinicopathologic correlations. *Pathol Annu* 1987;22:193–223.
66. Davies JA, Rees E, Hobson D, Karayiannis P. Isolation of *Chlamydia trachomatis* from Bartholin's ducts. *Br J Venereol Dis* 1978;54:409–413.
67. Josey WE. Viral infections of the vulva. *Clin Obstet Gynecol* 1978;21:1053–1059.
68. Brown D. Herpes zoster of the vulva. *Clin Obstet Gynecol* 1972;15:1010–1014.
69. Humphrey DC. Localized accidental vaccinia of the vulva. Report of three cases and a review of the world literature. *Am J Obstet Gynecol* 1963;86:460–469.
70. Portnoy J, Ahronheim GA, Ghibu F, Clecner B, Joncas JH. Recovery of Epstein-Barr virus from genital ulcers. *N Engl J Med* 1984;311:966–968.
71. Syrjanen KJ. *Human papillomavirus* (HPV) infections of the female genital tract and their associations with intraepithelial neoplasia and squamous cell carcinoma. *Pathol Annu* 1986;21:53–89.
72. Growdon WA, Fu YS, Lebherz TB, Rapkin A, Mason GD, Parks G. Pruritic vulvar squamous papillomatosis: evidence for human papillomavirus etiology. *Obstet Gynecol* 1985;66:564–568.
73. Ferenczy A, Mitao M, Nagai N, Silverstein SJ, Crum CP. Latent papillomavirus and recurring genital warts. *N Engl J Med* 1985;313:784–788.
74. Crum CP, Braun LA, Shah KV, Fu YS, Levine RU, Fenoglio CM, Richart RM, Townsend DE. Vulvar intraepithelial neoplasia: correlation of nuclear DNA content and the presence of a human papilloma virus (HPV) structural antigen. *Cancer* 1982;49:468–471.
75. Wade TR, Ackerman AB. The effects of resin of podophyllin on condyloma acuminatum. *Am J Dermatopathol* 1984;6:109–122.
76. Crum CP, Fu YS, Levine RU, Richart RM, Townsend DE, Fenoglio CM. Intraepithelial squamous lesions of the vulva: biologic and histologic criteria for the distinction of condylomas from vulvar intraepithelial neoplasia. *Am J Obstet Gynecol* 1982;144:77–83.
77. Friedrich EG Jr, Wilkinson EJ, Fu YS. Carcinoma *in situ* of the vulva: a continuing challenge. *Am J Obstet Gynecol* 1980;136:830–843.
78. Rhatigan RM, Saffos RO. Condyloma acuminatum and squamous carcinoma of the vulva. *South Med J* 1977;70:591–594.
79. Shafeek MA, Osman MI, Hussein MA. Carcinoma of the vulva arising in condylomata acuminata. *Obstet Gynecol* 1979;54:120–123.
80. Gupta J, Pilotti S, Rilke F, Shah K. Association of human papillomavirus type 16 with neoplastic lesions of the vulva and other genital sites by *in situ* hybridization. *Am J Pathol* 1987;127:206–215.
81. Pilotti S, Rilke F, Shah KV, Delle Torre G, De Palo G. Immunohistochemical and ultrastructural evidence of papilloma virus infection associated with *in situ* and microinvasive squamous cell carcinoma of the vulva. *Am J Surg Pathol* 1984;8:751–761.
82. Gissmann L, de Villiers EM, zur Hausen H. Analysis of human genital warts (condylomata acuminata) and other genital tumors

for human papillomavirus type 6 DNA. *Int J Cancer* 1982;29:143–146.

83. Rando RF, Sedlacek TV, Hunt J, Jenson AB, Kurman RJ, Lancaster WD. Verrucous carcinoma of the vulva associated with an unusual type 6 human papillomavirus. *Obstet Gynecol* 1986;67:70s–75s.

84. Durst M, Gissmann L, Ikenberg H, zur Hausen H. A papillomavirus DNA from a cervical carcinoma and its prevalence in cancer biopsy samples from different geographic regions. *Proc Natl Acad Sci USA* 1983;80:3812–3815.

85. Gissman L, Wolnik L, Ikenberg H, Koldovsky U, Schnurch HG, zur Hausen H. Human papillomavirus types 6 and 11 DNA sequences in genital and laryngeal papillomas and in some cervical cancers. *Proc Natl Acad Sci USA* 1983;80:560–563.

86. Ikenberg H, Gissmann L, Gross G, Grussendorf-Conen EI, zur Hausen H. Human papillomavirus type-16-related DNA in genital Bowen's disease and in bowenoid papulosis. *Int J Cancer* 1983;32:563–565.

87. Gross G, Hagedorn M, Ikenberg H, Rufli T, Dahlet C, Grosshans E, Gissmann L. Bowenoid papulosis. Presence of human papillomavirus (HPV) structural antigens and of HPV 16-related DNA sequences. *Arch Dermatol* 1985;121:858–863.

88. Lynch PJ. Molluscum contagiosum venereum. *Clin Obstet Gynecol* 1972;15:966–975.

89. Reed RJ, Parkinson RP. The histogenesis of molluscum contagiosum. *Am J Surg Pathol* 1977;1:161–166.

90. Gardner HL. Candidiasis. In: Gardner HL, Kaufman RH, eds. *Benign diseases of the vulva and vagina,* 2nd edition. Boston: GK Hall, 1981:217–242.

91. Scott RA, Gallis HA, Livengood CH. Phycomycosis of the vulva. *Am J Obstet Gynecol* 1985;153:675–676.

92. McKee PH, Wright E, Hutt MSR. Vulval schistosomiasis. *Clin Exp Dermatol* 1983;8:189–194.

93. Santa Cruz DJ, Martin SA. Verruciform xanthoma of the vulva. Report of two cases. *Am J Clin Pathol* 1979;71:224–228.

94. Rocamora A, Santonja C, Vives R, Varona C. Sebaceous gland hyperplasia of the vulva: a case report. *Obstet Gynecol* 1986;68:63s–65s.

95. Axe S, Parmley T, Woodruff JD, Hlopak B. Adenomas in minor vestibular glands. *Obstet Gynecol* 1986;68:16–18.

96. Buchler DA, Sun F, Chuprevich T. Case report. A pilar tumor of the vulva. *Gynecol Oncol* 1978;6:479–486.

97. Jackson R. Melanosis of the vulva. *J Dermatol Surg Oncol* 1984;10:119–121.

98. Friedman RJ, Ackerman AB. Difficulties in the histologic diagnosis of melanocytic nevi in the vulvae of premenopausal women. In: Ackerman AB, ed. *Pathology of malignant melanoma.* New York: Masson, 1981:119–127.

99. Daunt SO, Kotowski KE, O'Reilly AP, Richardson AT. Ulcerative vulvitis in Reiter's syndrome. A case report. *Br J Venereol Dis* 1982;58:405–407.

100. Dodson MG, Klegerman ME, Kerman RH, Lange CF, Tressler HH, O'Leary JA. Behcet syndrome. With immunologic evaluation. *Obstet Gynecol* 1978;51:621–625.

101. Davis J, Shapiro L, Baral J. Vulvitis circumscripta plasmacellularis. *J Am Acad Dermatol* 1983;8:413–416.

102. Kaufman RH, Gardner HL. Benign mesodermal tumors. *Clin Obstet Gynecol* 1965;8:953–981.

103. Kempson RL, Sherman AI. Sclerosing lipogranuloma of the vulva. *Am J Obstet Gynecol* 1968;101:854–856.

104. Tavassoli F, Norris HJ. Smooth muscle tumors of the vulva. *Obstet Gynecol* 1979;53:213–217.

105. Aneiros J, Beltran E, Garcia del Moral R, Nogales FF Jr. Epithelioid leiomyoma of the vulva. *Diagn Gynecol Obstet* 1982;4:351–355.

106. Messina AM, Strauss RG. Pelvic neurofibromatosis. *Obstet Gynecol* 1976;47:63s–66s.

107. Schreiber MM. Vulvar von Recklinghausen's disease. *Arch Dermatol* 1963;88:320–321.

108. Huang HJ, Yamabe T, Tagawa H. A solitary neurilemmoma of the clitoris. *Gynecol Oncol* 1983;15:103–110.

109. Woodruff JM, Marshall ML, Godwin TA, Funkhouser JW, Thompson NJ, Erlandson RA. Plexiform (multinodular) schwannoma. A tumor simulating the plexiform neurofibroma. *Am J Surg Pathol* 1983;7:691–697.

110. Altaras M, Jaffe R, Bernheim J, Ben Aderet N. Granular cell myoblastoma of the vulva. *Gynecol Oncol* 1985;22:352–355.

111. Slavin RE, Christie JD, Swedo J, Powell LC Jr. Locally aggressive granular cell tumor causing priapism of the crus of the clitoris. A light and ultrastructural study, with observations concerning the pathogenesis of fibrosis of the corpus cavernosum in priapism. *Am J Surg Pathol* 1986;10:497–507.

112. Gaffney EF, Majmudar B, Bryan JA. Nodular fasciitis (pseudosarcomatous fasciitis) of the vulva. *Int J Gynecol Pathol* 1982;1:307–312.

113. Kfuri A, Rosenshein N, Dorfman H, Goldstein P. Desmoid tumor of the vulva. *J Reprod Med* 1981;26:272–273.

114. di Sant'Agnese PA, Knowles DM II. Extracardiac rhabdomyoma: a clinicopathologic study and review of the literature. *Cancer* 1980;46:780–789.

115. Kaufman-Friedman K. Hemangioma of clitoris, confused with adrenogenital syndrome. Case report. *Plast Reconstr Surg* 1978;62:452–454.

116. Imperial R, Helwig EB. Angiokeratoma of the vulva. *Obstet Gynecol* 1967;29:307–312.

117. Jagadha V, Srinivasan K, Panchacharam P. Glomus tumor of the clitoris. *NY State J Med* 1985;85:611.

118. Kohorn EI, Merino MJ, Goldenhersh M. Vulvar pain and dyspareunia due to glomus tumor. *Obstet Gynecol* 1986;67:41s–42s.

119. Young AW Jr, Wind RM, Tovell HMM. Lymphangioma of vulva. Acquired following treatment for cervical cancer. *NY State J Med* 1980;80:987–989.

120. La Polla J, Foucar E, Leshin B, Whitaker D, Anderson B. Vulvar lymphangioma circumscriptum: a rare complication of therapy for squamous cell carcinoma of the cervix. *Gynecol Oncol* 1985;22:363–366.

121. Garcia JJ, Verkauf BS, Hochberg CJ, Ingram JM. Aberrant breast tissue of the vulva. Case report and review of the literature. *Obstet Gynecol* 1978;52:225–228.

122. O'Hara MF, Page DL. Adenomas of the breast and ectopic breast under lactational influences. *Hum Pathol* 1985;16:707–712.

123. Foushee JHS, Pruitt AB Jr. Vulvar fibroadenoma from aberrant breast tissue. Report of two cases. *Obstet Gynecol* 1967;29:819–823.

124. Rickert RR. Intraductal papilloma arising in supernumerary vulvar breast tissue. *Obstet Gynecol* 1980;55:84s–87s.

125. Hendrix RC, Behrman SJ. Adenocarcinoma arising in a supernumerary mammary gland in the vulva. *Obstet Gynecol* 1956;8:238–241.

126. Guerry RL, Pratt-Thomas HR. Carcinoma of supernumerary breast of vulva with bilateral mammary cancer. *Cancer* 1976;38:2570–2574.

127. Reyman L, Milano A, Demopoulos R, Mayron J, Schuster S. Metastatic vulvar ulceration in Crohn's disease. *Am J Gastroenterol* 1986;81:46–49.

128. Tatnall FM, Barnes HM, Sarkany I. Sarcoidosis of the vulva. *Clin Exp Dermatol* 1985;10:384–385.

129. Arul KJ, Emmerson RW. Malacoplakia of the skin. *Clin Exp Dermatol* 1977;2:131–135.

130. Paquin ML, Davis JR, Weiner S. Malacoplakia of Bartholin's gland. *Arch Pathol Lab Med* 1986;110:757–758.

131. Northcutt AD, Vanover MJ. Nodular cutaneous amyloidosis involving the vulva. Case report and literature review. *Arch Dermatol* 1985;121:518–521.

132. St. Clair JT, Majmudar B. Tumoral calcinosis masquerading as metastatic carcinoma. *Gynecol Oncol* 1980;10:69–74.

133. Kernen JA, Morgan ML. Benign lymphoid hamartoma of the vulva. Report of a case. *Obstet Gynecol* 1970;35:290–292.

134. Marwah S, Berman ML. Ectopic salivary gland in the vulva (choristoma): report of a case and review of the literature. *Obstet Gynecol* 1980;56:389–391.

135. International Society for the Study of Vulvar Disease. New nomenclature for vulvar disease. *Obstet Gynecol* 1976;47:122–124.

136. Wilkinson EJ, Kneale B, Lynch PJ. Report of the ISSVD terminology committee. *J Reprod Med* 1986;31:973–974.

137. Wallace HJ. Lichen sclerosus et atrophicus. *Trans St Johns Hosp Dermatol Soc* 1971;57:9–30.

138. Kaufman RH, Gardner HL. Vulvar dystrophies. *Clin Obstet Gynecol* 1978;21:1081–1106.
139. Buscema J, Stern J, Woodruff JD. The significance of the histologic alterations adjacent to invasive vulvar carcinoma. *Am J Obstet Gynecol* 1980;137:902–909.
140. Hart WR, Norris HJ, Helwig EB. Relation of lichen sclerosus et atrophicus of the vulva to development of carcinoma. *Obstet Gynecol* 1975;45:369–377.
141. Friedman RJ, Kopf AW, Jones WB. Malignant melanoma in association with lichen sclerosus on the vulva of a 14-year-old. *Am J Dermatopathol* 1984;6:253–256.
142. Meyrick Thomas RH, McGibbon DH, Munro DD. Basal cell carcinoma of the vulva in association with vulval lichen sclerosus et atrophicus. *J R Soc Med* 1985;78(suppl):16–18.
143. Kaufman RH, Gardner HL, Brown D Jr, Beyth Y. Vulvar dystrophies: an evaluation. *Am J Obstet Gynecol* 1974;120:363–367.
144. Friedrich EG Jr, Burch K, Bahr JP. The vulvar clinic: an eight-year appraisal. *Am J Obstet Gynecol* 1979;135:1036–1040.
145. Buscema J, Woodruff JD, Parmley TH, Genadry R. Carcinoma *in situ* of the vulva. *Obstet Gynecol* 1980;55:255–230.
146. Crum CP, Liskow A, Petras P, Keng WC, Frick HC II. Vulvar intraepithelial neoplasia (severe atypia and carcinoma *in situ*). A clinicopathologic analysis of 41 cases. *Cancer* 1984;54:1429–1434.
147. Abell MR. Intraepithelial carcinomas of epidermis and squamous mucosa of vulva and perineum. *Surg Clin North Am* 1965;45:1179–1198.
148. Andreasson B, Bock JE. Intraepithelial neoplasia in the vulvar region. *Gynecol Oncol* 1985;21:300–305.
149. Zaino RJ, Husseinzadeh N, Nahhas W, Mortel R: Epithelial alterations in proximity to invasive squamous carcinoma of the vulva. *Int J Gynecol Pathol* 1982;1:173–184.
150. Patterson JW, Kao GF, Graham JH, Helwig EB. Bowenoid papulosis. A clinicopathologic study with ultrastructural observations. *Cancer* 1986;57:823–836.
151. Ulbright TM, Stehman FB, Roth LM, Ehrlich CE, Ransburg RC. Bowenoid dysplasia of the vulva. *Cancer* 1982;50:2910–2919.
152. Benedet JL, Turko M, Fairey RN, Boyes DA. Squamous carcinoma of the vulva: results of treatment, 1938 to 1976. *Am J Obstet Gynecol* 1979;134:201–207.
153. Bartholdson L, Eldh J, Eriksson E, Peterson LE. Surgical treatment of carcinoma of the vulva. *Surg Gynecol Obstet* 1982;155:655–661.
154. Hacker NF, Berek JS, Lagasse LD, Leuchter RS, Moore JG. Management of regional lymph nodes and their prognostic influence in vulvar cancer. *Obstet Gynecol* 1983;61:408–412.
155. Figge DC, Tamimi HK, Greer BE. Lymphatic spread in carcinoma of the vulva. *Am J Obstet Gynecol* 1985;152:387–394.
156. Gosling JRG, Abell MR, Drolette BM, Loughrin TD. Infiltrative squamous cell (epidermoid) carcinoma of vulva. *Cancer* 1961;14:330–343.
157. Choo YC. Invasive squamous carcinoma of the vulva in young patients. *Gynecol Oncol* 1982;13:158–164.
158. Kennedy AW, Hart WR. Multiple squamous-cell carcinomas in Fanconi's anemia. *Cancer* 1982;50:811–814.
159. Way S. Carcinoma of the vulva. *Am J Obstet Gynecol* 1960;79:692–697.
160. Kneale BL. Microinvasive cancer of the vulva. Report of the ISSVD Task Force. *J Reprod Med* 1984;29:454–456.
161. Broders AC. Squamous-cell epithelioma of the lip. A study of five hundred and thirty-seven cases. *JAMA* 1920;74:656–664.
162. Jakobsson PA, Eneroth CM, Killander D, Moberger G, Martensson B. Histologic classification and grading of malignancy in carcinoma of the larynx. *Acta Radiol Oncol* 1973;12:1–7.
163. Magrina JF, Webb MJ, Gaffey TA, Symmonds RE. Stage I squamous cell cancer of the vulva. *Am J Obstet Gynecol* 1979;134:453–459.
164. Andreasson B, Bock JE, Visfeldt J. Prognostic role of histology in squamous cell carcinoma in the vulvar region. *Gynecol Oncol* 1982;14:373–381.
165. Wilkinson EJ, Rico MJ, Pierson KK. Microinvasive carcinoma of the vulva. *Int J Gynecol Pathol* 1982;1:29–39.
166. Hoffman JS, Kumar NB, Morley GW. Microinvasive squamous carcinoma of the vulva: search for a definition. *Obstet Gynecol* 1983;61:615–618.
167. Husseinzadeh N, Zaino R, Nahhas WA, Mortel R. The significance of histologic findings in predicting nodal metastases in invasive squamous cell carcinoma of the vulva. *Gynecol Oncol* 1983;16:105–111.
168. Podratz KC, Symmonds RE, Taylor WF, Williams TJ. Carcinoma of the vulva: analysis of treatment and survival. *Obstet Gynecol* 1983;61:63–74.
169. Hacker NF, Berek JS, Lagasse LD, Nieberg RK, Leuchter RS. Individualization of treatment for Stage I squamous cell vulvar carcinoma. *Obstet Gynecol* 1984;63:155–162.
170. Boice CR, Seraj IM, Thrasher T, King A. Microinvasive squamous carcinoma of the vulva: present status and reassessment. *Gynecol Oncol* 1984;18:71–76.
171. Dvoretsky PM, Bonfiglio TA, Helmkamp FB, Ramsey G, Chuang C, Beecham JB. The pathology of superficially invasive, thin vulvar squamous cell carcinoma. *Int J Gynecol Pathol* 1984;3:331–342.
172. Boyce J, Fruchter RG, Kasambilides E, Nicastri AD, Sedlis A, Remy JC. Prognostic factors in carcinoma of the vulva. *Gynecol Oncol* 1985;20:364–377.
173. Shimm DS, Fuller AF, Orlow EL, Dosoretz DE, Aristizabal SA. Prognostic variables in the treatment of squamous cell carcinoma of the vulva. *Gynecol Oncol* 1986;24:343–358.
174. Franklin EW III, Rutledge FD. Prognostic factors in epidermoid carcinoma of the vulva. *Obstet Gynecol* 1971;37:892–901.
175. Crissman JD, Azoury RS. Microinvasive carcinoma of the vulva. A report of two cases with regional lymph node metastasis. *Diagn Gynecol Obstet* 1981;3:75–80.
176. Iversen T, Abeler V, Aalders J. Individualized treatment of Stage I carcinoma of the vulva. *Obstet Gynecol* 1981;57:85–89.
177. Donaldson ES, Powell DE, Hanson MB, van Nagell JR Jr. Prognostic parameters in invasive vulvar cancer. *Gynecol Oncol* 1981;11:184–190.
178. Wilkinson EJ. Superficially invasive carcinoma of the vulva. In: Wilkinson EJ, ed. *Pathology of the vulva and vagina.* New York: Churchill Livingstone, 1987:103–117.
179. Dvoretsky PM, Bonfiglio TA. The pathology of vulvar squamous cell carcinoma and verrucous carcinoma. *Pathol Annu* 1986;21:23–45.
180. Lasser A, Cornog JL, Morris JM. Adenoid squamous cell carcinoma of the vulva. *Cancer* 1974;33:224–227.
181. Underwood JW, Adcock LL, Okagaki T. Adenosquamous carcinoma of skin appendages (adenoid squamous cell carcinoma, pseudoglandular squamous cell carcinoma, adenocanthoma of sweat gland of Lever) of the vulva. A clinical and ultrastructural study. *Cancer* 1978;42:1851–1858.
182. Copas P, Dyer M, Comas FV, Hall DJ. Spindle cell carcinoma of the vulva. *Diagn Gynecol Obstet* 1982;4:235–241.
183. Steeper TA, Piscioli F, Rosai J. Squamous cell carcinoma with sarcoma-like stroma of the female genital tract. Clinicopathologic study of four cases. *Cancer* 1983;52:890–898.
184. Kraus FT, Perez-Mesa C. Verrucous carcinoma. Clinical and pathologic study of 105 cases involving oral cavity, larynx, and genitalia. *Cancer* 1966;19:26–38.
185. Japaze H, Dinh TV, Woodruff JD. Verrucous carcinoma of the vulva: Study of 24 cases. *Obstet Gynecol* 1982;60:462–466.
186. Palladino VS, Duffy JL, Bures GJ. Basal cell carcinoma of the vulva. *Cancer* 1969;24:460–470.
187. Cruz-Jimenez PR, Abell MR. Cutaneous basal cell carcinoma of vulva. *Cancer* 1975;36:1860–1868.
188. Merino MJ, LiVolsi VA, Schwartz PE, Rudnicki J. Adenoid basal cell carcinoma of the vulva. *Int J Gynecol Pathol* 1982;1:299–306.
189. Jimenez HT, Fenoglio CM, Richart RM. Vulvar basal cell carcinoma with metastasis: a case report. *Am J Obstet Gynecol* 1975;121:285–286.
190. Leuchter RS, Hacker NF, Voet RL, Berek JS, Townsend DE, Lagasse LD. Primary carcinoma of the Bartholin gland: a report of 14 cases and review of the literature. *Obstet Gynecol* 1982;60:361–368.
191. Copeland LJ, Sneige N, Gershenson DM, McGuffee VB, Abdul-

Karim F, Rutledge FN. Bartholin gland carcinoma. *Obstet Gynecol* 1986;67:794–801.

192. Abrao FS, Marques AF, Marziona F, Abrao MS, Uchoajunqueira LC, Torloni H. Adenoid cystic carcinoma of Bartholin's gland: review of the literature and report of two cases. *J Surg Oncol* 1985;30:132–137.

193. Abell MR. Adenocystic (pseudoadenomatous) basal cell carcinoma of vestibular glands of vulva. *Am J Obstet Gynecol* 1963;86:470–482.

194. Dodson MG, O'Leary JA, Orfei E. Adenoid cystic carcinoma of the vulva. Malignant cylindroma. *Obstet Gynecol* 1978;51:26s–29s.

195. Dudley AG, Young RH, Lawrence WD, Scully RE. Endodermal sinus tumor of the vulva in an infant. *Obstet Gynecol* 1983;61:76s–79s.

196. Tang CK, Toker C, Nedwich A, Zaman ANF. Unusual cutaneous carcinoma with features of small cell (oat cell-like) and squamous cell carcinomas. A variant of malignant Merkel cell neoplasm. *Am J Dermatopathol* 1982;4:537–548.

197. Bottles K, Lacey CG, Goldberg J, Lanner-Cusin K, Hom J, Miller TR. Merkel cell carcinoma of the vulva. *Obstet Gynecol* 1984;63:61s–65s.

198. Copeland LJ, Cleary K, Sneige N, Edwards CL. Neuroendocrine (Merkel cell) carcinoma of the vulva: a case report and review of the literature. *Gynecol Oncol* 1985;22:367–378.

199. Chung AF, Woodruff JM, Lewis JL Jr. Malignant melanoma of the vulva. A report of 44 cases. *Obstet Gynecol* 1975;45:638–646.

200. Johnson TL, Kumar NB, White CD, Morley GW. Prognostic features of vulvar melanoma: a clinicopathologic analysis. *Int J Gynecol Pathol* 1986;5:110–118.

201. Podratz KC, Gaffey TA, Symmonds RE, Johansen KL, O'Brien PC. Melanoma of the vulva: an update. *Gynecol Oncol* 1983;16:153–168.

202. Warner TFCS, Hafez GR, Buchler DA. Neurotropic melanoma of the vulva. *Cancer* 1982;49:999–1004.

203. DiSaia PJ, Rutledge F, Smith JP. Sarcoma of the vulva. Report of 12 patients. *Obstet Gynecol* 1971;38:180–184.

204. Davos I, Abell MR. Soft tissue sarcomas of vulva. *Gynecol Oncol* 1976;4:70–86.

205. Santala M, Suonio S, Syrjanen K, Uronen MT, Saarikoski S. Malignant fibrous histiocytoma of the vulva. *Gynecol Oncol* 1987;27:121–126.

206. Taylor RN, Bottles K, Miller TR, Braga CA. Malignant fibrous histiocytoma of the vulva. *Obstet Gynecol* 1985;66:145–148.

207. Talerman A. Sarcoma botryoides presenting as a polyp on the labium majus. *Cancer* 1973;32:994–999.

208. Copeland LJ, Sneige N, Stringer CA, Gershenson DM, Saul PB, Kavanagh JJ. Alveolar rhabdomyosarcoma of the female genitalia. *Cancer* 1985;56:849–855.

209. Ulbright TM, Brokaw SA, Stehman FB, Roth LM. Epithelioid sarcoma of the vulva. Evidence suggesting a more aggressive behavior than extra-genital epithelioid sarcoma. *Cancer* 1983;52:1462–1469.

210. Hall JS, Amin UF. Fibrosarcoma of the vulva: case reports and discussion. *Int J Surg* 1981;66:185–187.

211. Bock JE, Andreasson B, Thorn A, Holck S. Dermatofibrosarcoma protuberans of the vulva. *Gynecol Oncol* 1985;20:129–135.

212. Hall DJ, Burns JC, Goplerud DR. Kaposi's sarcoma of the vulva: a case report and brief review. *Obstet Gynecol* 1979;54:478–483.

213. Reymond RD, Hazra TA, Edlow DW, Bawab MS. Haemangiopericytoma of the vulva with metastasis to bone 14 years later. *Br J Radiol* 1972;45:765–768.

214. Zakut H, Lotan M, Lipnitzky M. Vulvar hemangiopericytoma. A case report and review of previous cases. *Acta Obstet Gynecol Scand* 1985;64:619–621.

215. Shen JT, D'ablaing G, Morrow CP. Alveolar soft part sarcoma of the vulva: report of first case and review of literature. *Gynecol Oncol* 1982;13:120–128.

216. Robertson AJ, McIntosh W, Lamont P, Guthrie W. Malignant granular cell tumor (myoblastoma) of the vulva: report of a case and review of the literature. *Histopathology* 1981;5:69–79.

217. Brooks JJ, LiVolsi VA. Liposarcoma presenting on the vulva. *Am J Obstet Gynecol* 1987;156:73–75.

218. Steeper TA, Rosai J. Aggressive angiomyxoma of the female pelvis and perineum. Report of nine cases of a distinctive type of gynecologic soft-tissue neoplasm. *Am J Obstet Gynecol* 1983;7:463–475.

219. Begin LR, Clement PB, Kirk ME, Jothy S, McCaughey WTE, Ferenczy A. Aggressive angiomyxoma of pelvic soft parts. A clinicopathologic study of nine cases. *Hum Pathol* 1985;16:621–628.

220. Plouffe L Jr, Tulandi T, Rosenberg A, Ferenczy A. Non-Hodgkin's lymphoma in Bartholin's gland: case report and review of literature. *Am J Obstet Gynecol* 1984;148:608–609.

221. Labes J, Ring A. Ulcerating cutaneous Hodgkin's disease of the vulva. *Am J Obstet Gynecol* 1964;89:272–273.

222. Doss LL. Simultaneous extramedullary plasmacytomas of the vagina and vulva. A case report and review of the literature. *Cancer* 1978;141:2468–2474.

223. Swanson S, Innes DJ Jr, Frierson HF Jr, Hess CE. T-immunoblastic lymphoma mimicking B-immunoblastic lymphoma. *Arch Pathol Lab Med* 1987;111:1077–1080.

224. Rose PG, Johnston GC, O'Toole RV. Pure cutaneous histiocytosis X of the vulva. *Obstet Gynecol* 1984;64:587–590.

225. Dehner LP. Metastatic and secondary tumors of the vulva. *Obstet Gynecol* 1973;42:47–57.

226. Jones RE Jr, Austin C, Ackerman AB. Extramammary Paget's disease. A critical reexamination. *Am J Dermatopathol* 1979;1:101–132.

227. McKee PH, Hertogs KT. Endocervical adenocarcinoma and vulval Paget's disease: a significant association. *Br J Dermatol* 1980;103:443–448.

228. Tchang F, Okagaki T, Richart RM. Adenocarcinoma of Bartholin's gland associated with Paget's disease of vulvar area. *Cancer* 1973;31:221–225.

229. Powell FC, Bjornsson J, Doyle JA, Cooper AJ. Genital Paget's disease and urinary tract malignancy. *J Am Acad Dermatol* 1985;13:84–90.

230. Hart WR, Millman JB. Progression of intraepithelial Paget's disease of the vulva to invasive carcinoma. *Cancer* 1977;40:2333–2337.

231. Creasman WT, Gallager HS, Rutledge F. Paget's disease of the vulva. *Gynecol Oncol* 1975;3:133–148.

232. Lee RA, Dahlin DC. Paget's disease of the vulva with extension into the urethra, bladder and ureters. A case report. *Am J Obstet Gynecol* 1981;140:834–836.

233. Gunn RA, Gallager HS. Vulvar Paget's disease. A topographic study. *Cancer* 1980;46:590–594.

234. Lee SC, Roth LM, Ehrlich C, Hall JA. Extramammary Paget's disease of the vulva. A clinicopathologic study of 13 cases. *Cancer* 1977;39:2540–2549.

235. Helwig EB, Graham JH. Anogenital (extramammary) Paget's disease. A clinicopathologic study. *Cancer* 1963;16:387–403.

236. Nadji M, Morales AR, Girtanner RE, Ziegels-Weissman J, Penneys NS. Paget's disease of the skin. A unifying concept of histogenesis. *Cancer* 1982;50:2203–2206.

237. Ordonez NG, Awalt H, Mackay B. Mammary and extramammary Paget's disease. An immunocytochemical and ultrastructural study. *Cancer* 1987;59:1173–1183.

238. Koss LG, Brockunier A Jr. Ultrastructural aspects of Paget's disease of the vulva. *Arch Pathol Lab Med* 1969;87:592–600.

239. Demopoulos RI. Fine structure of the extramammary Paget's cell. *Cancer* 1971;27:1202–1210.

240. Parmley TH, Woodruff JD, Julian CG. Invasive vulvar Paget's disease. *Obstet Gynecol* 1975;46:341–346.

241. Meeker JH, Neubecker RD, Helwig EB. Hidradenoma papilliferum. *Am J Clin Pathol* 1962;37:182–195.

242. Woodworth H Jr, Dockerty MB, Wilson RB, Pratt JH. Papillary hidradenoma of the vulva: a clinicopathologic study of 69 cases. *Am J Obstet Gynecol* 1971;110:501–508.

243. Hashimoto K. Hidradenoma papilliferum. An electron microscopic study. *Acta Derm Venereol (Stockh)* 1973;53:22–30.

244. Cooper PH. Carcinomas of sweat gland. *Pathol Annu* 1987;22:83–124.

245. Rorat E, Wallach RC. Mixed tumors of the vulva: clinical outcome and pathology. *Int J Gynecol Pathol* 1984;3:323–328.

246. Young AW Jr, Herman EW, Tovell HMM. Syringoma of the vulva: incidence, diagnosis, and cause of pruritis. *Obstet Gynecol* 1980;55:515–518.
247. Neilsen NC. Hidroadenoma of the vulva. *Acta Obstet Gynecol Scand* 1973;52:387–389.
248. Wick MR, Goellner JR, Wolfe JT III, Su WPD. Vulvar sweat gland carcinomas. *Arch Pathol Lab Med* 1985;109:43–47.
249. Bondi R, Di Lollo S, Pagnini P. Il carcinoma delle ghiandole apocrine. *Arch De Vecchi Anat Pathol* 1974;59:429–446.
250. Griffin JE, Edwards C, Madden JD, Harrod MJ, Wilson JD. Congenital absence of the vagina. The Mayer-Rokitansky-Kuster-Hauser syndrome. *Ann Intern Med* 1976;85:224–236.
251. Varner RE, Younger JB, Blackwell RE. Mullerian dysgenesis. *J Reprod Med* 1985;30:443–450.
252. Evans TN, Poland ML, Boving RL. Vaginal malformations. *Am J Obstet Gynecol* 1981;141:910–920.
253. Sueldo CE, Rotman CA, Cooperman NR, Rana N. Transverse vaginal septum. A report of four cases. *J Reprod Med* 1985;30:127–131.
254. Sandberg EC. Benign cervical and vaginal changes associated with exposure to stilbestrol *in utero. Am J Obstet Gynecol* 1976;125:777–789.
255. Jefferies JA, Robboy SJ, O'Brien PC, Bergstralh EJ, Labarthe DR, Barnes AB, Noller KL, Hatab PA, Kaufman RH, Townsend DE. Structural anomalies of the cervix and vagina in women enrolled in the Diethylstilbestrol Adenosis (DESAD) Project. *Am J Obstet Gynecol* 1984;148:59–66.
256. Herbst AL, Ulfelder H, Poskanzer DC. Adenocarcinoma of the vagina. Association of maternal stilbestrol therapy with tumor appearance in young women. *N Engl J Med* 1971;284:878–881.
257. Robboy SJ, Taguchi O, Cunha GR. Normal development of the human female reproductive tract and alterations resulting from experimental exposure to diethylstilbestrol. *Hum Pathol* 1982;13:190–198.
258. Sonek M, Bibbo M, Wied GL. Colposcopic findings in offspring of DES-treated mothers as related to onset of therapy. *J Reprod Med* 1976;16:65–71.
259. O'Brien PC, Noller KL, Robboy SJ, Barnes AB, Kaufman RH, Tilley BC, Townsend DE. Vaginal epithelial changes in young women enrolled in the National Cooperative Diethylstilbestrol Adenosis (DESAD) project. *Obstet Gynecol* 1979;53:300–308.
260. Antonioli DA, Burke L. Vaginal adenosis. Analysis of 325 biopsy specimens from 100 patients. *Am J Clin Pathol* 1975;64:625–638.
261. Robboy SJ, Kaufman RH, Prat J, Welch WR, Gaffey T, Scully RE, Richart R, Fenoglio CM, Virata R, Tilley BC. Pathologic findings in young women enrolled in the National Cooperative Diethylstilbestrol Adenosis (DESAD) project. *Obstet Gynecol* 1979;53:309–317.
262. Robboy SJ, Hill EC, Sandberg EC, Czernobilsky B. Vaginal adenosis in women born prior to the diethylstilbestrol era. *Hum Pathol* 1986;17:488–492.
263. Hart WR, Townsend DE, Aldrich JO, Henderson BE, Roy M, Benton B. Histopathologic spectrum of vaginal adenosis and related changes in stilbestrol-exposed females. *Cancer* 1976;37:763–775.
264. Burke L, Antonioli D, Friedman EA. Evolution of diethylstilbestrol-associated genital tract lesions. *Obstet Gynecol* 1981;57:79–84.
265. Robboy SJ, Noller KL, O'Brien P, Kaufman RH, Townsend D, Barnes AB, Gundersen J, Lawrence WD, Bergstrahl E, McGorray S, Tilley BC, Anton J, Chazen G. Increased incidence of cervical and vaginal dysplasia in 3,980 diethylstilbestrol-exposed young women. Experience of the National Collaborative Diethylstilbestrol Adenosis Project. *JAMA* 1984;252:2979–2983.
266. Kurman RJ, Scully RE. The incidence and histogenesis of vaginal adenosis. An autopsy study. *Hum Pathol* 1974;5:265–276.
267. Robboy SJ, Welch WR. Microglandular hyperplasia in vaginal adenosis associated with oral contraceptives and prenatal diethylstilbestrol exposure. *Obstet Gynecol* 1977;49:430–434.
268. Robboy SJ, Young RH, Welch WR, Truslow GY, Prat J, Herbst AL, Scully RE. Atypical vaginal adenosis and cervical ectropion. Association with clear cell adenocarcinoma in diethylstilbestrol-exposed offspring. *Cancer* 1984;54:869–875.
269. Brown D Jr, Kaufman RH, Gardner HL. *Gardnerella vaginalis* vaginitis: The current opinion. *J Reprod Med* 1984;29:300–306.
270. Spiegel CA, Amsel R, Eschenbach D, Schoenknecht F, Holmes KK. Anaerobic bacteria in nonspecific vaginitis. *N Engl J Med* 1980;303:601–607.
271. Bergdoll MS, Schlievert PM. Toxic shock syndrome toxin. *Lancet* 1984;2:691.
272. Todd JK, Todd BH, Franco-Buff A, Smith CM, Lawellin DW. Influence of focal growth conditions on the pathogenesis of toxic shock syndrome. *J Infect Dis* 1987;155:673–681.
273. Larkin SM, Williams DN, Osterholm MT, Tofte RW, Posalaky Z. Toxic shock syndrome: clinical, laboratory, and pathologic findings in nine fatal cases. *Ann Intern Med* 1982;96:858–864.
274. Strate SM, Taylor WE, Forney JP, Silver FG. Xanthogranulomatous pseudotumor of the vagina: evidence of a local response to an unusual bacterium (mucoid *Escherichia coli*). *Am J Clin Pathol* 1983;79:637–643.
275. Chalvardjian A, Picard L, Shaw R, Davey R, Cairns JD. Malacoplakia of the female genital tract. *Am J Obstet Gynecol* 1980;138:391–394.
276. Okagaki T, Twiggs LB, Zachow KR, Clark BA, Ostrow RS, Faras AJ. Identification of human papillomavirus DNA in cervical and vaginal intraepithelial neoplasia with molecularly cloned type (group) specific DNA probes. *Int J Gynecol Pathol* 1983;2:153–159.
277. Okagaki T, Clark BA, Zachow KR, Twiggs LB, Ostrow RS, Pass F, Faras AJ. Presence of human papillomavirus in verrucous carcinoma (Ackerman) of the vagina. Immunocytochemical, ultrastructural, and DNA hybridization studies. *Arch Pathol Lab Med* 1984;108:567–570.
278. Shafer MA, Sweet RL, Ohm-Smith MJ, Shalwitz J, Beck A, Schachter J. Microbiology of the lower genital tract in postmenarchal adolescent girls: differences by sexual activity, contraception, and presence of nonspecific vaginitis. *J Pediatr* 1985;107:974–981.
279. Friedrich EG Jr. Vaginitis. *Am J Obstet Gynecol* 1985;152:247–251.
280. Gardner HL. Trichomoniasis. In Gardner HL, Kaufman RH, eds. *Benign diseases of the vulva and vagina.* 2nd edition. Boston: GK Hall, 1981:243–272.
281. Munguia H, Franco E, Valenzuela P. Diagnosis of genital amebiasis in women by the standard Papanicolaou technique. *Am J Obstet Gynecol* 1966;94:181–188.
282. Gardner HL. Desquamative inflammatory vaginitis: a newly defined entity. *Am J Obstet Gynecol* 1968;102:1102–1105.
283. Gardner HL, Fernet P. Etiology of vaginitis emphysematosa. Report of ten cases and review of literature. *Am J Obstet Gynecol* 1964;88:680–694.
284. Friedrich EG Jr, Siegesmund KA. Tampon-associated vaginal ulcerations. *Obstet Gynecol* 1980;55:149–156.
285. Danielson RW. Vaginal ulcers caused by tampons. *Am J Obstet Gynecol* 1983;146:547–549.
286. Givel JC, Hawker P, Allan RN, Alexander-Williams J. Enterovaginal fistulas associated with Crohn's disease. *Surg Gynecol Obstet* 1982;155:494–496.
287. Deppisch LM. Cysts of the vagina. Classification and clinical correlations. *Obstet Gynecol* 1975;45:632–637.
288. Pradhan S, Tobon H. Vaginal cysts: a clinicopathologic study of 41 cases. *Int J Gynecol Pathol* 1986;5:35–46.
289. Kjaeldgaard A, Fianu S. Classification and embryological aspects of ectopic ureters communicating with Gartner's cysts. *Diagn Gynecol Obstet* 1982;4:269–273.
290. Gardner HL. Cervical and vaginal endometrioisis. *Clin Obstet Gynecol* 1066;9:358–372.
291. Kurman RJ, Prabha AC. Thyroid and parathyroid glands in the vaginal wall: Report of a case. *Am J Clin Pathol* 1973;59:503–507.
292. Mathie JG. Vaginal deciduosis simulating carcinoma. *J Obstet Gynecol Br Emp* 1957;34:720–721.
293. Haines M. Hydatidiform mole and vaginal nodules. *J Obstet Gynecol Br Emp* 1955;62:6–11.
294. Elston CW. The histopathology of trophoblastic tumours. *J Clin Pathol* [Suppl] 1971;10:111–131.

295. Duckman S, Suarez J, Spitaleri J. Vaginal pregnancy presenting as a suburethral cyst. *Am J Obstet Gynecol* 1984;149:572–573.

296. Wood P. Persistence of vaginal vault granulation. *Lancet* 1986;2:918.

297. Silverberg SG, Frable WJ. Prolapse of fallopian tube into vaginal vault after hysterectomy. Histopathology, cytopathology, and differential diagnosis. *Arch Pathol Lab Med* 1974;97:100–103.

298. Wheelock JB, Schneider V, Goplerud DR. Prolapsed fallopian tube masquerading as adenocarcinoma of the vagina in a postmenopausal woman. *Gynecol Oncol* 1985;21:369–375.

299. Norris HJ, Taylor HB. Melanomas of the vagina. *Am J Clin Pathol* 1966;46:420–426.

300. Bottles K, Lacey CG, Miller TR. Atypical melanocytic hyperplasia of the vagina. *Gynecol Oncol* 1984;19:226–230.

301. Tobon H, Murphy AI. Benign blue nevus of the vagina. *Cancer* 1977;40:3174–3176.

302. Rodriguez HA, Ackerman LV. Cellular blue nevus. Clinicopathologic study of forty-five cases. *Cancer* 1968;21:393–405.

303. Nigogosyan G, de la Pava S, Pickren JW. Melanoblasts in vaginal mucosa. Origin for primary malignant melanoma. *Cancer* 1964;17:912–913.

304. Norris HJ, Taylor HB. Polyps of the vagina. A benign lesion resembling sarcoma botryoides. *Cancer* 1966;19:227–232.

305. Chirayil SJ, Tobon H. Polyps of the vagina: a clinicopathologic study of 18 cases. *Cancer* 1981;47:2904–2907.

306. Elliott GB, Elliott JDA. Superficial stromal reactions of lower genital tract. *Arch Pathol Lab Med* 1973;95:100–101.

307. Novak E, Woodruff JD, Novak ER. Probable mesonephric origin of certain female genital tumors. *Am J Obstet Gynecol* 1954;68:1222–1242.

308. Janovski NA, Kasdon EJ. Benign mesonephric papillary and polypoid tumors of the cervix in childhood. *J Pediatr* 1963;63:211–216.

309. Norris HJ, Bagley GP, Taylor HB. Carcinoma of the infant vagina. A distinctive tumor. *Arch Pathol Lab Med* 1970;90:473–479.

310. Sirota RL, Dickersin GR, Scully RE. Mixed tumors of the vagina. A clinicopathological analysis of eight cases. *Am J Surg Pathol* 1981;5:413–422.

311. Ulbright TM, Alexander RW, Kraus FT. Intramural papilloma of the vagina: evidence of mullerian histogenesis. *Cancer* 1981;48:2260–2266.

312. Chen KTK. Brenner tumor of the vagina. *Diagn Gynecol Obstet* 1981;3:255–258.

313. Spitzer M, Molho L, Seltzer VL, Lipper S. Vaginal glomus tumor: case presentation and ultrastructural findings. *Obstet Gynecol* 1985;66:86s–88s.

314. Pezeshkpour G. Solitary paraganglioma of the vagina—report of a case. *Am J Obstet Gynecol* 1981;139:219–221.

315. Tavassoli FA, Norris HJ. Smooth muscle tumors of the vagina. *Obstet Gynecol* 1979;53:689–693.

316. Gold JH, Bossen EH. Benign vaginal rhabdomyoma. A light and electron microscopic study. *Cancer* 1976;37:2283–2294.

317. Autio-Harmainen H, Apaja-Sarkkinen M, Martikainen J, Taipale A, Rapola J. Production of basement membrane laminin and type IV collagen by tumors of striated muscle: an immunohistochemical study of rhabdomyosarcomas of different histologic types and a benign vaginal rhabdomyoma. *Hum Pathol* 1986;17:1218–1224.

318. Allen PW. Nodular fasciitis. *Pathology* 1972;4:9–26.

319. Hertig AT, Gore H. Tumors of the female sex organs. *Atlas of tumor pathology,* part 2, section IX, fascicle 33. Washington, DC: Armed Forces Institute of Pathology, 1960:66–67.

320. Gold BM. Neurofibromatosis of the bladder and vagina. *Am J Obstet Gynecol* 1972;113:1055–1056.

321. Azzopardi JG, Eusebi V, Tison V, Betts CM. Neurofibroma with rhabdomyomatous differentiation: benign "Triton" tumor of the vagina. *Histopathology* 1983;7:561–572.

322. Proppe KH, Scully RE, Rosai J. Postoperative spindle cell nodules of genitourinary tract resembling sarcomas. A report of eight cases. *Am J Surg Pathol* 1984;8:101–108.

323. Snover DC, Phillips G, Dehner LP. Reactive fibrohistiocytic proliferation simulating fibrous histiocytoma. *Am J Clin Pathol* 1981;76:232–235.

324. Benedet JL, Sanders BH. Carcinoma *in situ* of the vagina. *Am J Obstet Gynecol* 1984;148:695–700.

325. Peters WA III, Kumar NB, Morley W. Carcinoma of the vagina. Factors influencing treatment outcome. *Cancer* 1985;55:892–897.

326. Lenehan PM, Meffe F, Lickrish GM. Vaginal intraepithelial neoplasia: biologic aspects and management. *Obstet Gynecol* 1986;68:333–337.

327. Petrilli ES, Townsend DE, Morrow CP, Nakao CY. Vaginal intraepithelial neoplasia: biologic aspects and treatment with topical 5-fluorouracil and the carbon dioxide laser. *Am J Obstet Gynecol* 1980;138:321–328.

328. Perez CA, Arneson AN, Dehner LP, Galakatos A. Radiation therapy in carcinoma of the vagina. *Obstet Gynecol* 1974;44:862–872.

329. Benedet JL, Murphy KJ, Fairey RN, Boyes DA. Primary invasive carcinoma of the vagina. *Obstet Gynecol* 1983;62:715–719.

330. Rubin SC, Young J, Mikuta JJ. Squamous carcinoma of the vagina: treatment, complications, and long-term follow-up. *Gynecol Oncol* 1985;20:346–353.

331. Beck I, Clayton JK. Vaginal carcinoma arising in vaginal condylomata. Case report. *Br J Obstet Gynaecol* 1984;91:503–505.

332. Hopkins MP, Morley GW. Squamous cell carcinoma of the neovagina. *Obstet Gynecol* 1987;69:525–527.

333. General Assembly of FIGO. Classification and staging of malignant tumours in the female pelvis. *Acta Obstet Gynecol Scand* 1971;50:1–7.

334. Peters WA III, Kumar NB, Morley GW. Microinvasive carcinoma of the vagina: a distinct clinical entity? *Am J Obstet Gynecol* 1985;153:505–507.

335. Ramzy I, Smout MS, Collins JA. Verrucous carcinoma of the vagina. *Am J Clin Pathol* 1976;65:644–653.

336. Melnick S, Cole P, Anderson D, Herbst A. Rates and risks of diethylstilbestrol-related clear-cell adenocarcinoma of the vagina and cervix. An update. *N Engl J Med* 1987;316:514–516.

337. Senekjian EK, Hubby M, Bell DA, Anderson D, Herbst AL. Clear cell adenocarcinoma (CCA) of the vagina and cervix in association with pregnancy. *Gynecol Oncol* 1986;24:207–219.

338. Robboy SJ, Scully RE, Welch WR, Herbst AL. Intrauterine diethylstilbestrol exposure and its consequences. Pathologic characteristics of vaginal adenosis, clear cell adenocarcinoma, and related lesions. *Arch Pathol Lab Med* 1977;101:1–5.

339. Dickersin GR, Welch WR, Erlandson R, Robboy SJ. Ultrastructure of 16 cases of clear cell adenocarcinoma of the vagina and cervix in young women. *Cancer* 1980;45:1615–1624.

340. Senekjian EK, Frey KW, Anderson D, Herbst, AL. Local therapy in Stage I clear cell adenocarcinoma of the vagina. *Cancer* 1987;60:1319–1324.

341. Ray J, Ireland K. Non-clear-cell adenocarcinoma arising in vaginal adenosis. *Arch Pathol Lab Med* 1985;109:781–783.

342. Hinchey WW, Silva EG, Guarda LA, Ordonez NG, Wharton JT. Paravaginal Wolffian duct (mesonephros) adenocarcinoma: a light and electron microscopic study. *Am J Clin Pathol* 1983;80:539–544.

343. Fukushima M, Twiggs LB, Okagaki T. Mixed intestinal adenocarcinoma-argentaffin carcinoma of the vagina. *Gynecol Oncol* 1986;23:387–394.

344. Okagaki T, Ishida T, Hilgers RD. A malignant tumor of the vagina resembling synovial sarcoma. A light and electron microscopic study. *Cancer* 1976;37:2306–2320.

345. Shevchuk MM, Fenoglio CM, Lattes R, Frick HC II, Richart RM. Malignant mixed tumor of the vagina probably arising in mesonephric rests. *Cancer* 1978;42:214–223.

346. Brooks JJ, Wheeler JE. Malignancy arising in extragonadal endometriosis. A case report and summary of the world literature. *Cancer* 1977;40:3065–3073.

347. Goldberg MI, Ng ABP, Belinson JL, Hutson ED, Nordqvist SRB. Clear cell adenocarcinoma arising in endometriosis of the rectovaginal septum. *Obstet Gynecol* 1978;51:38s–40s.

348. Kapp DS, Merino M, LiVolsi V. Adenocarcinoma of the vagina arising in endometriosis: long-term survival following radiation therapy. *Gynecol Oncol* 1982;14:271–278.

349. Berkowitz RS, Ehrmann RL, Knapp RC. Endometrial stromal

sarcoma arising from vaginal endometriosis. *Obstet Gynecol* 1978;51:34s–37s.

350. Copeland LJ, Sneige N, Ordonez NG, Hancock KC, Gershenson DM, Saul PB, Kavanagh JJ. Endodermal sinus tumor of the vagina and cervix. *Cancer* 1985;55:2558–2565.

351. Young RH, Scully RE. Endodermal sinus tumor of the vagina: a report of nine cases and review of the literature. *Gynecol Oncol* 1984;18:380–392.

352. Andersen WA, Sabio H, Durso N, Mills SE, Levien M, Underwood PB Jr. Endodermal sinus tumor of the vagina. The role of primary chemotherapy. *Cancer* 1985;56:1025–1027.

353. Chung AF, Casey MJ, Flannery JT, Woodruff JM, Lewis JL Jr. Malignant melanoma of the vagina. Report of 19 cases. *Obstet Gynecol* 1980;55:720–727.

354. Lee RB, Buttoni L Jr, Dhru K, Tamimi H. Malignant melanoma of the vagina: a case report of progression from preexisting melanosis. *Gynecol Oncol* 1984;19:238–245.

355. Socinski MA, Ershler WB, Belinson JL. Coexistent breast and vaginal granulocytic sarcoma. *Gynecol Oncol* 1983;16:299–304.

356. Osanto S, Valk P, Meijer CJLM, van Amstel WJ, Willemze R. Solitary plasmocytoma of the vagina. *Acta Haematol* 1981;66:140–144.

357. Chorlton I, Karnei RF Jr, King FM, Norris HJ. Primary malignant reticuloendothelial disease involving the vagina, cervix, and corpus uteri. *Obstet Gynecol* 1974;44:735–748.

358. Harris NL, Scully RE. Malignant lymphoma and granulocytic sarcoma of the uterus and vagina. A clinicopathologic analysis of 27 cases. *Cancer* 1984;53:2530–2545.

359. Dupree EL Jr, Lee RA. Histiocytosis X in the female genital tract. *Obstet Gynecol* 1973;42:201–204.

360. Hays DM, Shimada H, Raney RB Jr, Tefft M, Newton W, Crist WM, Lawrence W Jr, Ragab A, Maurer HM. Sarcomas of the vagina and uterus: the intergroup Rhabdomyosarcoma Study. *J Pediatr Surg* 1985;20:718–724.

361. Malkasian GD Jr, Welch JS, Soule EH. Primary leiomyosarcoma of the vagina. Report of 8 cases. *Am J Obstet Gynecol* 1963;86:730–736.

362. Davos I, Abell MR. Sarcomas of the vagina. *Obstet Gynecol* 1976;47:342–350.

363. Peters WA III, Kumar NB, Andersen WA, Morley GW. Primary sarcoma of the adult vagina: a clinicopathologic study. *Obstet Gynecol* 1985;65:699–704.

364. Webb MJ, Symmonds RE, Weiland LH. Malignant fibrous histiocytoma of the vagina. *Am J Obstet Gynecol* 1974;119:190–192.

365. Hiura M, Nogawa T, Nagai N, Yorishima M, Fujiwara A. Vaginal hemangiopericytoma: a light microscopic and ultrastructural study. *Gynecol Oncol* 1985;21:376–384.

366. Buscema J, Rosenshein NB, Taqi F, Woodruff JD. Vaginal hemangiopericytoma: a histopathologic and ultrastructural evaluation. *Obstet Gynecol* 1985;66:82s–85s.

367. Ulbright TM, Kraus FT. Endometrial stromal tumors of extrauterine tissue. *Am J Clin Pathol* 1981;76:371–377.

368. Zaleski S, Setum C, Benda J. Cytologic presentation of alveolar softpart sarcoma of the vagina. A case report. *Acta Cytol* 1986;30:665–670.

369. O'Toole RV, Tuttle SE, Lucas JG, Sharma HM. Alveolar soft part sarcoma of the vagina: an immunohistochemical and electron microscopic study. *Int J Gynecol Pathol* 1985;4:258–265.

370. Phillips GL, Prem KA, Adcock LL, Twiggs LB. Vaginal recurrence of adenocarcinoma of the endometrium. *Gynecol Oncol* 1982;13:323–328.

371. Bergman F. Carcinoma of the ovary: a clinicopathological study of 86 autopsied cases with special reference to mode of spread. *Acta Obstet Gynecol Scand* 1966;45:211–231.

372. O'Reilly AP, McLeod F, Craft I. Hypernephroma presenting as a vaginal metastasis. Case report. *Br J Obstet Gynaecol* 1984;91:812–815.

373. Jacobs AJ, Deppe G, Kessinger MA, Newland JR. Case report. Breast carcinoma metastatic to the vagina. *Acta Obstet Gynecol Scand* 1983;62:83–85.

374. Xiu-yu Y, Hong-zhao S, Yuan-e W, Min-yi T, Yan-ning Z. Vaginal metastasis of choriocarcinoma and invasive mole. Clinical and pathological characteristics, diagnosis and treatment. *Chin Med J* 1985;98:463–470.

375. Goldberg GL, Yon DA, Block B, Levin W. Gestational trophoblastic disease: the significance of vaginal metastases. *Gynecol Oncol* 1986;24:155–161.

Surgical Pathology of the Female Reproductive System and Peritoneum, edited by Stephen S. Sternberg and Stacey E. Mills. Raven Press, Ltd, New York © 1991.

CHAPTER 4

The Cervix

Christopher P. Crum and Gerard Nuovo

RELEVANT ANATOMY

The uterus and endocervix are formed by the fusion of the müllerian ducts, which distally meet with the vaginal epithelium to form the ectocervix (1). At the external os the ectocervix joins the endocervical canal, which, in turn, joins the isthmus or internal os. The original squamocolumnar (SC) junction exists in the region of the external os, where the squamous epithelium of the ectocervical portio joins the mucus-secreting columnar epithelium of the endocervix. During the reproductive years the original SC junction is located out on the ectocervix as a result of the process of "eversion." Eversion, or protrusion of the cervical lips, occurs as a consequence of hormonal factors that influence the conformation of the cervix during fetal life, puberty, and, particularly, pregnancy. Eversion of the anterior cervix is more pronounced and occurs twice as often as on the posterior lip (2). The endocervix is composed of stromal papillae lined with mucinous epithelium. The recesses between the papillae (crypts) are termed "glands," although they are not true glands.

An important anatomical change occurring during the reproductive years is the replacement, or transformation, of the endocervical columnar epithelium by squamous epithelium. This process occurs in the region of the original SC junction, delineating a circumferential zone around the external os, termed the "transformation zone" or "T-zone" (Fig. 1A). It occurs principally on the anterior and posterior cervical lips, in parallel with the site of most prominent cervical eversion. This transformation of columnar epithelium occurs either by ingrowth of portio epithelium into the region of columnar epithelium or replacement of the columnar cells from beneath by reserve cells that have undergone squamous differentiation (metaplasia) (Fig. 1B). The latter is a function of the dual potential of these reserve cells to differentiate into either squamous or glandular components. The squamous epithelium gradually replaces the endocervical columnar cells, bridging the endocervical papillae and producing a smooth surface with loss of the grape-like papillae. Moreover, this bridging phenomenon covers the necks of the endocervical crypts, producing distension of the crypt ("gland") proximally to form a nabothian cyst. The process of transformation begins with menarche and is considered a consequence of the acidic vaginal pH that is produced by the action of bacteria on the glycogenated squamous cells. Chronic inflammation and repair, produced by infectious or other stimuli, also contribute to squamous metaplasia and the development of the T-zone. The gradual reduction of cervical eversion, combined with the advancement of the T-zone, eventually places the squamocolumnar junction deep within the endocervical canal by menopause (3).

The T-zone is the principal site of origin for precancers and invasive squamous-cell carcinomas of the cervix. Predictably, these neoplasms occur most commonly on the anterior and posterior cervical lips (3).

PAPILLOMAVIRUS-RELATED CERVICAL INTRAEPITHELIAL NEOPLASIA

Background

Cervical cancer is closely linked to sexual behavior and the development of a noninvasive precursor lesion in the T-zone. The sexual factors that correlate strongest with cervical cancer are the number of sexual partners and, to a lesser extent, the age of first intercourse (4). An increasing number of sexual partners presumably increases the risk of acquiring an oncogenic factor. Patients who initiate intercourse at an early age also have a greater risk, possibly because the transformation zone is most susceptible at that time (4). Cervical cancer is also associated with a noninvasive intraepithelial precursor (termed "dysplasia-carcinoma *in situ*" or "cervical in-

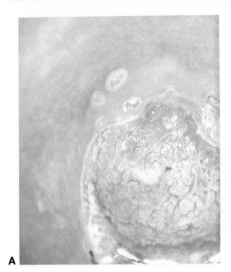

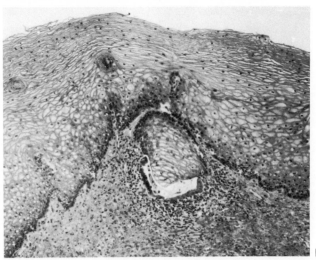

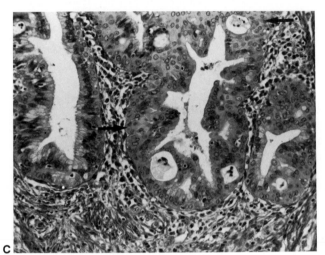

FIG. 1. The cervical transformation zone. **A:** A colpophotograph of the cervix illustrates the external os (*bottom right*) with the native portio squamous epithelium at the left and upper portion of the picture. A cervical eversion (erosion) is present centrally, exposing the grape-like papillae of the endocervix. The transformation zone is visible at the 12 o'clock position as a poorly defined, thin white epithelium just above the present squamocolumnar junction. The circular defects in this area are gland (crypt) openings surrounded by squamous epithelium, identifying where gland epithelium has become replaced by squamous mucosa. **B:** Mature transformation-zone squamous epithelium. The crypt opening has become occluded, and the gland neck has become partly replaced by mature squamous epithelium. **C:** Immature transformation-zone epithelium. Glandular epithelium is being replaced by immature squamous metaplasia (*arrows*).

traepithelial neoplasia"). The mean age of patients with intraepithelial abnormalities precedes that of cancer by over 20 years, and a proportion of patients with these abnormalities will develop cancer if not treated (3).

One of the first clues that papillomaviruses were associated with cancer and cancer precursors came in the 1950s. Koss and Durfee reported a cytologic abnormality termed "koilocytotic atypia," which consisted of a cytoplasmic halo and an abnormal nucleus in the superficial cells of some cervical dysplasias (5). However, at that time the viral origin of koilocytotic atypia was not recognized.

Interest in a viral oncogen increased in view of the epidemiologic data and the development of technology for analyzing the presence of viral DNA at the molecular level. Frenkel's discovery of herpesvirus nucleic acids in a squamous-cell carcinoma spurred interest in herpesviruses (6). However, in the 1970s Purola and Savia, as well as Meisels and Fortin, formalized the link between koilocytotic atypia and cervical papillomavirus infection and identified it as a highly prevalent infection (7,8). Meisels reported that as many as 2.5% of randomly screened yearly Papanicolaou smears from young women contained evidence of HPV infection (koilocytotic atypia), and retrospective studies have established that, from 1965 to 1978, the reported incidence of genital warts in men and women increased over 400% (9,10).

Koilocytotic atypia was also associated with higher-grade precancers and invasive carcinomas, prompting efforts to identify HPV in genital neoplasms as well as condylomata (10,11). Ultrastructural and immunhisto-chemical studies localized HPV capsid antigens or virions within some koilocytes, but these techniques yielded relatively little information about the relationship between HPV and genital neoplasia (12,13). The cloning of the first genital HPV DNA in 1980 initiated a second series of studies which established that most condylomata, squamous precancers, and carcinomas contained HPV DNA (14). Moreover, distinct types of HPV have been identified which are associated with specific clinical and pathologic characteristics (15).

Clinically, cervical precancers are now viewed from a different perspective because they have their genesis in a sexually transmitted HPV infection. First, the association between HPV and genital neoplasia points to the need for effective screening and removal of potential precancers (16). A second issue is latent or occult infection and its relevance to both diagnosis and therapy (17,18). A related issue is the importance of histologic criteria that will distinguish HPV infections from nonspecific abnormalities having no association with either HPV infection or neoplasia (19).

The process of identifying a cervical precancer involves two steps. The first is recognizing the abnormality and distinguishing it from nonspecific changes, and the second is selecting appropriate terminology for the clinician. For reasons that will be discussed below, the term "precursor" or "precancer" will be applied to both flat condyloma and CIN. Although most benign condyloma of the external genitalia can be distinguished from precancers, in the cervix this distinction may be difficult (20–22). Thus for practical reasons, it is presumed that any recognizable HPV-related lesion, either flat condyloma or CIN, must be removed. Identification of the lesion is facilitated by colposcopy; following this, sampling of the lesion and the endocervical canal is performed to exclude cancer (Fig. 2).

Before defining precursor lesions, it is useful to review five concepts that bear upon our understanding of these diseases:

1. *Precancers encompass several biologic and histologic entities.* The traditional approach to classifying

cancer precursors employs the dysplasia/carcinoma-*in-situ* classification, by which precursor lesions are classified based upon their maturational characteristics. Low-grade precancers (mild dysplasia or CIN grade I) are composed of mature epithelium in which cellular atypia is predominately superficial, frequently including koilocytotic atypia (Fig. 3A). In contrast, higher-grade precancers demonstrate less maturation, a higher nuclear-to-cytoplasmic ratio in all layers of the epithelium, and nuclear atypia in all layers of the epithelium as well (23–25) (Fig. 3B and C). The latter translates as anisonucleosis, polychromasia, loss of polarity, and a high mitotic index. The ultrastructural correlates of this histologic picture are the loss of cellular differentiation, including (a) a reduction or loss of glycogen, desmosomes, and tonofilaments and (b) an increase in the number of microvilli in the constituent cells (26). Investigators emphasized an aggressive approach to high-grade precancers because these lesions rarely regress and often progress to cancer if not treated (27,28). However, numerous follow-up studies (an excellent review of which can be found in a study by Nasielle et al.) have established that up to one-third of mild or moderate dysplasias may also progress to higher grades if not treated (29). Studies in which precancers were not altered by biopsy, and which required repeated abnormal smears for entry prior to follow-up reported high rates of progression (29,30).

Evidence that lesions which regress can be distinguished from those which persist or progress was supported by DNA microspectrophotometric studies which divided lesions into different categories based upon nuclear DNA content (23,31). In a retrospectively analyzed series of women who were treated with biopsy alone for cervical intraepithelial abnormalities, Fu et al. found that 85% of lesions which regressed were diploid or

TABLE 1. *Selection of criteria for cervical diagnosis*

Findings	Diagnosis	Management
Negative; no transformation zone seen	Descriptive	Repeat if indicated
Acanthosis; parakeratosis; nonspecific halos; atrophy	Descriptive	Follow
Severe inflammation; reparative atypia	Descriptive	Culture; follow
Koilocytosis; maturation; minimal basal atypia	CIN I (with koilocytosis)	Remove
Koilocytosis; maturation; diffuse atypia	CIN II (with koilocytosis)	Remove
Minimal koilocytosis or maturation; diffuse atypia	CIN III	Remove
Neoplastic epithelium in the ECC[a]	Strips of neoplastic squamous epithelium	Cone biopsy
Condyloma in the ECC	Strips of neoplastic squamous epithelium	Cone biopsy
Very scant condyloma or neoplastic epithelium in the ECC	Descriptive (determine if canal is involved clinically)	Repeat or cone

[a] ECC, endocervical curretage.

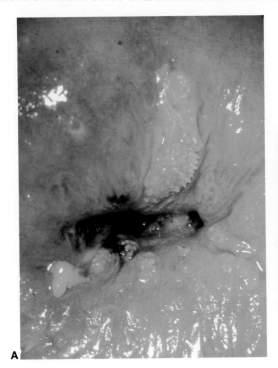
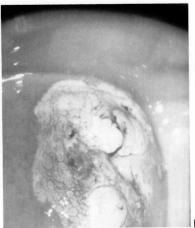

FIG. 2. Colposcopy of papillomavirus-related cervical precancers. **A:** This lesion contains thick white epithelium as well as small, evenly spaced papilla (asperites). **B:** This lesion consists of a mixture of flat, nodular, and papillomatous epithelium.

polyploid, in contrast to 90% of lesions persisting, which were aneuploid. All lesions which progressed to cancer were aneuploid in retrospect (23). Noteworthy in this study was the observation that the biologic behavior of a lesion correlated closely with its DNA content, which, in turn, correlated with the presence of abnormal mitotic figures and increasing severity of cytologic atypia (23). In retrospect, a portion of the subset of diploid/polypoid lesions which regressed consisted of typical flat condylomata (Fig. 3A) (23). Interestingly, some precursors contain features of both flat condylomata and aneuploid precancers. Because of this, some authors suggest that the pathway to cancer may involve the development of atypical flat condylomata which have a higher risk of evolving into high-grade precancers (carcinomas *in situ*) or invasive cancer than conventional condylomata (Fig. 3A and B) (23,32–34).

2. *Specific papillomaviruses predominate in certain types of cervical lesions.* With molecular hybridization technology, certain HPV types, including 6 and 11, have been recovered primarily from benign genital warts, principally those on the external genitalia (Fig. 3A) (35). In contrast, HPV 16 is the most commonly detected HPV type in invasive cancers (36), in addition to types 18, 31, 33, 35, and others (15). Moreover, HPV-16 DNA sequences have been found in approximately 70% of cervical lesions containing the morphologic features of aneuploidy (Fig. 3B and C) (25,37,38). The potential significance of HPV 16 was illustrated by a small fol-

low-up study by Campion et al., who found that 85% of mild atypias progressing to high-grade CIN contain HPV 16 (39). However, the association of HPV 16 with progression and cancer is not 100%. HPV 16 has been isolated from up to 8% of flat condylomata, and some cancers have been found to contain HPV-6 DNA (36–38,40). Moreover, Campion et al. found that a proportion of lesions progressing to CIN III contain HPV-6-related DNA sequences (39).

3. *HPV infection is a morphologic spectrum.* Several factors appear to contribute to the variable morphologies that characterize cervical precancers. They include: (a) the topography and maturational characteristics of the involved epithelium and (b) the underlying biologic process, which is related frequently to the HPV type present. First, portio lesions tend to be well differentiated, whereas lesions in metaplastic epithelium tend to be immature (41). Second, there is a spectrum of *morphologic atypia,* which is frequently greater in aneuploid lesions containing HPV 16 (21,23,38). Low-grade cervical lesions, including flat condylomata, may vary in degree of maturation but display relatively little variation in nuclear size, shape, and staining intensity within the lower epithelial layers (Fig. 4). In contrast, higher-grade precancers vary both in maturation and the severity of nuclear atypia, the latter often present in all layers of the epithelium (Fig. 5). This degree of morphologic heterogeneity in some precancers illustrates the difficulty of attempting to predict the biologic behavior of a given

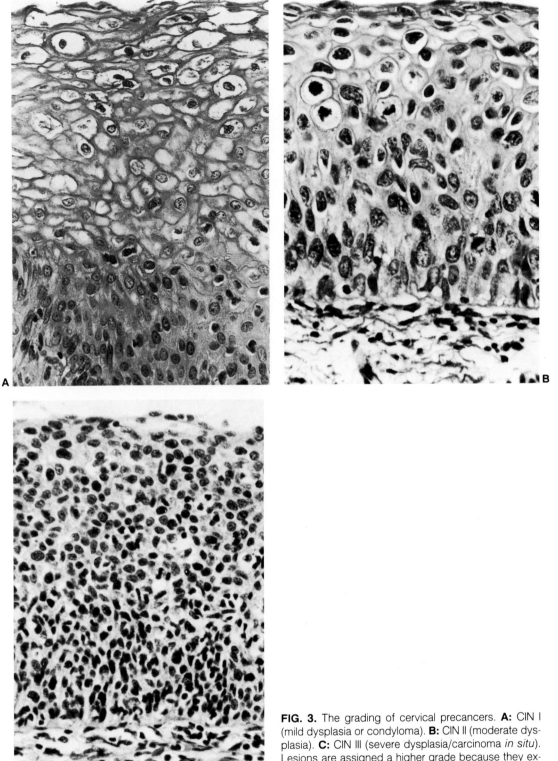

FIG. 3. The grading of cervical precancers. **A:** CIN I (mild dysplasia or condyloma). **B:** CIN II (moderate dysplasia). **C:** CIN III (severe dysplasia/carcinoma *in situ*). Lesions are assigned a higher grade because they exhibit less maturation and nuclear atypia in all layers of the epithelium.

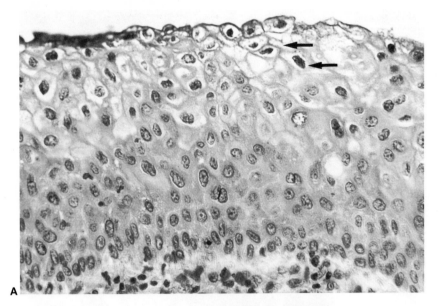

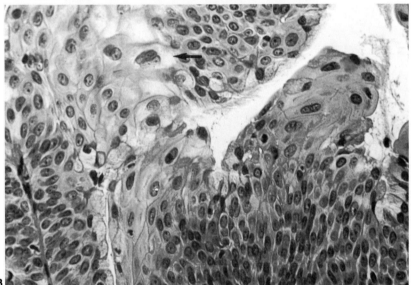

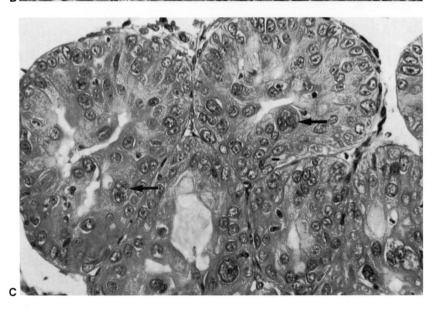

FIG. 4. The spectrum of flat condyloma (CIN I or mild dysplasia). **A:** This flat condyloma exhibits focal koilocytotic atypia (*arrows*). Note the minimal nuclear atypia in the parabasal cells. **B:** This flat condyloma occurring in metaplastic epithelium consists primarily of a proliferation of mildly atypical cells with focal koilocytotic atypia (*arrow*). **C:** Atypical immature metaplastic epithelium in glands. There is focal nuclear atypia in the most mature layers (*arrows*). Note the absence of mitoses. **D:** Condyloma (inverted) involving gland epithelium. As in the previous photographs, the epithelium is immature, demonstrates minimal nuclear crowding or atypia in the basal layers, and exhibits variable koilocytotic atypia (*arrow*).

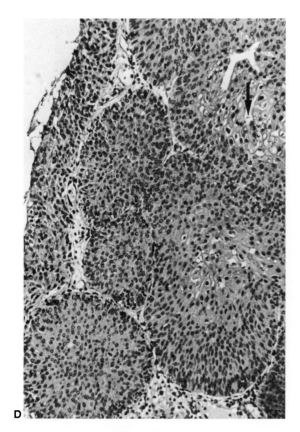

D

FIG. 4. *Continued*

lesion based upon a Papanicolaou smear or limited biopsy.

4. *Koilocytosis per se does not denote a benign process and is not uniformly associated with viral "infection".* Previous ultrastructural studies of warts localized virions to the koilocytotic nuclei, confirming the intimate relationship between this cytologic change and the presence of HPV virions (12). However, not all koilocytotic cells contain virions, capsid antigens, or abundant HPV DNA (42,43). This, combined with the ultrastructural studies, suggests that the koilocyte may be a marker for epithelium which has been altered or *transformed* by HPV but does not specifically indicate that a benign HPV *infection* is present. Appropriately, koilocytosis may be found in any HPV-related process, ranging from flat condyloma to invasive cancer (Fig. 6). Roy et al. demonstrated that nearly 14% of patients with high-grade CIN (carcinoma *in situ*) presented initially with Papanicolaou smears containing koilocytotic atypia alone (Roy et al., *personal communication*). Syrjanen et al. segregated and followed patients with cervical smears containing either koilocytotic atypia alone or koilocytosis with features of CIN. The progression rates of both groups to higher grades of CIN were essentially the same (44).

5. *The morphologic threshold for HPV infection (condyloma) has not been defined.* This is the result of two

problems. The first problem is that a significant proportion of women without abnormal Papanicoloau smears contain HPV in their genital tracts (45,46). This "latent" infection cannot be diagnosed by means other than molecular hybridization (17,18). The second problem is that there exists a spectrum of morphologic abnormalities in the genital tract. Some of these changes are nonspecific, including acanthosis, parakeratosis, and cytoplasmic halos. These changes can be interpreted as subtle or "early" flat condylomata (19) (Fig. 7), however, not all lesions with these subtle changes contain HPV DNA (19).

Diagnosis of Cervical Precancers

Because the distinction of precursors with low versus high risk is not always possible, the principal aim of the diagnostician is to recognize lesions that should be removed rather than being overly concerned with nuances of grading. However, flat or exophytic condylomata of the cervix will usually be classified in the low end of the spectrum (CIN I) (Fig. 3A), whereas lesions of higher risk will be diagnosed as higher-grade lesions (CIN II or CIN III) (Fig. 3B and C). What follows is an adaptation of the traditional classification system designed to place the majority of flat warts into the CIN I category and to place significant precursors into the CIN II and CIN III groups.

Condylomata (CIN I, Mild Dysplasia)

The typical cervical condyloma may vary in appearance: it may be flat to slightly raised, or it may resemble condyloma accuminata of the vulva. Accordingly, the degree of papillomatosis observed histologically will vary. The distinguishing features consist of epithelial thickening (acanthosis) and koilocytotic atypia in the mid- and upper portions of the epithelium. Koilocytotic atypia is defined as follows: nuclear atypia with variation in nuclear size and shape; wrinkling of nuclei; polychromatism; binucleate forms; and perinuclear halos. The halos tend to vary, as well, in appearance and shape, with a distinct zone of clearing between the nucleus and cytoplasmic membrane. Important features of flat condyloma/CIN I are as follows: modest nuclear atypia in the lower half of the epithelium, a low mitotic index, and absence of bizarre or abnormal mitoses. Maturation and koilocytotic atypia will vary as a function of the underlying epithelium, but the predominate finding is the presence of (a) mild atypia in areas of immaturity and (b) koilocytotic atypia in areas of maturation (Figs. 3A and 4) (8,33,41).

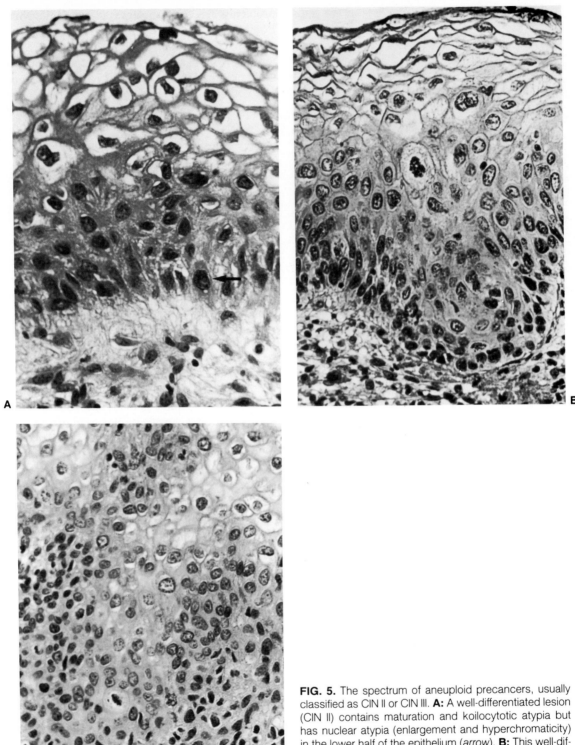

FIG. 5. The spectrum of aneuploid precancers, usually classified as CIN II or CIN III. **A:** A well-differentiated lesion (CIN II) contains maturation and koilocytotic atypia but has nuclear atypia (enlargement and hyperchromaticity) in the lower half of the epithelium (*arrow*). **B:** This well-differentiated lesion (CIN II) exhibits maturation but contains an abnormal mitotic figure centrally; it also demonstrates nuclear crowding with atypia in the lower third of the epithelium. **C:** This higher-grade CIN (III) exhibits focal surface maturation with loss of cell polarity and nuclear atypia throughout the thickness of the epithelium.

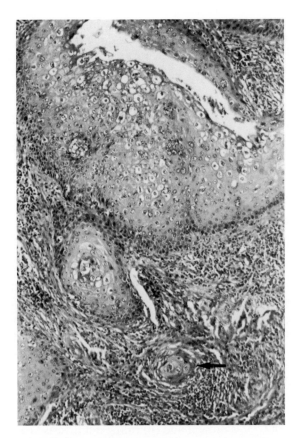

FIG. 6. Koilocytotic atypia associated with invasive squamous-cell carcinoma of the cervix (*arrow*).

CIN with Koilocytotic Atypia
(CIN II, Moderate Dysplasia)

Lesions in this category exhibit features of both condyloma and aneuploid epithelium. Mature cells are present in the upper half of the epithelium, usually with koilocytotic atypia. The koilocytes may be identical to those in flat condyloma, but they commonly differ by the presence of smaller, more concentric halos and dense, hyperchromatic, pleomorphic nuclei. The epithelial surface of CIN II and CIN III lesions frequently contains horizontally arranged parakeratotic cells with abnormal nuclei. In addition, nuclear atypia is present in the lower half of the epithelium in at least a portion of the lesion. The picture may be of a mixed lesion, with a combination of flat condyloma and CIN (21,25,33,34) (Figs. 3B and 5).

CIN without Koilocytotic Atypia
(CIN III, Severe Dysplasia-Carcinoma In Situ)

These lesions contain minimal evidence of maturation or koilocytotic atypia, although they may be combined with areas resembling CIN I or II. Cells with a high nuclear-to-cytoplasmic ratio are present throughout the epithelium. Paradoxically, high-grade CIN le-

sions often exhibit a more homogeneous population of neoplastic cells, with less variation in nuclear size and staining than lower-grade CIN lesions. However, the nuclei are crowded, enlarged, and hyperchromatic and contain a higher mitotic index than conventional basal cells (Figs. 3C and 5).

Differential Diagnosis

Nonspecific Cellular Changes Mimicking Koilocytotic Atypia

The increased emphasis on recognizing cervical HPV infections has brought with it the expected problems of differentiating HPV-specific changes from nonspecific halos in superficial cells. Because HPV may be present in completely normal epithelium, the morphologic threshold for identifying "condyloma" is, by definition, arbitrary. However, by requiring the presence of nuclear atypia for the diagnosis of koilocytosis, many nonspecific changes can be excluded (Figs. 3A, 4, and 7).

Inflammation and Infection

Acute and chronic cervicitis is caused by a variety of organisms; most commonly described are *Trichomonas*,

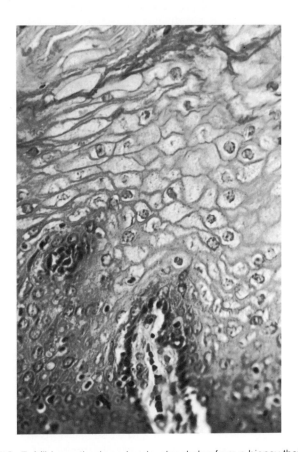

FIG. 7. Mild acanthosis and perinuclear halos from a biopsy that tested negative for papillomavirus DNA.

Candida, Hemophilus vaginalis, Chlamydia, and *Neisseria gonorrhea.* Less common forms of cervicitis include (a) those associated with viral diseases such as herpes genitalis and cytomegalovirus, (b) granulomatous cervicitis, and (c) chemical or traumatic irritation and systemic diseases (46–49). Iatrogenic causes include postoperative necrobiotic granulomas and reactions to Monsel's solution (50,51). The causative agent or organism may be unknown. The inflammatory reaction produced in either acute or chronic cervicitis is usually nonspecific, and the diagnosis is made following analysis of wet mounts, direct smear, or culture.

Cervicitis is characterized by ulceration, reparative atypia, and a mixed inflammatory infiltrate consisting of polymorphonuclear leukocytes, plasma cells, lymphocytes, and other lymphoreticular cells. Lymphoid follicles may also be present, prompting the diagnosis of follicular cervicitis. When severe inflammation is present and, in particular, when it consists of lymphoreticular cells, the diagnosis of chlamydia should be considered and excluded (52–54). Chlamydia infects endocervical columnar and immature metaplastic cells, executing its life cycle in inclusion vacuoles that eventually produce cell lysis. It is invariably associated with marked inflammation. Despite the fact that chlamydia produces cytoplasmic vacuoles in infected cells, the presence of cytoplasmic vacuoles in biopsies or Papanicolaou smears is not diagnostic, due to the nonspecific nature of such changes (Fig. 8D) (52–55). The diagnosis of chlamydia is confirmed either by culture or direct immunofluorescence for chlamydia organisms (52,56) (Fig. 8C).

Inflammation will induce epithelial changes with cytologic atypia, the most common of which is anaplasia of repair or reparative atypia. This is characterized by enlarged nuclei, inflammatory cells in the epithelium, and the presence of mitoses. In contrast to CIN, nucleoli are present and there is minimal nuclear crowding or overlap on the histologic section (Fig. 9) (3).

Other forms of reactive atypia which may or may not be associated with inflammation include acanthosis, parakeratosis, and, occasionally, perinuclear halos and mild nuclear atypia. These lesions may be difficult to distinguish from flat condyloma (Fig. 9).

Postmenopausal Patients

Other lesions that may be diagnostically confusing occur in postmenopausal women. In these patients there are three types of lesions associated with abnormal Papanicolaou smears. The first type involves *CIN of all grades.* Many postmenopausal patients are sexually active, and it is not uncommon to see such lesions in these patients. The second type consists of *atrophic lesions.* In contrast to precancers, atrophy is characterized by a uniform population of immature cells with a very low mitotic index (Fig. 10A and B) (3). The third type of lesion is that associated with *low-grade abnormalities* on the Papanicolaou smear, an unremarkable colposcopy exam, and a vaginal smear suggesting a high estrogen effect. The origin of these lesions is obscure. In our experience, many do not appear to be HPV-related, but they will be associated with repeated-low grade abnormal Papanicolaou smears and may be particularly frustrating to the clinician. Whether they represent epithelial alterations peculiar to menopause remains to be proven.

Management of Cervical Precancers

Terminology

Once a histologic diagnosis of papillomavirus infection or cervical intraepithelial neoplasia is made, the lesion should be removed. Although many conventional flat condylomas will probably regress, a proportion will progress to higher-grade CINs and it is virtually impossible to clearly distinguish all "benign" papillomavirus infections from those which are going to be associated with progression (3,21,38). In this context, the precise distinction of one grade from the other (i.e., CIN I versus CIN II) is not as important as (a) determining whether or not CIN is present and (b) ruling out invasive cancer (16). Whether the pathologist defines lesions as dysplasia/carcinoma *in situ,* CIN, or a combination of flat condyloma/CIN is unimportant, provided all lesions so classified are removed (Table 1). If a lesion is not recognized on the biopsy, the pathologist must ensure that the biopsy was taken from the region of the cervix which contains the T-zone. If metaplastic epithelium or endocervical glands are not identified, it cannot be assumed that the patient was adequately biopsied, and the pathologist should note on the report that the T-zone is not present (16) (Table 1).

Management of Inflammation

When confronted with a smear containing inflammation and equivocal biopsy results, the pathologist should review the biopsy and the Papanicolaou smear and determine whether the atypia in the smear can be explained by the biopsy. Depending upon the interpretation, empiric treatment with an antibiotic followed by a repeat exam or repeat colposcopy and biopsies will be recommended. Ideally, this approach will resolve many discrepancies between cytology and histology and will minimize the number of cases requiring repeat biopsy.

Management of Subtle Lesions

An unsettled issue is the precise morphological threshold for the diagnosis of HPV infection. As noted

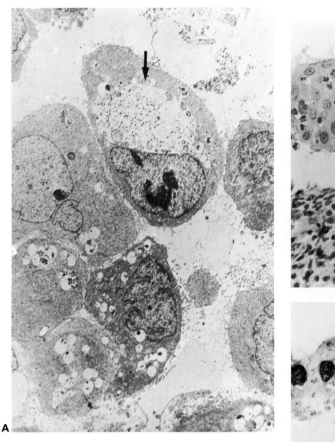

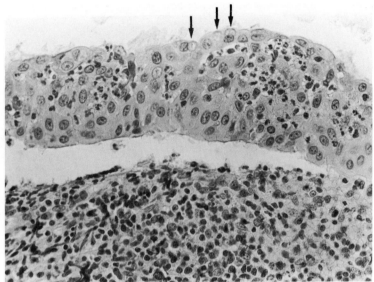

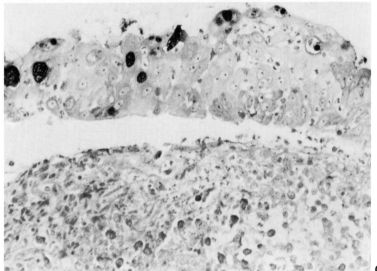

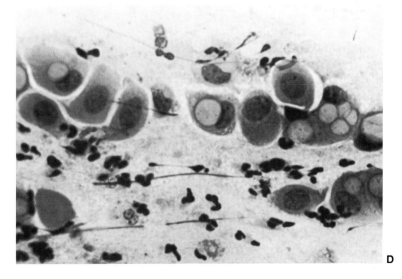

FIG. 8. Chlamydia infection of the cervix. **A:** An electron micrograph of a chlamydia-infected cell illustrates an inclusion vacuole with chlamydial particles (*arrow*). (Photograph provided courtesy of Dr. Jan Lindenman of Delft, Holland). **B:** Arrows denote subtle vacuoles containing chlamydia organisms, which stain intensely with antichlamydial antiserum as in part **C.** Note the intense underlying inflammation, which is frequently associated with this infection. **D:** ''Pseudoinclusions'' in endocervical cells in a Papanicolaou smear. These changes are not specific for chlamydia.

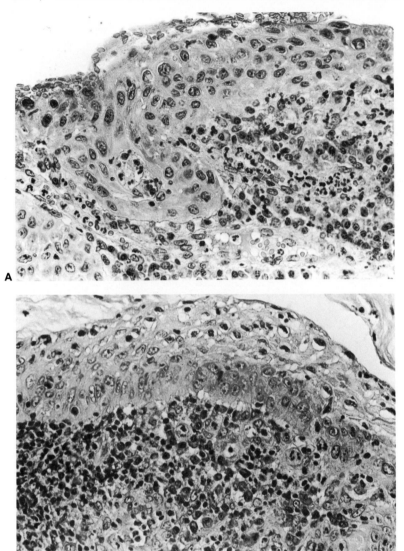

FIG. 9. Reactive and inflammation-associated changes in transformation-zone epithelium. **A:** Reparative atypia. **B:** Inflamed metaplastic epithelium. Note the cytoplasmic halos, which may be confused with koilocytotic atypia.

and illustrated above, there exists a spectrum of subtle cervical changes including acanthosis, parakeratosis, some perinuclear halos, and mild nuclear atypia, which may represent nonspecific abnormalities (Fig. 7). The appropriate approach to these lesions is to use descriptive terms, indicating that the diagnosis of condyloma has not been fulfilled. Such patients should be followed with Papanicolaou smears and treated only in the presence of clear-cut flat condyloma (CIN I) or higher-grade CIN. Likewise, in the postmenopausal patient with abnormal Papanicolaou smears and a negative exam, 4 to 6 weeks of intravaginal estrogen therapy may make it possible to distinguish atrophy from a bonafide CIN lesion.

The Role of Viral Diagnosis

At present it is possible to screen Papanicolaou smears and tissue samples for the presence of specific HPV types (45,57,58). This technology may have applications for determining the biologic potential of a given lesion and, in the case of clinically negative patients, determining if they carry occult HPV in their genital tract. However, determining the HPV type in a lesion that will ultimately be removed is of questionable value. Preliminary follow-up studies of precancers with specific HPV types support the association of HPV 16 with progression but do not exclude progression in some lesions containing other HPVs (39). Moreover, the wisdom of screening a large population of asymptomatic, cytologically normal women is debatable. One potentially useful aspect of DNA screening may be in evaluating patients with borderline Papanicolaou smears and/or histologically equivocal lesions. However, given the potential false-negative rate of a single sample, negative results would have to be viewed carefully, with repeat analyses. At present, HPV DNA typing is a research tool, and its clinical use awaits a more thorough under-

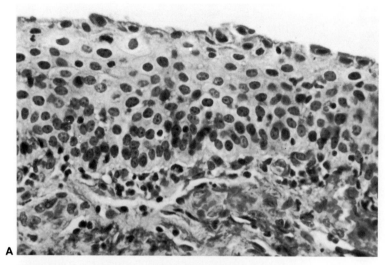

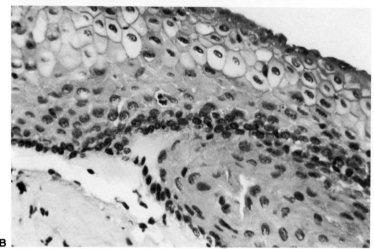

FIG. 10. Epithelial changes found in biopsies from postmenopausal patients. **A:** Atrophy, characterized by loss of maturation, uniformity of nuclear size and staining, absence of nuclear crowding, and a very few or no mitoses. **B:** Partial maturation with perinuclear halos, resembling condyloma.

standing of latent infection and the natural history of cervical HPV infection in general.

The Positive Endocervical Curettage

The clinical management of cervical precancers depends upon both the identification of disease which must be removed and the exclusion of invasive cancer. This can be accomplished if the colposcopic appearance of the lesion is consistent with the Papanicolaou smear and biopsy (16). However, if the precancer or condyloma extends deeply into the endocervical canal, invasion cannot be ruled out and cone biopsy is necessary. The suspicion of canal involvement is corroborated by the endocervical curettage. If it contains free strips of neoplastic squamous epithelium, cone biopsy is necessary (Fig. 11). If the curettage contains strips of condyloma, conization should be considered seriously because associated invasive cancer cannot be excluded. One possible exception is the curettage that contains very small amounts of neoplastic or condylomatous epithelium in the context of a clinically negative endocervical canal. In

such a case, inadvertent sampling of a portio lesion must be excluded (16). Resolving this issue and planning therapy requires consultation with the gynecologist, with whom the therapy can be decided.

Conization should also be considered if there is any question of microinvasion in either the Papanicolaou smear, the colposcopic examination, or the biopsies.

The Pregnant Patient

The incidence of HPV infection, either clinical or occult, in pregnant women ranges from 10% to 29% (59; Gissman et al., *personal communication*). The primary management goal is to exclude invasive cancer, which is achieved by sequential Papanicolaou smears and, when necessary, directed cervical biopsies. A limited cone biopsy will occasionally be necessary when lesions extend deeply into the endocervix and the Papanicolaou smear suggests cancer. In such cases it is useful to review the smear results before proceeding to cone biopsy. This will minimize the possibility of misdiagnosing an inflammatory atypia, which may mimic cancer when as-

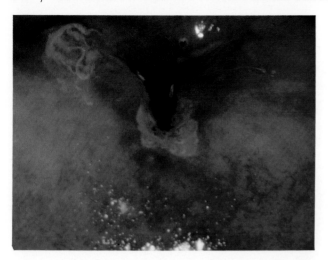

FIG. 11. Endocervical involvement by precancer: Colpophotograph illustrating a small lesion extending into the endocervical canal.

sociated with high-grade CIN. If invasive cancer is not suspected, a complete colposcopic exam can be performed 2 months post-partum.

MICROINVASIVE SQUAMOUS-CELL CARCINOMA

Introduction

Approximately 4% to 7% of CIN lesions are associated with superficial invasion (60,61). The basis for designating a subset of invasive cervix carcinoma as microinvasive is the assumption that a portion of "early" invasive cancers can be identified reproducibly and can be approached differently from conventional invasive cancer. Radical hysterectomy or radiation therapy is the treatment of choice for Stage 1B carcinoma of the cervix. Identification of a subset which carries no risk of lymph-node metastases (Stage IA) and which can be treated by simple hysterectomy carries a decided advantage. Currently, approximately 10% of invasive carcinomas are microinvasive when diagnosed (62–64).

There are several issues of importance or interest concerning microinvasive carcinoma of the cervix. They include (a) identifying invasion, (b) distinguishing it from mimics, and (c) applying correctly the criteria for microinvasion. It is important to emphasize that the diagnosis of microinvasion is histologic and can only be made on a cone specimen. The specimen must have negative margins, and the pathologist must examine a sufficient number of sections, usually one for every 2 mm of cone thickness and preferably with three levels from each block.

Diagnosis of Invasion

Identifying invasion in the routine biopsy specimen is the most important step in the proper management of

the patient. The classic criteria for invasion include the following: a desmoplastic response in the adjacent stroma; focal conspicuous maturation of the neoplastic epithelium with prominent nucleoli; blurring of the epithelial stromal interface; and loss of nuclear palisading at the epithelial-stromal border. Two additional and related features include (a) scalloping of the margins at the epithelial-stromal interface and (b) apparent "folding or duplication" of neoplastic epithelium. These features are helpful when faced with an intense inflammatory response that may obscure desmoplasia and blur the epithelial-stromal interface (Fig. 12) (65).

Differential Diagnosis of Invasion

In a review of 265 cases of presumed microinvasion sent to the Gynecologic Oncology Group, it was found that nearly 40% were overdiagnosed examples of intraepithelial lesions (66). The most important mimics of microinvasion are: gland involvement that is tangentially sectioned; cautery or crush artifact; and previous biopsy sites. As mentioned above, intraepithelial neoplasm associated with underlying inflammation, either from secondary infection or previous biopsy, may exhibit fragmentation of the epithelial-stromal interface (Fig. 13).

Diagnosis of Microinvasion

Cone biopsy is necessary if the lesion does not appear grossly invasive clinically or colposcopically and if it is not clearly deeper than 3 mm in the original biopsy. Once the cone biopsy is performed, the measurement of depth of invasion should be made from the most superficial epithelial-stromal interface of the adjacent intraepithelial process. This is best accomplished using an ocular micrometer. It is not always possible, however, to accurately estimate depth, because of specimen distortion (Fig. 13).

Three issues of potential concern when considering microinvasion are tumor depth, confluence of growth pattern, and capillary-lymphatic space invasion. Although microinvasion was originally defined as any lesion less than 5 mm in depth, the risk of lymph-node metastases increases with depths over 3.0 mm. The risk is 0% to 0.9% for lesions invading 3.0 mm or less, in contrast to 0% to 13.9% for lesions invading between 3.1 and 5.0 mm (67–70). Hence, a diagnosis of microinvasion requires that the lesion extend 3.0 mm or less into the stroma.

Despite a report emphasizing the prognostic importance of confluent patterns of invasion, some authors have not found that confluence is an independent factor once depth of invasion is controlled (67,69,70). Moreover, there are few studies that have clearly defined the

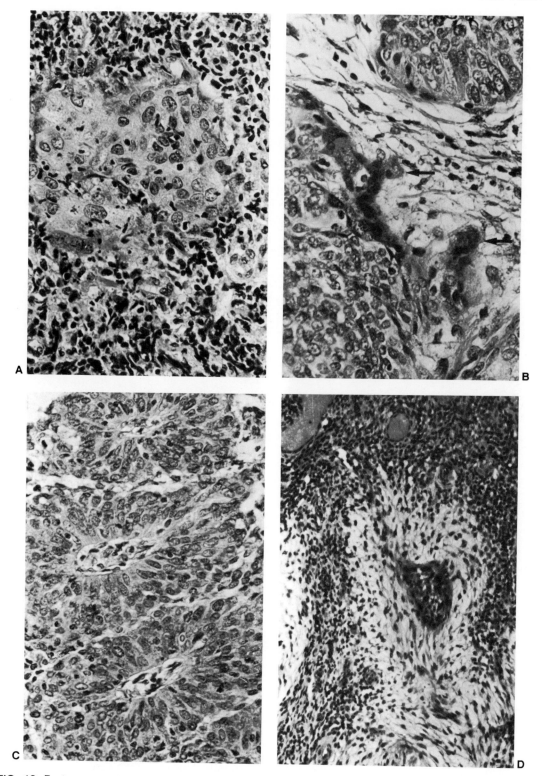

FIG. 12. Features associated with invasion. **A:** Loss of palisade, nuclear enlargement, and maturation at the stromal/epithelial interface. **B:** Angulation and scalloping of the epithelial borders (*arrows*). **C:** Folding or duplication of the epithelium with no intervening stroma. **D:** Desmoplastic stromal response.

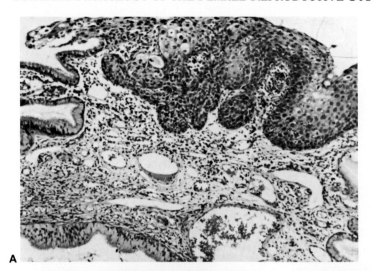

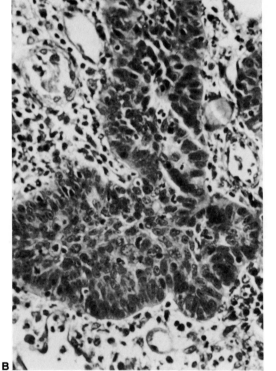

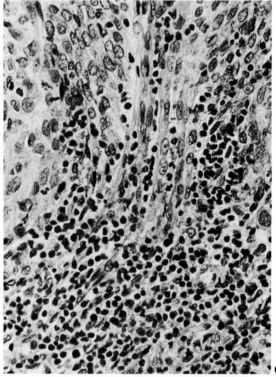

FIG. 13. Differential diagnosis of invasion. **A:** Irregularity of the epithelial-stromal interface may occur with CIN. Note, however, the smooth border and absence of desmoplasia or loss of nuclear palisade. **B:** Reparative atypia at the biopsy site. This tongue of epithelium appears to extend into the stroma. However, loss of cell polarity, desmoplasia, and nuclear changes characteristic of invasion are absent. **C:** Interruption of the interface by intense inflammation. This feature by itself is insufficient for a diagnosis of invasion.

criteria for confluence. However, lesion width may be important and will be discussed below (66,71).

The significance of capillary-lymphatic (CL) space invasion is controversial. CL space invasion increases in frequency as a function of lesion depth and, by itself, increases the risk of lymph-node metastases. However, it has not been established clearly whether CL space invasion is a critical factor in lesions of 3.0 mm depth or less (68–70). Van Nagell et al. (68) found that none of 17 patients with CL space invasion and lesions invading less than 3.0 mm had lymph-node metastases. Despite this, the nomenclature committee of the SGO does not accept the diagnosis of microinvasion if CL space invasion is present. In standard practice, most oncologists

will request that the presence of CL space invasion be reported, and they will probably opt for an aggressive approach if it is seen. Thus, it is important to ensure that CL space invasion is not overcalled, because such reports may result in radical therapy for lesions < 3.0 mm in depth. This requires a careful distinction between (a) CL space invasion and (b) artifacts resulting from inflammation or retraction (Fig. 14) (69).

The concept of tumor volume as a more accurate predictor of recurrence and metastases has been proposed by Burghardt and Holzer (71). They have found that lesions less than 420 mm^3 rarely recur. Unfortunately, determining tumor volume is tedious and not universally accepted. In lieu of this approach, the great-

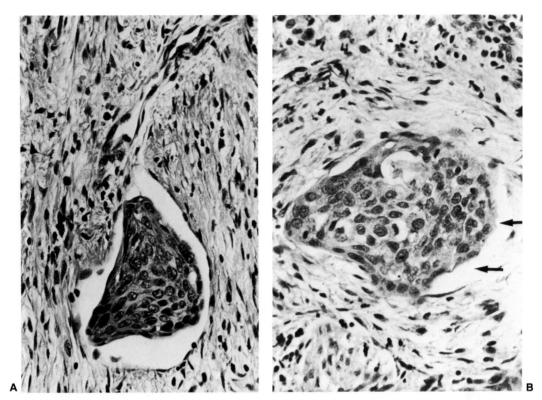

FIG. 14. Capillary-lymphatic space involvement and its mimic. **A:** A defined endothelial-lined space is identified. **B:** Retraction artifact (*arrows*) creates the appearance of a vascular space. The desmoplastic response in the surrounding stroma argues against the neoplastic epithelium being confined to a vascular space.

est width of the lesion can be determined and reported by examining the histological sections. There is an association between width, recurrence, and metastases, although the precise limits are unclear. A width of 10 mm is proposed by some as a limit for conservative therapy with lesion less than 3.0 mm in depth (2).

In summary, a diagnosis of microinvasive carcinoma requires an invasive lesion ≤ 3.0 mm in depth with no evidence of CL space invasion and free margins on the cone biopsy. Determination of greatest width is also advisable, although the precise width which should serve as a cutoff is unclear.

SQUAMOUS-CELL CARCINOMA AND ITS VARIANTS

Conventional Squamous-Cell Carcinoma

Introduction

The majority of squamous-cell carcinomas evolve from a precancerous lesion. Up to two-thirds of CIN III lesions will progress to cancer if untreated, and the time course for this evolution has been estimated to range from 3 to over 20 years (72,73). Squamous-cell carcinoma developing rapidly, without a defined precursor, has also been reported rarely (74). The mean age for

patients with cancer is approximately 51 years, in contrast to approximately 28 years for those with CIN III. A subset of invasive cancers is termed *occult carcinoma.* These are clinically inapparent Stage Ib lesions > 3.1 mm in depth. The mean age for this group has been estimated at 43 years, and the 5-year survival of 96% distinguishes this group from clinical Stage IB invasive carcinoma (86% 5-year survival) (60). Accordingly, patients with occult disease can be managed with radical hysterectomy and lymph-node dissection.

Survival is most closely related to the stage of disease when diagnosed (Table 2), which correlates closely with the risk of regional lymph-node metastases. Spread occurs principally through the lymphatics of the cervix, which consist of superficial and deep lymphatics draining to the iliac and obturator, hypogastric and common iliac, and sacral lymph nodes, as well as lymph nodes in the posterior bladder wall (1). Approximately two-thirds of invasive squamous carcinomas are Stage I or II when diagnosed. The actuarial 5-year survival drops abruptly from over 70% for Stage II to 30% to 35% for Stage III neoplasms (2).

Diagnosis

Squamous-cell carcinomas have been classified according to degree of squamous differentiation (Grades

TABLE 2. *Clinical staging of cervical cancer (FIGO)*

Stage 0:	Carcinoma *in situ* (intraepithelial neoplasia)
Stage I:	Carcinoma confined to the cervix
Ia:	Microinvasive carcinoma
Ib:	Other stage I disease, including occult
Stage II:	Extension of the carcinoma beyond the cervix without extension to the lower third of the vagina or pelvic wall
IIa:	No parametrial involvement
IIb:	Parametrial involvement
Stage III:	Extension of the carcinoma to the pelvic wall and/or lower third of the vagina. Cases with hydronephrosis or nonfunctioning kidney are included unless proven to be of other cause
IIIa:	No extension to the pelvic wall
IIIb:	Extension to the pelvic wall and/or hydronephrosis or nonfunctioning kidney
Stage IV:	Carcinoma extends beyond the true pelvis or involves the urinary bladder or rectum
IVa:	Spread to adjacent organs
IVb:	Spread to distant organs

I–III) or according to cell type. Reagan et al. subdivided squamous cancer of the cervix into (a) large-cell keratinizing carcinoma, (b) large-cell nonkeratinizing carcinoma, and (c) small-cell carcinoma (75). The basis for this distinction has been the observation that large-cell keratinizing carcinomas are radioresistant relative to nonkeratinizing carcinomas and that small-cell carcinomas have the worst overall prognosis. In a review of five large series by Reagan and Fu, the average 5-year survival for Stage I tumors treated by radiation therapy was 54%, 84%, and 42% for keratinizing, nonkeratinizing, and small-cell carcinomas, respectively (76). The distinction between large-cell keratinizing and nonkeratinizing squamous-cell carcinoma is based primarily upon the presence of intercellular bridges and keratin pearls in the former, although focal individual-cell keratinization may be present in the latter (77). The small-cell group has been more precisely defined and now consists of neoplasms that are morphologically and functionally identical to small-cell undifferentiated carcinoma (oat-cell carcinoma, argyrophilic carcinoma, neuroendocrine carcinoma).

Excepting small-cell undifferentiated carcinoma, classification according to cell type is not universally accepted. Not all authors have observed differences in survival between keratinizing and nonkeratinizing tumors. Randall et al. found that keratinizing tumors had a greater tendency to recur locally after radiotherapy but that the frequency of distant metastases was the same for both cell types (77). An alternative, but accepted, approach to grading is to classify squamous-cell carcinomas into the categories well, moderately, and poorly differentiated (Fig. 15A).

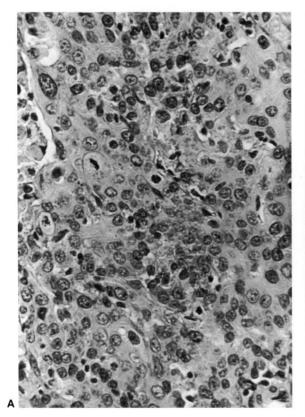 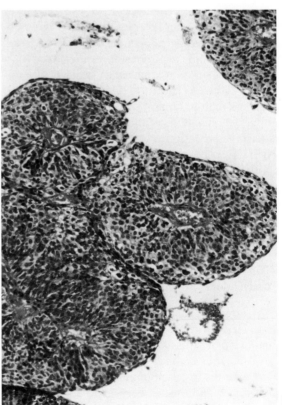

A   B

FIG. 15. Variants of squamous-cell carcinoma. **A:** Conventional moderately differentiated (large-cell nonkeratinizing) squamous-cell carcinoma. **B:** Papillary carcinoma.

Basaloid Carcinoma

A subset of squamous-cell carcinoma includes *basaloid carcinoma.* These lesions resemble basal-cell carcinomas of the skin. They are extremely rare in the cervix but have histologic features that may distinguish them from conventional squamous-cell carcinoma. The patients are older, the origin is often the cervical portio, and the tumors invade without a desmoplastic reaction. The diagnosis requires finding the following: infiltrative growth; nests or cords of small basaloid cells; peripheral palisading of the cells in the tumor nests; no desmoplasia; and no squamous-cell carcinoma (78). These lesions must be differentiated from adenoid cystic carcinoma (which possesses hyaline cylinders and a cribriform pattern) and small-cell undifferentiated carcinoma (which consists of a similar cell population). However, small-cell carcinomas demonstrate a loss of cellular cohesion, geographic zones of necrosis, and marked nuclear pleomorphism (see below).

Papillary and Verrucous Variants of Squamous Carcinoma

Verrucous Carcinoma

These are very rare lesions (79). The criteria for diagnosis are the same as in the vulva, and the diagnosis is one of exclusion. Verrucous carcinoma usually presents as a large sessile lesion resembling condylomata. Histologically, it consists of a hyperplastic-appearing lesion lacking the more delicate architecture of condylomata and demonstrating, instead, columns of well-differentiated epithelium expanding the underlying stroma. The pattern of invasion is blunt, with minimal nuclear atypia at the epithelial-stromal interface. An intense inflammatory infiltrate has been associated with verrucous carcinoma of the cervix but is, in itself, nonspecific. The differential diagnosis includes large exophytic condylomata with crypt involvement and well-differentiated squamous-cell carcinomas. The latter usually exhibit finger-like or angulated invasive tongues. The presence of filiform papillary projections or marked nuclear atypia at the epithelial-stromal interface rules out verrucous carcinoma. Given the extreme rarity of this lesion, the diagnosis of verrucous carcinoma must be made with caution.

Because verrucous carcinomas present grossly as large, sessile, wart-like growths, the diagnosis may be difficult without multiple biopsies or hysterectomy. Local excision is not usually possible, and extension into the adjacent pelvic tissues may occur. Very few cases are available to determine metastatic potential, although the few reported cases did not metastasize to lymph nodes. Human papillomavirus DNA sequences, including types 6 and 16, have been isolated from verrucous carcinomas, primarily in the vulva and larynx (80,81).

Papillary Neoplasms

Papillary lesions have been described in the cervix, ranging from those resembling transitional-cell papillomas to those diagnosed as papillary carcinoma *in situ* (82–84). Although the former are not invariably associated with invasive cancer, a number of filiform cervical papillomas have been observed in which deeper sampling disclosed invasive cancer (84,85). For this reason, any diagnosis of transitional papilloma should be made carefully and should be based upon local excision of the lesion, to rule out invasion. Papillary lesions containing marked squamous atypia (carcinoma *in situ*) may be associated with invasion and probably should be considered invasive until proven otherwise. The differential diagnosis, as with verrucous carcinoma, includes condylomata, although the latter do not exhibit delicate finger-like proliferations. An occasional diagnostic problem is the presence of immature metaplasia either overlying endocervical papillae or in association with condylomata. In this case, the diagnosis of papillary neoplasia can be excluded by the presence of endocervical columnar cells in the lesion, identifying an origin in metaplastic epithelium rather than denoting a papillary neoplasm (Fig. 15B).

Deep Endocervical/Endometrial Condylomata with Invasive Cancer

Rare reports have described classical(or almost classical)-appearing condylomata extending deeply into the endocervical canal or endometrium, some of which have been associated with invasive cancer (86; B. Steinberg, B. W. Winkler, *personal communication*). Another rare variant is CIN extending into the endometrial cavity (87). Lesions of this type are usually picked up on the endocervical or endometrial curettage. Hence, if the ECC contains abundant fragments of condyloma, or any papillary neoplasm, a cone biopsy or hysterectomy should be strongly considered to confirm or exclude invasive cancer.

GLANDULAR NEOPLASIA OF THE CERVIX

Adenocarcinoma *In Situ*

General

Adenocarcinoma *in situ* (ACIS) of the uterine cervix is uncommon and comprises less than 5% of true cervical intraepithelial neoplasms (88). The frequency of ACIS (2–to 7%) is much lower than that of squamous-cell carcinoma *in situ,* which accounts for 57% to 70% of cervical neoplasms (88). There are very few series that contain large numbers of cases, have clarified the epidemiology of the disease, or have calculated the transit time from adenocarcinoma *in situ* to invasive adenocarcinoma.

Between 40% and 100% of ACIS lesions are associated with a cervical intraepithelial neoplasm (89). This raises questions concerning the origin of these lesions. Whether they are due to some venereally transmitted oncogen has been debated. One study has linked a high incidence of herpes antibodies with adenocarcinoma of the cervix (90). The strongest evidence is the presence of HPV sequences in some adenocarcinomas (91).

Little is known about the relationship of ACIS to invasive adenocarcinoma. The incidence of ACIS is actually less than that of invasive adenocarcinoma of the cervix, possibly representing the difficulty of detecting ACIS relative to invasive cancer (88). Expansion and refinement of cytological criteria for the diagnosis of ACIS may alter the frequency with which glandular precursors are detected (92,93).

Diagnosis

The histologic features of ACIS are generally easily recognized and consist of partial or complete replacement of endocervical crypts or surface glandular epithelium by stratified cells with variable nuclear size and mitotic figures. Careful examination of virtually every ACIS will uncover individual large, hyperchromatic nuclei, which are always associated with mitoses. These two features will distinguish ACIS from its benign mimics. The degree of stratification may be so great that cribriform patterns are produced, but these should be limited to glandular lumens and should not form an extensive, confluent lesion extending into the stroma. Evaluation of endocervical curettings should be made with care because large fragments of cribriform epithelium may tempt the pathologist to make a diagnosis of invasion without clear-cut evidence of stromal infiltration (Fig. 16).

Differential Diagnosis

The differential diagnosis of ACIS, as well as the distinguishing features of ACIS, includes the following:

1. *Microglandular hyperplasia* has classically been described in pregnant patients or those receiving exogenous hormones (94). Microglandular hyperplasia may occur alone or in concert with endocervical polyps. It is characterized by a regularly irregular interlacing pattern of endocervical glandular epithelium. Distinction from

ACIS is based upon the regular pattern, minimal stratification, and rare mitoses (Fig. 17A). Focal, individual, hyperchromatic nuclei characterizing reactive change may be present, and confusion with adenocarcinoma has been observed (94).

2. The term *adenomatous hyperplasia of the endocervix* has been used to describe confluent microcystic endocervical glands often associated with nabothian cysts (95). The lining of these cysts is that of a flattened glandular epithelium, which contradicts the diagnosis of adenomatous hyperplasia. This lesion should not be confused with ACIS nor should it be diagnosed as adenomatous hyperplasia.

3. *Ciliated-cell metaplasia and endometriosis* may be confused with ACIS since the epithelium may be pseudostratified and may contain mild cytological atypia. However, the presence of cilia, the absence of large hyperchromatic nuclei, and the uniform polarity of the cells should distinguish this epithelium from a neoplasm (Fig. 17B). Endometriosis is similar to ciliated-cell metaplasia, since a pseudostratified epithelium is present with mitotic figures and some cilia. Endometrial stroma may or may not be conspicuous.

4. *Mesonephric* (Gartner's duct) *remnants* are usually located in the lateral wall of the cervix deep to the endocervical glands. However, they may rarely occur near the lumen of the cervix. Mesonephric remnants can be distinguished by their single layer of cuboidal epithelium, rare or absent mitoses, minimal cytologic atypia, and intraluminal eosinophillic material (Fig. 17C). Differentiating rare cases of mesonephric hyperplasia from ACIS or invasive cancer may be more difficult, although the predominately deep location of the lesion is an important factor in making this distinction.

5. *Reactive changes,* which may also cause diagnostic problems, include rare Aria-Stella phenomenon, viral infections, and inflammatory lesions. The primary distinguishing features in these cases are a low mitotic index and, principally, confinement of the cytological atypia to only a few cells in the epithelium.

Distinction of ACIS from invasive adenocarcinoma may be difficult. "Microinvasive" adenocarcinoma is not a recognized entity, and any infiltrative lesion must be considered a full-fledged invasive cancer, irrespective of depth of invasion. Important clues to invasion include the following: (a) numerous small neoplastic glands arranged in monotonous groups or parallel rows which are juxtaposed with little intervening stroma; (b) neoplastic glands which extend significantly deeper than the normal adjacent endocervical glands; (c) poorly formed glands which infiltrate in irregular cords; and (d) desmoplasia. In our experience, the desmoplastic reaction may be absent in these lesions (Fig. 18).

If ACIS is confirmed on conization, simple hysterectomy is justified. In the young patient, cone biopsy alone

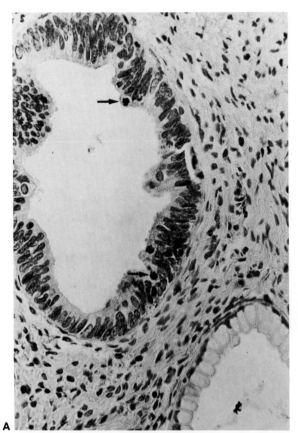

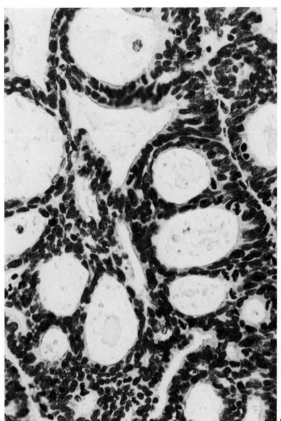

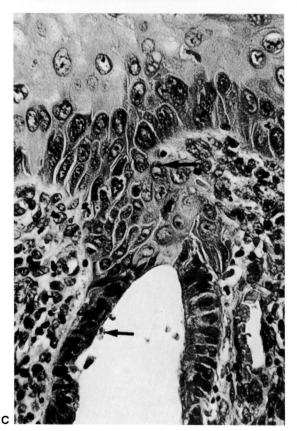

FIG. 16. Adenocarcinoma *in situ* (ACIS). **A:** In contrast to normal gland (*below*), ACIS contains a stratified epithelium with discrete nuclear enlargement, atypia, and mitoses (*arrows*). **B:** Cribriform arrangement of neoplastic glandular cells in a crypt. This pattern by itself is not diagnostic of invasion. **C:** Merging of ACIS (*small arrow, bottom*) and CIN (*large arrow, top*).

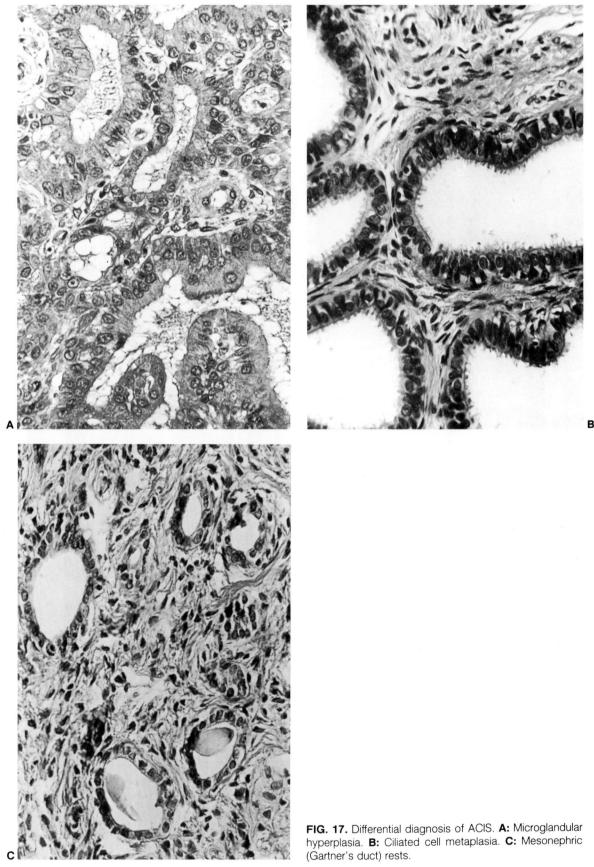

FIG. 17. Differential diagnosis of ACIS. **A:** Microglandular hyperplasia. **B:** Ciliated cell metaplasia. **C:** Mesonephric (Gartner's duct) rests.

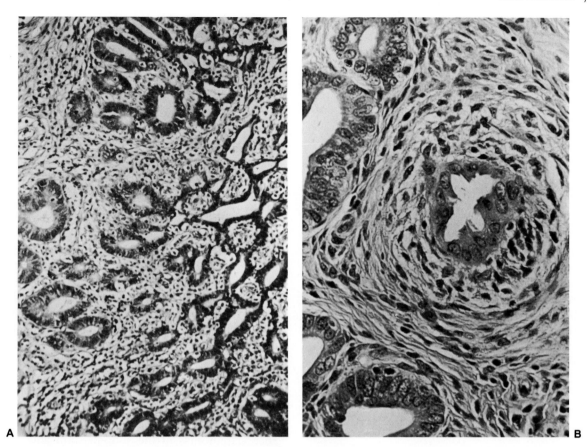

FIG. 18. Invasive adenocarcinoma. **A:** Closely packed, small irregular glands. **B:** Periglandular desmoplasia.

may be considered if the margins are free, if invasive carcinoma can be excluded, and if the patient is amenable to careful follow-up. It is obvious that each case must be individualized, and it must be kept in mind that the biologic nature and distribution of ACIS is unclear, particularly with respect to its curability by conization.

Adenocarcinoma and Its Variants

Introduction

Adenocarcinoma accounts for 3% to 7% of primary epithelial malignancies of the uterine cervix (96–99). The relative incidence of cervical adenocarcinoma has been increasing, apparently because of a decrease in squamous-cell carcinoma as well as an absolute increase in the rate of adenocarcinoma (93,99,100). About 50% of cervical adenocarcinomas are primary, and a nearly equal percentage represent extensions from an endometrial source (101). The majority of women with cervical adenocarcinoma (73–84%) are symptomatic, and most have vaginal bleeding (99,102). About 85% will have disease limited to the cervix (Stage I) or extending into the parametrium or vagina (Stage II) at the time of diagnosis (99,102,103). The mean age is in the mid- to late

forties to the early fifties, similar to that for squamous cell carcinoma (98,99,102,104).

The pathogenesis of the disease is unclear. On one hand, it shares with endometrial adenocarcinoma certain risk factors such as being nulligravid, obese, hypertensive, and/or diabetic (99,105). Consistent with these nonvenereal risk factors is the observation by Menczner et al. of a higher incidence in those ethnic groups of Israeli women who had a low risk for squamous-cell carcinoma (106). Another nonvenereal association is that of minimal deviation adenocarcinoma with Peutz-Jeghers syndrome (107). Further, there are many reports of the disease in infants and children (99,108–110). Clear-cell carcinoma has a relationship to *in utero* exposure to diethylstilbesterol, though not as strong as for the vagina (109–111). A possible association with oral contraceptives has not been substantiated by other, more recent studies (99). There may, however, be a subset of cervical adenocarcinomas that are related to venereal factors. This is suggested by the presence of squamous intraepithelial neoplasia (which is highly correlated with venereal factors) in about 24% of all cases and the detection of human papillomavirus nucleic acids in some adenocarcinomas (89,91,99).

The sensitivity of cytologic exam of cervical swabs in detecting endocervical adenocarcinoma is approximately 90% (108). This high sensitivity has been observed both in screening asymptomatic patients and in detecting recurrent disease (93,108).

In a recent review, Moberg et al. noted 5-year survival rates of 84%, 50%, and 9% for Stages I, II, and III, respectively (104). This is lower than the corresponding survivals for squamous-cell carcinoma.

Histologic Types

Mucin-secreting adenocarcinoma

The most common pattern is that of a well- to moderately differentiated mucin-secreting tumor (98,99,112). Typically, the cells are columnar with variable amounts of mucin secretion. The nuclei may be basally situated or pseudostratified with slight to moderate chromatin clumping, pleomorphism, one or more nucleoli, and mitoses. The pattern of growth is usually that of abnormally crowded, complex, branching acinar structures lacking the lobular architecture characteristic of normal endocervical glands. Up to 43% will contain foci of carcinoma in situ (113), implying that they evolve from the latter. There may be abrupt transitions within glands from normal to neoplastic epithelium.

Minimal-deviation adenocarcinoma (adenoma malignum)

This form of cervical adenocarcinoma presents diagnostic difficulties as reflected in the high rate of missed diagnoses in initial biopsies (93,114). The nuclear atypia characteristic of an adenocarcinoma is absent, but, in most cases, hyperchromatic nuclei can be found. The primary distinguishing feature is a pattern of growth that is distinct from normal endocervical glandular epithelium. This includes branching, irregularly oriented, "claw-like" glands that penetrate deeper into the stroma than do the adjacent endocervical crypts. Another, less obvious feature is the presence of some mitotic activity, albeit rare (Fig. 19A) (115,116).

Several recent studies have found that histochemical staining for carcinoembryonic antigen will differentiate a high proportion of minimal-deviation adenocarcinomas from benign endocervical gland proliferations. Michael et al. and Steeper et al. found that all minimal-deviation adenocarcinomas studied stained positively for CEA; in contrast, none of the benign lesions stained positively for CEA (114,116). Staining may be both intracellular and luminal, the latter occurring when cellular debris is released into the extracellular space.

The majority of investigators have observed a poor prognosis for minimal-deviation adenocarcinoma (85). However, Silverberg and Hurt challenged this claim, citing the fact that poor prognosis is probably due to advanced disease in many patients (117).

Endometrioid carcinoma

The second most common histologic type is endometrioid, having an appearance indistinguishable from its uterine counterpart (98,99) (Fig. 19B). In the series of Saigo et al., this pattern was noted in 24% of cases, as compared to 47% for the endocervical mucin-producing type (99). The 5-year survival rate for endometrioid carcinoma is approximately 57%, which is slightly better than that for endocervical adenocarcinoma in general (85,98,100,118).

Clear-cell carcinoma

Approximately 75% of clear-cell carcinomas of the cervix and vagina have occurred in women exposed in utero to diethylstilbestrol or related compounds (119,120). The affected patients are usually in their late teens when diagnosed, in contrast to women without a history of DES exposure, who are usually in their forties. Interestingly, only 39% of black women with clear-cell carcinoma have a history of DES exposure (121). In general, about 50% of cervical clear-cell carcinomas can be linked to a history of DES exposure (119,120).

Clear-cell carcinomas presumably have their origin in müllerian-derived epithelium, analogous to clear-cell adenocarcinomas of the endometrium and ovary. In DES-exposed patients, over 50% of cervical neoplasms have been associated with vaginal adenosis (111).

The morphology of clear-cell carcinoma parallels its counterpart in the endometrium and includes tubular, papillary, microcystic, and solid patterns (111). The characteristic cytologic changes consist of either clear or "hobnail" cells lining gland-like spaces or papillary stalks. The stroma of the stalks exhibits an eosinophillic, homogeneous appearance (Fig. 19C).

The differential diagnosis of clear-cell carcinoma includes (a) mesonephric hyperplasia and (b) microglandular hyperplasia. Mesonephric remnants have a distinct location in the lateral cervical wall. Despite the presence of clear cells, they do not exhibit hobnail patterns or cytological atypia and should not normally be confused with clear-cell neoplasms. Microglandular hyperplasia is distinguished by the regularity of pattern and associated squamous metaplasia.

Over 85% of clear-cell carcinomas are Stage I or II when diagnosed, and approximately 70% of patients in the study by Herbst et al. were free of disease (120). In contrast, others have reported an approximately 40% 5-year survival for older patients without a DES history (98,122).

Adenosquamous carcinoma

Adenosquamous carcinoma accounts for approximately 15% of adenocarcinomas; because of its poor

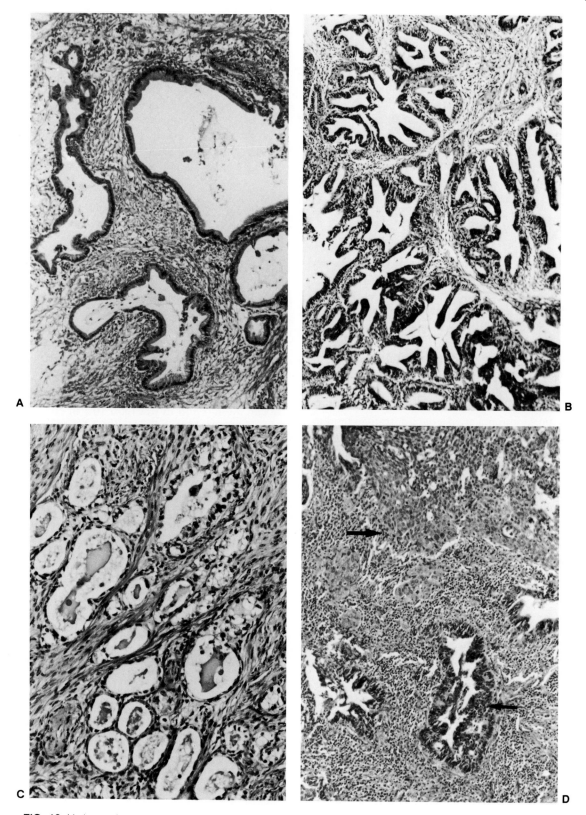

FIG. 19. Variants of endocervical adenocarcinoma. **A:** Minimal deviation adenocarcinoma (adenoma malignum). **B:** Endometrioid carcinoma. **C:** Clear-cell adenocarcinoma. **D:** Adenosquamous carcinoma.

prognosis, it deserves to be considered separately (99,123,124). Interestingly, this tumor is seen in both elderly and young women, with 17% diagnosed during or following pregnancy (125–127).

Adenosquamous carcinoma can be divided histologically into the mature, mixed, and signet-ring types (Fig. 19D). The latter contains a mixture of signet-ring cells and squamous cells (100). Glassy-cell carcinoma has also been included under adenosquamous carcinomas, although it is listed under undifferentiated carcinomas in this chapter.

Adenoid cystic carcinoma

Whether adenoid cystic carcinoma of the cervix deserves designation as a separate entity is a matter of debate. Unlike adenoid cystic carcinomas of the salivary gland or Bartholin's gland, cervical "adenoid cystic carcinoma" does not arise in sweat glands, is associated with either squamous neoplasia (60%) or adenocarcinoma (16%), has an age distribution similar to adenocarcinoma of the cervix, and does not display the characteristic nerve sheath invasion of its counterparts in other sites. On the other hand, neoplasms containing adenoid cystic carcinoma are deeply infiltrative, tend to recur, often metastasize to bone or lung, and are radioresistant, behaviors similar to those of their salivary gland analogues. These features, coupled with the distinct histologic pattern of adenoid cystic carcinoma, appear to warrant its recognition in surgical specimens. Adenoid cystic carcinoma has a poorer prognosis than conventional squamous-cell carcinoma (128,129).

Adenoid cystic carcinoma is exceedingly rare, and, as of 1980, fewer than 40 well-documented cases had been reported in the world literature. In contrast to squamous-cell carcinoma, adenoid cystic carcinoma occurs in older patients with a mean age in the sixties. Only 5% occur in patients less than 40 years of age. The presumed origin of adenoid cystic carcinoma is the undifferentiated reserve cells of the transformation zone. The most common symptom is vaginal bleeding, and the mass may be clinically exophytic or endophytic. Approximately 60% are Stage I at the time of diagnosis.

The characteristic features of adenoid cystic carcinoma of the salivary gland or Bartholin's gland apply to their counterpart in the cervix. Small, uniform, basaloid cells are arranged in a variety of patterns, including anastomosing cords, pseudoglands, and cribriform nests. As mentioned above, nerve-sheath invasion has not been demonstrated, but lymphatic invasion is almost always present. Adenoid cystic carcinoma carries at least a 50% mortality, and well-documented, tumor-free survivals occur in approximately 33% of cases. As expected, prognosis is linked to stage, although a significant percentage of patients with Stage I neoplasia die of

their disease. At present, the overall survival of Stage I neoplasms cannot be determined, since there has been a relatively short follow-up in most reported cases.

It is generally accepted that radiotherapy is suboptimal for cervical adenoid cystic carcinoma and that this feature, coupled with its frequent deep invasion, justifies radical hysterectomy and lymph-node dissection. Whatever the specific choice of therapy, adenoid cystic carcinoma should be approached as an aggressive variant of cervical carcinoma (128–130).

Differentiation of endometrial and endocervical adenocarcinoma

This is a frequent problem, since (a) about 50% of adenocarcinomas of the cervix are from extension of an endometrial primary and (b) the second most common type of primary endocervical adenocarcinoma is the endometrioid variant (99,101). Clinical correlation and, of course, study of the hysterectomy specimen will often resolve the problem. When the distinction cannot be made, immunoperoxidase studies for carcinoembryonic antigen may be of value. Cells containing this protein are detected in approximately 80% of endocervical adenocarcinomas and in less than 10% of endometrial carcinomas (131,132). All cases of adenosquamous carcinomas of the endometrium were positive, but only in the areas of squamous metaplasia (132).

Metastatic adenocarcinoma to the cervix

Metastatic adenocarcinoma to the cervix from extrauterine sites is rare, accounting for only about 1% of cervical adenocarcinomas (133). The majority are adenocarcinomas primary in the ovary or colon.

UNDIFFERENTIATED CARCINOMAS OF THE CERVIX

Small-Cell Undifferentiated Carcinoma

Interest in this group has increased in recent years, primarily because it exhibits specific histologic features and may be associated with peptide hormone production, a phenomenon commonly found in oat-cell carcinoma of the lung. Moreover, this carcinoma, like its counterpart in the lungs, appears to have a propensity for rapid metastasis and radiosensitivity and carries a high mortality (134).

Cervical small-cell carcinoma also shares many of the histologic features of small-cell carcinoma of the lung. It is composed of a small, uniform cell population with hyperchromatic nuclei and a very high nuclear-to-cytoplasmic ratio. The tumor cells form irregular, loose aggregates, often with little cohesion. The nuclei contain a coarse chromatin pattern, and, because there is little cytoplasm, they often appear to "mold" as they are artifactually compressed in tissue sections (Fig. 20A). The lesions tend to be small, but they extensively infiltrate the underlying cervical stroma. Hence, they may appear more as an indurated mass than as a fungating lesion. Additional histologic features that distinguish this entity are vascular invasion, observed in up to 93% of cases by Van Nagell et al., and conspicuous lack of coexisting inflammation, in contrast to most cases of conventional squamous-cell carcinoma (134). Furthermore, by virtue of their rapid growth, these neoplasms are often characterized by broad zones of necrosis (134).

One of the more intriguing aspects of small-cell carcinoma is its association with peptide hormone production, which can be exhibited by ultrastructural or immunohistochemical techniques in a portion of the neoplasms (135). Such neoplasms have been termed "argyrophilic carcinoma," "oat-cell carcinoma," "neuroendocrine carcinoma," or "poorly differentiated carcinoids" (136–139). These observations have led to the assumption that both small-cell undifferentiated carcinoma of the cervix and carcinoid tumors of the cervix are similar to other neoplasms capable of amine precursor uptake and decarboxylation (APUD) (141). These so-called APUDomas are characterized by peptide hormone production, the propensity to take up silver salts in special stains (argyrophilia), and, in a portion, dense-core granules on electron microscopy (138). As a result of peptide hormone production, APUDomas have the ability to induce certain clinical syndromes. The best known of these is the carcinoid syndrome caused by the production of serotonin, but neoplasms of the cervix, like their counterparts elsewhere, may also produce ACTH, insulin, parathormone, and other substances (136,140).

The origin of these neoplasms has been a matter of debate. Originally, it was thought that all APUDomas arise from cells with a common embryonic source—the neural crest (140). Evidence that this process could occur in the cervix was supported by Fox's observation of such cells as normal cervical inhabitants (141). Two other observations suggest, however, that small-cell undifferentiated carcinomas of the cervix, including those functional neoplasms, not only do not arise from preexisting, normal argyrophilic cells but also do not arise from cells originating in the neural crest. First, certain neoplasms occurring *de novo* may contain argyrophilic cells, including mucinous cystadenomas of the ovary that contain intestine-like epithelium (140). Second, carcinoids and small-cell carcinomas of the cervix have been observed in association with conventional neo-

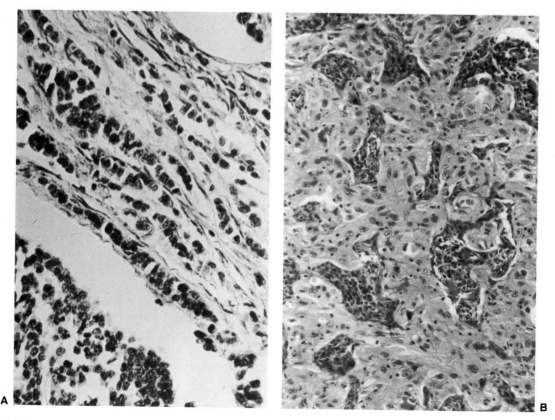

FIG. 20. Undifferentiated carcinoma of the cervix. **A:** Small-cell undifferentiated carcinoma. **B:** Glassy-cell carcinoma.

plasms, including adenocarcinoma *in situ,* invasive adenocarcinoma, and cervical intraepithelial neoplasms (142). Thus, it appears that, rather than originating from a specific argyrophilic cell, small-cell carcinomas and carcinoids probably represent "selective differentiation," often within a preexisting, more conventional carcinoma. This observation has been supported by findings in other organs where conventional carcinomas blend with the argyrophilic neoplasms (143).

Although certain small-cell neoplasms of the cervix may exhibit functional characteristics, the major criterion for distinguishing them from conventional squamous-cell carcinomas is histologic. Small-cell morphology is not itself the most important consideration in making the diagnosis of small-cell carcinoma. Many squamous-cell carcinomas are composed of relatively small cells, but these maintain the infiltrating pattern of a conventional squamous-cell cancer. In contrast, small-cell undifferentiated carcinoma not only is composed of small cells but also has the cellular characteristics and pattern of infiltration described above. Intermediate and well-differentiated (carcinoid) variants have also been described; however, with the exception of anecdotal reports, the prognosis is poor (85,137).

It is important to emphasize that Grimelius stains are not uniformly positive in small-cell carcinoma and that ultrastructural studies may not demonstrate dense-core cytoplasmic granules associated with these neoplasms (135,137). Positive immunohistochemical staining for neuron-specific enolase, chromogranin, and synaptophysin has been described in neuroendocrine tumors, but the sensitivity and specificity of these stains remains to be established for similar tumors in the genital tract (144–147). In most instances, application of histologic criteria alone will identify small-cell carcinomas. The recognition of this tumor is important, given its radiosensitivity, potential chemosensitivity, and metastatic potential.

Other Rare Variants

Glassy-cell carcinoma is an unusual variant composed of cells with "ground-glass" cytoplasm, prominent eosinophilic, PAS-positive cell membranes, and prominent nucleoli. It likely represents a variant of poorly differentiated adenocarcinoma or adenosquamous carcinoma, and, as would be expected, the prognosis is poor (Fig. 20B) (126,148). Another variant is *lymphoepithelioma-like carcinoma,* which resembles its nasopharyngeal counterpart and is composed of uniform, undifferentiated cells with eosinophillic cytoplasm, oval vesicular nuclei, and an intense stromal inflammatory-cell infiltrate (149). Too few cases have been reported to determine if this neoplasm has a prognosis distinguishing it from squamous-cell carcinoma of the cervix.

SOFT-TISSUE NEOPLASMS
Polyps

The differential diagnosis of polypoid masses on the cervix includes:

1. *Endocervical polyps.* These are not actually neoplasms but are, instead, a hamartomatous hyperplasia of both stroma and epithelium. Endocervical polyps are common lesions, most often occurring in the fourth to sixth decades in multigravidas (150,151). When symptomatic, they usually cause a profuse mucoid discharge or abnormal bleeding. They are usually small (up to 1 cm in size) and single, though cases of large polyps protruding into the canal and thus mimicking a malignant tumor have been reported (152). Histologically, many different patterns may be observed. The most common has a preponderance of glands lined by tall, mucin-secreting cells admixed with a fibrous stroma and large, thick-walled blood vessels. In addition, there is frequently squamous metaplasia and/or microglandular hyperplasia, as well as a mixed stromal inflammatory infiltrate containing plasma cells. Variations include polyps containing nabothian cysts. The distinction between these and simple nabothian cysts may be arbitrary. The stroma of endocervical polyps may be very vascular, mimicking a vascular tumor, or in some cases may be sufficiently cellular to suggest stromal sarcoma (153). Finally, especially in cases of pressure-induced trauma, granulation tissue may be a predominant finding. Carcinomas arising in an endocervical polyp are very rare and, if confined to the polyp, carry a very good prognosis (101).

2. *Fibroepithelial polyps.* Occasionally, fibroepithelial polyps occur on the cervical portio and consist of a prominent connective tissue base with normal to acanthotic overlying epithelium. The differential diagnosis includes condyloma, which is distinguished by the characteristic epithelial changes, and vaginal polyps, which contain atypical stromal cells (154).

3. *Polyps of endometrial origin.* These include (a) endometrial polyps, which extend through the endocervical canal, and (b) decidual polyps, which occur in pregnancy. Mixed polyps containing both endocervix and endometrium may also be seen, in which the diagnosis of polyp of mixed type is appropriate.

4. *Endometriosis.* Cervical endometriosis usually presents as one or more discolored, blue, raised lesions measuring a few millimeters in diameter. The histologic diagnosis requires the presence of endometrial-type glands surrounded by cervical stroma. Endometrial stroma will be variable and, like endometriosis at other sites, will contain evidence of old hemorrhage.

5. *Submucosal leiomyomas.* The most common benign neoplasm of the cervix is a leiomyoma, accounting for about 8% of all uterine leiomyomas (95). They may protrude from the endocervical canal and thus mimic an

endocervical polyp, although they are typically firmer and have a whorled appearance on cut section. As would be expected, their histologic features are similar to those of uterine corpus leiomyomas, with mitotic activity being the most useful predictive factor for malignant potential. As is true of leiomyomas in general, cervical leiomyomas are frequently associated with the thick walls of blood vessels, suggesting a site of origin for these lesions.

6. *Other rare variants.* These include (a) *mesonephric papilloma,* which has been reported in children, and (b) *papillary adenofibroma* (155,156). The latter is similar in appearance to adenofibroma of the endometrium and typically occurs in postmenopausal women. Histologically, it is characterized by blunt and branching stromal papillae covered with benign endocervical epithelium. The differential diagnosis includes (a) endocervical polyps, which lack the characteristic stromal papillary changes and stromal proliferation, and (b) adenosarcoma, which contains a higher stromal mitotic index (157).

Other Benign Soft-Tissue Neoplasms

Benign vascular tumors are rarely identified in the cervix. These include *capillary or cavernous hemangiomas,* although it is often difficult to differentiate such lesions from arteriovenous malformations with microvascular proliferation (158,159). Other rare benign tumors that have been reported in the cervix include *lipomas, blue nevi, glioma,* and *lymphangioma* (160–164). These lesions are usually reported as incidential findings at hysterectomy.

MALIGNANT SOFT-TISSUE NEOPLASMS

Sarcomas of the uterine cervix are very rare. They usually present in the fourth to sixth decade as a protruding cervical mass and/or postmenopausal or postcoital bleeding. The different types reported include *stromal sarcoma, leiomyosarcoma,* and *malignant mixed mesodermal tumors,* hence paralleling sarcomas of the uterine corpus (165,166). The most common variant is stromal sarcoma, which predominates in postmenopausal women and may present as a cervical polyp. The histologic features include sheets of round to spindle-shaped cells with a high nuclear-to-cytoplasmic ratio and mitoses. With the exception of low-grade stromal sarcoma, these tumors appear to have a poor prognosis. Stromal sarcoma can usually be differentiated from small-cell carcinoma and lymphoma by growth pattern alone, although stains for reticulin should exclude these entities.

Other types of cervical sarcoma include *embryonal rhabdomyosarcoma* of childhood (sarcoma botyriodes), *Wilms' tumor,* and *adenosarcoma* (167–169). Cervical embryonal rhabdomyosarcoma usually occurs in the first two decades and generally is associated with a better prognosis than sarcomas (including rhabdomyosarcomas) occurring in older women. Cervical adenosarcoma may also occur in adolescents and has a favorable prognosis. These tumors contain benign-appearing glands and a stroma which may resemble stromal sarcoma, or they may contain rhabdomyoblasts or cartilage. Chen emphasized the importance of distinguishing adenosarcomas with rhabdomyoblastic elements from embryonal rhabdomyosarcomas and mixed müllerian tumors, because adenosarcomas have a better prognosis (169,170).

Most of the different subtypes of *lymphoma* have been identified in the cervix, usually as a manifestation of systemic disease, although primary lymphoma of the cervix has been reported (171–173). Lymphomas usually present as a polypoid mass with the typical soft, gray-white "fish flesh" appearance on cut section. Microscopically, they infiltrate stroma without destroying the native glandular architecture, a feature which, in part, distinguishes them from carcinoma. Lymphoid-specific immunohistochemical markers such as leukocyte common antigen will allow recognition of diagnostically problematic cases. The prognosis is usually a function of the histologic subtype for the non-Hodgkin's lymphomas. When documented, lymphoma limited to the cervix is associated with a favorable prognosis (171,172).

ACKNOWLEDGMENTS

This work was supported, in part, by grants from the National Institutes of Health (grant no. AI00628) and from the American Cancer Society (to CPC). Dr. Crum is a recipient of a Physician Scientist Award from the National Institutes of Health.

REFERENCES

1. Krantz KE. The anatomy and the human cervix, gross and microscopic. In: Blandau RJ, Moghissi K, eds. *The biology of the cervix.* Chicago: University of Chicago Press, 1973:57–69.
2. Ferenczy A. Anatomy and histology of the cervix. In: Blaustein A, ed. *Pathology of the female genital tract.* New York: Springer-Verlag, 1982;119–135.
3. Richart RM. Cervical intraepithelial neoplasia. In: Sommers SC, ed. *Pathology annual.* New York: Appleton-Century-Crofts, 1973:301–328.
4. Kessler II. Perspectives on the epidemiology of cervical cancer with special reference to the herpes virus hypothesis. *Cancer Res* 1974;34:1091–1110.
5. Koss L, Durfee GR. Unusual patterns of squamous epithelium of the uterine cervix: cytologic and pathologic study of koilocytotic atypia. *Ann NY Acad Sci* 1956;63:1245–1261.
6. Frenkel N, Roizman B, Cassai E, Nahmias AJ. DNA fragment of

herpes simplex 2 and its transcription in human cervical cancer tissue. *Proc Natl Acad Sci USA* 1974;69:3780–3787.

7. Purola E, Savia E. Cytology of gynecologic condyloma accuminatum. *Acta Cytol* 1977;21:26–31.

8. Meisels A, Fortin R. Condylomatous lesions of the cervix and vagina. I. Cytologic patterns. *Acta Cytol* 1976;20:505–509.

9. Meisels A, Morin C. Human papillomavirus and cancer of the uterine cervix. *Gynecol Oncol* 1981;12:s111–s123.

10. *MMWR* 1983;32:306–308.

11. Syrjanen KI. Condylomatous epithelial changes in the uterine cervix and their relationship to cervical carcinogenesis. *Int J Obstet Gynecol* 1980;17:415–420.

12. Reid R, Laverty CR, Coppleson M, et al. Noncondylomatous cervical wart virus infection. *Obstet Gynecol* 1980;55:476–483.

13. Shah KH, Lewis MG, Jenson AB, et al. Papillomavirus and cervical dysplasia. *Lancet* 1980;2:1190.

14. deVilliers E-M, Gissman L, zur Hausen H. Molecular cloning of viral DNA from human genital warts. *J Virol* 1981;40:932–935.

15. Broker TR, Botchan M. Papillomaviruses: retrospectives and prospectives. In: Botchan M, Grodzicker T, Sharp PA, eds. *Cancer cells 4: DNA tumor viruses.* Cold Spring Harbor Laboratory, 1986:17–35.

16. Richart RM, Crum CP, Townsend DE. Workup of the patient with the abnormal Papanicoloau smear. *Gynecol Oncol* 1981;s265–s276.

17. Steinberg BM, Topp WC, Schneider PS, et al. Laryngeal papillomatosis infection during clinical remission. *N Engl J Med* 1983;308:1261–1264.

18. Ferenczy A, Mitao M, Nagai N, et al. Latent papillomavirus and recurring genital warts. *N Engl J Med* 1985;313:784–788.

19. Nuovo G, Nuovo M, Cottral S, et al. Histological correlates of clinically occult human papillomavirus infection of the uterine cervix. *Am J Surg Pathol* 1988;12:198–204.

20. Kaufmann R, Kurman RJ, Koss LG, et al. Statement of caution in the interpretation of papillomavirus-associated lesions. *Am J Obstet Gynecol* 1983;146:269–270.

21. Mitao M, Nagai N, Levine RU, et al. Human papillomavirus type 16 infection of the uterine cervix. A morphological spectrum with evidence of late gene expression. *Int J Gynecol Pathol* 1986;5:287–296.

22. Crum CP, Fu YS, Levine RU, et al. Intraepithelial squamous lesions of the vulva: biologic and histologic criteria for the distinction of condylomas from vulvar intraepithelial neoplasia. *Am J Obstet Gynecol* 1982;144:77–83.

23. Fu YS, Reagan JW, Richart RM. Definition of precursors. *Gynecol Oncol* 1981;12:s220–s231.

24. Fujii T, Crum CP, Winkler B, Fu YS, et al. Human papillomavirus infection and cervical intraepithelial neoplasia; histopathology and DNA content. *Obstet Gynecol* 1984;63:99–104.

25. Crum CP, Mitao M, Levine RU, Silverstein S. Cervical papillomaviruses segregate within morphologically distinct precancerous lesions. *J Virol* 1984;54:675–681.

26. Ferenczy A, Richart RM. *Female reproductive system: dynamics of scan and transmission electron microscopy.* New York: John Wiley & Sons, 1974.

27. Weid GL, ed. *Proceedings of the first international congress exfoliative cytology.* Philadelphia: JB Lippincott, 1961:287.

28. Koss LG, Stewart FW, Foote FW, et al. Some histological aspects of behavior of epidermoid carcinoma *in situ* and related lesions of the uterine cervix. A long-term prospective study. *Cancer* 1962;9:1160–1211.

29. Nasiell K, Nasiell M, Vaclavinkova V. Behavior of moderate cervical dysplasia during long term follow-up. *Obstet Gynecol* 1983;61:609–614.

30. Richart RM, Barron BA. A followup study of patients with cervical dysplasia. *Am J Obstet Gynecol* 1969;105:386–393.

31. Wilbanks GD, Richart RM, Terner JY. DNA content of cervical intraepithelial neoplasia studied by two-wavelength Feulgen cytophotometry. *Am J Obstet Gynecol* 1967;98:792–799.

32. Meisels A, Roy M, Fortier R. Human papillomavirus infection of the cervix: the atypical condyloma. *Acta Cytol* 1981;25:7–16.

33. Fu YS, Braun L, Shah KV, et al. Histologic, nuclear DNA and human papillomavirus study of cervical condylomas. *Cancer* 1983;52:1705–1711.

34. Winkler B, Crum CP, Fujii T, et al. Koilocytotic lesions of the cervix: the relationship of mitotic abnormalities to the presence of papillomavirus antigens and nuclear DNA content. *Cancer* 1984;53:1081–1087.

35. Gissman L, Wolnick L, Ikenberg H, et al. Human papillomavirus type 6 and 11 DNA sequences in genital and laryngeal papillomas and in some cervical cancers. *Proc Natl Acad Sci USA* 1983;80:560–563.

36. Durst M, Gissman L, Ikenberg H, et al. A papillomavirus DNA from a cervical carcinoma and its prevalence in cancer biopsy samples from different geographic regions. *Proc Natl Acad Sci USA* 1983;80:3812–3815.

37. Crum CP, Ikenberg H, Richart RM, Gissman L. Human papillomavirus type 16 in early cervical neoplasia. *N Engl J Med* 1984;310:880–883.

38. Reid R, Greenberg M, Jenson AB, et al. Sexually transmitted papillomaviral infection I. The anatomic distribution and pathological grade of neoplastic lesions associated with different viral types. *Am J Obstet Gynecol* 1987;156:212–222.

39. Campion MJ, Cuzich J, McCance DJ, Singer A. Progressive potential of mild cervical atypia: prospective cytological, colposcopical and virological study. *Lancet* 1986;2:237–240.

40. Rando RF, Sedlacek TV, Hunt J, et al. Verrucous carcinoma of the vulva associated with an unusual type 6 human papillomavirus. *Obstet Gynecol* 1986;67:70s–75s.

41. Crum CP, Egawa K, Fu YS, et al. Atypical immature metaplasia (AIM): a subset of human papillomavirus infection of the cervix. *Cancer* 1983;51:2214–2219.

42. Kurman R, Shah KH, Lancaster WD, et al. Immunoperoxidase localization of papillomavirus antigens in cervical dysplasias and vulvar condylomas. *Am J Obstet Gynecol* 1981;140:931–935.

43. Crum CP, Nagai N, Levine RU, Silverstein S. *In situ* hybridization analysis of HPV 16 DNA in early cervical neoplasia. *Am J Pathol* 1986;123:174–182.

44. Syrjanen K, Valkrynen M, Saarikoski S, et al. Natural history of cervical human papillomavirus (HPV) infection based upon prospective followup. *Br J Obstet Gynecol* 1986;92:1086–1092.

45. Lorincz AT, Temple GF, Patterson JA, et al. Correlation of cellular atypia and human papillomavirus DNA sequences in exfoliated cells of the uterine cervix. *Obstet Gynecol* 1986;68:508–512.

46. Ng ABP, Reagan JW, Yen SSC. Herpes genitalis: clinical and cytopathological experience with 256 patients. *Obstet Gynecol* 1970;36:645–651.

47. Schaefer C. Tuberculosis of the female genital tract. *Clin Obstet Gynecol* 1970;13:965–998.

48. Reagan JW, Fu YS. The uterine cervix. In: Silverberg S, ed. *Principles and practice of surgical pathology.* New York: John Wiley & Sons, 1983:1219–1263.

49. Wenckebach GFC, Curry B. Cytomegalovirus infection of the female genital tract. *Arch Pathol Lab Med* 1976;100:609–612.

50. Evans CS, Goldman RL, Klein HZ, Kohout ND. Necrobiotic granulomas of the uterine cervix. A probable postoperative reaction. *Am J Surg Pathol* 1984;8:841–844.

51. Davis JR, Steinbronn KK, Graham AR, Dawson BV. Effects of Monsel's solution in uterine cervix. *Am J Clin Pathol* 1984;82:332–335.

52. Kiviat NB, Paavonen JA, Brockway J. Cytologic manifestations of cervical and vaginal infection. I. Epithelial and inflammatory cellular changes. *JAMA* 1985;253:989–996.

53. Crum CP, Mitao M, Winkler B, et al. Localizing chlamydial infection in cervical biopsies with the immunoperoxidase technique. *Int J Gynecol Pathol* 1984;3:191–197.

54. Winkler BW, Crum CP. *Chlamydia trachomatis* infection of the female genital tract: pathogenetic and clinico-pathologic correlations. In: Rosen PP, Fechner R, eds. *Pathology annual.* New York: Appleton-Century-Crofts, 1985:193–223.

55. Giampaolo C, Murphy J, Benes S, McCormack WM. How sensitive is the Papanicolaou smear in the diagnosis of *Chlamydia trachomatis? Am J Clin Pathol* 1983;80:844–849.

56. Tam MR, Stamm WE, Handsfeld HH, et al. Culture-independent diagnosis of *Chlamydia trachomatis* using monoclonal antibodies. *N Engl J Med* 1984;310:1146–1149.

57. Wagner D, Ikenberg H, Boehm N, et al. Type specific identifica-

tion of human papillomavirus in cells obtained from cervical swabs by DNA *in-situ* hybridization—a cytologic-virologic correlation study. *Obstet Gynecol* 1984;64:767–772.

58. Schneider A, Kraus H, Schumann R, et al. Papillomavirus infection of the lower genital tract: detection of viral DNA in gynecologic swabs. *Int J Cancer* 1985;35:443–448.

59. Fife KH, Rogers RE, Zwickl BW. Symptomatic and asymptomatic cervical infection with human papillomavirus during pregnancy. *J Infect Dis* 1987;156:904–911.

60. Boyes DA, Worth AJ, Fidler HK. The results of treatment of 4389 cases of preclinical squamous cell carcinoma. *J Obstet Gynaecol Br Commonwealth* 1973;77:769–780.

61. Savage EW. Microinvasive carcinoma of the cervix. *Am J Obstet Gynecol* 1972;113:708–717.

62. Ng ABP, Reagan JW. Microinvasive carcinoma of the uterine cervix. *Am J Clin Pathol* 1969;52:511–529.

63. Rubio CA, Soderberg G, Einhorn N. Histological and followup studies in cases of microinvasive carcinoma of the uterine cervix. *Acta Path Microbiol Scand* [A] 1974;82:397–410.

64. Leman MH, Benson WL, Kurman RJ, et al. Microinvasive carcinoma of the cervix. *Obstet Gynecol* 1976;48:571–578.

65. Wilkinson EJ, Komorowski RA. Borderline microinvasive carcinoma of the cervix. *Obstet Gynecol* 1977;51:472–476.

66. Sedlis A, Sall S, Tsukada Y, et al. Microinvasive carcinoma of the uterine cervix: a clinicopathologic study. *Am J Obstet Gynecol* 1979;133:64–74.

67. Hasumi K, Sakamoto A, Sugano H. Microinvasive carcinoma of the uterine cervix. *Cancer* 1980;45:928–931.

68. Van Nagell JR, Greenwell N, Powell DF. Microinvasive carcinoma of the cervix. *Am J Obstet Gynecol* 1983;145:981–991.

69. Benson WL, Norris HJ. A critical review of the frequency of lymph node metastasis and death from microinvasive carcinoma of the cervix. *Obstet Gynecol* 1977;49:632–638.

70. Roche WD, Norris HJ. Microinvasive carcinoma of the cervix. The significance of lymphatic invasion and confluent patterns of growth. *Cancer* 1975;36:180–186.

71. Burghardt E, Holzer E. Diagnosis and treatment of microinvasive carcinoma of the uterine cervix. *Obstet Gynecol* 1977;49:641–653.

72. Fidler HK, Boyes DA, Worth AJ. Cervical cancer detection in British Columbia. *J Obstet Gynecol Br Commonwealth* 1968;75:392–404.

73. Barron BA, Cahill MC, Richart RM. A statistical model of the natural history of cervical neoplastic disease: the duration of carcinoma *in situ*. *Gynecol Oncol* 1978;6:196–205.

74. Schiller W, Daro AF, Gollin HA, et al. Small pre-ulcerative invasive carcinoma of the cervix-the spray carcinoma. *Am J Obstet Gynecol* 1953;65:1088–1098.

75. Reagan JW, Mamonic MS, Wentz WB. Analytical study of the cells in cervical squamous cell cancer. *Lab Invest* 1957;6:241–250.

76. Reagan JW, Fu YS. Histologic types and prognosis of cancers of the uterine cervix. *Int J Radiol Oncol Biol Phys* 1979;5:1015–1020.

77. Randall ME, Constable WC, Hahn SS, et al. Results of the radiotherapeutic management of carcinomas of the cervix with emphasis on the influence of histologic classification. *Cancer* 1988 (*in press*).

78. Daroca PJ, Dhurandhar HN. Basaloid carcinoma of the uterine cervix. *Am J Surg Pathol* 1980;4:235–239.

79. Spratt DW, Lee SC. Verrucous carcinoma of the cervix. *Am J Obstet Gynecol* 1977;129:699–670.

80. Abramson A, Brandsma J, Steinberg B, et al. Verrucous carcinoma of the larynx. Possible human papillomavirus etiology. *Arch Otolaryngol* 1985;111:709–715.

81. Gissman L, de Villiers E-M, zur Hausen H. Analysis of genital warts and other genital tumors for human papillomavirus type 6 DNA. *Int J Cancer* 1982;29:143–146.

82. Kister RW, Hertig AT. Papillomas of the uterine cervix—the malignant potentiality. *Obstet Gynecol* 1955;6:147–161.

83. Qizilbash A. Papillary squamous tumors of the uterine cervix. A clinical and pathological study of 21 cases. *Am J Clin Pathol* 1974;61:508–520.

84. Randall ME, Andersen WA, Mills SE, et al. Papillary squamous cell carcinoma of the uterine cervix. A clinicopathologic study of nine cases. *Int J Gynecol Pathol* 1986;5:1–10.

85. Walker AN, Mills SE. Unusual variants of uterine cervical carcinoma. *Pathol Annu* 1987:277–310.

86. Venkataseshan VS, Woo TH. Diffuse viral papillomatosis (condyloma) of the uterine cavity. *Int J Gynecol Pathol* 1985;4:370–377.

87. Ferenczy A, Richart RM, Okagaki T. Endometrial involvement by cervical carcinoma *in-situ*. *Am J Obstet Gynecol* 1971;110:590–592.

88. Christopherson WM, Nealon N, Gray LA. Non-invasive precursor lesions of adenocarcinoma and mixed adenosquamous carcinoma of the cervix uteri. *Cancer* 1979;44:975–983.

89. Maier RC, Norris HJ. Coexistence of cervical intraepithelial neoplasia with primary adenocarcinoma of the endocervix. *Obstet Gynecol* 1980;56:361–364.

90. Menczer J, Yaron-Schiffer O, Leventon-Criss S. Herpes virus Type 2 and adenocarcinoma of the uterine cervix: a possible association. *Cancer* 1981;48:1497–1499.

91. Smotkin D, Berek J, Fu Y-S, et al. Human papillomavirus DNA in adenocarcinoma and adenosquamous carcinoma of the uterine cervix. *Obstet Gynecol* 1986;68:241–244.

92. Bousfield L, Pacey F, Young Q. Expanded cytologic criteria for the diagnosis of adenocarcinoma *in-situ* of the cervix and related lesions. *Acta Cytol* 1980;24:283–295.

93. Betsill WL, Clark AH. Early endocervical glandular neoplasia. Histomorphology and cytomorphology. *Acta Cytol* 1986;30:115–126.

94. Leslie KO, Silverberg SG. Microglandular hyperplasia of the cervix: unusual clinical and pathological presentations and their differential diagnosis. *Pathol Annu* 1982:95–114.

95. Fluhman CF. *The cervix and its diseases*, 1st edition. Philadelphia: WB Saunders, 1961.

96. Davis JR, Moon LB. Increased incidence of adenocarcinoma of the uterine cervix. *Obstet Gynecol* 1975;45:79–83.

97. Tamimi HK, Figge DC. Adenocarcinoma of the uterine cervix *Gynecol Oncol* 1982;13:335–344.

98. Hurt WG, Silverberg SG, Frable WF, et al. Adenocarcinoma of the cervix: histopathologic and clinical features. *Am J Obstet Gynecol* 1977;129:304–313.

99. Saigo PE, Cain JM, Kim WS, et al. Prognostic factors in adenocarcinoma of the uterine cervix. *Cancer* 1986;57:1584–1593.

100. Fu YS, Reagan JW, Hsiu JG, et al. Adenocarcinoma and mixed carcinoma of the uterine cervix. I. A clinicopathologic study. *Cancer* 1982;49:2560–2570.

101. Abell MR, Gosling JRG. Gland cell carcinoma (adenocarcinoma) of the uterine cervix. *Am J Obstet Gynecol* 1962;83:729–755.

102. Weiss RJ, Lucas WE. Adenocarcinoma of the uterine cervix. *Cancer* 1986;57:1996–2001.

103. Abell MR. Invasive carcinomas of uterine cervix. In: Norris HJ, Hertig AT, Abell MR, eds. *The uterus.* International Academy of Pathology Monograph. Baltimore: Williams & Wilkins, 1973:13–456.

104. Moberg PJ, Einhorn N, Silfversward C, Soderberg G. Adenocarcinoma of the uterine cervix. *Cancer* 1986;57:407–410.

105. Milsom I, Friberg LG. Primary adenocarcinoma of the uterine cervix: a clinical study. *Cancer* 1983;52:942–947.

106. Menczner J, Modan B, Oelsner G, et al. Adenocarcinoma of the uterine cervix in Jewish women. A distinct epidemiological entity. *Cancer* 1978;41:2464–2467.

107. Kaku T, Hachisuga T, Toyoshima S, et al. Extremely well-differentiated adenocarcinoma ("adenoma malignum") of the cervix in a patient with Peutz-Jeghers syndrome. *Int J Gynecol Pathol* 1985;4:266–273.

108. Saigo PE, Wolinska WH, Kim KS, Hadju SI. The role of cytology in the diagnosis and followup of patients with cervical adenocarcinoma. *Acta Cytol* 1985;29:785–794.

109. Senekjian EK, Hubby M, Bell DA, et al. Clear cell adenocarcinoma (CCA) of the vagina and cervix in association with pregnancy. *Gynecol Oncol* 1986;24:207–219.

110. Pollack RS, Taylor HC. Carcinoma of the cervix during the first two decades of life. *Am J Obstet Gynecol* 1947;53:135–141.

111. Scully RE, Robboy SJ, Welch WR. Pathology and pathogenesis of diethylstilbesterol—related disorders of the female genital tract. In: Herbst AL, ed. *Intrauterine exposure to diethylstilbesterol in the human.* Chicago: American College of Obstetrics and Gynecologists, 1978:8–22.

112. Sorvari TE. A histochemical study of epitheial mucosubstances in endometrial and cervical adenocarcinoma. With reference to normal endometrium and cervical mucosa. *Acta Pathol Microbiol Scand [Suppl]* 1969;207:1–85.

113. Abell MR. Invasive carcinomas of uterine cervix. In: Norris HJ, Hertig AT, Abell MR, eds. *The uterus.* International Academy of Pathology Monograph. Baltimore: Williams & Wilkins, 1973:413–456.

114. Steeper TA, Wick MR. Minimal deviation adenocarcinoma of the uterine cervix ("adenoma malignum"): an immunohistochemical comparison with microglandular endocervical hyperplasia and conventional endocervical adenocarcinoma. *Cancer* 1986;58:1131–1138.

115. Kaminski PF, Norris HJ. Minimal deviation carcinoma (adenoma malignum) of the cervix. *Int J Gynecol Pathol* 1983;2:141–152.

116. Michael H, Grawe L, Kraus FT. Minimal deviation endocervical adenocarcinoma: clinical and histologic features, immunohistochemical staining for carcinoembryonic antigen, and differentiation from confusing benign lesions. *Int J Gynecol Pathol* 1984;3:261–276.

117. Silverberg SG, Hurt WG. Minimal deviation adenocarcinoma (adenoma malignum) of the cervix: a reappraisal. *Am J Obstet Gynecol* 1983;121:971–975.

118. Rombout RP, Charles D, Murphy A. Adenocarcinoma of the cervix. A clinicopathologic study of 47 cases. *Cancer* 1966;19:891–900.

119. Herbst AL, Cole P, Norusis MJ, et al. Epidemiologic aspects and factors related to survival in 384 registry cases of clear cell adenocarcinoma of the vagina and cervix. *Am J Obstet Gynecol* 1979;135:876–886.

120. Herbst AL, Robboy SL, Scully RE. Clear cell adenocarcinoma of the vagina and cervix in girls. Analysis of 170 Registry cases. *Am J Obstet Gynecol* 1974;119:713–724.

121. Johnston GA Jr, Anderson D, Herbst AL, et al. Clear cell carcinoma of the vagina and cervix in black females. *J Natl Med Assoc* 1982;74:361–363.

122. Kaminski PF, Maier RC. Clear cell adenocarcinoma of the cervix unrelated to diethylstilbestrol exposure. *Obstet Gynecol* 1983;62:720–727.

123. Cherry CP, Glucksmann A. Histopathology of carcinomas of the uterine cervix and survival rates in pregnant and nonpregnant patients. *Surg Gynecol Obstet* 1961;113:763–776.

124. Wheeless CR, Graham RM, Graham JB. Prognosis and treatment of adenoepidermoid carcinoma of the cervix. *Obstet Gynecol* 1970;35:928–932.

125. Glucksmann A. Relationships between hormonal changes in pregnancy and the development of mixed carcinoma of the uterine cervix. *Cancer* 1957;10:831–837.

126. Glucksman A, Cherry CP. Incidence, histology, and response to radiation of mixed carcinomas (adenoacanthomas) of the uterine cervix. *Cancer* 1956;9:971–979.

127. Steiner G, Friedell GH. Adenosquamous carcinoma *in-situ* of the cervix. *Cancer* 1965;18:807–810.

128. Fowler WC, Miles PA, Surwit EA, et al. Adenoid cystic carcinoma of the cervix: report of 9 cases and a reappraisal. *Obstet Gynecol* 1978;52:337–342.

129. Hoskins WJ, Averette AG, Ng ABP, et al. Adenoid cystic carcinoma of the cervix uteri: report of 6 cases and review of the literature. *Gynecol Oncol* 1979;7:371–384.

130. Prempree T, Villa Santa U, Tang CK. Management of adenoid cystic carcinoma of the uterine cervix (cylindroma). *Cancer* 1980;46:1631–1635.

131. Cohen C, Shulman G, Budgeon LR. Endocervical and endometrial adenocarcinoma: an immunoperoxidase and histochemical study. *Am J Surg Pathol* 1982;6:151–157.

132. Wahlstrom T, Lindgren J, Korhonen M, et al. Distinction between endocervical and endometrial adenocarcinoma with immunoperoxidase staining of carcinoembyonic antigen in routine histological specimens. *Lancet* 1979;1159–1160.

133. Lemoine NR, Hall PA. Epithelial tumors metastatic to the uterine cervix. A study of 33 cases and review of the literature. *Cancer* 1986;57:2002–2005.

134. Van Nagell JR, Donaldson ES, Wood EG, et al. Small cell cancer of the uterine cervix. *Cancer* 1977;40:2243–2249.

135. Barrett RJ, Davos I, Leuchter RS, Lagasse LD. Neuroendocrine features in poorly differentiated and undifferentiated carcinomas of the cervix. *Cancer* 1987;60:2325–2325.

136. Albores-Saavedra J, Larraza P, Poucell S, et al. Carcinoids of the uterine cervix: additional observations in a new tumor entity. *Cancer* 1976;38:2328–2342.

137. Groben P, Reddick R, Askin F. The pathologic spectrum of small cell carcinoma of the cervix. *Int J Gynecol Pathol* 1985;4:42–57.

138. Mullins JD, Hilliard GD. Cervical carcinoid ("argyrophil cell carcinoma") associated with an endocervical adenocarcinoma: a light and ultra-structural study. *Cancer* 1981;47:785–790.

139. MacKay B, Osborne BM, Wharton JT. Small cell tumor of the cervix with neuroepithelial features: ultrastructural observations in two cases. *Cancer* 1979;43:1138–1145.

140. Pearce AGE. The APUD cell concept and its implications in pathology. *Pathol Annu* 1974;9:27–41.

141. Fox H, Kazzaz B, Langley FA. Argyrophil and argentaffin cells in the female genital tract and in ovarian mucinous cysts. *J Pathol Bacteriol* 1964;88:479–488.

142. Stassart J, Crum CP, Yordan EL, et al. Argyrophilic carcinoma of the cervix: a report of a case with coexisting cervical intraepithelial neoplasia. *Gynecol Oncol* 1982;13:247–251.

143. Taxi JB, Tischler AS, Insalaco SJ, et al. "Carcinoid" tumor of the breast. A variant of breast cancer? *Hum Pathol* 1981;12:170–179.

144. Gould VE, Wiedenmann B, Lee I, et al. Synaptophysin expression in neuroendocrine neoplasms as determined by immunocytochemistry. *Am J Pathol* 1987;126:243–257.

145. Said JW, Vimadalal S, Nash G, et al. Immunoreactive neuron-specific enolase, bombesin, and chromogranin as markers for neuroendocrine lung tumors. *Hum Pathol* 1985;16:236–240.

146. Inoue M, Ueda G, Nakajima T. Immunohistochemical demonstration of neuron-specific enolase in gynecologic malignant tumors. *Cancer* 1985;55:1686–1690.

147. Fujii S, Konishi I, Ferenczy A, et al. Small cell undifferentiated carcinoma of the uterine cervix: histology, ultrastructure, and immunohistochemistry of two cases. *Ultrastruct Pathol* 1986;10:337–346.

148. Littman P, Clement PB, Henriksen B, et al. Glassy cell carcinoma of the cervix. *Cancer* 1976;37:2238–2246.

149. Mills SE, Austin MB, Randall ME. Lymphoepithelioma-like carcinoma of the uterine cervix. A distinctive, undifferentiated carcinoma with inflammatory stroma. *Am J Surg Pathol* 1985;9:883–889.

150. Aaro LA, Jacobsen LJ, Soule E. Endocervical polyps. *Obstet Gynecol* 1963;21:659–665.

151. Dougherty CM, Moore WR, Cotten N. Histological diagnosis and clinical significance of benign lesions of the nonpregnant cervix. *Ann NY Acad Sci* 1962;97:683–702.

152. Lippert LJ, Richart RM, Ferenczy A. Giant benign endocervical polyp: report of a case. *Am J Obstet Gynecol* 1974;118:1140–1141.

153. Cachaza JA, Caballero JJL, Fernandez JA, Salido E. Endocervical polyp with pseudosarcomatous pattern and cytoplasmic inclusions: an electron microscopic study. *Am J Clin Pathol* 1986;85:633–635.

154. Chirayil SJ, Tobon H. Polyps of the vagina: a clinicopathologic analysis of 18 cases. *Cancer* 1981;47:2904–2907.

155. Selzer I, Nelson H. Benign papilloma (polypoid tumor) of the cervix uteri in children. *Am J Obstet Gynecol* 1962;84:165–169.

156. Abell MR. Papillary adenofibroma of the uterine cervix. *Am J Obstet Gynecol* 1971;110:990–993.

157. Zaloudek CJ, Norris HJ. Adenofibroma and adenosarcoma. A clinical and pathological study of 35 benign and low grade variants of mixed mesodermal tumor of the uterus. *Cancer* 1981;48:354–366.

158. Gusdon JT. Hemangioma of the cervix. *Am J Obstet Gynecol* 1965;91:204–209.

159. Nuovo GJ, Nagler HM, Fenoglio JJ. Arteriovenous malformation of the bladder presenting as gross hematuria. *Hum Pathol* 1986;17:94–97.

160. Rilke F, Cantaboni A. Lipomas of the uterus. Presentation of 2 cases and a review of the recent literature. *Ann Obstet Gynecol.* 1964;86:645.

161. Patel DS, Bhagavan BS. Blue nevus of the uterine cervix. *Hum Pathol* 1985;16:79–86.

162. Dundore W, Lamas C. Benign nevus (ephelis) of the uterine cervix. *Am J Obstet Gynecol* 1985;152:881–882.

163. Luevano-Flores E, Sotelo J, Tena-Suck M. Glial polyp (glioma) of the uterine cervix, report of a case with demonstration of glial fibrillary acidic protein. *Gynecol Oncol* 1985;21:385–390.

164. Stout AP. Hemangioendothelioma: a tumor of blood vessels featuring vascular endothelial cells. *Ann Surg* 1943;118:445–464.

165. Jaffe R, Altaras M, Bernheim J, Aderet NB. Endocervical stromal sarcoma—a case report. *Gynecol Oncol* 1985;22:105–108.

166. Abell MR, Ramirez JA. Sarcomas and carcinosarcomas of the uterine cervix. *Cancer* 1973;31:176–192.

167. Williamson HO, McIver FA. Sarcoma botryoides of the cervix treated by vaginal hysterectomy and subtotal vaginectomy. *Obstet Gynecol* 1968;31:689–694.

168. Bell DA, Shimm DS, Gang DL. Wilms' tumor of the endocervix. *Arch Pathol Lab Med* 1985;109:371–373.

169. Chen KTK. Rhabdomyosarcomatous uterine sarcoma. *Int J Gynecol Pathol* 1985;4:146–152.

170. Hart WR, Craig JR. Rhabdomyosarcomas of the uterus. *Am J Clin Pathol* 1978;70:217–223.

171. Lathrop JC. Views and reviews. Malignant pelvic lymphomas. *Obstet Gynecol* 1967;30:137–145.

172. Volpe R, Tirelli U, Tumolo S, et al. Stage IIe diffuse small cleaved cell lymphoma of the cervix. *Pathologica* 1983;75:887–892.

173. Freeman C, Berg JW, Cutler SJ. Occurrence and prognosis of extranodal lymphomas. *Cancer* 1972;29:252–260.

Surgical Pathology of the Female Reproductive System and Peritoneum, edited by Stephen S. Sternberg and Stacey E. Mills. Raven Press, Ltd, New York © 1991.

CHAPTER 5

The Uterine Corpus

Michael R. Hendrickson and Richard L. Kempson

EVALUATION OF ENDOMETRIAL AND MYOMETRIAL SPECIMENS

Endometrial Samples

The most commonly employed endometrial sampling techniques are the dilation and curettage (D&C) and the endometrial biopsy. The D&C is, in essence, an excisional biopsy of the endometrium (1–3). This is the most complete sampling technique, if done correctly, although mechanically distorting lesions such as leiomyomas and polyps may occasionally shield some portion of the endometrial tissue from the curet. The D&C requires anesthesia, and there is a small but definite risk of uterine perforation or secondary amenorrhea and subsequent postcurettage adhesions (Asherman's syndrome) (4,5). The endometrial biopsy, in contrast, is an inexpensive office procedure and does not require anesthesia (6). The chief disadvantages of the endometrial biopsy are the limited sample that is obtained (usually not a problem) and its unsuitability for the diagnosis and removal of such focal lesions as endometrial polyps. In a patient suspected of having a malignant neoplasm, a negative biopsy does not exclude that possibility, and it is mandatory to perform a curettage on such patients if the biopsy does not contain malignancy (7–11). Patients who are being evaluated for infertility should be biopsied well into the presumed luteal phase, as determined by the shift in basal-body temperature or hormonal assays (12,13). The optimal time for biopsy is postovulatory day 8 to 10, although some have advocated biopsy at the onset of uterine bleeding (13a). Usually, biopsies are recommended for at least two consecutive cycles.

The importance of correlating the morphologic features of an endometrial biopsy with the clinical findings cannot be overemphasized. A morphologically normal endometrium may be associated with a variety of abnormal clinical states. For example, a morphologically normal late proliferative endometrium is obviously abnormal during what should be a patient's late luteal phase. The minimal clinical information should include the patient's age, the last menstrual period (and its characteristics), the previous menstrual period (and its characteristics), whether or not the patient is taking steroidal medication, and an explanation of the current chief complaint and physical findings. In general, progestational agents should not be administered prior to a diagnostic curettage, particularly in a postmenopausal patient. These agents can mask important features necessary to identify abnormal endometrial proliferative states, including adenocarcinoma.

Hysterectomy Specimens

An outline containing suggestions for the handling of hysterectomy specimens received for various reasons is supplied in Tables 1 and 2. The sections taken are very much dependent upon the clinical questions being asked (explicitly or implicitly) and the gross abnormalities encountered in sectioning the specimen.

Myomectomy Specimens

The gross appearance of these specimens is particularly important in regard to the question of possible leiomyosarcoma. Almost all leiomyosarcomas deviate from the characteristic gross features of leiomyomas by being soft, hemorrhagic, and/or necrotic. Sections must be suitable for mitotic counts, i.e., thin and well stained (Table 3).

APPROACH TO UTERINE CORPUS DIAGNOSIS (14)

Even in the absence of any prior information, the range of differential diagnostic possibilities is narrowed

TABLE 1. *Approach to the hysterectomy specimen for uterine corpus disease*

Uterus removed for non-neoplastic disease

No gross pathology present
  One section of the anterior or posterior fundal
    endometrium and subjacent myometrium
  Standard cervix sections (see Chapter 47)
Gross pathology discovered
  See Table 2 (gross differential diagnosis) for
    recommendations

Uterus removed for neoplastic disease

1. *Endometrial carcinoma*
  Questions that motivate the examination:
    1. What is the histologic type and (if appropriate) grade
      of the carcinoma?
    2. What is surgical Stage?
  Sectioning of the endometrium
    Confirm the prehysterectomy diagnosis
      • Special variant?
      • Grade? (if not a special variant)
  Assessing the depth of myometrial invasion
    • Record gross impression (sections should include
      what grossly appears to be the deepest extent of the
      myoinvasion)
    • Record microscopic impression (in 1/2's or 1/3's)
    • Check vascular invasion or psammoma bodies
      (UPSC) (particularly with high-grade carcinomas)
      N.B: Mimics of myoinvasion
        • Carcinoma involving an irregular
          endomyometrial junction (i.e., basalis)
        • Carcinoma involving foci of adenomyosis
        • Involvement of the mucosa of the intramural
          portion of the fallopian tube by carcinoma
  Assessment of the cervix (if involvement is documented—
    i.e., surgical Stage II—additional therapy may be
    warranted)
    • Sections should include the high cervical canal and
      the lower uterine segment. Check the deep lymphatics!
    • With extensive involvement of the cervix, give some
      thought to a cervical primary secondarily involving the
      uterine corpus
    • Simultaneous primary cervical and uterine corpus
      neoplasms is also a possibility raised by the finding of
      divergent histologies in the two sites
    • Are the vaginal and cervical margins of the specimen
      free of carcinoma?
  Assessment of the adnexa
    • If the endometrial carcinoma is a high-risk variant
      (e.g., UPSC), carefully check the hilar lymphatics (the
      ovaries may well be grossly normal)
    • Check if low-grade endometrioid carcinoma is
      present in the ovary and if the uterine corpus
      carcinoma is not myoinvasive
    • May be a simultaneous primary Stage I ovarian and
      Stage I endometrial (rather than a Stage III
      endometrial carcinoma)
2. Uterine sarcoma
  Questions that motivate examination:
    1. What is the histologic type of sarcoma?
    2. What is the surgical Stage?
    • Protocol is much the same as for endometrial
      adenocarcinoma detailed above
    • If the histologic type is in doubt, more sections of tumor
      may be required than for cases of adenocarcinoma
    • Check margins of resection

initially by the overall low-power appearance of the endometrium. Most specimens fall into one of six "low-power groups." In our view, it is very helpful in formulating differential diagnoses to examine the endometrium at low-power magnification and attempt to place it into one of the following six categories.

Pattern 1. Proliferations Composed of Glands and Supportive Non-neoplastic Stroma

This is the most common type of pattern encountered in endometrial pathology. The low-power evaluation of the ratio of glands to stroma leads to a further general low-power sorting into three categories: (i) A normal, roughly one-to-one glands-to-stroma ratio is exhibited by most normal cycling endometria and is also encountered in the majority of endometria associated with dysfunctional uterine bleeding and infertility. (ii) Endometria marked by a shift in the glands-to-stromal ratio in favor of glands include some fully developed late secretory and menstrual endometria, endometrial hyperplasias, and carcinomas. (iii) Endometria featuring a predominance of stroma include normal decidua, some examples of atrophy, and all of the pattern-3 monophasic stromal proliferations listed below.

Glands

The next step in narrowing the differential diagnosis involves an examination of the cytology and the architecture of the constituent glands. Proliferating glands are lined by columnar epithelium exhibiting nuclear pseudostratification, mitotic figures, high nucleus-to-cytoplasm ratios, and elongate ovoid nuclei with dense basophilic chromatin. Cytologic atypia in such glands is manifest by an increase in nuclear (and cell) size, an increase in the nucleus-to-cytoplasm ratio, increasing prominence of nucleoli, rounding of nuclei, and a tendency of the cells to become stratified. In many carcinomas the epithelium tends to grow in a complex stratified sheet-like pattern punctuated by sharply rounded spaces (cribriform pattern). Atrophic and weakly proliferative glands are lined by low cuboidal to columnar cells with sparse or absent mitotic figures.

Secretory epithelia can be broadly divided into those exhibiting early secretory changes and those exhibiting late secretory changes. In early secretion a large cytoplasmic vacuole is present in either the subnuclear or the supranuclear position. In the fully developed secretory gland the epithelium is low columnar to cuboidal and the cells possess an oval-to-round vesicular, usually basilar nucleus, with a small but discernible nucleolus. The cytoplasm is eosinophilic to clear. Well-developed secretory glands are dilated and frequently show luminal secretion and luminal border fraying. Marked cytoplasmic vacuolization associated with nuclear hyperchro-

TABLE 2. *Differential diagnosis of gross findings in the uterus*

Focally polypoid endometrium
Endometrial polyp
  Multicystic cut surface
  May be sessile or pedunculated
Submucous leiomyoma
  Firm whorled cut surface
  Thin, focally hemorrhagic
    lining mucosa
Atypical polypoid adenomyoma
  Usually located in lower uterine segment
  Compressive margin
Adenofibroma
  Firm, multicystic
  Not necrotic
  N.B: Multiple sections to distinguish from adenosarcoma
Polypoid malignancy
  Firm, friable
  Focal necrosis
  Check for myoinfiltration
    Neoplasms to consider:
      Adenocarcinoma (unusual presentation)
      Malignant mixed müllerian tumor (common presentation)
      Adenosarcoma (common presentation)
 	
Diffusely thickened endometrium
Secretory endometrium
  Lush, polypoid
  No necrosis
  May be hemorrhagic if close to menstruation
Gestational endometrium or florid decidual reaction
  Look for evidence of pregnancy
    Placental fragments
    Gestational sac
	Hyperplastic-carcinomatous endometrium
	  Lush, polypoid endometrium
	  Presence of yellowish necrotic areas should raise the
	    possibility of adenocarcinoma
	  Examine and section the uterus as if a carcinoma were
	    known to be present (see below)
	
	Space occupying intramural lesions
	Leiomyoma (with/without "degeneration")
	  Shells out, bulging, trabeculated
	  Often multiple
	  Wide variety of appearances
	  N.B: Sample all smooth-muscle neoplasms with a
	    deviant gross appearance; take at least one
	    section per centimeter of diameter of any tumor
	    which has unusual microscopic features.
	Leiomyosarcoma
	  Fish-flesh consistency; hemorrhage and necrosis common
	  Infiltrative margins
	  Usually solitary mass with extension rather than one of
	    multiple masses
	Adenomyosis
	  Trabeculated smooth muscle; may be nodular
	  Merges with surrounding myometrium
	  Resists shelling out (unlike leiomyoma)
	Adenomatoid tumor
	  Subserosal cornual region
	  May be yellow
	
	Grossly visible tumor within vessels
	• Low-grade stromal neoplasm
	• Smooth-muscle neoplasms (usually intravenous
	  leiomyomatosis)

masia and pleomorphism in absence of mitotic figures is characteristic of Arias-Stella reaction. The epithelial cells of disintegrating glands often contain karyorrhectic fragments.

Architecturally, the normal endometrial gland is a nonbranched, coiled structure. Branching and budding of varying degrees of complexity are the hallmark of

TABLE 3. *Caveats concerning mitotic activity (1)*

1. Sections thin, well stained
2. Strict criteria for accepting mitotic figures
   (a) Separation of chromatin
   (b) Clear or eosinophilic cytoplasm with distinct cell membrane
   (c) Differential diagnosis: lymphocytes, mast cells, stripped nuclei, degenerated cells, precipitated hemotoxylin. If in doubt, don't accept it as a mitotic figure.
3. Perform counts in a compulsive fashion
4. Begin in area of highest mitotic activity
5. Four sets of 10 fields per section, and take the highest counts.
6. Counts are usually performed with a binocular microscope utilizing 10× or 15× wide-field eyepieces and 40× high dry objectives. Minor variations in eyepiece and objectives do not significantly affect diagnostic interpretation.

endometrial hyperplasia and carcinoma. Occasionally, secretory changes will be superimposed on the budding pattern of hyperplasia or even carcinoma.

Stroma

Characteristically, endometrial stromal cells are either oblong to spindled with scant hard-to-discern cytoplasm or they show varying degrees of deciduation. *Deciduation* refers to the transformation of a proliferative-phase stromal cell with a dense nucleus and sparse ill-defined cytoplasm to one with large ovoid-to-round vesicular nuclei and abundant well-defined eosinophilic to clear cytoplasm. Lesser degrees of this transformation are known as predecidua and are characteristic of the normal late secretory phase.

Vessels

The hallmark of the normal developing endometrium is a synchronous proliferation of blood vessels, glands, and stroma. The delicate arborizing vasculature characteristic of the normal proliferative endometrium is the hallmark of endometrial stromal neoplasms. During the normal secretory phase of the menstrual cycle the vessels become coiled into easily recognized spiral-like structures. This is particularly evident near the surface of the endometrium.

Pattern Uniformity

The hallmark of a normal endometrium is a uniformity of development from one portion of the stratum functionalis to another. In curettage or biopsy specimens this implies uniformity of one fragment to another. There are two important exceptions: (i) The region around the internal cervical os (lower uterine segment) is typically less responsive to hormonal stimulation than the functionalis in the fundus. Fragments from the lower uterine segment are very commonly present in endometrial samples and can be identified by their spindled stromal cells with intercellular collagen and the presence of hybrid endometrial-endocervical glands. (ii) The second frequently encountered "out-of-step" fragment derives from the stratum basalis. This endometrial zone maintains an essentially constant appearance throughout the menstrual cycle and does not exhibit the striking glandular and stromal changes of the cycling functionalis. The basalis is composed of small caliber, minimally torturous, weakly proliferative glands embedded in a cellular stroma. This stroma frequently intermingles with wisps of superficial myometrium.

Pattern 2. Biphasic Proliferations Composed of Glands and Abundant (Possibly Neoplastic) Stroma

Entities that figure in the differential diagnosis of this pattern include endometrial polyps, atypical polypoid adenomyomas, mixed müllerian proliferations, and some of the patterns with prominent stroma in Pattern 1 above.

Pattern 3. Predominately Monophasic Spindle-Cell Proliferations

This pattern figures prominently in the evaluation of hysterectomy or myomectomy specimens; occasionally, an endometrial sample will contain fragments of spindled stroma devoid or largely devoid of glands. The major differential diagnostic considerations raised by this low-power pattern are smooth-muscle neoplasms, endometrial stromal neoplasms, and spindled epithelial neoplasms.

Epithelial Versus Mesenchymal Differentiation

Strategies useful in separating spindled epithelial neoplasms from spindled mesenchymal neoplasms include (a) additional H&E sections to search for less equivocal epithelial differentiation and (b) reticulin stains to demonstrate reticulin around groups of cells (epithelial feature) or around single cells (mesenchymal feature). Immunohistochemical staining for keratin or muscle antigens is sometimes useful, but it should be remembered that some classes of keratin are present in normal and neoplastic smooth-muscle cells. Today we rarely, if ever, use electron microscopy for this purpose.

Smooth Muscle Versus Stromal Versus Heterologous Differentiation

Under the assumption that a proliferation is mesenchymal, a number of strategies may be useful in distinguishing these possibilities. These are set out in Table 4. This is further discussed in the introductory section of the text devoted to smooth-muscle neoplasms.

Pattern 4. Sheet-like Proliferations Composed of Large, Round, Undifferentiated Cells

A cluster of differential diagnostic problems are conveniently treated under this heading. These include leukemia, lymphoma, stromal sarcoma, malignant mixed müllerian tumor, metastatic carcinoma (particularly extragenital), and Grade III adenocarcinoma (15–17). Our usual approach to this problem is summarized below.

More H&E Sections

The most useful maneuver in sorting out this differential diagnosis in our experience is submitting more tissue if it is available, and if not, cutting deeper sections from the block.

Reticulin Stain

The usual reticulin staining pattern of carcinoma is that of reticulin around groups of cells, whereas the usual pattern of sarcoma features reticulin around individual cells. A biphasic pattern is typical of malignant mixed müllerian tumor. Unfortunately, these reticulin patterns are most dramatic when least needed, i.e., when the diagnosis is obvious on routine H&E sections.

Chloracetate Esterase Preparations

Rarely, acute myelogenous leukemia will present as a tumor mass in the endometrium, and the esterase preparation is useful in identifying this process. It must be remembered that mast cells and non-neoplastic polymorphs are also esterase-positive.

TABLE 4. *Comparison of differentiating features for endometrial stromal cells and smooth muscle cells*

Technique	Endometrial stromal cell	Usual smooth muscle cell	Epithelioid smooth muscle
Light microscopy Architecture	Reticulin around individual cells		Reticulin around single cells or groups of cells
	Haphazardly arranged cells (cf. normal proliferative endometrium)	Cells arranged in looping intersecting fascicles	Clusters and/or cords of cells compartmentalized by hyalin
	Complex plexiform vascular pattern not prominent	Vascular component	Rounded or polygonal cells with moderate amount of cytoplasm
	Hyalin often abundant		Foci of neoplasm often exhibit standard smooth-muscle features
Cytological features Nucleus	Blunt, fusiform, uniform, bland	Elongate, cigar-shaped	Round, crumpled
Cytoplasm	Scanty (on H&E and trichrome)	Moderate amount (on H&E and trichrome), typically fibrillar	Clear (vacuolated) to eosinophilic cytoplasm
			Glycogen+, slightly over half of cases
			PAS with diastase (−)
			Mucin (−) in all cases
			Lipid (−) except for slight positivity in some
Ultrastructure	Undifferentiated mesenchymal cells	Abundant, 6.0–8.0 nm, longitudinally arranged myofilaments parallel to long axis of cell; some filaments at oblique angles to these	Some cases lack ultrastructural features of smooth muscle
	No myofilaments or dense bodies		8.0–9.0-nm myofilaments with marginal dense bodies in some cells
	Intercellular collagen	Marginal spindle-shaped to oval dense bodies adjacent to plasma lemma (plaques) or along the trajectory of the filaments	Rare pinocytotic vesicles
	No basal lamina		No basement membrane materials around individual cells
	No micropinocytotic vesicles	Micropinocytotic vesicles adjacent to plasma membrane	Vacuoles probably derived from swollen mitochondria
	Complex cytoplasmic processes	Occasional cilia	
		Interrupted basal lamina around individual cells	
		(These features are variably present in tumors)	
Immunohistochemistry	Vimentin only	Muscle-specific actin	Largely unknown for uterine tumors
		Desmin	
		Cytokeratin	
		(Some tumors do not express these)	

From ref. 217.

Immunohistochemistry

The most useful procedure in identifying lymphoma in paraffin-embedded sections is a common leukocyte antigen immunohistochemical stain. Keratin, desmin, and muscle-specific actin stains may also be helpful, but their specificity is largely unknown for uterine tumors. S-100 and melanoma "specific" antibodies can be utilized when metastatic malignant melanoma is a consideration.

Clinical History and Additional Clinical Studies

When a proliferation's histologic appearance raises the possibility of a metastatic neoplasm, clinical history and additional clinical studies are often indicated. We have encountered several cases of cytologically bland, undifferentiated tumors infiltrating the endometrial stroma, which caused abnormal endometrial bleeding; a history of lobular carcinoma of the breast was elicited in each of these cases.

Usually, these five maneuvers serve to narrow the possibilities to one or two processes, and examination of the hysterectomy specimen most often establishes the diagnosis. It is obviously important to identify leukemia, lymphoma, and metastatic carcinomas, and it is rare for the procedures listed above not to do so. There are occasions when even complete sampling of a malignant uterine primary neoplasm fails to reveal the direction of differentiation of the tumor. Of some comfort is the clinical fact that failure to distingush high-grade sarcomas from malignant mixed müllerian tumor and poorly differentiated carcinoma is usually of little consequence.

Pattern 5. Samples That Feature Extensive Necrosis, Inflammation, or Disintegration

Extensive necrosis in endometrial samples should always raise the possibility of a malignancy, especially carcinoma. A careful search should be made for individual cytologically malignant cells in such a sample. Inflammatory cells and necrosis are a normal finding in the postpartum endometrium, but sheets of polymorphs (pus) should raise the possibility of a postpartum bacterial infection. Necrotic endometrial samples are obtained when cervical stenosis and pyometra are present.

Disintegrating endometria may be encountered in a variety of settings most commonly at the time of menstruation. The features of menstrual endometrium are familiar. Glands exhibit secretory exhaustion surrounded by a halo of disintegrating, swollen predecidual cells; often both are suspended in fibrin and blood. Karyorrhectic fragments are often present in epithelial cells. Nonsecretory endometria, including hyperplastic endometria, may also disintegrate. On occasion, the degenerative changes produced in the epithelial and stromal cells of these endometria raise the possibility of malignancy. For the same reason that a diagnosis of malignancy should be avoided in *cytologic* specimens composed of degenerated cells, so a diagnosis of malignancy should be avoided in this setting. If the specimen exhibits degeneration and disintegration, and when carcinoma is a possibility, we recommend repeat tissue sampling.

Pattern 6. Scanty Samples That Raise the Question of Sampling Adequacy

Scanty endometrial samples are commonly encountered. There are a number of diagnostic possibilities. Occasionally, this may be due to inadequate sampling because of an obstructing lesion, but more commonly there is little or no endometrium at the time of sampling either because the endometrium was atrophic or because of prior endometrial shedding or removal. When

neoplasm is suspected, inquiries about the thoroughness and extent of the curettage should be made.

SPECIFIC PATTERNS AND THEIR DIFFERENTIAL DIAGNOSIS

The Normal Menstrual Cycle Endometrium (12,18–20)

It is important in the evaluation of an infertile patient's endometrial biopsy not only to ascertain whether the endometrium is morphologically normal, but also to assign a morphologic menstrual date (21–24). The nomenclature used to describe the menstrual cycle is undergoing revision. The first day of the menstrual cycle has traditionally been defined as the first day of menstrual flow. Menses usually lasts for less than 5 days and is followed by the endometrial proliferative phase, the length of which exhibits great variation (9–20 days), but on average it lasts for 10 days. After ovulation, the coordinated and highly predictable series of stromal and glandular changes characteristic of the secretory (luteal) phase takes place. The traditional view is that the length of this phase is constant (14 days), and it is this alleged constancy that provides the basis for endometrial dating. The morphologic pattern associated with a particular postovulatory day is assigned the number of that day. For example, postovulatory day 10 refers to the pattern seen on the tenth postovulatory day of the "standard" cycle. Recently, advantage has been taken of the great technological advances in the measurement of serum levels of gonadotrophic and steroid hormones, and as a result there is a growing tendency to use as the point of reference the midcycle surge of luteinizing hormone (LH) which initiates ovulation rather than the first day of menstrual flow (25). The precise details of the morphologic patterns corresponding to standard cycle dates are presented in Table 5 and Fig. 1.

Recent studies of reproductively successful women by Johannisson and associates, comparing biopsies and serum hormone levels, have shown not only the length of the proliferative phase varies as previously reported (9–21 days) but also that the length of the secretory phase varies from 9 to 17 days (18,26). As a result of this and other studies, the validity of assigning a *functional* postovulatory date on the basis of endometrial *morphology* alone has been questioned. Pathologists are still expected to assign morphologic dates to cycling endometria, but the biopsy findings should then be correlated with serum hormone levels. It is important to emphasize that the changes occurring from day to day are continuous, resulting in overlapping morphologic patterns that in our view preclude assigning postovulatory dates within a period of less than 48 hours (e.g., postovulatory day 10–11).

Usually, the most important question to be answered by an endometrial biopsy performed on the infertile pa-

TABLE 5. *Decision tree for endometrial dating*[a]

What type of gland is present?
A. Proliferative gland (early proliferative, midproliferative, late proliferative, interval)
  Is the gland straight or coiled?
    Straight: Early proliferative
    Coiled: Midproliferative, late proliferative, interval
    Is there stromal edema?
      Yes: Midproliferative
      No: Late proliferative, interval
    Are there scattered subnuclear vacuoles present, but with less than 50% of the glands exhibiting uniform subnuclear vacuolization?
      No: Late proliferative
      Yes: Interval—consistent with but not diagnostic of POD 1

B. Secretory gland-vacuolated (early secretory)
  POD 2: Subnuclear vacuolization uniformly present, leading to exaggerated nuclear pseudostratification; mitotic figures frequent (>50% of the glands exhibit uniform subnuclear vacuolization)
  POD 3: Subnuclear vacuoles and nuclei uniformly aligned; scattered mitotic figures
  POD 4: Vacuoles assume luminal position; mitotic figures rare
  POD 5: Vacuoles infrequent; secretion in lumen of gland, nonvacuolated cells have nonvacuolated secretory appearance

C. Secretory gland-nonvacuolated (midsecretory, late secretory, menstrual)
  Is there stromal predecidualization?
    No: Midsecretory
      POD 6: Secretion prominent
      POD 7: Beginning stromal edema
      POD 8: Maximal stromal edema
    Yes: Late secretory, menstrual
  Is there crumbling of the stroma?
    No: Late secretory
      POD 9: Spiral arteries first prominent
      POD 10: Thick periarterial cuffs of predecidua
      POD 11: Islands of predecidua in superficial compactum
      POD 12: Beginning coalescence of islands of predecidua
      POD 13: Confluence of surface islands; stromal granulocytes prominent
      POD 14: Extravasation of red cells in stroma; prominence of stromal granulocytes
    Yes: Menstrual
      Crumbling stroma, hemorrhage
      Intravascular fibrin thrombi
      Stromal granulocytes prominent
      Polymorphs present
      Late menstrual: Regenerative changes prominent

[a] From *Surgical Pathology of the Uterine Corpus,* M.R. Hendrickson and R. L. Kempson. Major Problems in Pathology Series, Vol. 12, James L. Bennington, consulting editor. Philadelphia, W. B. Saunders, 1980.

tient is whether or not the patient has ovulated. The characteristic postovulatory secretory changes in the endometrium lag behind actual ovulation by at least 1 day. A biopsy at the time of ovulation (interval pattern) will show spotty, nonuniform subnuclear vacuolization. Such vacuolization may be seen in late proliferative endometria as well as in other types of nonsecretory endometria and is, for this reason, not diagnostic of ovulation. Because of the ambiguous morphologic picture in the early postovulatory period, it is imperative that endometrial biopsies be obtained well into the presumed luteal phase of the cycle (13). We require uniform subnuclear vacuolization in most of the endometrial sample before "diagnosing" the earliest morphologic evidence of ovulation.

Accurate endometrial dating requires attention to a number of details (12). Dating criteria should be sought only in fragments of endometrial functionalis, which are lined by surface epithelium. Fragments of basalis and lower uterine segment should be ignored. The assigned date should be of the most developed area and should be based on features near the surface epithelium (the "egg's eye view" of Noyes) (12). Accurate dating is not possible in the presence of extensive inflammation, hyperplasia, metaplasia, or other patterns not encountered in the normal cycling endometrium. Thus, a precondition for applying the dating criteria is that one is dealing with a "roughly normal" endometrial pattern. This assessment is both a low-power one based upon pattern uniformity and the absence of branching and budding of glands, and a high-power one assessing the shape and appearance of the glandular nuclei as well as detecting the presence of inflammation and necrosis.

Normal Proliferative Endometrium (Fig. 2)

Description. The functionalis of the normally cycling proliferative endometrium is characterized by non-branching, nonbudded, similarly shaped glands evenly distributed throughout a stroma composed of monomorphous undifferentiated stromal cells supplied by a uniformly developed arborizing vasculature. Early in proliferation the glands are tubular and of narrow caliber, but as proliferation continues they become increasingly coiled and their caliber increases. Normal proliferative endometria are further marked by pseudostratified, mitotically active, elongate epithelial cells with dense chromatin and mitotically active stromal cells. Most of the vessels are inconspicuous and capillary-like, particularly near the endometrial surface.

CPC. A normal proliferative pattern may also be seen associated with anovulatory cycles and with exogenous estrogen therapy.

Interval Endometrium

Description. In essence, an interval endometrium is a late proliferative endometrium in which the glands are coiled and the epithelial cells feature spotty nonuniform

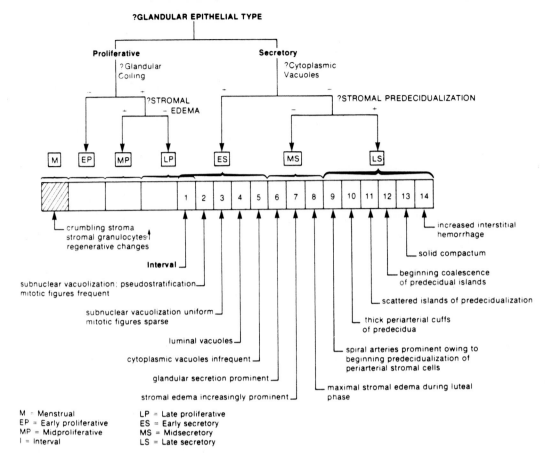

FIG. 1. Decision tree for endometrial dating. This diagram should be used in conjunction with Table 5.

subnuclear vacuolization. By convention, less than half of the glands exhibit uniform subnuclear vacuolization.

CPC. The presence of this pattern is no guarantee that ovulation has occurred even though the normal first postovulatory day endometrium has this appearance.

Normal Early Secretory Endometrium Postovulatory Days 2 to 4

Description. This endometrium features coiled glands composed of cells resembling those found in the

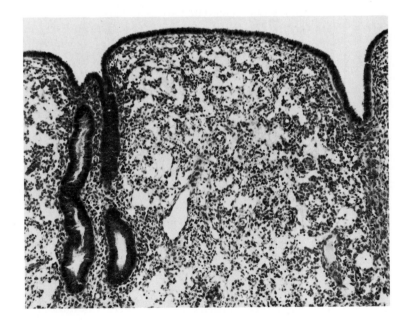

FIG. 2. Normal midproliferative endometrium. This endometrium can be identified as proliferative because elongate dense pseudostratified nuclei line the glands. The stroma is edematous, thereby causing the stromal cell nuclei to be spaced apart. This can be confused with a predecidual pattern in which the nuclei are widely spaced by virtue of their cytoplasm. Such an error can be avoided by attending to the nuclear features of the glandular cells, specifically the elongate dense nuclei characteristic of proliferative phase endometrium, and by insisting that predecidual cells have distinct cytoplasm often with cytoplasmic margins.

proliferating phase, but they contain relatively large cytoplasmic vacuoles. The glands are set within a nonpredecidualized stroma. The precise date assigned to such patterns depends upon the location of the cytoplasmic vacuole (subnuclear, supranuclear) and the number of mitotic figures present.

CPC. This pattern may be accompanied by a clinical history of midcycle spotting and Mittelschmerz.

Normal Midsecretory Endometrium
Postovulatory Days 5 to 9

Description. The endometrium is characterized by fully coiled secretory glands lined by cells with round, often vesicular nuclei. The cytoplasm of such cells does not contain large cytoplasmic vacuoles, but luminal secretions may well be present. The stroma has not begun to undergo predecidualization. The fine tuning of the postovulatory date within 48 hours in this segment of the secretory phase depends upon an evaluation of the extent of stromal edema and the prominence of the glandular luminal secretion.

CPC. Implantation occurs during this part of the cycle. This *morphologically* normal pattern may be *clinicopathologically* (functionally) abnormal depending upon the time of ovulation.

Normal Late Secretory Endometrium
Postovulatory Days 10 to 14

Description. At this time in the cycle, low-power examination reveals the spiral arteries to be prominent due in part to the thickness of their walls but also in large part to the cuffs of predecidualized stromal cells around them. Predeciduation begins initially around spiral arteries (POD 10) and then extends to form islands in the superficial reaches of the endometrial stroma. At the end of the late secretory phase, these decidual islands become confluent and then, as menstruation becomes imminent, they are dissected by interstitial hemorrhage.

Menstrual Endometrium (19)

Description. The menstrual period is characterized by disintegrating fragments of fully developed secretory endometrium. The glandular epithelium exhibits secretory exhaustion, and the stroma is fully predecidualized. Karyorrhectic fragments are present in the subnuclear location of some glands, the cell margins are frayed, the epithelioid nuclei are pyknotic, and fibrin thrombi are present in vessels and sometimes within the stroma. As menstruation proceeds, the glands break up into strips, the stroma crumbles, and the endometrial cells lose cohesion.

CPC. Menstrual shedding should be distinguished from shedding of abnormal endometrial tissue, e.g., premature shedding of proliferative endometria, shedding of hyperplastic endometria, and disintegrating fragments of carcinoma.

Differential Diagnosis

Listed below are some of the more common problems that we have encountered in evaluating and dating normal cycling endometria.

Compact late proliferative stroma versus predecidualized stroma

Predeciduation begins around spiral arteries and only later becomes confluent. It is invariably accompanied by thick-walled prominent spiral arteries rather than the thin-walled capillary-like vessels of the late proliferative endometrium. Proliferative phase stromal cells have indistinct cell margins and scant cytoplasm, while decidual cells have abundant cytoplasm and, most often, distinct cell margins. When edema is prominent, proliferative stromal-cell nuclei may be spread apart and appear to have abundant cytoplasm. Attention to cell margins and the vascular pattern will help avoid misclassifying such proliferative stromal changes as secretory.

Interval versus early secretory

The importance of this distinction is that an early secretory pattern (postovulatory day 2) is required before a definitive morphologic statement about ovulation can be made. We require that at least 50% of the glands show uniform subnuclear vacuolization before asserting that ovulation has occurred. The reason for this is that scattered subnuclear vacuoles may be seen in a wide variety of nonsecretory settings, including endometrial hyperplasia and well-differentiated (secretory) carcinoma. With sensible timing of the biopsy, this "50% rule" should only rarely have to be invoked.

Midsecretory versus late secretory

In late secretory endometria, predecidua first forms cuffs around vessels then coalesces to form islands in the superficial endometrium. Later these islands become confluent.

For details of the following differential diagnoses, see the sections concerning other secretory patterns or the section on gestational endometrium below: (a) normal secretory versus underdeveloped secretory, (b) normal secretory versus early gestational, (c) normal secretory versus endometrium associated with ectopic gestation, and (d) secretory changes superimposed on abnormal nonsecretory patterns.

Other Secretory Patterns (21,27–33)

Deviations from the patterns expected in normal secretory phase endometria may occasionally be encountered, particularly in infertile women (23). The pathogenesis and significance of these changes are controversial. Some believe these endometria are the result of an inadequate corpus luteum, while others implicate a defect in the endometrium itself. Indeed, some of these patterns, particularly underdeveloped (out of phase) endometria, may be normal variations because recent studies based on serum hormone levels at various

times during the menstrual cycle have cast doubt on the constancy of the length of the post-ovulatory portion of the menstrual cycle in fertile women and hence the validity of inferring functional date from morphologic date. Patients with unusual secretory patterns may present with oligomenorrhea or hypomenorrhea, as well as infertility.

Underdeveloped Secretory (Fig. 3)

Description. This term is used in two senses: (i) an endometrium in which the glands are inadequately developed. This may take the form of inadequate coiling (suggesting deficiencies in the proliferative phase), or the secretory changes may be incomplete (deficient luteal phase); (ii) the morphologic pattern is normal but is

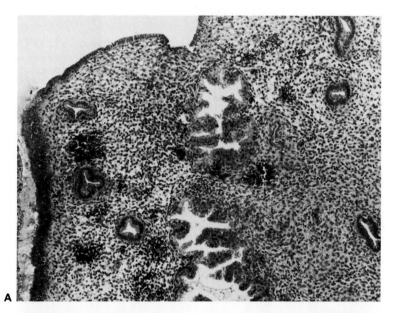

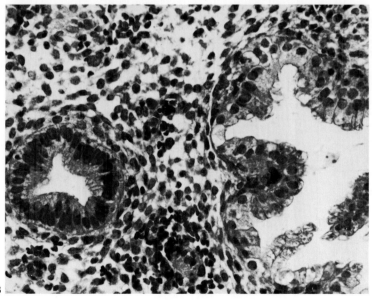

FIG. 3. Incomplete secretory reaction. **A:** In this field there is an extensively coiled secretory gland in addition to tubular proliferative glands. The secretory reaction is incomplete because not all of the glands have undergone secretory change. **B:** Higher magnification demonstrating elongate dense nuclei in the proliferative gland on the left, and the round, mainly basilar nuclei in the secretory gland on the right. Nuclear changes are very helpful in dating the endometrium.

inappropriately delayed when compared with some nonmorphologic determination of the time of ovulation.

CPC. This is the morphologic correlate of the somewhat controversial clinical entity of "inadequate luteal phase" (28,34,35). Patients alleged to suffer from this disorder are said to have an increased incidence of spontaneous early abortion. They frequently seek the care of a physician because of infertility, and some have abnormalities of pituitary-ovarian hormone secretion.

Mixed Secretory Patterns (36)

Description. This term is used when there is more than 2 days' disparity in the development of the secretory endometrium from region to region in the functionalis.

CPC. The clinical significance of this pattern is unknown.

Secretory Change Superimposed on Abnormal Nonsecretory Patterns

Description. Secretory change may be superimposed on a disordered proliferative endometrium, endometrial hyperplasia, or carcinoma. The diagnostic importance of this phenomenon is that the features used to distinguish atypical hyperplasia from well-differentiated carcinoma may be lost or substantially altered in these circumstances. Secretory change in well-differentiated endometrial adenocarcinoma is referred to as "secretory carcinoma."

CPC. Secretory changes of this sort may be produced by spontaneous ovulation or prebiopsy administration of progestational agents. Combination progestational agents typically produce a weakly secretory pattern characterized by underdeveloped noncoiled glands set within a spindled, vaguely predecidualized stroma (37,38). A fully developed decidual response is sometimes seen, and occasionally the stromal cells may be atypical (39).

Differential Diagnosis (37–39)

Atypical hyperplasia with secretory change versus secretory carcinoma

Although secretory carcinomas are very low grade, the architectural and cytologic features of well-differentiated carcinoma must be present before making that diagnosis. These include a rather extensive cribriform pattern, some degree of nucleomegaly, nuclear rounding, and chromatin abnormalities, and mitotic figures. If most of these features are not present but the architecture is complex, we designate the process as "atypical

hyperplasia with superimposed secretory effect" and specify the degree of cytologic atypia.

Gestational Endometrium (40)

Following implantation, the secretory changes in the endometrium become more pronounced, and the gestational endometrium can usually be recognized on the basis of the features discussed below. However, such changes in the endometrium can be seen in patients harboring an ectopic pregnancy, as well as in patients receiving progestogen therapy.

Early Gestational Endometrium

Description. Hertig described changes which he considered to be indicative but not diagnostic of early gestation (40). These are the coincidence of (a) prominent glandular luminal secretion, (b) prominent predeciduation, and (c) prominent stromal edema. In the cycling endometrium, these changes assume their maxima in a sequential fashion. In early gestational endometria, their maximal development is simultaneous.

CPC. When these changes are encountered in an endometrial biopsy, they are highly suggestive of early gestation, but because there is considerable overlap with late secretory changes in the cycling endometrium they are not diagnostic. Obviously, extrauterine as well as intrauterine pregnancy also can cause such endometrial changes. Surprisingly, biopsy at this early stage of gestation only infrequently leads to abortion of the gestation (13).

Fully Developed Gestational Endometrium

Description. The fully developed gestational endometrium is characterized by sheets of decidua surrounding glands lined by relatively low cuboidal or flattened cells (47a). Some of the glands may be tubular or gaping rather than coiled. Glandular cells with cleared chromatin can be seen in the presence of trophoblasts. Although they resemble nuclei infected with herpes virus, there is no evidence that virus is present in such cells (41). Associated findings in curettage specimens depend, of course, on the age of the gestation, and they range from primary villi and anchoring cytotrophoblastic tissue to, in more advanced gestations, fetal parts and placental fragments. Intermediate trophoblasts infiltrate the endometrium and the underlying myometrium in normal gestation, and these often large bizarre-appearing cells must not be misconstrued as evidence of a gestational trophoblastic neoplasm.

CPC. The unequivocal diagnosis of intrauterine pregnancy requires, in our opinion, the presence of chorionic villi, fetal parts, or unambiguous trophoblastic cells. The latter may be identified by immunohisto-chemical techniques.

Arias-Stella Reaction (42–46)

Description. This change is marked by hypersecretory glands lined by large cells with abundant clear to eosinophilic cytoplasm and irregularly shaped, hyperchromatic, smudged, enlarged nuclei exhibiting striking pleomorphism (Fig. 4). Mitotic figures, if present at all, are very rare. The stroma is often decidualized. Arias-Stella reaction may be focal, and the remainder of the endometrium may or may not exhibit a secretory reaction.

CPC. The Arias-Stella phenomenon may be found in the endometrium in a variety of settings, including normal pregnancy, gestational trophoblastic disease, ectopic gestation, and in association with the administration of exogenous hormones. In these circumstances, this glandular reaction may also develop in extra endometrial sites such as the cervix, fallopian tubes, and in foci of endometriosis.

Gestational Pattern without Placental Tissue or Fetal Parts

Description. Endometrial samples composed entirely of decidua and secretory glands with or without Arias-Stella reaction but *unassociated* with fetal or placental tissues are *not* diagnostic of intrauterine pregnancy. On occasion, such endometria may be shed intact (decidual cast). Typically, the secretory development is florid and characterized by dilated glands and inspissated secretions.

CPC. These changes are not infrequently found in the endometia of patients who have spontaneously aborted an intrauterine gestation. They may also be seen in the endometrium associated with ectopic gestations, in the endometrium associated with a corpus luteum cyst or persistent corpus luteum, or in endometria that have responded to the administration of progestational agents.

Subinvolution of Placental Site

The myometrium beneath an implantation site is invaded by trophoblasts shortly after implantation occurs. This phenomenon has been labeled "syncytial metritis" (erroneously, since the reaction is not inflammatory). The trophoblasts have enlarged nuclei which may be arranged in a syncytium, they contain mitotic figures, including abnormal forms, and they may invade blood vessels. Intermediate, cyto- and syncytial trophoblasts are all present in varying numbers. The resemblance to a malignant neoplasm is striking, particularly if the infiltration is composed predominantly of intermediate trophoblasts. The latter often resemble smooth muscle cells.

Other features of subinvolution include patchy chronic inflammation and distended spiral arteries whose walls are composed, in part, of hyalinized decidua. These vessels (rather than retained placental fragments) are usually the culprits in postpartum hemorrhage. The chronic inflammation routinely encountered in this setting does not indicate clinically significant infection. Distinguishing choriocarcinoma from an implantation site is based on the large numbers of cytotrophoblasts and syncytial trophoblasts in the former, as well as their often striking, bizarre nuclear forms. Extensive hemorrhagic necrosis is also a feature of choriocarcinoma. Placental-site trophoblastic tumor (PSTT) is composed of intermediate trophoblasts and shares many

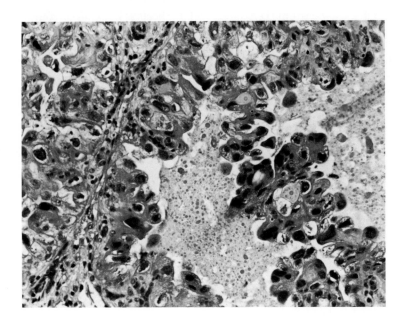

FIG. 4. Arias-Stella reaction. The endometrial glands are lined by enlarged cells with markedly hyperchromatic pleomorphic nuclei. However, the chromatin is smudged, and mitotic figures are not present. Knowledge of the age of the patient and finding accompanying decidua almost always allows this morphologic change to be distinguished easily from clear-cell carcinoma.

features with an implantation site. Distinction from the latter is based on the presence of confluent masses of intermediate trophoblasts in PSTT and the fact that villi are not present in PSTT. Syncytial trophoblasts and cytotrophoblasts produce predominantly HCG, while intermediate trophoblasts express larger amounts of placental lactogen. Human chorionic gonadotropin (HCG) is absent in, or only expressed in small quantities by, the latter cells. Antibodies against these hormones are available, so they can be detected in cells in tissue sections.

Differential Diagnosis

Arias-Stella reaction versus clear-cell carcinoma. Patients with Arias-Stella reaction are in the childbearing years, and they will have had a recent or a current pregnancy event, an HCG-producing tumor, or hormonal therapy. However, the patient may be unaware of a pregnancy, especially if it is ectopic. HCG-producing tumors may also be silent. Patients with clear-cell carcinoma of the endometrium are almost always postmenopausal. The cells in Arias-Stella reaction are not dividing, and the chromatin is smudged rather than angulated. A stromal decidual reaction is often associated with the glands demonstrating the Arias-Stella reaction but not with the tumor glands of clear-cell carcinoma unless the patient has received progestogen therapy.

Infiltrating normal trophoblastic cells versus mimics. Normal trophoblasts invading beneath an implantation site can mimic malignant neoplasms, particularly leiomyosarcoma and choriocarcinoma. The clinical history will usually allow accurate interpretation, but occasionally immunohistochemical stains for HCG, placental lactogen, and muscle filaments will be indicated. An implantation site must be distinguished from choriocarcinoma (characterized by a lamellar pattern of syncytial trophoblasts and cytotrophoblasts as well as extensive hemorrhage and necrosis), invasive hydatidiform mole (villi are present), and placental-site trophoblastic tumor (there will be a mass composed mainly of intermediate trophoblasts). These neoplasms are further discussed in the chapter on placental trophoblastic disease (see Chapter 44).

Inflammation, Necrosis, and Infections

Endometritis

General comments. The endometrium is normally populated by a variety of "inflammatory" cells. These include lymphocytes, occasionally organized into follicles and germinal centers, and cells that resemble neutrophils or eosinophils. The latter infiltrate the stroma of late secretory, menstrual, and gestational endometria

and probably represent modified endometrial stromal cells ("stromal or metrial granulocytes") and produce the polypeptide hormone relaxin (47a). These observations imply that specific morphologic criteria must be present before diagnosing clinically significant endometrial inflammation. These criteria are discussed in the following sections.

Acute Endometritis (47)

Description. This diagnosis requires confluent aggregates of polymorphonuclear cells (microabscesses), as well as infiltration and destruction of glandular epithelium. The diffuse infiltration of the endometrium by stromal neutrophils during menstruation should not be construed as evidence of acute endometritis.

Chlamydial endometritis may be an acute or a mixed inflammatory process (48,49).

Nonspecific Chronic Endometritis (50–54)

Description. This diagnosis requires the presence of more than rare plasma cells. In convincing examples, lymphocytes, lymphoid follicles, and histiocytes are also usually present. The stroma often is fibrous, and there may be glandular destruction. Xanthomatous endometritis is a form of chronic endometritis characterized by sheets of xanthoma cells.

CPC. The most frequent situations in which chronic endometritis (as defined above) is encountered include pelvic inflammatory disease, the presence of an IUD, and endometria associated with retained products of conception. "Chronic endometritis" is also present in the immediate postpartum endometrium, but in this circumstance it is considered a normal finding (55). Most patients with chronic endometritis have menstrual abnormalities, and one-half of them will have pelvic pain. Xanthomatous endometritis is seen most frequently in the elderly and is almost exclusively associated with cervical stenosis and pyometra (56,57). Tuberculous endometritis, characterized by a granulomatous inflammatory response, is rare in the United States (58,59).

Specific Infections

See Table 6.

Nonsecretory Endometrial Patterns Other than Normal Proliferative Including Endometrioid Adenocarcinoma (Fig. 5)

Differential diagnosis is at the end of this section following the discussion of endometrioid carcinoma.

TABLE 6. *Unusual uterine disease processes**

Specific infections

- Actinomycosis (317)
- Bilharzia (318)
- Chlamydia (48, 49, 319)
- Coccidiomycosis (320)
- Cytomegalovirus (321–323)
- Enterobiasis (324)
- Herpes (325, 326)
- Toxoplasmosis (327, 328)
- Human papilloma virus (329)

Specific non-neoplastic patterns

- Congenital intramural cysts (330)
- Giant-cell arteritis (331)
- Glial implants (332, 333)
- Herpetic pseudo-inclusions (334)
- Histiocytic endometritis (335)
- Malakoplakia (336)
- Pneumopolycystic endometritis (337)
- Radiation reaction (338)
- Sarcoid (339)
- Xanthomatous endometritis (56)

Neoplasms

Benign and teratomatous
- Brenner tumor (340)
- Peritoneal foreign-body reaction to keratin of endometrial origin (161)
- Glioma (341, 342)
- Lipoleiomyomas, lipomas (276–278)
- Osseous and cartilagenous metaplasia (343, 344)
- Teratoma (345)

Malignant
Epithelial
- Pure squamous-cell carcinoma (162, 163)
- Spindle-cell squamous carcinoma (312)
- Small-cell carcinoma (346–349)
- Carcinomas with trophoblastic differentiation and/or HCG secretion (350, 351)
- Verrucous carcinoma (165, 166)

Mesenchymal
- Alveolar soft parts sarcoma (352)
- Angiosarcoma (353)
- Chondrosarcoma (354, 355)
- Lipoleiomyosarcoma (356)
- Malignant Fibrous Histiocytoma (357, 358)
- Osteoclastic Sarcoma (359, 360)
- Osteosarcoma (356, 361, 362)
- Rhabdomyosarcoma (356, 363–366)

Miscellaneous
- Carcinofibroma (367)
- Lymphoma/granulocytic sarcoma (368, 369)
- Primitive neurectodermal tumor (370)
- Wilms' tumor (371)

Metastasis and local extension of cervical squamous carcinoma
- Metastasis (15–17)
- Squamous carcinoma *in situ* (166, 167)

---

* Numbers in parenthesis are reference citations.

Introduction

Nonsecretory patterns other than normal proliferation in which stroma plays a supportive role are often encountered in endometrial specimens. With the exception of hyperplasias and carcinomas, these patterns are normal in certain clinical settings. For example, an atrophic endometrium is normal for the prepubertal girl and the elderly postmenopausal woman; however, it is distinctly abnormal during the reproductive years unless the patient has been treated with hormones. The clinical significance of many of these histopathologic patterns emerges only after clinicopathologic correlation. Patients with nonsecretory-type endometria may be asymptomatic, but if not they most often have experienced abnormal uterine bleeding. If abnormal uterine bleeding occurs during the reproductive years and is not associated with a detectable uterine abnormality, it is termed "dysfunctional uterine bleeding" (60,61). Uterine bleeding is termed abnormal if it is excessive or scanty or if it occurs at the wrong time. The clinical diagnosis of "dysfunctional uterine bleeding" should be made only after excluding other causes of uterine bleeding. These include focal abnormalities (such as submucous leiomyomas and polyps), carcinoma and other malignant neoplasms, gestational sequelae, endometritis, and systemic coagulation abnormalities. Exclusion of these other abnormalities usually requires tissue sampling, and tissue examination is mandatory for the woman in the peri- and postmenopausal years who has abnormal uterine bleeding (7–11). For women with dysfunctional uterine bleeding, curettage is usually both diagnostic and curative (1).

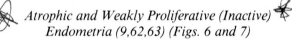

Atrophic and Weakly Proliferative (Inactive) Endometria (9,62,63) (Figs. 6 and 7)

Description. Both of these terms refer to the appearance (and inferred activity) of the epithelium lining the glands of these endometria. The epithelium tends to be mitotically inactive and cytologically bland. The glands are embedded in a similarly "inactive" spindled stroma which exhibits varying degrees of collagenization and practically no mitotic activity. The glands-to-stroma ratio is near unity, although pattern uniformity is variable. The glandular architecture may be cystic or budded, and the buds may even be closely packed, as in hyperplastic endometria; however, typically the glands are tubular. Occasionally the epithelium may be metaplastic. Weakly proliferative endometria differ from those that are atrophic by virtue of cells with pseudostratified, elongate, densely basophilic nuclei rather than the cuboidal or flattened nuclei characteristic of the cells which populate an atrophic endometrium. Cystic atrophy is the term applied to endometria composed predominantly of cystically dilated glands lined by cuboidal to flattened (and consequently atrophic) epithelial cells.

CPC. Atrophy and weakly proliferative patterns are normal in post- and perimenopausal as well as prepubertal patients. Such patterns are distinctly abnormal during the reproductive years unless there is a history of hormonal medication.

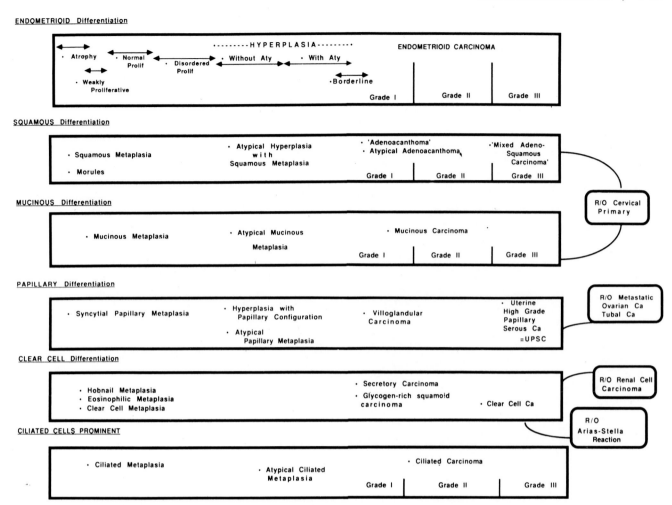

FIG. 5. The differential diagnosis of nonsecretory endometrial patterns. The epithelium of nonsecretory endometrial proliferations may have a variety of appearances. Best known is a differentiated appearance reminiscent of normal proliferative endometrium ("endometrioid"). Alternative differentiated epithelial types are frequently encountered and include "squamous," "mucinous," "papillary," "clear-cell," and epithelial with a "prominence of ciliated cells." Often these patterns are mixed in a single proliferation. These differentiated epithelial types can further be stratified in accordance with their architectural and/or cytologic atypia. These designations are indicated in the top "endometrioid" strip and are bracketed by "atrophy" on the left and "Grade III" carcinoma on the right. The designations corresponding to these are indicated in the other strips and include "metaplasia" for the benign proliferations and special variant carcinomas for the malignant ones. In short, this diagram can be thought of as a map of endometrial nonsecretory patterns: Differentiated epithelial type is indicated in the vertical direction (*y*-axis), and the composite degree of architectural complexity and cytologic atypia are indicated in the horizontal direction (*x*-axis).

Disordered Proliferative Endometrium *(11,60,64,65) (Fig. 8)*

Description. The disordered proliferative endometrium resembles the normal proliferative one in consisting of glands lined by cytologically bland, pseudostratified, proliferative, mitotically active epithelium and in having a roughly normal (unitary) glands-to-stroma ratio or only a modest shift in this ratio in favor of the glands. It differs from the normal proliferative endometrium in its lack of synchronous growth, which results in substantial variation in glandular architecture from place to place throughout the sample. Some of the glands in this pattern may be cystically dilated, others may demonstrate varying degrees of shallow budding while yet others are tubular. Metaplastic epithelium is commonly encountered. No significant cytologic atypia is present. Disordered proliferation differs from hyperplasia without cytologic atypia by virtue of its near-unitary glands-to-stroma ratio. Thus, disordered proliferation serves as a morphologic "bridge" between normal proliferation and hyperplasia. Most of the changes encompassed by the terms "cystic hyperplasia" and "simple hyperplasia" are included by us in the category of disordered proliferation.

CPC. This is a common and normal pattern in perimenarchal and postmenopausal years. The functional correlates are anovulatory cycles and exogenous estrogen therapy (66). There is no evidence that patients with

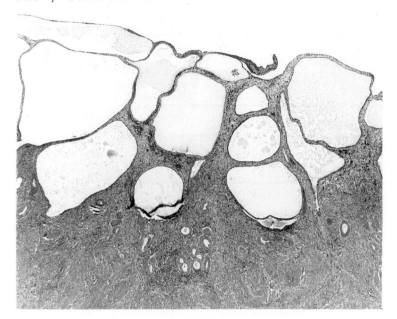

FIG. 6. Cystic atrophy. The apparent shift in the glands-to-stroma ratio has come about because the glands are cystically dilated. However, there is no evidence of budding growth, and the epithelium lining the spaces is flattened. Cystic atrophy is probably secondary to inspissated secretions, and it should not be confused with hyperplasia with cystically dilated glands. In the latter, the epithelium is at least proliferative, if not atypical.

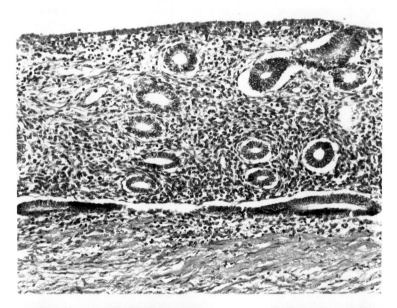

FIG. 7. Weakly proliferative endometrium. The endometrium is thin and is populated by tubular glands lined by cells with pseudostratified nuclei. Mitotic figures are absent. Such endometria differ from normal proliferation by virtue of the absence of mitotic figures and the absence of glandular development. They differ from atrophic endometria because the cells are pseudostratified rather than cuboidal or flattened. This is a common and normal pattern in the peri- and postmenopausal years.

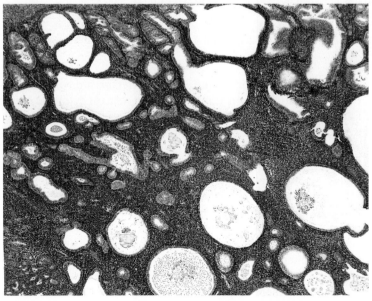

FIG. 8. Disordered proliferative endometrium. The glands-to-stroma ratio is near unity, but the constituent glands are not synchronously developed. Some are dilated and budding, whereas others are tubular. The epithelium lining the glands is composed of unremarkable mitotically active pseudostratified proliferative cells. Disordered proliferation is common during anovulatory cycles, particularly in the perimenopausal years. We do not think this pattern should be considered to be hyperplasia.

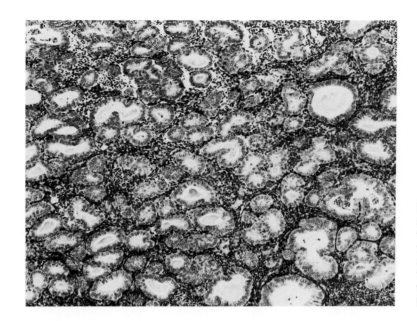

FIG. 9. Endometrial hyperplasia without cytologic atypia. This is designated as hyperplasia because of the significant shift in the glands-to-stroma ratio in favor of the glands, but it is in the neighborhood of our architectural threshold for distinguishing hyperplasia from disordered proliferation. Compare with Fig. 8, which shows a disordered proliferative pattern with a lower glands-to-stroma ratio.

disordered proliferative endometria have a significantly increased risk of developing endometrial carcinoma. For this reason, and because disordered proliferation is a normal pattern in the perimenopausal years coupled with the clinicians' tendency to equate "hyperplasia" with precancer, we do not think it should be labeled as a form of hyperplasia.

Hyperplasia (14,67–74) (Figs. 9–12)

Description. Endometrial hyperplasia connotes a proliferating endometrium featuring glandular architectural abnormalities which take the form either of glandular cystic dilatation or glandular budding. The latter leads to complex glandular structures with branching channels and papillary infoldings. Villoglandular pat-terns may also be encountered. We further require that the glandular proliferation in hyperplasia must be pronounced enough to cause a substantial shift in the glands-to-stroma ratio in favor of the glands. The epithelium exhibits at least prominent pseudostratification and the cells may, in some cases, be stratified. The constituent cells may resemble those of a proliferative endometrium or they may exhibit varying degrees of nuclear atypia, including nuclear enlargement, chromatin abnormalities, and prominent nucleoli.

The morphologic changes encountered in hyperplasia range from (a) endometria which contain only slightly more glands than in disordered proliferation to (b) endometria which approach the architectural complexity and cytological atypia of well-differentiated adenocarcinoma (75–77). Many taxonomic schemes have been

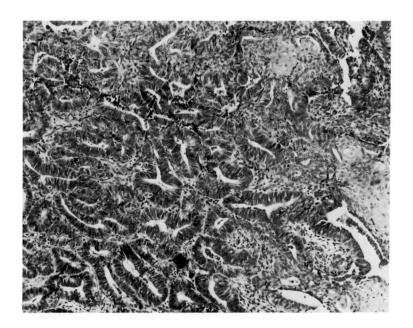

FIG. 10. Endometrial hyperplasia with morules. Many of the glands have an abnormal configuration and they are crowded, but the cells are not significantly atypical. The islands of morules are composed of stratified bland cells. Although carcinoma cells stratify, they also demonstrate nuclear features of carcinoma not present in this endometrium.

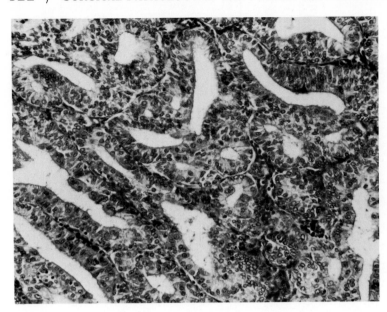

FIG. 11. Endometrial hyperplasia with moderate atypia and ciliary metaplasia. The glands are complex and focally developed into cribriform patterns. However, the nuclei are not atypical. The cytoplasm is eosinophilic, a feature of ciliary cells.

proposed to subdivide this continuum, but none enjoys universal acceptance. As a result, a number of different terms are used for the same patterns. Moreover, some, but not all, forms of hyperplasia have been shown to be associated with an increased risk of developing endometrial adenocarcinoma. We think any terminology for hyperplasia should clearly distinguish between proliferations that represent an increased risk to the patient and those that do not. Recent studies provide evidence that the degree of cytologic atypia is the best predictor of a significantly increased risk of developing a subsequent carcinoma (73,78). Thus, for purposes of clinical decision-making, we think hyperplasia is best classified into two categories: (i) hyperplasia without cytologic atypia and (ii) hyperplasia with cytologic atypia. The degree of

cytologic atypia can be specified as minimal, moderate, and severe. The International Society of Gynecologic Pathologists is proposing a three-tiered classification as follows: (i) simple hyperplasia (which roughly corresponds to "cystic" hyperplasia and in our definition still requires a significant shift in the glands to stroma ratio in favor of the glands), (ii) complex hyperplasia (hyperplasia without cytologic atypia but with architectural complexity), and (iii) atypical hyperplasia (the constituent cells demonstrate cytologic atypia).

In most instances, hyperplastic endometria have an increased volume. However, on occasion the architectural and cytologic abnormalities (definitional of hyperplasia) may be present only focally in an endometrium. The term "focal hyperplasia" would seem reasonable for

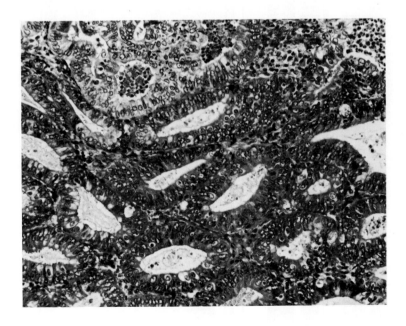

FIG. 12. Endometrial hyperplasia with severe atypia (a borderline lesion). In this endometrial proliferative process, most of the glands are discrete, but at the 11 o'clock position there is a cribriform area. The constituent cells are round and have prominent nucleoli, and chromatin abnormalities are present. If a more extensive cribriform pattern could be found, this would be designated as adenocarcinoma. Because of the very focal nature of the cribriform growth, we think it should be categorized as severely atypical hyperplasia, or it could be labeled a borderline lesion.

this finding. In other instances the features of hyperplasia are present throughout a thin endometrium (or scanty curetting). The prognostic and therapeutic implications are probably those that would attach to a more abundant proliferation with these features.

The term "epithelial metaplasia" denotes the presence of epithelial cells expressing differentiated features not usually encountered to any noticeable degree in endometrial cells. This phenomena is most often encountered in hyperplastic endometria with any degree of atypia; the details of specific metaplastic cell types and their relationship to hyperplasia are discussed in the section concerning the metaplasias.

CPC. Hyperplastic endometria without atypia and those with minimal atypia can usually be successfully treated by curettage and hormonal manipulation. *Peri- and postmenopausal women* with severe or even moderate cytologic atypia are usually treated by hysterectomy. Thus, the pathologist need not label borderline, worrisome lesions "adenocarcinoma" in order to have the uterus removed. Occasionally, curettings will contain only atypical hyperplasia, while adenocarcinoma is found in the hysterectomy specimen. No harm has been done in this circumstance by the diagnosis of atypical hyperplasia because the carcinoma would have been treated in an identical manner. *Premenopausal* women with atypical hyperplasia who desire uterine preservation may be treated by (a) hormonal eradication of the lesion, (b) recurettage, and (c) induction of ovulation (79).

Although there is little doubt that atypical hyperplasia is a marker for an increased risk of developing adenocarcinoma, the magnitude of that risk is a subject of controversy (71,73,74,80–83). Most studies have indicated that the greater the degree of atypia and the longer the hyperplasia is in place, the greater the risk. In a recent study by Kurman and associates, approximately 30% of women with hyperplasia characterized by glands with marked architectural complexity and crowding in addition to some degree of cytologic atypia progressed to adenocarcinoma (73). In their study, once a patient had atypical hyperplasia, no further insight into risk was provided by grading the degree of atypia; i.e., varying degrees of cytologic atypia were not reflected in a greater or lesser risk of developing adenocarcinoma once the endometrium was architecturally complex and the glands were lined by cytologically atypical cells. This observation notwithstanding, we continue to grade atypia, and the degree of atypia usually determines, to some extent, the kind of therapy administered.

Endometrial Polyp

Description. The usual endometrial polyp is a grossly pedunculated lesion whose bulk is made up predominantly of collagenized fibrous stroma populated by cys-

tically dilated and occasionally crowded glands lined by inactive atrophic to weakly proliferative endometrium. However, all types of endometria, including hyperplastic types, can be seen in polyps, and occasionally adenocarcinoma or even malignant mixed müllerian tumor will be found focally or diffusely in an otherwise characteristic polyp (84,85). The central portion of a polyp contains thick-walled coiled blood vessels, and metaplastic epithelium may be present. Rarely, polyps may be sessile. Polyps containing cycling endometrium are designated "functional polyps." If the stroma contains smooth muscle but the glands are not atypical, the term "adenomyoma" is often used.

CPC. Endometrial polyps are often asymptomatic incidental findings, but they may produce clinically significant bleeding or spotting. They are thought to be foci of retained endometrium that over several cycles has become pedunculated and fibrotic.

Atypical Polypoid Adenomyoma (86,87) (Fig. 13)

Description. Atypical polypoid adenomyoma is a lesion that, like adenofibroma, is biphasic. The glandular component has the features of atypical hyperplasia, and morules and/or squamous metaplasia are present in 75% of cases. The architectural complexity and the cytologic atypia are often severe enough to cause confusion with carcinoma. The stroma is composed of bundles of smooth muscle which interdigitate between the complex crowded glands.

CPC. Atypical polypoid adenomyoma is a potentially recurring but noninvasive and nonmetastasizing process that almost invariably occurs in premenopausal women.

Usual Endometrioid Adenocarcinoma (Figs. 14–20)

General description (26,72,88–91). Usual or "endometrioid" adenocarcinomas arising in the endometrium exhibit a range of appearances. This continuum is bracketed at one end by proliferations difficult to distinguish from atypical endometrial hyperplasia and is bracketed at the other end by sheet-like proliferations of malignant cells difficult to distinguish from uterine sarcomas. Endometrioid adenocarcinomas most often form endometrial-like glands in which the cells stratify into cribriform patterns, but these architectural arrangements can be lost in high-grade carcinomas to the extent that glands or spaces are not present at all. Besides forming gland-like spaces, the tumor cells may also be disposed along delicate, attenuated, fibrovascular stalks —a pattern we designate as "villoglandular" instead of "papillary" to distinguish it from high-grade uterine papillary serous carcinoma (UPSC). In general, increasing architectural complexity and increasing cytologic

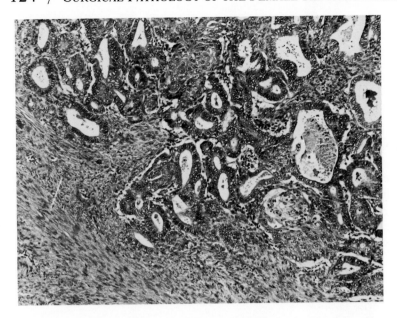

FIG. 13. Atypical adenomyoma. Crowded glands, some of which contain morules, can be seen in the upper right-hand portion of the photomicrograph. The stroma is spindled and resembles smooth muscle. Atypical endometrial hyperplasia (often with morules) within a smooth-muscle stroma is characteristic of atypical adenomyoma.

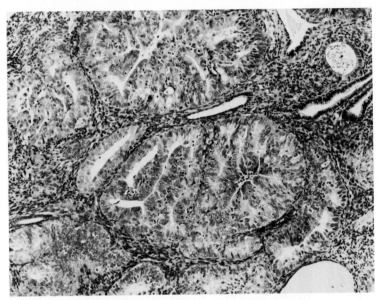

FIG. 14. Grade I (very well differentiated) endometrioid adenocarcinoma (low-power features). The islands of carcinoma cells have developed cribriform patterns. Compare the carcinoma glands with the nearby weakly proliferative glands. This lesion is just over our threshold for well-differentiated adenocarcinoma.

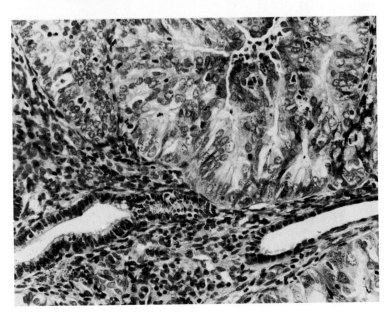

FIG. 15. Grade I (very well differentiated) endometrioid carcinoma (high-power features). This is the same neoplasm as in Fig. 14. The nucleomegaly, the rounding of the nuclei, and the jumbled stratification can be appreciated. Compare the enlarged open tumor nuclei to the dense nuclei in the weakly proliferative gland at the bottom of the photomicrograph.

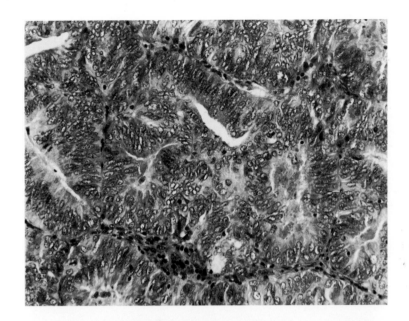

FIG. 16. Grade I adenocarcinoma. This proliferation is clearly an adenocarcinoma based on nuclear features, but it is still well differentiated. The nuclei are round, enlarged, and open, and stratification is present. Tangential cutting is evident, giving rise to areas that might be confused with the sheet-like growth of high-grade carcinoma. The prominent nuclear clearing is characteristic of many endometrial adenocarcinomas.

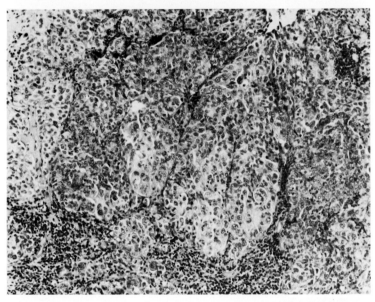

FIG. 17. Grade III endometrioid adenocarcinoma. In this example the tumor cells are growing as solid sheets compartmentalized by narrow bands of fibrous tissue. Gland formation is not evident. In addition to sheet-like growth, we think that high-grade carcinomas should have nuclei with obviously malignant changes.

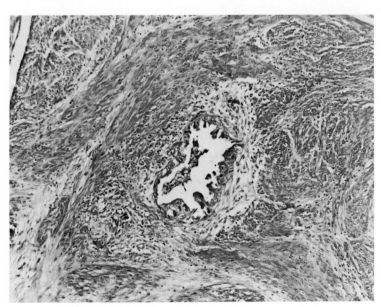

FIG. 18. Endometrial adenocarcinoma with myoinvasion. The inflamed granulation tissue around this carcinomatous gland aids in identifying it as myoinvasive and helps distinguish invasion from carcinomatous involvement of adenomyosis or tangential cutting of the endometrial/myometrial junction. Such a host reaction should be searched for before interpreting a carcinoma of the endometrium as invasive, although these changes are not always present around invasive foci.

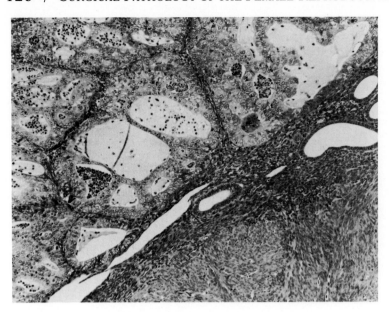

FIG. 19. Adenomyosis involved by well-differentiated adenocarcinoma. This is a deep myometrial focus containing malignant glands, but it also contains normal endometrial glands and stroma, thus identifying it as adenomyosis. Involvement of adenomyosis by adenocarcinoma is not an adverse prognostic finding and should not be construed as evidence of myoinvasion. Helpful features include the rounded appearance of the tumor mass, as well as the endometrial stroma and glands.

atypia are positively correlated in endometrioid adenocarcinoma. It is conventional to include carcinomas with areas of squamous or morular differentiation in the "endometrioid" or usual group.

Many clinicopathologic studies have shown that the grade of endometrial endometrioid adenocarcinomas is correlated with relapse-free survival. A number of grading schemes have been suggested. The one proposed by the International Federation of Gynecology Obstetrics (FIGO) is a three-tiered scheme and is based on an evaluation of the low-power architectural features of the neoplasm. Other published grading schemes less widely employed are those of Broder and the World Health Organization. Both of these require an evaluation of both architectural and cytologic features. We employ a three-tiered grading scheme which incorporates both architectural and cytologic features. We assign more weight to cytology than to architecture because of the difficulty in distinguishing squamoid or morular differentiation from sheet-like undifferentiated areas in a carcinoma at low-power magnification and because carcinomas featuring cells growing on papillary stalks may be either low grade or high grade (villoglandular versus uterine papillary serous carcinoma). The presence of vascular invasion should be recorded.

CPC (88,92,93). Almost all patients with adenocarcinomas of the endometrium are over the age of 40 at the time of diagnosis. Even if adenocarcinoma develops in a woman under 40, it is most often well differentiated and confined to the endometrium (94–98). Young women with adenocarcinoma of the endometrium frequently have a history of anovulatory cycles or exogenous estro-

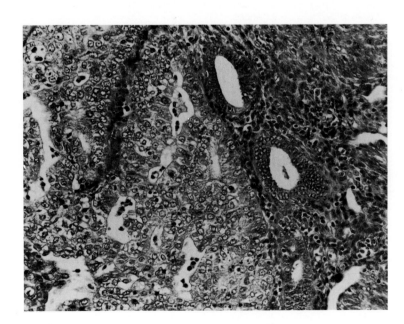

FIG. 20. Well-differentiated adenocarcinoma involving adenomyosis. Here the enlarged and stratified tumor cells can be compared to the proliferative glands embedded in the endometrial stroma in this focus of adenomyosis.

gen therapy; rarely, they may have a functioning ovarian tumor (99–103). We think a conservative approach is warranted for young women with well-differentiated (Grade I) adenocarcinoma who desire uterine preservation because such tumors are rarely aggressive. Those infrequent women in the reproductive years with Grade II and Grade III carcinomas should be treated as an older patient with high-grade carcinoma. Estrogen therapy also has been linked to an increased risk of developing adenocarcinoma of the endometrium for peri- and postmenopausal women. Almost all of these carcinomas are well differentiated (104–115).

The outlook for patients with endometrial adenocarcinoma depends primarily upon four factors: (i) the grade of the tumor and the histologic subtype; (ii) the depth of myometrial invasion; (iii) the stage; and (iv) the age of the patient (older women generally do worse than younger women) (90,93,116–121). To obtain this information, it is essential to examine and section the hysterectomy specimen in a way which unambiguously reveals whether invasion of the myometrium is present or not. If invasion is present, sections must be cut so that the maximum depth of invasion of the carcinoma into the myometrial wall can be determined. Histologic sectioning must also include areas of the tumor with the highest grade, as well as sufficiently complete sampling of the cervix and lower uterine segment, to determine whether carcinoma is present. Vascular invasion and serosal involvement adversely affect prognosis (122).

Determining whether an adenocarcinoma of the endometrium is myoinvasive is not always a straightforward task. The normal endometrial-myometrial junction is irregular and it often dips down deeply into the myometrium (123,124). Carcinomatous involvement of deep basalis, unlike myoinvasion, does not worsen the prognosis. Likewise, involvement of adenomyosis by carcinoma should be distinguished from myoinvasion since this finding does not imply a worse prognosis than carcinoma strictly limited to the endometrium. Careful sectioning to identify residual benign endometrial glands and/or endometrial stroma in suspected foci of myoinvasion is a useful way of proving the tumor is still confined to the endometrium or to an area of adenomyosis. Invasive adenocarcinomas typically infiltrate the myometrium in the form of jagged, irregular branching glands, and inflamed granulation tissue often forms around these invasive foci (Fig. 18). In contrast, neoplastic glands within deep invaginations of the endometrium or in adenomyosis form a mass with a blunted advancing front (Figs. 19 and 20). Foci of adenomyosis are often surrounded by hyperplastic struts of myometrium, a feature not present around myoinvasive foci. If there is uncertainty whether invasion is present or not, we think it better to express this uncertainty rather than erring on the side of "invasive carcinoma," particularly if the tumor is well differentiated.

Endocervical curettage is often performed on patients with endometrial carcinoma prior to hysterectomy in an attempt to determine whether the cervix is involved (125). Contamination of such specimens by carcinoma actually originating from the endometrium is a common phenomenon. Consequently, we do not think cervical involvement should be diagnosed unless the carcinoma actually involves cervical tissue either as growth along the surface or by invading into cervical stroma (126). If fragments of endometrial adenocarcinoma and fragments of normal cervix are present but separate from each other in the endocervical specimen, and the adenocarcinoma is primary in the endometrium, the prognostic implications seem to be the same as if the endocervical curettage did not contain the adenocarcinoma.

Occasionally, endometrioid adenocarcinomas will be present in both the endometrium and the ovary. Whether these are considered to be metastatic to one site or the other (and hence high stage) or whether they are better considered to be simultaneous primaries has significant therapeutic importance. When both tumors are well differentiated and the endometrial one is not myoinvasive, we think the available published evidence supports simultaneous primaries. This construable interpretation implies that adjuvant therapy will not be needed (93,127,129).

The final surgical pathologic stage assigned to an endometrial carcinoma patient is based on an examination of the hysterectomy specimen as well as the operative findings. A modified version of the FIGO staging scheme can be found in Table 7. Nearly three-quarters of patients with adenocarcinoma of the endometrium have tumors limited to the corpus at the time of hysterectomy (Stage I). Another 10% have cervical involvement (Stage II), while the remainder are fairly evenly divided between Stages III and IV (130–132). Somewhere around 10% of patients thought clinically to be Stage I have cervical and/or occult lymph-node metastasis detected at the time of hysterectomy. These are almost exclusively patients with Grade II or Grade III carcinomas. While patients with high-stage (Stages III and IV) neoplasms have a poor prognosis, patients with Stage I or II endometrial adenocarcinoma of the usual type have an excellent outcome (Stage I survival is better than 90%, Stage II approximately 80%) (125,133,134). These survival figures are higher if the carcinoma is Grade I. Thus, grade and depth of myometrial invasion are the parameters used to gauge prognosis, and they determine the need for adjuvant therapy (92, 121,134–136).

There has been intense interest concerning the correlation between the level of progesterone and estrogen receptors in endometrial adenocarcinoma cells and clinical outcome under current therapies. The results of numerous studies to date are inconclusive, and, in gen-

TABLE 7. *FIGO classification of endometrial carcinoma*

Stage		
	IA G123	Tumor limited to endometrium
	IB G123	Invasion of less than half of the myometrium
	IC G123	Invasion of more than half of the myometrium
	IIA G123	Endocervical glandular involvement only
	IIB G123	Cervical stromal invasion
	IIIA G123	Tumor invades serosa and/or adnexae and/or positive peritoneal cytology
	IIIB G123	Vaginal metastases
	IIIC G123	Metastases to pelvic and/or paraaortic lymph nodes
	IVA G123	Tumor invasion of bladder and/or bowel mucosa
	IVB	Distant metastases including intraabdominal and/or inguinal lymph node

Histopathology: Degree of differentiation

Cases of carcinoma of the corpus should be grouped according to the degree of differentiation of the adenocarcinoma as follows:
G1 = 5% or less of a nonsquamous or nonmorular solid growth pattern
G2 = 6% to 50% of a nonsquamous or nonmorular solid growth pattern
G3 = more than 50% of a nonsquamous or nonmorular solid growth pattern

Approved by FIGO, October 1988, Rio de Janeiro.

The grading scheme applies to endometrioid mucinous and ciliary carcinomas. Clear-cell, UPSC, and adenosquamous carcinomas are Grade III by definition. Secretory carcinoma is Grade I by definition.

eral, the level of receptor protein does not appear to be superior to morphologic grading as a prognostic variable (137–140).

Grade I Endometrioid Adenocarcinoma (76,77,141) (Figs. 14–16)

Description. The typical Grade I adenocarcinoma consists almost entirely of epithelium with very little intervening stroma. Usually the tumor has a complex glandular pattern featuring budding and branching of neoplastic glands which result in the formation of side channels and papillary infoldings. Less commonly, the tumor has a low-power papillary pattern with neoplastic cells growing on delicate fibrous cores ("villoglandular" pattern). In at least some areas, we require true stratification of the epithelial lining cells to be present; most often, sharply punched out spaces appear within the sheets of stratified cells ("cribriform" pattern). Cytologic features in carcinoma include nucleomegaly, prominent nucleoli, high nucleus-to-cytoplasm ratios, chromatic abnormalities, and easily found mitotic figures. Squamous differentiation is often present; in Grade I carcinoma, squamous elements are cytologically bland ("adenoacanthoma"). An extensive cribriform pattern is typically seen in Grade I carcinoma and is a most useful feature in recognizing the lesion as malignant. We require both the architectural features (stratification, abnormal glands, villoglandular growth, and/or an extensive cribriform pattern) and the cytologic features (nucleomegaly, nuclear rounding, chromatin abnormalities, and easily found mitotic figures which may be abnormal) described above to be present before making a diagnosis of well-differentiated adenocarcinoma. Abnormal glands infiltrating a granulation tissue-like fibrous stroma are indicative of carcinoma, but great care must be taken to distinguish this diagnostically important finding from inflamed endometrial stroma unassociated with carcinoma, the stroma of the lower uterine segment, and the fibrous stroma found in polyps. We often find this distinction to be a most difficult one, and consequently we place less reliance on it than others. Moreover, such stroma is most common in our experience in high-grade carcinomas rather than difficult-to-recognize well-differentiated carcinomas. Large masses of squamous epithelium are also more commonly found in carcinoma than in benign endometria. Foam cells may be present in either hyperplastic endometria or in those harboring adenocarcinoma, and thus their presence is not a useful discriminating feature.

CPC. Grade I adenocarcinomas of the endometrium are almost always Stage I, and the vast majority are not myoinvasive. In the Stanford series, the overall survival for Grade I, Stage I patients was nearly 95% (93). The figure is essentially 100% for patients whose Grade I, Stage I tumors are confined to the endometrium. Hysterectomy is the treatment of choice for patients with Grade I endometrioid adenocarcinoma, and we do not think preoperative radiation should be administered. Adjuvant radiation therapy is often used for those rare patients whose Grade I adenocarcinoma has invaded beyond 50% of the thickness of the uterine wall.

Grade II Endometrioid Adenocarcinoma

Description. Architecturally, the usual Grade II adenocarcinoma has all of the features of a Grade I adenocarcinoma, but, in addition, over 10% of the tumor is composed of a sheet-like proliferation of malignant cells in which glands are poorly, or not at all, formed. Almost always the cells have cytologic features easily recognized as malignant.

Care must be taken to distinguish between the sheet-like proliferation of essentially undifferentiated carcinoma cells required for grading and the cytologically bland sheet-like formations produced by squamous differentiation in otherwise Grade I adenocarcinomas. (See section on squamous differentiation below.)

CPC. Patients with Grade II carcinomas are treated initially by hysterectomy at our institution. Postoperative adjuvant radiation therapy is given for patients with invasion beyond 30% of the thickness of the myometrial wall. Because the behavior of Grade II and Grade III adenocarcinomas of the endometrium is distinctly more aggressive than for Grade I, there have been suggestions that carcinomas of the endometrium be divided into two groups, namely, those that are low grade and those that are high grade. The latter would encompass Grades II and III. We prefer to still use the three-tiered grading scheme. However, it should be realized that Grade II carcinomas with significant myometrial invasion are frequently aggressive.

Grade III Endometrioid Adenocarcinoma (Fig. 17)

Description. The usual case of Grade III adenocarcinoma features extensive areas of the solid or sheet-like growth of cytologically high-grade undifferentiated cells with a minor component of gland-forming tumor; even the latter are usually poorly formed. The constituent cells are easily recognized as malignant.

CPC. Most Grade III carcinomas have deeply invaded the myometrium by the time of hysterectomy. We think any degree of myometrial invasion by a Grade III carcinoma warrants adjuvant therapy.

Differential Diagnosis: Nonsecretory Patterns

Atrophic versus insufficient for diagnosis. At times, the endometrial sample may contain only fragments of lower uterine segment. The glands in such a specimen are similar to those found in endometrial atrophy. Misinterpretation of such fragments as "atrophy" would mislead the clinician into believing that the endometrium had been adequately sampled when in fact it had not. This error can be avoided by paying attention to the prominent fibrotic stroma characteristic of the lower uterine segment. Even if the specimen consists entirely of atrophic endometrium, a scanty specimen may not be a representative sample of the entire endometrium. In each instance, the diagnosis should be "insufficient for evaluation of the endometrium."

Atrophic versus weakly proliferative. In the usual case, weakly proliferative glands are tubular and lined by pseudostratified, elongate, bland cells with densely basophilic nuclei. Mitoses are distinctly rare or absent. Atrophic glands are lined by flattened to cuboidal cells and may be tubular or cystically dilated. Both of these patterns are common in the perimenopausal and postmenopausal years and may be seen in endometria of patients experiencing abnormal uterine bleeding. It is of no importance to distinguish between atrophic and weakly proliferative endometria. Of importance, however, is ensuring that the sample is representative and that nothing else is present in curettings with this pat-

tern. In this regard, it should be remembered that many cases of high-grade carcinoma in postmenopausal women are unaccompanied by hyperplastic endometria. In some cases of uterine papillary serous carcinoma, for example, the only evidence of the malignant neoplasm in curettings will be individual malignant cells scattered amongst otherwise atrophic endometrial fragments.

Disordered proliferative versus normal proliferative. Both of these patterns are encountered in patients who are experiencing sporadic anovulation during the perimenopausal and preperimenarchal. The normal proliferative pattern is, of course, the normal follicular-phase pattern found during the reproductive years. In addition, both of these patterns are commonly found in patients receiving exogenous estrogens. Distinguishing disordered proliferative endometria from proliferative endometria is of no particular importance. The essential information is that the patient has not ovulated, that neither atypical hyperplasia nor carcinoma are present, and that the specimen is judged to be representative of the uterine lining. Curettage is usually sufficient to control bleeding and eradicate the lesion, especially if the estrogenic stimulus is removed. Morphologic features to distinguish these two patterns have been presented above. Weakly proliferative endometria lack the mitotic activity found in both disordered proliferative and normal proliferative endometria, and the constituent nuclei are smaller and thinner.

Hyperplasia: Non-atypical versus atypical (Figs. 9–11). The term "atypical hyperplasia" implies there is *both* architectural complexity with crowded glands ("architectural atypia") and cytologic atypia. Although cytologic atypia can be found in relatively simple non-crowded glands ("simple atypical hyperplasia"), this is rare in our experience. Endometria demonstrating architectural complexity (architectural atypia) *without* cytologic atypia apparently are not a significant risk for the development of carcinoma. Thus, recognition of cytologic atypia in a complex endometrium is the important observation when evaluating hyperplastic endometria, and only endometria with cytologic atypia are labeled by us as "atypical hyperplasia." Cytologic atypia entails finding most of the following features: nucleomegaly, rounding of nuclei, prominent nucleoli, chromatin clearing, hyperchromatism, and a tendency for the cells to appear piled up with loss of polarity. Cells with minimal atypia deviate only very little from those in proliferative endometria in being larger but still elongate and having increased chromatin, while cells demonstrating severe atypia have many, but not all, of the features found in carcinoma cells. Our moderate and severe categories of atypia roughly correspond to the complex atypical hyperplasia of Kurman et al. (73).

Atypical hyperplasia versus Grade I adenocarcinoma. The diagnostic decision-making problems in the range of atypical hyperplasia-to-Grade I adenocarcinoma are notoriously difficult and fully discussed elsewhere (72,76,77,141,142). It is important to remember that there are no abrupt biochemical, cellular, kinetic, chromosomal, ultrastructural, or light-microscopic discontinuities as one travels along the morphologic continuum from significantly atypical hyperplasias into proliferations whose light-microscopic features would compel a diagnosis of malignancy by all observers (75,143–145). Criterial line-drawing is as much dependent on patient values, risks of current therapies, and medical-legal considerations as it is on "objectively evaluated" morphologic features of these proliferations. There is nothing wrong with declaring a very atypical endometrial proliferation to be borderline between severely atypical hyperplasia and well-differentiated adenocarcinoma and suggesting the uterus be removed if the patient is an operative candidate and beyond the childbearing years. The morphologic features of atypical hyperplasia and well-differentiated adenocarcinoma have been presented above. Kurman and Norris have observed that large masses of squamous epithelium, extensive papillary (including villoglandular) growth, and cribriform patterns are features of carcinoma (141). While we agree these are often found in carcinoma, they can also be found in hyperplasia, and we suggest that the nuclear changes of carcinoma also be present before making a diagnosis of carcinoma. These investigators also point out that a fibroblastic stroma around neoplastic glands is a feature of carcinoma. In our experience, this pattern of growth is most frequently limited to cases of obvious carcinoma. In the range where a diagnosis of carcinoma is difficult, crowded glandular growth and villoglandular patterns are far more common than infiltration of fibrous stroma by neoplastic glands. We have also had some difficulty in distinguishing a "neoplastic-type" fibrous stroma from a residual inflamed and edematous endometrial stroma.

Disintegrating endometria versus adenocarcinoma. This might seem a trivial differential diagnostic problem, but in reality it is a common and sometimes difficult problem. When the stroma of endometria with a variety of different patterns disintegrates and collapses, the glands may remain intact and come to lie close to one another. This pattern can simulate a significant shift in the glands-to-stroma ratio and thus imitate the changes seen in hyperplasia and carcinoma. Careful attention to the nuclei usually allow distinction of this pattern from carcinoma. In menstrual endometria, a search for evidence of secretory changes in either glands or stroma is helpful (see above).

Polypoid fragments of endometrium versus endometrial polyp. Normal endometria, particularly secretory endometria, may have grossly polypoid areas, but these are histologically indistinguishable from surrounding nonpolypoid fragments. Microscopically, we require a fibrous stroma containing large thick-walled vessels before diagnosing an endometrial polyp.

Endometrial polyp versus adenofibroma versus atypical polypoid adenomyoma. Adenofibromas and some adenosarcomas (see the section on mixed müllerian tumors) usually have a gross papillary architecture manifest microscopically either as long epithelial-lined clefts extending into the stroma or as rounded papillae, some of which may be inserted into cystic spaces. Endometrial polyps do not have this architecture. Adenomyomas have a smooth muscle rather than fibrous stroma. Atypical polypoid adenomyomas have a smooth-muscle stroma, and the glandular elements are architecturally and cytologically atypical. Morules and squamous differentiation are frequently encountered in atypical polypoid adenomyoma.

Grading of adenocarcinoma: Grade I versus Grade II. The delimiting of endometrial carcinoma grades is as arbitrary as the delimiting of atypical hyperplasia and well-differentiated adenocarcinoma. The statistics relating grade to prognosis are summary statistics that reflect the behavior of the majority of cases that concentrate toward the "centers" of the groups; it is doubtful that those statistics would change significantly with shifting ambiguous cases from one side to the other of the Grade I-II or II-III line. We are nevertheless called upon to assign an unambiguous grade to a malignancy, and our conventions for doing so have been indicated above.

Grade III adenocarcinoma versus other neoplasms featuring sheet-like proliferation of malignant cells. Grade III adenocarcinomas are, by definition, largely undifferentiated. This raises a number of differential diagnostic difficulties that are discussed under the heading of "sheet-like" malignant proliferations encountered in uterine curettings. (See Pattern 4 above.)

Endometria with Alternative Differentiated Epithelium: Metaplasias and Special Variant Carcinomas (72,146,147) (Fig. 5)

Introduction

At times, benign cells with differentiation more commonly encountered elsewhere in the female genital tract may be discovered in endometrial proliferations. Similarly, carcinomas arising in the endometrium may, on occasion, demonstrate differentiation found more commonly in neoplasms arising in other parts of the female genitalia. The concept of the extended müllerian system (EMS) is a useful construct for understanding these observations. The ovarian surface "epithelium," fallopian tubes, uterus, and the upper third of the vagina share a common embryologic history, and all of these structures act, in many ways, as a single extended organ system. Many of these components show similar changes during pregnancy, develop a common set of epithelial metaplasias, and share a common set of differentiated neoplasms. Furthermore, multiple neoplasms (often of identical histologic type) may arise in different components of the müllerian system metachronously or synchronously. Although the full range of müllerian epithelial neoplasms may develop at any particular site within the female genitalia, the frequency of a particular differentiated type varies from one anatomic site to another. For example, all of the carcinomas that arise in the ovary may also be primary in the endometrium; however, in the endometrium, endometrioid carcinomas are by far the most common type; in the ovary, endometrioid carcinomas identical to those arising in the uterus are less common than serous and mucinous types. In general, there is nothing in the intrinsic histology of a müllerian neoplasm that pinpoints its anatomic site of origin. Papillary serous carcinoma looks much the same whether it arises in the endometrium (an infrequent occurrence) or in the ovary (a common occurrence).

These considerations have certain important implications for the histopathologist. First, clinicopathologic correlation is often required to establish the primary site of a gynecologic malignancy. In the endometrium, this is particularly true for neoplasms exhibiting mucinous (endocervical primary?) or papillary serous (ovarian primary?) differentiation. Secondly, the diagnosis of benign or malignant, given a particular type of differentiation, may depend on primary site. Considerably more cytologic atypia, mitotic activity, and epithelial stratification is allowed in benign endometrial proliferations with mucinous areas (mucinous metaplasia) than in benign endocervical proliferations with mucinous areas. Finally, the occurrence of synchronous, primary, müllerian neoplasms in multiple sites in the female genital tract has important implications for staging, prognosis, and therapy.

Endometrial epithelial metaplasias (76,146)

In a variety of circumstances, benign endometrial cells may exhibit epithelial differentiation other than the well-known differentiated patterns seen in proliferative and secretory endometria. The commonly encountered alternative epithelial types ("metaplasias") will be discussed below. It is important to realize that these benign alternative epithelial types may be present in association with any of the nonsecretory endometria (i.e. atrophic, weakly proliferative, disordered proliferative, hyperplastic, including atypical hyperplasia, and carcinoma). This is indicated in Fig. 5 (148). The clinical significance that attaches to these patterns is, as far as we know, that of the underlying associated nonsecretory pattern. For example, patients with atypical hyperplasia and squamous metaplastic areas presumably have the same risk of developing carcinoma as those patients with hyperplasia with the same degree of cytologic atypia but uncomplicated by this feature. Benign metaplastic cells often cause diagnostic difficulties because of their un-

usual appearance and because they may grow in architectural arrangements also found in carcinoma. In particular, they may stratify (morules) or they may have cribriform patterns (ciliary metaplasia). When benign metaplastic cells are present in an endometrium which also houses carcinoma, the metaplastic cells do not change the classification of the carcinoma. The classification of the carcinoma is based on the changes in the carcinomatous epithelium. However, cells with aberrant differentiation may themselves be malignant, and when this occurs, the term "metaplasia" is no longer appropriate; rather, the term "special variant carcinoma" is used.

Special variant carcinomas

The endometrium gives rise to a wide variety of differentiated carcinomas, but over 80% are glandular neoplasms that resemble the epithelium found in endometrial hyperplasia. Squamous or squamoid ("morular") differentiation is commonly encountered in this usual or "endometrioid" carcinoma. Other müllerian differentiated types make up the remainder of endometrial carcinomas, the "special variants." Papillary serous carcinoma and clear-cell carcinoma are important because of their notorious aggressiveness. Mucinous carcinoma raises localization problems since both the cervix and the endometrium give rise to mucinous neoplasms, and the treatment of carcinomas in these two sites differs. Ciliated carcinomas are a curiosity.

Specifics about Various Types of Differentiation

Squamous differentiation

Squamous differentiation in the endometrium takes many forms, ranging from (a) highly keratinized epithelia that exfoliate anucleate squames to (b) sheet-like proliferations of cells with indistinct cytoplasmic margins, no obvious keratinization, and oftentimes a rounded contour ("morules"). (Figs. 21–23) (149). Occasionally the sheet-like morules may feature either abrupt central hyaline keratinization or a central accumulation of granular necrotic material. Sometimes morular cells are spindled (Fig. 23). None of these differentiating features in and of themselves is diagnostic of malignancy.

The nuclear features of squamous cells encountered in the endometrium range from completely bland to obviously malignant. Cytologically bland squamous elements may be seen in association with normal endometrial glands, hyperplasias, and glandular proliferations with the features of carcinoma. The latter has been referred to as "adenoacanthoma" (see below). Cytologically malignant squamous elements may, on extremely rare occasions, be present in isolation (pure squamous

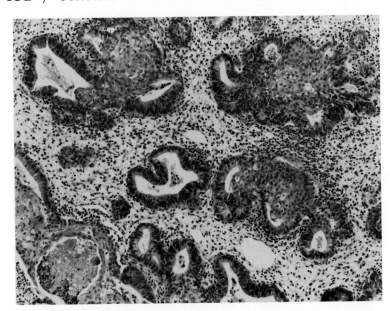

FIG. 21. Morules in a disordered proliferative endometrium (low magnification). Note the sheet-like growth and bland nuclei. Although morular cells stratify, this should not be construed as evidence of malignancy. Necrosis, seen at the 1 o'clock position, is a frequent occurrence in morules.

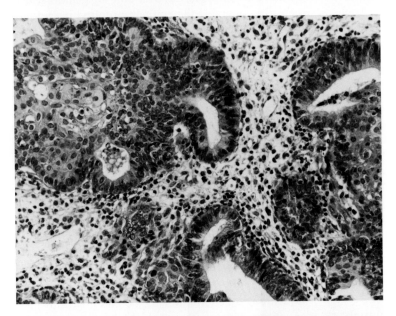

FIG. 22. Morules (high magnification). Sheet-like growth of cells with bland nuclei is the key feature of morules. At the 10 o'clock position the cells have a squamoid appearance. Morules may be found both in benign and malignant glandular proliferations, so the glandular elements must be used to determine whether the proliferation is malignant or not since the morules are noninformative.

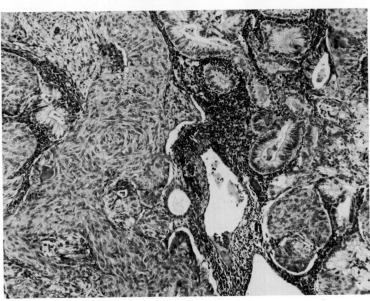

FIG. 23. Spindled morules. Morular cells may become spindled and thus come to resemble mesenchymal cells. A reticulin stain often clarifies the situation.

carcinoma), but they are more commonly seen in association with high-grade carcinomatous glandular elements (adenosquamous carcinoma). When the squamous or morular elements lack malignant cytologic features, the prognostic and therapeutic implications of proliferations containing squamous elements are essentially those that attach to the associated glandular part of the process. That is, proliferations containing benign squamous or morular elements mixed with neoplastic glands will behave as the glandular component.

Squamous metaplasia associated with benign glandular elements. This may be seen in association with foreign-body reactions, chemical irritants, and endometritis but is seen most commonly, and most extensively, in hyperestrogenic states, particularly endometrial hyperplasia (150,151). Ichthyosis uteri refers to the complete replacement of the endometrium by benign squamous epithelium.

Carcinoma with squamous elements. Squamous differentiation is commonly encountered in endometrial carcinomas. Two views have been taken of this phenomenon. The traditional view, which can be labeled as the "two-disease" school, has it that endometrioid carcinomas with cytologically bland squamous elements represent one distinct disease entity ("adenoacanthoma"), whereas endometrioid carcinomas with cytologically malignant squamous elements ("mixed adenosquamous carcinoma") represent another distinct disease entity (152–155) (Fig. 24). Workers supporting this view concede that the glandular components in the former disease are typically low grade, whereas the glandular components in the second disease are typically high grade. An intermediate group of "atypical" adenoacanthomas with "atypical" but not malignant squamous elements has been isolated by Christopherson and co-workers; the behavior of this group is indistinguishable from that of carcinoma with bland squamous elements (156). Adenoacanthomas have a prognosis comparable to (and possibly better than) Grade I endometrioid carcinomas without squamous elements, whereas mixed adenosquamous carcinomas are thought to be a highly aggressive malignancy comparable to (or possibly worse than) Grade III endometrioid carcinomas without squamous elements. A differential diagnostic corollary of this view is that it is important to distinguish Grade III endometrioid carcinomas from adenosquamous carcinomas with large-cell nonkeratinizing areas.

The second view is that the squamous elements encountered in endometrioid carcinoma exhibit a spectrum of cytologic atypia, ranging from cytologically "benign" to cytologically "malignant" squamous proliferations of the high-grade, large-cell nonkeratinizing type (157–159, 159a). Supporters of this position note that the cytologic atypicality of the squamous elements more or less correlates with that of the glandular elements. They see no reason to postulate the existence of two separate diseases, and they further suggest that all of the clinically relevant information is conveyed by a simple statement of overall grade. We take this latter view. Accordingly, we do not make any special effort to distinguish Grade III endometrioid carcinomas from adenosquamous carcinomas of large-cell nonkeratinizing type. However, when we diagnose Grade III adenocarcinoma with squamous or nonkeratinizing large-cell elements, we point out that such neoplasms are classified by some as "adenosquamous carcinoma" because clinicians are attuned to this term. Following Christopherson et al., we consider "glassy-cell carcinoma" to be a variant of mixed adenosquamous carcinoma (160). Carcinomas of the endometrium with squamous differentiation can be associated with a foreign-body reaction on the peritoneum in the absence of metastases, apparently secondary to discharge of keratin through the fallopian tubes (161).

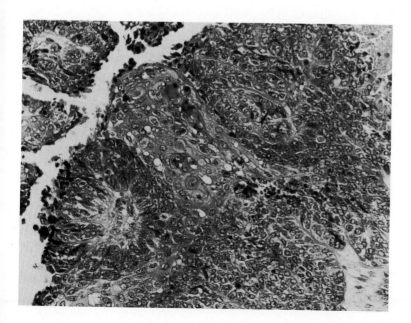

FIG. 24. Adenosquamous carcinoma. Here the squamous element is cytologically malignant, as are the large-cell undifferentiated cells. In low-grade carcinomas with squamous metaplasia (adenoacanthomas), the squamous or morular elements are cytologically bland and are the same as in squamous or morular metaplasia in benign endometrial proliferations. Compare the cytologic features of the squamous cells in this high-grade carcinoma with those in the morules in Fig. 22.

Differential Diagnosis

Not all endometrial proliferations with squamous elements are malignant. The differential diagnosis of bland squamous elements includes squamous metaplasia and morular metaplasia. The distinction between *atypical hyperplasia with squamous metaplasia and well-differentiated adenocarcinoma* with bland squamous elements rests on an evaluation of the glandular component; the squamous component in this situation is noninformative as to whether the proliferation is benign or malignant. Most cytologically atypical squamous proliferations of the endometrium are intimately admixed with atypical or neoplastic endometrial glandular elements. When this is not the case, the possibility of a *primary squamous-cell carcinoma* should be considered. The recovery of pure squamous-cell carcinoma in a curettage specimen always raises the possibility of a cervical primary, and suitable clinical localizing studies should be undertaken. While a handful of cases of pure squamous-cell carcinoma primary in the endometrium have been reported, this is indeed a rare event (162–165). Even more of a curiosity is the primary verrucous carcinoma primary of the endometrium. On rare occasions there may be extension of cervical carcinoma *in situ* into the uterine fundus (166,167).

Sheet-like growth of poorly differentiated carcinoma versus sheet-like growth of morules. This is an important consideration, both in deciding between benign and malignant proliferations and (particularly if one uses the FIGO grading scheme) in establishing the grade of carcinoma. The distinction is a cytologic one. High-grade carcinomas with sheet-like architecture have malignant nuclear features and easily found mitotic figures. In contrast, the constituent cells of morules lack malignant features, and mitotic figures are very difficult to find. Central necrosis of morules is common whether the glandular proliferation is benign or malignant. When there is uncertainty as to whether the squamous elements are malignant (high grade), the glandular elements can be used for grading. Most lesions containing squamous cells which are ambiguous as to whether the squamous cells are benign or malignant are low grade.

The recovery of abundant bland squamous elements unassociated with glands in an endometrial sample. This problem occasionally arises and, while more often than not, carcinoma is discovered in the hysterectomy specimens of such patients, this finding by no means establishes that diagnosis. Endometria ranging from atrophic to atypical hyperplasia may be associated with large zones of squamous metaplasia.

Mucinous Differentiation (72,146)

Mucinous differentiation is relatively common in the endometrium and may be encountered in association with the entire spectrum of nonsecretory endometrial patterns. Mucinous differentiation takes many different forms. On occasion the epithelium may be highly reminiscent of normal endocervix, and when such fragments are encountered in an endometrial curettage they may masquerade as an endocervical fragment. On other occasions, endometrial cells containing cytoplasmic mucin are arranged on delicate fibrovascular stalks. When mucinous differentiation occurs in glands with a tubuloalveolar pattern, acute inflammatory cells are commonly embedded in the pools of mucin—a useful low-power marker of mucinous differentiation. Predominantly mucinous carcinomas occur in the endometrium and, on occasion, resemble those more commonly encountered in the endocervix or ovary. This histologic similarity raises the sometimes difficult localization problems discussed below:

1. Mucinous metaplasia (168,169) (Fig. 25)

Mucinous metaplasia is most often encountered in hyperestrogenic settings and may, on rare occasions when associated with some element of cervical stenosis, produce a dramatic mucometra (169). Diffuse or focal mucinous metaplasia is commonly present in endometrial polyps and is not uncommon in postmenopausal endometria, usually in association with other metaplasias.

2. Mucinous carcinoma (170–172)

Description. When searched for, focal mucinous differentiation is common in the usual endometrioid carcinoma. When carcinoma cells with intracytoplasmic mucin are prominent and extensive (greater than 50%), the term "mucinous carcinoma" is appropriate.

CPC. The clinicopathologic profile of patients with mucinous carcinoma of the endometrium is essentially indistinguishable from patients with endometrioid carcinoma of the usual sort. The importance of this variant lies in the localization problems it presents. Localization studies utilizing differential curettage are usually required to distinguish primary endometrial from primary endocervical mucinous carcinoma. This distinction is important because the therapeutic approach is quite different for carcinomas arising from these two sites. There are no reliable histochemical or immunohistochemical techniques to distinguish these two possibilities in an individual case, although CEA-containing carcinoma cells are more commonly found in primary endocervical carcinomas than in endometrioid carcinomas. (173,174). Metastatic mucinous carcinomas to the endometrium are rare but should be excluded. Primary mucinous endometrial carcinoma must be distinguished from metaplasia of the endometrium. The distinction is made using the same cytologic and architectural features used to distinguish atypical hyperplasia from well-differentiated adenocarcinoma of the usual sort (171).

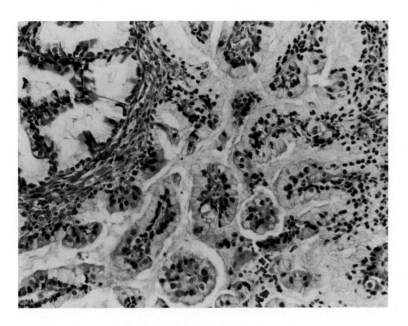

FIG. 25. Mucinous metaplasia. These bland endometrial cells demonstrate mucinous differentiation and have come to resemble endocervical cells. A digested PAS stain was strongly positive. The lesions demonstrate no evidence of carcinoma, although mucinous carcinomas do occur in the endometrium. The latter are recognized on the basis of complex growth and nuclear features.

Differential Diagnosis

Atypical mucinous metaplasia versus mucinous carcinoma. The usual cytologic and architectural features used to distinguish atypical hyperplasia from the usual endometrioid carcinoma are also used in this setting (171).

Rule out cervical primary by differential curettage.

Argyrophilic cells in carcinomas of the endometrium (175–181)

Argyrophilic cells are ubiquitous in the endometrium, both in benign and malignant proliferations. The presence of these cells has no particular clinical significance. Rarely, a small-cell carcinoma with neuroendocrine features arises in the endometrium (346–349). As in other sites, these are aggressive neoplasms.

Patterns featuring papillary architecture

All of the proliferations listed under this heading have in common a papillary architecture with or without fibrovascular connective tissue cores.

Syncytial papillary metaplasia (182) (Figs. 26–28). This is a phenomenon that is probably closely related to morule formation. It characteristically involves the surface of the endometrium or that portion of the gland that opens onto the endometrial surface. Syncytial papillary metaplasia features a sheet-like syncytium of cytologically bland cells. Focally, these cells pile up into columns, but no fibrovascular stromal cores are present. The constituent cells are cytologically bland, although some nuclei may be pyknotic and mitotic figures are infrequent. The sheets of cells are usually infiltrated with polymorphs.

Villoglandular endometrial hyperplasia. On some oc-

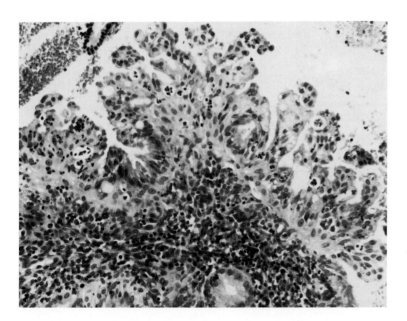

FIG. 26. Papillary syncytial metaplasia. This process usually is seen along the endometrial surface or in the orifices of the endometrial glands. The cells stratify into pillars, but fibrous cores usually are not identified. The nuclei are smudged, and acute inflammatory cells are characteristic. The resemblance to morules is quite striking.

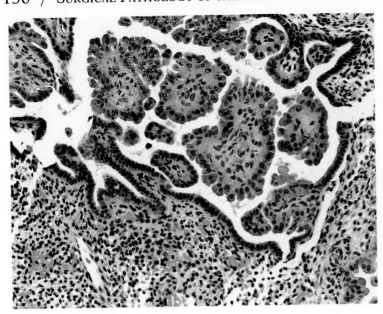

FIG. 27. Papillary metaplasia with fibrovascular stalks. The cells lining the fibrous stalks are bland. Compare with villoglandular carcinoma (Figs. 29 and 30) and with UPSC (Figs. 31 and 32). This photomicrograph emphasizes that not all papillary processes in the endometrium are malignant.

casions, endometrial hyperplasia may have a low-power papillary configuration, featuring bland stratified columnar cells disposed over fine fibrovascular stalks (villoglandular pattern).

Villoglandular (Grade I) carcinoma (183) (Figs. 29 and 30). Well-differentiated (Grade I) endometrioid adenocarcinomas may occasionally have a low-power papillary architecture, either focally or diffusely, in which tumor cells grow on delicate fibrovascular stalks. Bland squamous differentiation is commonly encountered in this pattern of carcinoma. Some pathologists label this type of carcinoma "papillary." If this practice is adopted, then high-grade uterine papillary serous carcinoma (UPSC) must be labeled in a way that clearly distinguishes it from low-grade endometrioid carcinoma with a villoglandular pattern. This can be done by using

the "villoglandular"-"UPSC" terminology, as we do, or by appending the modifiers "low-grade" or "high-grade" to the label "papillary." The unmodified label "papillary" is unacceptably ambiguous. We consider villoglandular carcinoma to be part of the spectrum of endometrioid carcinomas, and we do not classify it separately nor do we specify it in the diagnosis line. However, it is important to (a) recognize that low-grade adenocarcinomas of the endometrium may have this pattern and (b) distinguish this pattern from high-grade papillary carcinoma (UPSC).

Uterine papillary serous carcinoma (high-grade papillary carcinoma, serous adenocarcinoma) (183–187) (Figs. 31 and 32). Uterine papillary serous carcinoma (UPSC) in its differentiated features resembles ovarian serous carcinoma. In the usual case the neoplasm is

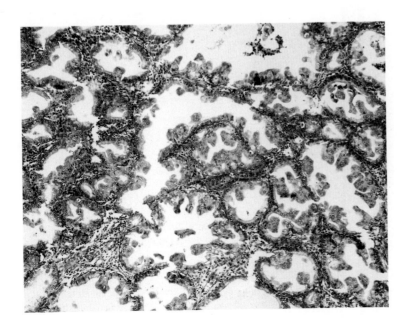

FIG. 28. Mixed papillary and ciliated-cell metaplasia. Another example of a benign papillary process in which eosinophilic ciliated cells are producing a micropapillary pattern.

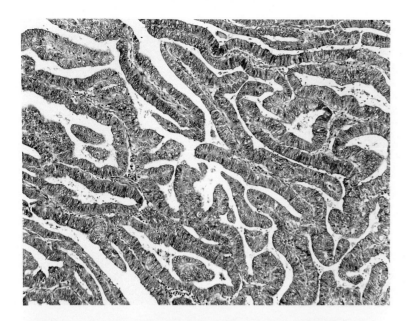

FIG. 29. Villoglandular endometrioid carcinoma (low magnification). Not infrequently, endometrioid carcinomas grow on thin, delicate fibrous stalks. Compare this photomicrograph with that of uterine papillary serous carcinoma, Fig. 31.

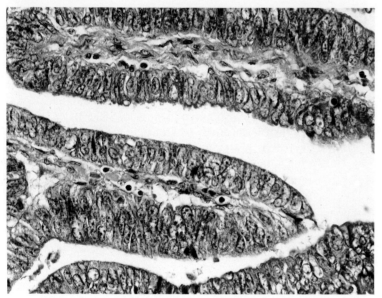

FIG. 30. Villoglandular endometrioid carcinoma (high magnification). Although the constituent cells are neoplastic, they do not show the marked cytologic atypia seen in uterine papillary serous carcinoma. In addition, the fibrous stalks are thin and delicate. We include villoglandular carcinomas within the category of endometrioid carcinomas.

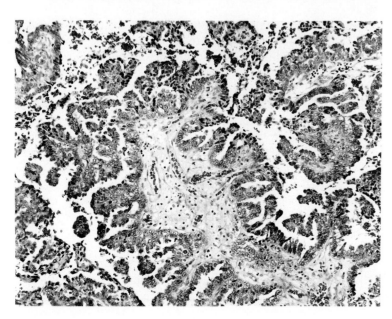

FIG. 31. Uterine papillary serous carcinoma (low magnification). The broad fibrous papillary stalk is a hallmark of UPSC, as is the tufted stratification.

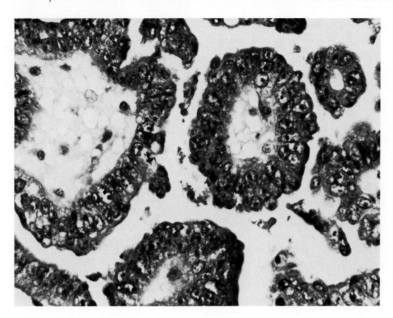

FIG. 32. Uterine papillary serous carcinoma (high magnification). The enlarged tumor cells have macronucleoli and irregular nuclear shapes. The combination of broad stalks, tufting, and high-grade cytology are the identifying hallmarks of uterine papillary serous carcinoma.

composed of coarse fibrovascular stalks layered with large, highly malignant-appearing cells. Nuclear pleomorphism is marked, nucleoli tend to be prominent, and mitotic figures are easily found. Tumor giant cells and abnormal mitotic figures are frequently encountered; in one-third of cases, psammoma bodies are present (188). Myoinvasion is commonly present at the time of diagnosis. This may take the form of gaping, i.e., empty tumor glands embedded in granulation tissue-like fibroblastic stroma within the myometrium. Uterine papillary serous carcinomas have a propensity for vascular and lymphatic invasion; at times, such invasion is so subtle that a careful search of the myometrium and serosa will be required to find the small clusters of tumor cells within vascular spaces. Similarly, the vasculature of the cervix and ovary may be involved by UPSC without gross evidence of tumor. Myometrial and vascular invasion may be quite extensive without uterine enlargement. Clinically inapparent peritoneal involvement is frequently discovered at the time of staging laparotomy.

Up to 10% of clinical Stage I carcinomas of the endometrium are uterine papillary serous carcinomas. As a rule, patients who develop UPSC are older than patients with the usual endometrioid carcinoma, and they are less likely to have been on hormone replacement therapy. The diagnosis of carcinoma can sometimes be made on cervical/vaginal smears because tumor cells are easily shed and easily recognized as malignant, but placing the tumor clearly into the UPSC category usually requires a tissue specimen. Although UPSC accounted for approximately 10% of the surgical Stage I carcinomas reviewed at Stanford, this was the histologic type in 50% of the patients who relapsed (184). Most relapses occurred within 2 years of the hysterectomy. After adjustment for stage and depth of myometrial invasion, the prognosis of patients in the Stanford series for UPSC was significantly worse than for the combined group of

patients with Grade II and Grade III endometrioid carcinomas. More recently, it has become apparent that preoperative clinical understaging is common when patients have UPSC. In recent reviews, up to 60% of clinical Stage I patients with UPSC have been found to have a higher surgical stage; in fact, 50% of clinical Stage I patients are promoted to surgical Stage III or IV.

When a diagnosis of UPSC is made on a biopsy or curettage specimen, we urge the surgeon to perform a meticulous staging operation at the time of hysterectomy. This should include careful inspection and biopsy of all of the surfaces normally examined during the course of ovarian staging procedures. Most patients with UPSC will require postoperative therapy. The form this therapy should take is as yet not standardized.

Differential Diagnosis

Because of the prognostic and therapeutic implications of a diagnosis of uterine papillary serous carcinoma, this neoplasm must be distinguished from other papillary proliferations that arise in the endometrium. UPSC combines papillary architecture (which, at least focally, has broad, often hyalinized, stalks) with high-grade cytology. These features serve to distinguish UPSC from other papillary proliferations such as hyperplasia with villoglandular architecture, endometrioid carcinoma with villoglandular architecture, and syncytial papillary metaplasia. Both syncytial papillary metaplasia and hyperplasia feature bland cytology, but syncytial papillary metaplasia typically lacks fibrovascular cores. A minority of papillary carcinomas have cytologic features intermediate between "villoglandular" carcinoma and UPSC; we think it is reasonable to assume that these will have an intermediate behavior, although published information on this point is not available.

Clear-cell carcinoma and UPSC have in common high-grade cytology, and clear-cell carcinomas may have papillary areas. Distinction between these two is arbitrary and, in our opinion, of no clinical significance—both are high-grade, clinically aggressive neoplasms that can spread over peritoneal surfaces. Occasionally, the epithelial component of a malignant mixed müllerian tumor will have UPSC features. The distinction between the two rests on identifying a sarcomatous component in malignant mixed müllerian tumors. Serous carcinomas arising primarily in the ovary or fallopian tube and involving the endometrium have an appearance identical to primary uterine papillary serous carcinoma. The fact that the ovary or tube is involved may not be apparent until the time of laparotomy. Fortunately, the managerially important fact is that a high-grade serous carcinoma (site not otherwise specified) involves both ovary and uterus. The identity of the primary site is always tentative and, in general, is clinically irrelevant.

Syncytial papillary metaplasia and villoglandular hyperplasia versus endometrioid adenocarcinoma with villoglandular architecture. Proliferations featuring syncytial growth with small papillary-like columns of stratified cells are very commonly encountered in the endometrium, and most are clinically benign metaplastic processes. These are composed of cells with small bland nuclei, and nucleoli are typically inconspicuous. Papillary carcinomas, on the other hand, are composed of cells with malignant features.

Both hyperplasia and carcinoma with villoglandular architecture share the pattern of epithelial cells arranged upon a delicate fibrovascular core; they are distinguished by employing the usual cytologic criteria for distinguishing atypical hyperplasia from well-differentiated adenocarcinoma (see section on hyperplasia-carcinoma).

Villoglandular endometrioid carcinoma versus uterine papillary serous carcinoma (UPSC). It is usually an easy task to distinguish these two entities because UPSC is a high-grade carcinoma featuring nucleomegaly, macronucleoli, abnormal mitotic figures, and highly abnormal chromatin, whereas villoglandular carcinomas are most often Grade I, although a few will be Grade II. Moreover, the stalks in UPSC tend to be broad and fibrous or hyalinized in comparison to the thin fibrovascular stalks found in villoglandular carcinoma.

Ovarian or fallopian tube primary with secondary involvement of the endometrium. See section on papillary differentiation above.

UPSC versus clear-cell carcinoma. See section on papillary differentiation above.

Patterns Featuring a Prominence of Ciliated Cells

Scattered ciliated cells are normal constituents of the proliferative endometrium. In hyperestrogenic settings, ciliated cells sometimes become more numerous, and when they become interspersed with nonciliated cells the pattern is strikingly reminiscent of normal tubal epithelium. While the majority of endometrial proliferations that feature a prominence of ciliated cells are clinically benign, rare cases of myoinvasive carcinomas composed of numerous ciliated cells have been reported.

Ciliary metaplasia (72,146,189) (Fig. 33). This term is used when endometrial glands are lined entirely, or nearly entirely, by ciliated cells which characteristically have eosinophilic or cleared cytoplasm. The usual endometrium with this pattern is hyperplastic and exhibits some degree of architectural complexity and cytologic atypia. Ciliated cells often stratify, resulting in cribriform patterns. However, the eosinophilic cytoplasm of the cells and the cilia, if they are intact, alert the observer to the ciliary differentiation. Sometimes the cilia are visible within cytoplasmic microcystic structures. The nuclear atypia in ciliary metaplasia is never as great as is seen in ciliary carcinoma, and the cribriform areas are more often dissected by fibrous tissue than those typically seen in carcinoma, i.e., they are smaller.

Ciliated-cell carcinoma (190). Scattered occasional ciliated cells may be seen in ordinary endometrioid carcinomas. When carcinomas are composed almost entirely of ciliated cells, the term "ciliated-cell carcinoma" is appropriate. These are very rare, and most are Grade I adenocarcinomas, although occasional carcinomas with a prominent solid component will be encountered. In ciliary carcinoma the cells, although producing cilia, are obviously malignant and ciliated-cell differentiation accounts for the microcystic cytoplasmic inclusions found in some of the tumor cells.

Differential Diagnosis

Ciliary metaplasia versus well-differentiated adenocarcinoma. Architecturally complex ciliated-cell proliferations are frequently mistaken for well-differentiated adenocarcinoma chiefly because the cytology of the constituent cells deviates from that of the usual proliferative-type endometrial cell. Indeed, early illustrations of so-called carcinoma *in situ* of the endometrium depict large nonstratified cells with rounded nuclei containing prominent nucleoli and set within (reportedly) eosinophilic cytoplasm. Importantly, the luminal borders of these cells were prominently lined by cilia. When nonstratified cells such as these line complexly branching glands, the resemblance to well-differentiated carcinoma is striking. However, complex ciliated metaplasia lacks the extensive cribriform architecture and cytologic atypia of carcinoma. In addition, mitotic figures are generally difficult to find and no abnormal mitotic figures are present. As a rule, if cilia are prominent in a proliferation, it is highly unlikely that the process will be

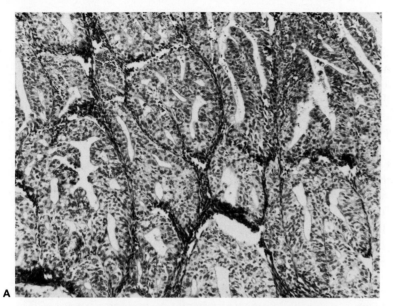

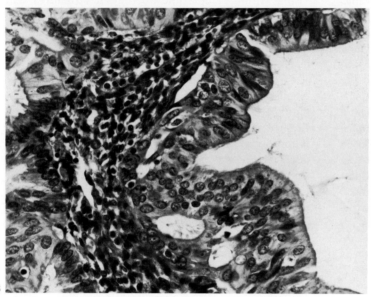

FIG. 33. Ciliary metaplasia. **A:** Although the architecture is complex and cribriform areas are noted, the nuclei are bland. **B:** At higher magnification the bland nuclei can be appreciated. Cilia are present on some of the cells.

myoinvasive or behave in a clinically malignant fashion. There is no evidence that ciliary metaplasia is a preinvasive lesion, i.e., adenocarcinoma *in situ*. Rather, we prefer to regard ciliary metaplasia with atypical architectural patterns and atypical nuclei in the same light as we do atypical endometrial hyperplasia, and we recommend similar treatment.

Patterns featuring a prominence of cleared cells or cells with prominent eosinophilic cytoplasm, but without visible cilia

A variety of differentiated cell types in the endometrium may have cleared cytoplasm. In addition to the entities discussed below, these include the following which have been discussed previously: normal secretory endometria, Arias-Stella reaction, cells containing intra-cytoplasmic mucin, and squamous cells containing abundant glycogen.

Clear-cell, hobnail, and eosinophilic metaplasia (146). Occasionally, benign cells in nonsecretory endometria will feature prominent clearing in the cytoplasm without demonstrable mucin or glycogen. This change we label "clear-cell metaplasia" if such cells are reasonably numerous. Rarely, endometrial cells may have a nonstratified hobnail (or pear-shaped) appearance with or without cleared cytoplasm (hobnail metaplasia). Another peculiar cell type occasionally encountered in the endometrium has striking cytoplasmic eosinophilia. Not infrequently these cells are focally stratified to produce a cribriform architecture. We suspect many such cells are ciliated cells which have lost their cilia. Whether they have cleared or eosinophilic cytoplasm, they lack the cytologic features of malignancy.

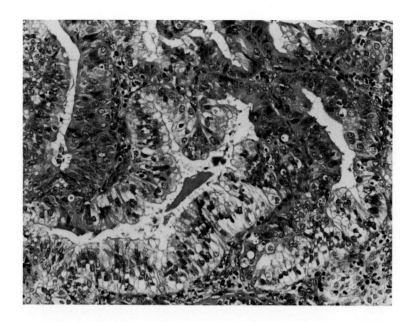

FIG. 34. Secretory carcinoma. Note the vacuolated cytoplasm and compare with Fig. 35. The vacuoles in this tumor are generally subnuclear and therefore the pattern mimics that of an early secretory endometrium. However, the nuclear features of carcinoma are present.

Secretory endometrioid carcinoma and glycogen-rich squamoid carcinoma (Fig. 34). Some well-differentiated endometrioid Grade I carcinomas show a striking uniform subnuclear vacuolization reminiscent of normal early secretory endometrium. Such carcinomas may be encountered in patients who have not received progestational agents. These neoplasms, which must have the cytologic features of carcinoma, have a prognosis essentially identical to that of Grade I adenocarcinomas unassociated with this feature. For this reason we consider them to be a morphologic variant of endometrioid carcinoma. Occasionally, carcinomas composed of well-differentiated glandular elements and bland squamous elements will have zones of strikingly cleared squamoid cells. On PAS preparations, these cells are usually found to contain glycogen.

Clear-cell carcinoma (see also section on uterine papillary serous carcinoma) (191–196) (Fig. 35). Primary clear-cell carcinoma of the endometrium is histologically indistinguishable from clear-cell carcinoma occurring in the ovary or in the cervix or vagina of DES-exposed individuals. This neoplasm combines high-grade cytology with (at least focally) cytoplasmic clearing. The architecture may be papillary, glandular, or sheet-like. There is no known association between the development of endometrial clear-cell carcinoma and diethylstilbestrol (DES) exposure. In fact, the clinical profile of patients with clear-cell carcinoma is similar to that of patients with uterine papillary serous carcinoma in that most patients are over 50 years of age, but the majority have not been taking estrogen. As with UPSC, a prehysterectomy diagnosis of clear-cell carcinoma should prompt a complete surgical staging of the abdomen.

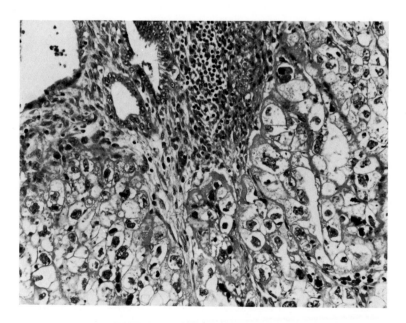

FIG. 35. Clear-cell carcinoma. The tumor cells have clear cytoplasm and bizarre enlarged nuclei. Compare the nuclear features of the carcinoma cells with the cells composing the nearby normal endometrial glands. The cells forming this particular carcinoma are growing in sheets, but papillary and tubular alveolar architectural patterns can also be found in clear-cell carcinoma.

Differential Diagnosis

Clear-cell carcinoma versus other proliferations featuring cleared cells. The distinction between secretory carcinoma and clear-cell carcinoma is a cytologic one: clear-cell carcinoma features high-grade cytology, whereas the cells are relatively bland in secretory carcinoma. Clear-cell carcinoma might be confused with Arias-Stella reaction, but attention to the clinical setting and the histologic features will almost invariably serve to distinguish the two. Most patients with Arias-Stella reaction are in the reproductive years; this change is often associated with decidual reaction elsewhere, and, as would be expected in a secretory setting, glandular mitotic figures are rare or absent. Metastatic renal-cell carcinoma should be a consideration in the differential diagnosis of clear-cell carcinoma.

Clear-cell carcinoma versus uterine papillary serous carcinoma (see section on UPSC). Clear-cell areas may be encountered in uterine papillary serous carcinoma; both are high-grade lesions, and the distinction between the two is of no clinical significance.

Clear-cell carcinoma: primary cervix versus primary endometrium. Almost all women with clear-cell carcinoma of the cervix are below the age of 30 years, and most have a history of exposure *in utero* to diethylstilbestrol. Women with clear-cell carcinoma of the endometrium are almost exclusively postmenopausal. Thus the age of the patient will almost always suggest the primary.

Mixed Müllerian Neoplasia (197–199)

Introduction

Mixed müllerian neoplasms are biphasic epithelial-mesenchymal proliferations that exhibit a range of clinical behaviors from benign (adenofibroma) to highly malignant (malignant mixed müllerian tumor).

The taxonomy of mixed müllerian neoplasms is based upon an assessment of both the epithelial and mesenchymal components. Assignment of each of these to a morphologically "benign" or morphologically "malignant" category results in a fourfold classification. The term "adenofibroma" is used for neoplasms with "benign" epithelium and "benign" proliferating abundant stroma; the term "adenosarcoma" is used for neoplasms with "benign" epithelium and "malignant" stroma; and the term "malignant mixed müllerian tumor" is used for neoplasms composed of "malignant" epithelium and "malignant" stroma. The combination of malignant epithelium and benign stroma is usually ascribed to a concomitant non-neoplastic proliferation of fibroblastic-like stroma in association with a carcinoma (e.g., the stalk stroma of uterine papillary serous carcinoma). Only rarely has it been considered an integral part of the neoplasm. In the past, all tumors containing malignant epithelium but with benign stroma have been classified as "carcinomas." Recently the term "carcinofibroma" has been proposed for tumors in which the stroma is deemed to be "neoplastic" rather than reactive. Convincing cases of this type are rare.

We present below the clinicopathologic profile of typical cases of the three established mixed müllerian tumors. An alternative view of mixed müllerian neoplasia is that these three "disease entities" represent concentrations of cases along what is in reality a morphologic spectrum.

Adenofibroma (198–202) (Figs. 36 and 37)

Description. Adenofibroma mimics both grossly and microscopically its namesake in the ovary. The neo-

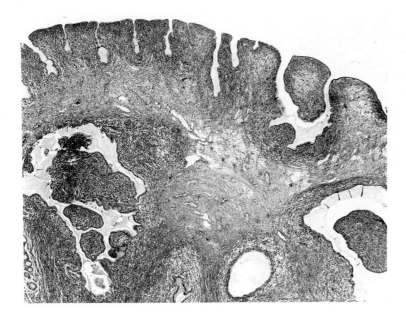

FIG. 36. Adenofibroma of the endometrium (low power). Note the papillary architecture formed by clefts running into the stroma, as well as papillae inserted into spaces. Another feature of both adenofibroma and adenosarcoma is the condensation of the stroma around the glands found in this photomicrograph.

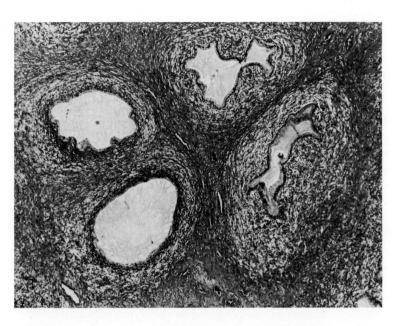

FIG. 37. Adenofibroma (medium power). This photomicrograph emphasizes the condensation of stroma around the benign glands, a feature of both adenofibroma and adenosarcoma. Distinction between the two is based on mitotic counts and morphologic features as described in the text.

plasm is papillary and most often sessile. Histologically, the highlights are cytologically bland epithelium layered over mitotically inactive paucicellular hyalinized fibrous stroma. The stroma may resemble mitotically inactive endometrial stroma. The archetypic microarchitectural themes are papillary structures invaginated into cystic epithelial-lined spaces or blunt broad papillae continuous with deep epithelial stromal invaginations. The epithelial lining may be mucinous, serous, or endometrioid (including endometrial cells with secretory activity), or it may be simple nondescript cuboidal-to-columnar. Squamous metaplasia may be present.

CPC. Adenofibroma is a benign neoplasm that arises in the cervix or endometrium of, by and large, postmenopausal women. It is cured by hysterectomy, which is often necessary to establish the diagnosis (199). Diagnostic difficulties arise when this neoplasm is present in a curettage because the cellularity and mitotic activity of the stroma varies considerably from area to area in the chief differential diagnostic consideration, namely, adenosarcoma—so ruling out a more aggressive neoplasm by examination of the hysterectomy specimen is mandatory. Fortunately, uterine conservation is generally not a problem in the age group where this lesion most frequently occurs.

Adenosarcoma (198,199,202–205)

Description. Adenosarcoma is a polypoid or sessile, often multicystic, neoplasm that characteristically is only minimally myoinvasive. Microscopically, individual cases fall into two general groups. One group of neoplasms has the typical low-power appearance of adenofibroma but differs from that lesion in that the stroma is more cellular and mitotically active, particularly the cuff immediately adjacent to glandular ele-

ments. Distinguishing this pattern of adenosarcoma from adenofibroma is based on an evaluation of stromal mitotic counts. Zauolodek and Norris advocate four mitotic figures (mf) per 10 high-power fields (hpf) as the dividing line between adenofibroma and adenosarcoma; Clement and Scully suggest a dividing line in the neighborhood of two mf per 10 hpf (198,199,199a). We use the 4 mf/10 hpf criterion to make a diagnosis of adenosarcoma, but we consider tumors with particularly cellular stroma and/or borderline mitotic counts as being of uncertain malignant potential. Cellular and mitotically active areas may be focal, so thorough sectioning is indicated (a minimum of one section for each centimeter of tumor diameter). The second commonly encountered pattern is that of an easily diagnosed sarcoma containing large numbers of scattered benign glandular elements which are typically enlarged and dilated. Characteristically, the stroma is cellular and the spindled stromal cells condense around the glands. The differential diagnosis suggested by this pattern is either a leiomyosarcoma or high-grade uterine sarcoma secondarily incorporating non-neoplastic glandular endometrial components. Heterologous sarcoma may also be encountered. The mitotic counts in this pattern are almost always well over four per 10 hpf. Rarely, the stromal cells may arrange themselves in cord-like patterns reminiscent of the structures seen in the uterine tumors resembling ovarian sex-cord tumors and endometrial stromal tumors (206). The stroma in bland adenosarcomas may dedifferentiate to high-grade sarcoma with recurrence.

CPC. Patients with adenosarcoma are usually postmenopausal. Hysterectomy is curative unless the neoplasm is deeply myoinvasive or has extended beyond the uterine corpus or unless the sarcoma is highly anaplastic.

Malignant mixed müllerian tumor (carcinosarcoma) (198,199,207,209–214,216a,220)

Description. Almost all malignant mixed müllerian tumors are easily recognized as high-grade malignant neoplasms upon microscopic examination, regardless of whether the specimen is obtained by a curettage, endometrial biopsy, or hysterectomy, but the biphasic pattern may be inconspicuous, particularly in curettage or biopsy specimens. These neoplasms are almost invariably fleshy, necrotic, hemorrhagic, polypoid growths that fill the uterine cavity. Cervical and extrauterine involvement at the time of hysterectomy is common. Gross sectioning of the uterus typically reveals extensive myometrial invasion.

Microscopically, both the high-grade nuclear features and the biphasic pattern of this neoplasm are obvious in the typical case. However, in many instances, one or the other component predominates, particularly in curettings. The epithelial component may be any type of müllerian carcinoma—mucinous, squamous, endometrioid, high-grade papillary, clear-cell, undifferentiated, or mixtures of these—although endometrioid is the most common. It is traditional to divide the stromal components into homologous (leiomyosarcoma, stromal sarcoma, "fibrosarcoma") and heterologous (chondrosarcoma, rhabdomyosarcoma, osteosarcoma) types, although the prognostic usefulness of this ritual has not been proved and the therapeutic utility of such a subclassification is nonexistent.

CPC (215,216). The clinical course of patients with malignant mixed müllerian tumor is that of a high-grade aggressive malignant neoplasm. Prior to the era of multiagent chemotherapy, almost all patients with myoinvasive lesions died of their disease within 2 years. Aggressive chemotherapy has resulted in a few remissions and somewhat better survivals, but rarely long survival. There are no consistent survival differences between homologous and heterologous malignant mixed müllerian tumors and neither the number of mitotic figures nor the degree of anaplasia and pleomorphism of the stromal component predict survival. In clinical Stage I disease the following features are associated with a high frequency of metastasis: carcinoma that is high grade uterine papillary (UPSC), high grade endometrioid or clear cell, deep myometrial invasion, lymphvascular space involvement, and tumor involvement of the cervical isthmus or the cervix (216a).

Differential Diagnosis

Polyp versus adenofibroma versus adenomyoma versus atypical polypoid adenomyoma. This problem has been discussed in the differential diagnosis section that can be found immediately following the discussion of endometrioid adenocarcinoma (page 1616).

Adenofibroma versus adenosarcoma. When the entire uterus is available for examination, the distinction between these two can usually be made using the criteria described above, even though there is some controversy regarding the level of mitotic activity which indicates a "significant" potential for aggressive behavior in the absence of obviously malignant stromal cells. The resolution to this line-drawing problem varies from center to center. Zaloudek and Norris present evidence to support a four mitotic figures per 10-hpf threshold, whereas Clement and Scully employ a two-mitotic-figures-per-10-hpf threshold (198,199,199a). Our policy has been described above.

Adenosarcoma versus malignant mixed müllerian tumor. This distinction revolves around whether the epithelial component is malignant or benign. Ambiguous cases are unusual, but when there is uncertainty on this point in a curettage or biopsy specimen, resolution may have to await hysterectomy. The behavior of the neoplasms can be predicted by the most anaplastic areas.

Adenosarcoma versus pure sarcoma invading nonneoplastic endometrium and leaving remnant glands. In adenosarcoma the benign glands are typically evenly distributed throughout the tumor and they are large and cystic; in fact, they are sometimes visible grossly. In addition, the stroma often condenses in concentric layers around the glands to form a cambium-like layer. In contrast, residual glands trapped by pure sarcoma are small, they are an inconspicuous focal feature, and usually they do not possess a cambium layer.

Adenosarcoma versus endometrial stromal neoplasm with glandular elements. Occasionally, distinguishing low-grade endometrial stromal sarcoma with glands from adenosarcoma is a problem. By convention, the former features a very minor component of poorly circumscribed small tubular glands or cords of epithelial-like cells, whereas in adenosarcoma the glandular component is prominent, often cystic, and uniformly distributed throughout the tumor. Also helpful is a search for more characteristic features of low-grade endometrial stromal sarcoma such as (a) intravascular growth, (b) a monomorphous population of uniform cells resembling those found in the normal proliferative endometrium, (c) osteoid-like collagen matrix, and (d) an arborizing vasculature.

Malignant mixed müllerian tumor versus sheet-like proliferations of malignant undifferentiated cells. This arises as a differential diagnostic problem most commonly with endometrial biopsy or curettage specimens. At least two problems may be encountered. In some cases, unequivocal carcinoma is identified, but it is associated with areas of undifferentiated tumor cells that are not definitely sarcomatous so that the question of a pure high-grade carcinoma versus a malignant mixed müllerian tumor arises. Sometimes reticulin preparations help resolve this question since reticulin is more often disposed around groups of cells in carcinomas while it is usually formed around individual cells in sarcomas. More often than not the reticulin preparation is ambiguous, and resolution of the problem must await hysterectomy. Immunohistochemical techniques may be useful, but they will fail to identify many sarcomas, and more than a few high-grade carcinomas will not react with keratin antibodies (208). Given this uncertain state of affairs, it is fortunate that clinically very little depends on distinguishing between malignant mixed müllerian tumor and anaplastic carcinoma prior to hysterectomy.

The second situation involves an endometrial sample composed of sheets of undifferentiated malignant cells without a discernible carcinomatous epithelial component. Five possibilities need to be considered: (i) pure poorly differentiated carcinoma, (ii) pure sarcoma, (iii) lymphoma or leukemia, (iv) a malignant mixed müllerian tumor in which only the undifferentiated areas have been sampled, and (v) metastatic carcinoma. (See discussion of pattern 4, page 1594.)

Endometrial Stromal Tumors (198,217–220) (Table 8)

Endometrial stromal differentiation connotes a monomorphous population of blunt spindled to oblong cells with scanty cytoplasm and relatively small uniform nuclei embedded in an abundant reticulin framework. A highly characteristic feature of endometrial stromal dif-

TABLE 8. *Pathological characteristics of endometrial stromal neoplasms (neoplasms differentiating as endometrial stroma)*

I. Stromal nodule
  (a) Histologic and cytologic features identical to low-grade stromal sarcoma
  (b) Circumscribed with pushing margins, often small
  (c) Fewer than 10 mitoses in 10 hpf
  (d) No lymphatic or vascular invasion
  (e) Confined to the uterus
II. Low-grade stromal sarcoma (endolymphatic stromal myosis; endometrial stromatosis)
  (a) Cells bland and resemble proliferative-phase endometrial cells; plexiform vascular pattern; hyalin often prominent
  (b) Infiltrating margins
  (c) Vascular and lymphatic involvement common; grossly visible vascular intrusion gives rise to distinctive "worm-like" appearance
  (d) May extend beyond the uterus and can metastasize
  (e) Up to 15 normal mf/10 hpf
III. Uterine tumors resembling ovarian sex-cord tumors
  (a) Predominantly or exclusively composed of cells arranged in cords, trabeculae, or tubules resembling the structures found in ovarian sex-cord stromal tumors.
    Focal areas of "gland formation" or epithelial cords or tubules may be found in tumor Types I, II, or III above. Such tumors should not be classified as "sex-cord-like tumors."
  (b) Aggressive potential to be evaluated by using the criteria listed in I, II, and III above.

ferentiation is the delicate arborizing vasculature reminiscent of that found in the normal proliferative endometrium. Sometimes the arborizing vessels are hyalinized. Predicting the behavior of a neoplasm with this differentiation depends upon an evaluation of (a) the interface between the proliferation and the surrounding normal uterine structures (in particular, whether the proliferation is circumscribed or infiltrative, and whether or not it is present within vascular spaces) and (b) the mitotic index usually expressed as the number of mitotic figures per 10 hpf in the most mitotically active areas of the tumor. A classification of endometrial stromal neoplasm is presented in Table 8.

Stromal Nodule (221)

Description. The stromal nodule is a circumscribed, noninfiltrative, typically spherical mass of endometrial stromal cells without an intravascular component. The cells are identical to those found in proliferative endometria and in low-grade endometrial stromal sarcoma. Mitotic figures are, in general, difficult to find but may be present as high as 15 mf/10 hpf. Stromal nodules usually occur in the endometrium, but they also may involve the myometrium.

CPC. Because distinction from low-grade endometrial stromal sarcoma depends on evaluating the presence or absence of myometrial infiltration or vascular invasion, stromal nodules can only rarely be reliably distinguished from low-grade stromal sarcoma in curettings. Therefore, unfortunately, a hysterectomy is usually needed to make this distinction.

Low-Grade Endometrial Stromal Sarcoma (198,217,218,222–228) (Figs. 38–41)

Description. Low-grade stromal sarcoma may occur at any age and, by definition, features infiltrative margins and/or intravascular tumor. These tumors are composed of uniform cells that resemble proliferative phase endometrial stromal cells. Hyalinization and an arborizing vascular pattern are usual features of this tumor. Specifically excluded are sarcomas with significant atypia, anaplasia and pleomorphism. Foam cells and deciduallike reactions may be a part of this neoplasm. A few glands or tubules may present in low grade stromal sarcomas, but cases with more numerous tubules are conventionally assigned to the category of uterine tumor resembling ovarian sex-core tumor, while those with numerous cysticly dialated glands are classified as adenosarcoma (199a). In most low grade endometrial sarcomas mitotic features are few and far between but occasionally tumors will have easily found division figures.

Since the publication of Norris and Taylor's classic study on endometrial stromal tumors in 1966, it has been customary to divide endometrial stromal sarcomas

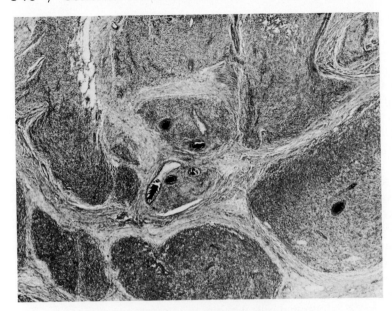

FIG. 38. Low-grade endometrial stromal sarcoma (low power). The photomicrograph shows the extensive vascular intrusion characteristic of this tumor. In this example, as in many others, the vascular spaces are inconspicuous because the plugs of tumor fill them almost completely.

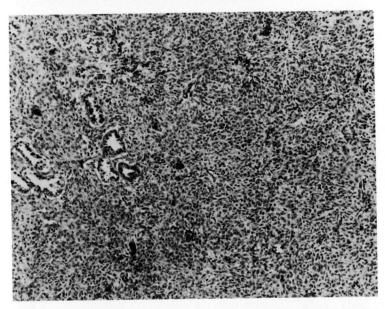

FIG. 39. Low-grade endometrial stromal sarcoma (medium power). Endometrial stromal sarcomas are composed of uniform cells resembling those found in proliferative-phase endometria. Inconspicuous small glands may be found in endometrial stromal sarcoma.

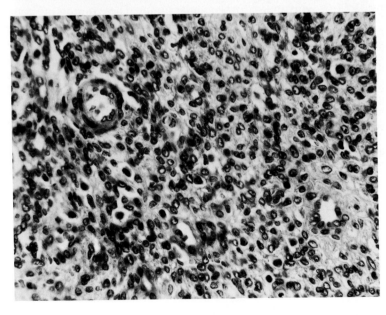

FIG. 40. Low-grade endometrial stromal sarcoma (high power). The resemblance to proliferative phase endometrial cells can be appreciated as can the prominent blood vessels. Mitotic figures are absent and the cells are uniform with inconspicuous cytoplasm.

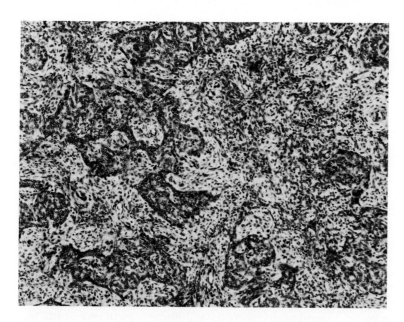

FIG. 41. Low-grade endometrial stromal sarcoma with epithelioid elements. Sometimes the cells in low-grade endometrial stromal sarcomas arrange themselves in epithelial-like islands. The surrounding stroma is paucicellular. This pattern blends imperceptively into the so-called uterine tumors resembling ovarian sex-cord tumors. The latter contain variable numbers of tubules and cords of cells set in a similar stroma.

into low and high grade types on the basis of mitotic counts (220). These investigators drew the line between low-grade and high-grade stromal sarcomas at 10 mitotic figures per 10 hpf. More recently, Evans has suggested a division into categories labeled "undifferentiated endometrial sarcoma" and "endometrial stromal sarcoma" based not on mitotic counts but, instead, on the pattern of differentiation (219). Those endometrial stromal neoplasms composed of relatively bland monomorphous, oblong to spindled cells resembling proliferative-phase endometrial stromal cells independent of the mitotic counts are considered by Evans to be endometiral stromal sarcomas, while those lacking such features he places in the undifferentiated endometrial sarcoma group. The latter generally are anaplastic and contain large numbers of mitotic figures, some of which may be abnormal. The main difference between the two points of view is that some lesions that would be classified as high-grade stromal sarcoma by the criteria of Norris and Taylor because of mitotic counts of 10 or more per 10 hpf are placed in the endometrial stromal sarcoma (low-grade endometrial stromal sarcoma) category by Evans on the basis of differentiation and patient outcome. A study at Stanford of 109 cases of endometrial stromal sarcoma supports Evans' conclusions (222). Not only did we find that mitotic counts over 10mf/10hpf did not predict outcome for patients with Stage I endometrial stromal sarcomas, a paucity of mitotic figures was no guarantee of a cure. Consequently, we no longer utilize a category of "highgrade" stromal sarcoma, rather, we place all neoplasms that meet the morphologic definition of endometrial stromal sarcoma into that category. However, we continue to use the term "lowgrade" as a modifier to endometrial stromal sarcoma to avoid confusion with undifferentiated (and hence high grade) uterine sarcomas.

CPC. Low-grade endometrial stromal sarcomas, including those few with a characteristic histologic pattern but with up to 15 normal mitotic figures per 10 hpf, are indolent slowly progressing neoplasms. Small tumors completely removed by hysterectomy are most often cured by the hysterectomy, but some tumors may recur, particularly those that are larger. Recurrences and metastases are observed 20 to 30 years after the primary tumor has been removed (229,230). Metastatic neoplasms may respond to progestational therapy, but the role of progesterones in an adjuvant setting is not settled (231–235). Low-grade endometrial stromal sarcomas can, on rare occasions, arise from extrauterine sites including the ovary, vagina, and peritoneum (236–242).

Undifferentiated Uterine Sarcoma (219,220,243)

Description. We prefer the term "undifferentiated uterine sarcoma" for anaplastic neoplasms that bear little resemblance to proliferative phase endometrial stroma. Continuing to label them "endometrial stromal sarcoma" when they don't resemble endometrial stromal cells causes confusion—more confusion than changing the nomenclature. Undifferentiated uterine sarcoma is much less common than low-grade stromal endometrial sarcoma once one has carefully excluded leukemia, lymphoma, high-grade carcinoma, malignant mixed müllerian tumors, and differentiated pure sarcomas. Undifferentiated uterine sarcomas are composed of undifferentiated cells with a high mitotic rate, and often the tumor has a sarcomatous appearance. Usually it lacks the characteristic arborizing vasculature and the areas of hyalinization characteristic of low-grade endometrial stromal sarcoma. All pure undifferentiated sarcomas of the uterus, including the giant-cell variety, can for convenience be placed in this category. Pure sarcomas containing cells differentiating along recognizable mesenchymal lines are given names depending on the direction of their differentiation, i.e., leiomyosarcoma, osteosarcoma, rhabdomyosarcoma, etc.

CPC. Almost all undifferentiated uterine sarcomas behave in a highly aggressive fashion, a pattern of behavior identical to that of pure sarcomas demonstrating heterologous differentiation.

Uterine Neoplasms with Sex-Cord-like Elements (199,244,245) (Fig. 38)

Description. Clement and Scully first drew attention to these unusual neoplasms in 1976 (244). The neoplastic cells are arranged in cords, hollow tubules, trabeculae, and/or sheets resembling epithelial cells, and they most often have scant cytoplasm, indistinct cell margins, and round nuclei. However, in some tumors the constituent cells may have abundant eosinophilic or clear cytoplasm. The stroma between the epithelioid structures varies from paucicellular and fibroblastic to an appearance similar to normal proliferative endometrial stroma. Hyaline matrix may be prominent. Most tumors have pushing margins, but vascular intrusion has been observed in some cases. Because in some tumors some of the constituent cells resemble endometrial stromal cells, we consider these neoplasms to be a subset of endometrial stromal neoplasms.

CPC. Most of these neoplasms are benign, but some have recurred and/or metastasized. Too few have been studied to know if there are morphologic features that would predict aggressive behavior. At the present time we use the same criteria to distinguish benign sex-cord-like tumors from the malignant variety as we do to distinguish stromal nodule from low-grade endometrial stroma sarcoma; i.e., only tumors with circumscribed borders, low mitotic activity, and uniform cells are considered to be benign.

Differential Diagnosis

Low-grade endometrial stromal sarcoma versus stromal nodule. The distinction between these two can

usually be made only with the entire uterus in hand and is based on the presence of infiltrating margins and/or vascular invasion in the former but not in the latter.

Low-grade stromal sarcoma versus lymphoma/leukemia versus carcinoma (see pattern 4, page 1594) (Fig. 42). Because the constituent cells of low-grade endometrial stromal sarcoma have few discernible differentiated cytologic features, identification of these tumors is mainly based on (a) the resemblance of the constituent cells to normal proliferative endometrial stroma, (b) the arborizing vascular pattern, (c) the characteristic osteoid-like hyalin, and (d) the intrusion of tumor cells into vascular spaces. When these features are muted, the differential diagnostic possibilities are numerous. Lymphoma and leukemia can closely mimic low-grade endometrial stromal sarcoma, and we advocate liberal use of common leukocyte antigen and esterase stains in any doubtful case. Poorly differentiated carcinomas, particularly metastatic lobular carcinoma from the breast, are a constant diagnostic consideration when considering a diagnosis of low-grade endometrial stromal sarcoma (Fig. 42). PAS, reticulin, and keratin immunohistochemical stains are often useful, as is a complete clinical history. This differential diagnostic problem is complicated by the observation that the cells forming the glands or tubules in endometrial stromal tumors may express keratin, as do smooth muscle cells (199,246,247). Tumor present within large vascular spaces is a characteristic feature of low-grade endometrial stromal sarcoma but not the other neoplasms under consideration in this differential diagnosis section (see the discussion on low-grade endometrial stromal sarcoma versus smooth muscle tumor, below).

Low-grade stromal sarcoma versus inflammation, fragmented lymphoid nodules, and immunoblasts. Follicular center cells in lymphoid nodules and sheets of immunoblasts can come to resemble neoplastic endo-

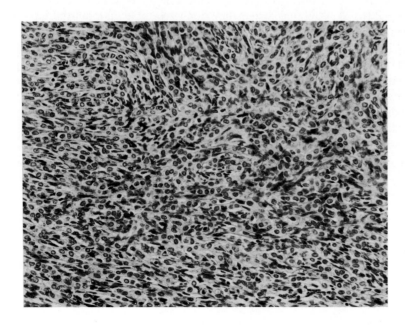

FIG. 42. Metastatic lobular carcinoma to the endometrium. The resemblance of this carcinoma to low-grade endometrial stromal sarcoma and to epithelioid smooth-muscle tumors is awe inspiring. Whenever a diagnosis of low-grade stromal sarcoma or epithelioid smooth muscle tumor is contemplated, the possibility of metastatic lobular carcinoma should be considered. The mimicry is heightened by the uniformity of the tumor cells, the paucity of mitotic figures, and the failure of the tumor cells to differentiate into glandular or tubular structures.

metrial stromal cells, particularly in endometrial biopsies and curettings. Searching on the one hand for the characteristic endometrial stromal features discussed above and, on the other hand, for features of inflammatory processes such as follicular center cells in intact lymphoid follicles, numerous plasma cells and acute inflammatory cells should help clarify the situation.

Low-grade endometrial stromal sarcoma versus smooth muscle tumor, particularly epithelioid smooth-muscle tumors. This problem is discussed in the introduction to the section devoted to smooth muscle neoplasms. It is an important differential consideration because both smooth muscle and endometrial stromal neoplasms intrude into vessels and because the two neoplasms can closely resemble one another.

Low-grade endometrial sarcoma versus high-grade uterine sarcomas. See the discussion of high-grade endometrial stromal sarcoma immediately above.

Stromal nodule and low-grade stromal sarcoma versus sex-cord-like tumor. By definition, stromal nodule and low-grade endometrial stromal sarcoma can only contain infrequent small, scattered glands, cords, or tubular structures, whereas these structures are numerous or predominant in sex-cord-like tumors.

Adenofibroma and adenosarcoma versus sex-cord-like tumor. Adenofibroma and adenosarcoma feature benign, and most often cystically dilated, glands uniformly distributed throughout the tumor rather than the cords, trabeculae, or tubules characteristic of the sex-cord-like tumors. Moreover, a papillary architecture is absent in sex-cord-like tumors. In adenosarcoma, the mesenchymal component must meet the histologic or mitotic criteria for sarcoma, and spindled stromal cells often condense in a concentric cambium-like layer around the dilated glands.

Myometrium: Non-neoplastic Conditions (248–252)

Adenomyosis

Description. Endometrial tissue is considered ectopic in the uterus if it is present on the uterine serosa (endometriosis) or if it is located "excessively" deep in the myometrium (adenomyosis). The definition of "excessively" is a subject of a minor but continuous controversy in gynecologic pathology. In noncontroversial cases the uterus is grossly abnormal. When focal, adenomyosis mimics a leiomyoma in being a roughly spherical intramural space-occupying lesion but differs from leiomyoma in that the mass cannot be shelled out easily from the surrounding uninvolved myometrium. When involvement is diffuse the uterus is enlarged in a "globoid" fashion. In both situations the cut surface of the myometrium bulges and is coarsely trabecular; microscopically, foci of basalis-type endometrial glands and stroma are delimited by hypertrophied bands of smooth

muscle. Controversy arises when no gross abnormality is present, and the diagnosis is based entirely upon microscopical findings. The source of this definitional difficulty is the normal irregularity of the endometrial-myometrial junction and the tendency of tangential cuts of this region to produce convincing imitations of adenomyosis. Various strategies have been offered to distinguish this situation from "true adenomyosis." We make the diagnosis of adenomyosis when there is clear smooth muscle hypertrophy around foci of endometrial glands and stroma and, in the absence of that finding, when endometrial glands and stroma lie within the outer two-thirds of the uterine wall.

CPC. Patients with classic adenomyosis frequently present with abnormal uterine bleeding. The clinical significance, if any, of microscopically diagnosed "pathologist's adenomyosis" is unknown, but it is undoubtedly minimal.

On occasion, endometrial carcinoma may be present within foci of adenomyosis. This is usually accompanied by a coexistent endometrial carcinoma arising in the uterine lining. The difficulties in assessing whether myometrial invasion is present in this setting are described in the section on endometrial carcinoma.

Changes of Pregnancy

Description. The physiologic hypertrophy and hyperplasia of the myometrium during pregnancy, as well as the characteristic trophoblastic infiltration at the implantation site, are well known. Most of the differential diagnostic difficulties presented by curettage specimens obtained during or just after gestation relate to gestational trophoblastic disease and its mimics (see Chapter 44; see also the section on gestational changes in the endometrium). The physiologic "chronic endometritis" that occurs during this period has been described in the section on endometritis. Clinically important postpartum bacterial infections are accompanied by the production of pus and its microscopic correlate, namely, sheets of polymorphs admixed with disintegrating endometrium.

Differential Diagnosis

The diagnosis of endometrial carcinoma or an endometrial stromal sarcoma should be embarked upon with great caution in a young woman, particularly if decidua or other clues of a gestational setting are identified. Occasionally, gestational trophoblastic disease may mimic a nongestational uterine malignancy. In particular, placental-site trophoblastic tumor can closely resemble leiomyosarcoma. Whenever a diagnosis of leiomyosarcoma is contemplated in a woman in her reproductive years, the possibility of PSTT should be considered.

TABLE 9. *Definitions of smooth muscle tumors*

I. Usual histological patterns of smooth muscle
  A. Usual leiomyoma
    1. Morphological
      (a) Cells arranged in bundles with elongate nuclei and moderate amount of cytoplasm
      (b) Usually circumscribed but may have irregular or infiltrating margins
    2. Mitotic counts
      (a) Fewer than 2 mf/10 hpf, regardless of nuclear enlargement or cellular pleomorphism (no abnormal mitotic figures or tumor-cell necrosis)
      (b) Fewer than 5 mf/10 hpf if neoplasm is cellular, but without pleomorphism or significant cytologic atypia
  B. Leiomyoma with increased mitotic figures
    1. Morphological: bland spindle cells, paucicellular well-differentiated smooth-muscle neoplasm without tumor-cell necrosis, nuclear atypia, anaplasia, abnormal mitotic figures, or giant-cell forms
    2. Mitotic counts: 5–15 mf/10 hpf
  C. Uncertain malignant potential category includes smooth muscle neoplasms with:
      (a) Cytologic atypia and 2–5 mf/10 hpf
      (b) Hypercellularity in the absence of significant cytologic atypia or pleomorphism and 5–10 mf/10 hpf
      (c) Paucicellular, absence of cytologic atypia and pleomorphism, and greater than 15 mf/10 hpf
      (d) Smooth muscle tumors with counts less than those above but containing abnormal mitotic figures or tumor-cell necrosis
  D. Leiomyosarcoma
    1. Morphological: generally elongate cells, but may be all shapes and sizes; cells usually anaplastic and bizarre; almost always hypercellular. Tumor-cell necrosis and abnormal mitotic figures common. Infiltrating margins frequent. Vascular invasion may be found.
    2. Mitotic counts:
      (a) Greater than 10 mf/10 hpf for cellular neoplasms
      (b) Greater than 5 mf/10 hpf for tumors demonstrating anaplasia, pleomorphism, giant cells, or epithelioid patterns
II. Unusual histological patterns
  A. Cellular leiomyoma
    1. Morphological: contains more cells per unit area than the surrounding myometrium
    2. Mitotic counts: same as for leiomyoma
  B. Epithelioid smooth muscle tumors
    1. Morphological: round (epithelial-like) cells in sheets and/or cords; may blend into area of characteristic smooth muscle
      (a) Leiomyoblastoma = perinuclear clearing
      (b) Plexiform tumor = crumpled nuclei and cords within dense hyaline stroma
      (c) Clear cell
    2. Mitotic counts
      (a) Epithelioid leiomyoma (leiomyoblastoma): fewer than 2 mf/10 hpf
      (b) Epithelioid tumor of uncertain malignant potential: 2–5 mf/10 hpf
      (c) Epithelioid leiomyosarcoma: greater than 5 mf/10 hpf

  C. Symplastic ("atypical") smooth muscle tumors
    1. Morphological: giant cells, either multinucleated or hyperlobated and/or cells with enlarged hyperchromatic nuclei. Intranuclear inclusions common
    2. Mitotic counts:
      (a) Symplastic leiomyoma: fewer than 2 mf/10/hpf
      (b) Uncertain malignant potential: 2–5 mf/10 hpf
      (c) Leiomyosarcoma: greater than 5 mf/10 hpf
  D. Neurilemmoma-like leiomyoma
    1. Morphological: same as for leiomyoma except nuclei are palisaded and separated by hyalin, thereby causing resemblance to Verocay bodies
    2. Mitotic counts: same as for leiomyoma
  E. Lipoleiomyoma
    1. Morphological: leiomyoma with variable numbers of fat cells; when tumor is exclusively composed of fat cells, the term "lipoma" is appropriate
    2. Mitotic counts: same as for leiomyoma
  F. Leiomyoma with tubules
    1. Morphological: leiomyoma with focal tubular differentiation
    2. Mitotic counts: same as for leiomyoma
III. Unusual growth patterns
  A. Leiomyoma with vascular invasion
    1. Morphological: vascular intrusion is not visible grossly but is a microscopic finding and is within the confines of a leiomyoma
    2. Mitotic counts:
      (a) Leiomyoma with vascular invasion: fewer than 2 mf/10 hpf
      (b) Intravascular smooth muscle tumor of uncertain malignant potential: 2–5 mf/10 hpf
      (c) Leiomyosarcoma with vascular invasion: greater than 5 mf/10 hpf
  B. Intravenous leiomyomatosis
    1. Morphological: grossly visible fragments of smooth muscle extending into vascular spaces and/or microscopic extension of smooth muscle into vascular spaces outside the confines of a leiomyoma
    2. Mitotic counts:
      (a) Intravenous leiomyomatosis: fewer than 2 mf/10 hpf
      (b) Intravascular smooth muscle tumor of uncertain malignant potential: 2–5 mf/10 hpf
      (c) Leiomyosarcoma with vascular invasion: greater than 5 mf/10 hpf
  C. Benign metastasizing leiomyoma
    1. Morphological: deposits of benign smooth muscle in lymph nodes, lung, and other organs associated with a uterine smooth muscle tumor. The uterine smooth muscle tumor and the purported metastases are composed of bland, well-differentiated smooth muscle without anaplasia, significant pleomorphism, tumor-cell necrosis, or abnormal mitotic figures. No evidence of a smooth muscle tumor in another organ which could conceivably be the source of the metastases.
    2. Mitotic counts: fewer than 5 mf/10 hpf in purported metastases and the uterine smooth muscle tumor
  D. Disseminated peritoneal leiomyomatosis
    1. Morphological: numerous small (less than 2.0 cm) nodules of bland smooth muscle cells, often

TABLE 9. *Continued*

arranged in a whorled pattern. Decidual cells are frequent. Pregnancy or functional ovarian tumors are commonly associated.
   2. Mitotic counts:
      (a) Fewer than 5 mf/10 hpf
      (b) Uncertain malignant potential: 5–9 mf/10 hpf
      (c) Leiomyosarcoma: greater than 10 mf/10 hpf
E. Parasitic leiomyoma
   1. Morphological: uterine serosal leiomyoma which becomes detached from the uterus and derives blood supply from omentum, peritoneum, or other pelvic structures
   2. Mitotic counts:
      (a) Fewer than 2 mf/10 hpf
      (b) Uncertain malignant potential: 2–5 mf/10 hpf
      (c) Leiomyosarcoma: greater than 5 mf/10 hpf
F. Infiltrating leiomyoma
   1. Morphological: a characteristic leiomyoma with infiltrating margins
   2. Mitotic counts:
      (a) Fewer than 5 mf/10 hpf
      (b) Uncertain malignant potential: 5–9 mf/10 hpf

Smooth-Muscle Neoplasms (Table 9)

Introduction (198,217,218,228,253)

The vast majority of uterine smooth muscle neoplasms are easily recognized as being composed of cells differentiated as smooth muscle, and the benignancy or malignancy of these neoplasms is a glance diagnosis. However, an important minority of smooth muscle neoplasms present difficulties for one or more of the following reasons: (a) they are clinically benign neoplasms with a peculiar gross appearance; (b) they are clinically benign neoplasms with an unusual anatomic distribution; (c) they are clinically benign neoplasms with aberrant cytologic features; (d) they are clinically malignant neoplasms which resemble leiomyoma by virtue of their relative histologic blandness; (e) they are lesions whose smooth muscle differentiation is not obvious.

Before evaluating the benignancy or malignancy of a purported smooth muscle proliferation in the uterus, it is imperative to ensure that the constituent cells do indeed demonstrate smooth muscle differentiation. For most smooth muscle tumors, this is a straightforward task because the tumor cells resemble normal myometrial cells. However, smooth muscle cells can come to resemble epithelial cells (epithelioid smooth muscle tumors) or endometrial stromal cells. In the former circumstance, the blending of the epithelioid smooth muscle cells into more obvious areas of smooth muscle differentiation in the tumor, if such are present, is the best indicator that the neoplasm in question is indeed a smooth muscle tumor. A reticulin stain may be helpful because reticulin is typically abundant and is wrapped around individual smooth muscle cells in uterine smooth muscle tumors, but it is wrapped around groups of cells in carcinomas and other epithelial lesions. However, not all epithelioid smooth muscle tumors produce abundant reticulin. Immunohistochemical stains utilizing antikeratin antibodies have been suggested in such cases, but it must be remembered that normal smooth-muscle cells can express some types of keratin (246,247). Smooth muscle cells can also come to resemble endometrial stromal cells by losing much of their characteristic fibrillary cytoplasm and developing round to oblong nuclei of the type more often observed in endometrial stromal cells. At times, a trichrome stain will bring out the fibrillar brick-red cytoplasm characteristic of such altered smooth muscle cells. Antibodies against desmin and muscle-specific actin are available, but the specificity and sensitivity of these reagents for smooth muscle cells is unclear at this time (254,255). Our practice is to place tumors for which cellular differentiation still remains ambiguous after all reasonable maneuvers have been tried into the endometrial stromal category for purposes of determining therapy.

After the decision has been made that a uterine tumor demonstrates smooth muscle differentiation, the next step is to evaluate prognostically relevant features and assign the tumor to a category that will predict its behavior. The morphologic definitions we use for the various categories of uterine smooth muscle tumors are presented in Table 9 and Fig. 43. The term "uncertain malignant potential" appears throughout the table. It is used to designate a morphologically heterogeneous group of uterine smooth muscle tumors about which we have insufficient information to predict clinical outcome. So far in our experience, most of the cytologically bland uterine smooth muscle tumors deemed to be of uncertain malignant potential category solely on the basis of borderline mitotic counts have behaved in a benign fashion. On the other hand, smooth muscle neoplasms designated as uncertain malignant potential because of low mitotic counts but that also feature tumor-cell necrosis, cellular atypia, and/or abnormal mitotic figures have behaved aggressively in a significant number of cases. The observations needed to employ the classification in Table 9 include (a) the mitotic index (number of mitotic figures per 10 hpf), (b) the presence or absence of abnormal mitotic figures, (c) the relationship of the neoplasm to surrounding normal structures, (d) the architectural and cytologic features of the constituent tumor cells, and (e) the presence or absence of tumor-cell necrosis or extensive myxoid change (256–260).

Usual Leiomyoma (72,73,261)

Grossly, the usual leiomyoma is circumscribed and white, and it has a whorled trabecular appearance on cut section. Deviations from this typical pattern are rather

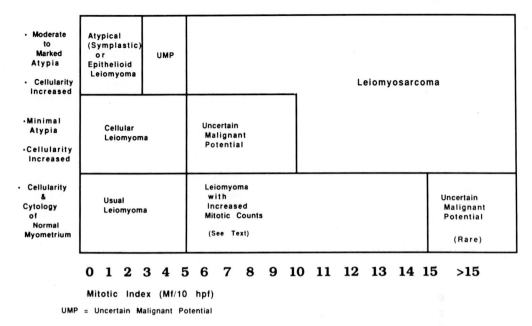

FIG. 43. Morphologic definition of uterine smooth muscle neoplasms. "Benign," "uncertain malignant potential" and "malignant" are morphologically defined using both cytologic-architectural features and mitotic index (see text).

common and result from the replacement of muscle fibers by various substances, including hyalin, collagen, blood, calcium, mucopolysaccharide, or combinations of these (262). Sampling is an important problem in detecting leiomyosarcoma. We think that when three or fewer tumors resembling leiomyomas are present in a uterus, all should be sampled. When there are more than three present, we randomly sample at least the three largest tumors if the gross appearance of all the tumors in the uterus is characteristic of leiomyoma. Any tumor that deviates from the characteristic whorled appearance expected in a leiomyoma should be sampled. We think a minimum of one section per centimeter of diameter of tumor should be taken from any smooth muscle tumor that does not have the characteristic histologic appearance of a leiomyoma.

Microscopically, the usual leiomyoma is easily recognized because the tumor cells resemble the smooth muscle cells that form the myometrium. In general, leiomyomas are slightly more cellular and composed of cells slightly larger than those found in the surrounding myometrium. Significant variation from this pattern should be recognized, and the possibility of leiomyosarcoma, or even another tumor, should be considered.

The margins of most leiomyomas are microscopically circumscribed, but occasional benign tumors will demonstrate apparent infiltration. Consequently, infiltration is not a malignant criterion for smooth muscle tumors. Submucous leiomyomas may well display extensive necrosis, often with acute inflammatory cells, if they protrude into the endometrial cavity. Not infrequently, there will be increased mitotic activity in the tumor cells near the areas of necrosis. On the other hand, tumor-cell necrosis, which is rather common in leiomyosarcoma, is

not associated very often with acute inflammation; in addition, the mitotic figures seen in conjunction with inflammatory necrosis are small and normal, whereas they may be large and abnormal in leiomyosarcoma. Hyaline degeneration is characterized by eosinophilic waxy-appearing material which replaces smooth muscle cells (263). Occasionally, ghost outlines of smooth muscle cells can be seen within areas of hyalin, and this can come to resemble the tumor-cell necrosis seen in leiomyosarcoma. However, nuclear chromatin is very difficult to identify in the ghost cells in hyaline degeneration, whereas a considerable part of the nucleic acid remains visible in most examples of tumor-cell necrosis. When hyalin liquifies, cysts may be produced (cystic degeneration). Myxoid and mucinous degenerations occur in leiomyomas; they are characterized by an increase in the mucopolysaccharide content of the stroma. The result can be in pools of mucinous material separating individual muscle fibers. This benign change must be distinguished from myxoid leiomyosarcoma, in which the tumor cells infiltrate the surrounding myometrium and almost always demonstrate some degree of pleomorphism and nucleomegaly, at least focally, even though the mitotic activity may be very low (see myxoid leiomyosarcoma below). The clinical features of patients with leiomyomas, as well as the natural history of these neoplasms, are described elsewhere (217).

Leiomyoma Variants (217,218)

Cellular leiomyoma

Description. A leiomyoma with a moderate to marked increase in the number of nuclei per unit area

TABLE 10. *Morphologic features that lower the threshold for leiomyosarcoma from 10 mf/10 hpf to something less[a]*

Architectural features
    Intravascular growth
    Tumor-cell necrosis (see text)
    Myxoid stroma
Cytologic features
    Abnormal mitotic figures
    Epithelioid histology
    Anaplasia: Atypia, hyperchromasia, pleomorphism

[a] See text and Table 9 for explanation of individual features.

relative to the surrounding normal myometrium is labeled "cellular leiomyoma."

CPC. Almost all leiomyosarcomas are hypercellular; hence, we always examine cellular leiomyomas carefully, looking for mitotic activity, tumor-cell necrosis, pleomorphism, and/or cellular atypia. Cellular leiomyomas can usually be recognized grossly because they are softer than the usual leiomyoma. Increased cellularity per se does not cause us to lower the mitotic counts for a diagnosis of leiomyosarcoma (see Table 10). Leiomyomas in older women often have closely approximated nuclei that can simulate hypercellularity. This overestimation of cellularity can be avoided by comparing the cells in the leiomyoma to those in the surrounding myometrium which should also be atrophic with closely approximated nuclei. Cellular leiomyomas have the same clinical behavior as ordinary leiomyomas.

Symplastic leiomyoma (217,264,265) (Fig. 44)

Description. This is the appellation we use for leiomyomas that contain cells with enlarged and pleomorphic nuclei. Oftentimes, enlarged multinucleated giant cells are part of this landscape. Definitionally, symplas-

tic leiomyomas do not have abnormal mitotic figures nor can mitotic figures be present in numbers in excess of 4 per 10 hpf. Symplastic smooth muscle tumors of uncertain malignant potential contain 2 to 4 mf/10 hpf.

CPC. Although benign smooth muscle tumors of the uterus may contain enlarged cells and atypical cells, this is a relatively uncommon phenomena in our experience. We lower the mitotic counts for a diagnosis of leiomyosarcoma from 10 mf/10 hpf to 5 mf/10 hpf when symplastic features are present. Uterine smooth muscle tumors demonstrating the cellular features found in symplastic leiomyomas but that also have areas of tumor cell necrosis and/or contain abnormal enlarged division figures should never be interpreted as completely benign; rather, we suggest the term "uncertain malignant potential" be applied, even if mitotic figures are not identified. One also should not interpret a symplastic smooth muscle tumor as being completely benign when the abnormal cells are distributed throughout the entire tumor because this is most frequently a feature of leiomyosarcoma. Again, "uncertain malignant potential" would seem the appropriate term in this circumstance if mitotic counts are below 5 mf/10 hpf. It is apparent that great care must be used when a diagnosis of symplastic leiomyoma is contemplated. Mitotic figures, abnormal mitotic figures, tumor cell necrosis, and vascular invasion are all very disturbing features in any smooth muscle tumor, particularly when the tumor contains enlarged cells, and pleomorphism is easily appreciated and extensive.

Mitotically active leiomyoma (leiomyoma with increased mitotic figures)

Description. This term is used by us for leiomyomas that contain more than 10 *normal* mitotic figures per 10 hpf but that are otherwise bland in microscopic and

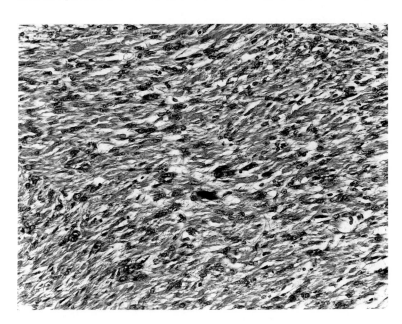

FIG. 44. Symplastic changes in a leiomyoma. Note the pleomorphism which imitates that seen in leiomyosarcoma. Mitotic activity was nonexistent in this lesion. However, as is emphasized in the text, great care should be taken in diagnosing symplastic leiomyomas.

gross appearance. It is imperative that this diagnosis *not* be used for neoplasms that exhibit nuclear pleomorphism nor for those that contain abnormal mitotic figures, demonstrate zones of tumor cell necrosis without inflammatory cells, or are hypercellular.

CPC. In recent years it has become apparent that clinically benign uterine smooth muscle tumors may contain more than 10 *normal* mitotic figures per 10 hpf. Increased mitotic activity has been seen by us in submucous leiomyomas that are necrotic and inflamed, as well as in the smooth muscle tumors of patients who have been receiving progestogens or have been pregnant (262,265,266). However, patients with none of these findings may also, on occasion, have mitotically active leiomyomas. Great care should be taken when contemplating a diagnosis of leiomyoma with increased mitotic figures to be sure that the tumor in question is a completely characteristic leiomyoma in which the *only* deviation from the usual leiomyoma is increased numbers of *normal* mitotic figures. If the specimen has been removed by myomectomy, it is also extremely comforting to know the lesion was easily and completely removed ("shelled out") from the myometrium rather than infiltrating the myometrium.

Epithelioid leiomyoma (Table 4; Figs. 45 and 46) (267)

Description. This is a uterine smooth muscle neoplasm composed predominantly or completely of non-spindled, rounded cells with an epithelial-like appearance. The cytoplasm of these cells may be cleared or eosinophilic. By definition, epithelioid leiomyomas have mitotic counts of fewer than 2 mf/10 hpf, whereas tumors with 2 to 4 mf/10 hpf in this category are designated as epithelioid smooth muscle tumors of uncertain malignant potential.

CPC. A number of histologic patterns have been described under the heading of "epithelioid leiomyoma." These include tumors composed of cells featuring perinuclear clearing, cells with peripheral cytoplasmic clearing, and cells with completely clear cytoplasm. The latter have also been designated as "clear-cell leiomyomas" (267–269). Plexiform tumors are sometimes included in this group and are composed of cells with crumpled nuclei and indistinct cytoplasm arranged in cords or rows (Fig. 46). Plexiform tumors are usually incidental findings at the endometrial myometrial junction, although they can be large (270). The direction of differentiation of the plexiform tumor has been controversial because the cells share features of both smooth muscle cells and endometrial stromal cells (271,272). Most ultrastructural studies suggest smooth muscle differentiation (273,274).

Differential diagnosis. Most epithelioid leiomyomas look like smooth muscle tumors grossly. Distinction of epithelioid leiomyoma from carcinoma may sometimes be a problem. The cells of epithelioid leiomyoma fail to produce convincing glands and lack the cytologic atypia and mitotic activity of carcinoma. Immunohistochemical stains for keratin may be unreliable discriminators since smooth muscle cells may express keratin. Apparently, most carcinoma cells do not express desmin or muscle-specific actin, but at this time the specificity of these two antibodies is largely unknown. Probably the best strategy is to cut more H&E sections searching for areas of more characteristic smooth muscle differentiation within the tumor. Unlike epithelioid leiomyoma, uterine tumors resembling ovarian sex-cord tumors, adenosarcomas, and adenofibromas lack a smooth

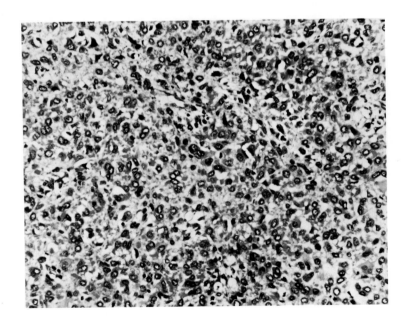

FIG. 45. Epithelioid smooth muscle neoplasm. In this tumor the cells are not spindled as would be expected in the usual smooth muscle tumor, but the rather abundant cytoplasm can be appreciated. The differential diagnosis includes epithelial neoplasms as described in the text.

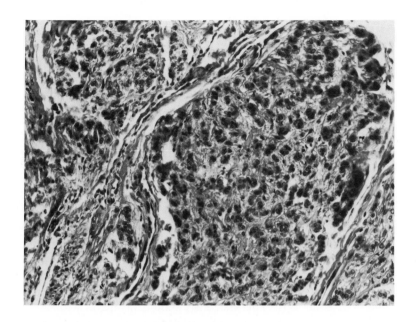

FIG. 46. Plexiform tumor. This lesion features rows and cords of cells with crumpled nuclei set in hyalin. Most often it is a small incidental finding at the endometrial/myometrial junction, but occasionally it can be large. We think the plexiform tumor is a smooth-muscle neoplasm.

muscle component and possess convincing tubular or glandular structures (275).

Lipoleiomyoma (including uterine lipoma) (276–278) (Fig. 47)

Description. This odd but easily recognized neoplasm is composed of an intimate admixture of mature adipocytes and smooth muscle cells. It is mitotically inactive. The term "lipoleiomyoma" covers a spectrum of lesions whose fat content ranges from being a minor component in what is otherwise a leiomyoma to being a neoplasm composed entirely of mature adipocytes.

CPC. This lesion is benign, and the only problem for the pathologist could be puzzlement over the unexpected presence of fat in a uterine tumor. Rarely, intravenous leiomyomatosis may have a fatty component (see below).

Neurilemmoma-like leiomyoma (275,279)

Description. Uterine neoplasms composed of spindle cells, some of which exhibit neurilemmoma-like palisading, are designated neurilemmoma-like leiomyomas. Neoplasms with this pattern are more common in the gastrointestinal tract than in the uterus.

CPC. Most are benign; however, prognosis is based on the same mitotic and morphologic criteria used for more typical uterine smooth muscle neoplasms.

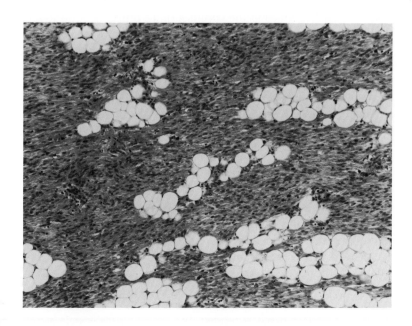

FIG. 47. Lipoleiomyoma. This uterine curiosity is easily recognized because of the fat cells interspersed among the smooth muscle cells. The term "lipoleiomyoma" also includes those neoplasms that are entirely composed of benign adult fat.

Leiomyomatosis (280)

Description. This is a multinodular diffuse proliferation of bland mitotically inactive smooth muscle throughout the myometrium that causes the uterus to become symmetrically enlarged when it is extensive. Microscopically, the process is manifest as small islands of hypercellular smooth muscle interspersed among areas of normal cellular smooth muscle. Within the nodules, smooth muscle cells may be condensed around vessels.

CPC. This is a rare benign process whose apparent infiltration and diffuse distribution should not be construed as evidence of leiomyosarcoma.

Disseminated peritoneal leiomyomatosis (DPL) (281–286)

Description. This rare lesion is characterized by multiple peritoneal nodules composed of an admixture of fibroblasts and smooth muscle cells. The nodules are invariably small (less than 2 cm), and they stud the surface of the peritoneum. There may be an associated decidual reaction.

CPC. DPL is a very rare condition usually discovered incidentally at the time of cesarean section. To the surgeon, DPL may appear as metastases, and the possibility of DPL should be considered whenever peritoneal nodules are encountered in a young woman, particularly if she is pregnant. Postpartum spontaneous regression is the rule.

Benign metastasizing leiomyoma

Description. Women with histologically benign uterine smooth-muscle tumors may, on rare occasions, develop mitotically inactive, cytologically bland extrauterine smooth muscle deposits (usually in the lymph nodes or in the lungs) in the absence of a primary smooth muscle malignancy in the gastrointestinal tract, retroperitoneum, or other nonuterine areas (287–290). Because one explanation for this phenomena is the spread of histologically benign smooth muscle from the uterine leiomyomas to distant sites, this process has been labeled "benign metastasizing leiomyoma."

CPC. The criteria for this improbable diagnosis are understandably strict, and an absolute minimal criterion is that all of the smooth muscle tumors must have been thoroughly examined histologically and judged to be unquestionably benign morphologically. The implication of this diagnosis is that available criteria for identifying leiomyosarcoma are inadequate to pick out those very rare smooth muscle neoplasms that are capable of involving other organs in addition to the uterus but are morphologically noninformative about this potential. While the "metastatic" bland smooth muscle deposits develop most commonly in lymph nodes or the lung, it is rare for the benign smooth muscle deposits to be found initially in abdominal lymph nodes and subsequently in the lungs. Because a few women with benign pulmonary smooth muscle tumors have not had uterine tumors, some investigators believe the pulmonary process is unrelated to the presence of uterine smooth muscle tumors; instead, they consider the lung nodules to be separate smooth muscle proliferations. The pulmonary nodules usually progress slowly, sometimes to the point of producing pulmonary insufficiency. These nodules may respond to hormonal manipulation.

Parasitic leiomyomas

Description. On rare occasions, leiomyomas have been reported to "detach" themselves from their initial subserosa location and "attach" themselves to some other pelvic site. This presumably is through the mediation of a combination of infarction and inflammatory adhesions. This diagnosis should be made with great caution since clinically malignant smooth muscle neoplasms arising in the retroperitoneum or large bowel are notorious for being bland and having a low mitotic index.

CPC. We have never seen a convincing "parasitic" leiomyoma.

Intravenous (intravascular) leiomyomatosis and leiomyoma with vascular intrusion (291,292,292a)

Description. These terms are used to describe localized or disseminated cytologically bland and mitotically inactive smooth muscle within vascular channels. Three situations are distinguished: (i) a solitary, otherwise unremarkable leiomyoma associated with a microscopic focus of intravascular neoplasm within the confines of the leiomyoma, (ii) grossly visible worm-like intravascular masses of cytologically benign smooth muscle, or (iii) microscopic intrusion of a benign smooth muscle into vessels outside the confines of an otherwise unremarkable leiomyoma. The first of these is designated "leiomyoma with vascular intrusion," while the latter two are designated "intravenous (or better, intravascular) leiomyomatosis." Usually smooth muscle tumors involving vascular spaces are composed of bland cells easily recognized as showing smooth muscle differentiation, but some neoplasms may be cellular or they may demonstrate epithelioid, symplastic, myxoid, or fatty features (292a).

CPC. Leiomyomas with vascular intrusion are benign and do not recur. Microscopic intravenous leiomyomatosis (situation iii above) is also, in general, a clinically benign lesion, but there exists a remote possibility of intravascular recurrence outside the uterus. Grossly visible intravenous leiomyomatosis confined to the uterus is generally cured by excising the involved organs, but occasionally it may recur within pelvic, abdominal, thoracic, or femoral vessels. It will recur more often if it has extended into extrauterine vessels at the time of hysterectomy (293,294). In rare instances, continuous extension from the uterus, through the inferior vena cava and into the heart, has been described (295,296). In this circumstance, the patients may be thought to have a primary cardiac neoplasm if the presence of tumor in the uterus and/or the vena cava is not appreciated. The definition of intravenous leiomyomatosis requires any extrauterine benign smooth muscle to remain within vascular lumens or within the chambers of the heart. The presence of morphologically benign smooth muscle within parenchymal organs excludes intravenous leiomyomatosis and raises the possibility of benign metastasizing leiomyoma or low-grade leiomyosarcoma.

Differential Diagnosis

Intravenous leiomyomatosis versus low-grade endometrial stromal sarcoma

In most cases the distinction between these two entities is straightforward and amounts to distinguishing endometrial stromal differentiation from smooth muscle differentiation (Table 4). In some cases, differentiation is ambiguous. Little is known about the natural history of such cases; in our study ambiguous cases tended to behave as low–grade endometrial stromal sarcoma. Thus, for management and prognostic purposes, we assign cases with ambiguous differentiation to the low-grade endometrial stromal sarcomas group.

Leiomyosarcoma (198,218,267,297,305a) (Figs. 48–50)

Leiomyosarcomas may be divided morphologically into three types: (i) the usual type, which includes tumors whose constituent cells can easily be recognized as showing smooth muscle differentiation, as well as those tumors in which smooth muscle differentiation can be demonstrated only focally; (ii) the epithelioid type characterized by tumor cells that take on the appearance of epithelial cells; and (iii) a myxoid type. The latter two types are unusual. Almost all leiomyosarcomas deviate from the usual white whorled macroscopic appearance of a leiomyoma, although not all grossly peculiar smooth muscle tumors are malignant. Consequently, all uterine tumors that have deviant gross appearances must be sampled. Typical and epithelioid leiomyosarcomas are usually hemorrhagic and soft and possess the celebrated fish-flesh texture, while the myxoid variety has a mucoid consistency.

Usual leiomyosarcoma

Description. The usual leiomyosarcoma is easily recognized as malignant in the vast majority of cases, and most often there is no difficulty in identifying it as a smooth-muscle neoplasm. It is common for the mitotic counts to be in the range of 15 to 30 mg/10 hpf and for abnormal division figures to be abundant. In addition, leiomyosarcomas rather frequently have infiltrating borders, they may invade into vessels, and they sometimes have extended beyond the confines of the uterus at the time of diagnosis. However, there is a small subset of leiomyosarcomas that are clearly composed of smooth-muscle cells but that are difficult to distinguish from leiomyoma because mitotic counts are low and the cells are relatively bland. There is another small set of leiomyosarcomas that are anaplastic with only rare tumor cells demonstrating smooth muscle differentiation.

Our conventions for separating uterine smooth muscle tumors into benign, uncertain malignant potential or malignant categories are presented in Fig. 43. As indicated, this classification depends upon an evaluation of

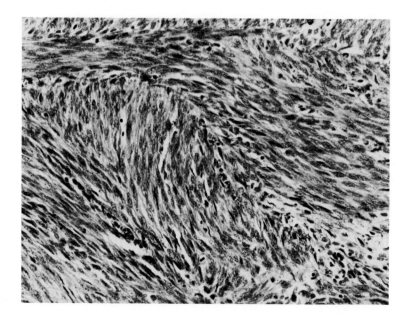

FIG. 48. Low-grade leiomyosarcoma. The spindled tumor cells resemble smooth muscle cells, but the chromatin is more granular and the cells are larger than those found in most leiomyomas.

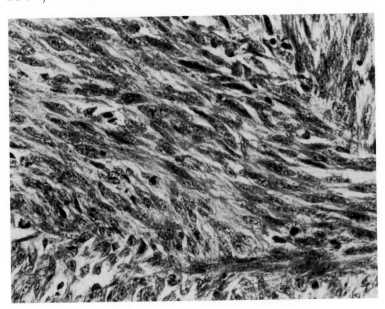

FIG. 49. Low-grade leiomyosarcoma (high power). The chromatin abnormalities and the nuclear enlargement can be appreciated, as can the mitotic figures. It is very unusual for a leiomyosarcoma (even those that are low grade) not to demonstrate at least some nuclear abnormalities.

cytoplasmic features (high nucleus-to-cytoplasm ratios, epithelioid features), nuclear features (hyperchromatism, chromatin patterns, abnormal mitotic figures, and pleomorphism), and, most importantly, mitotic counts (256–260,298–300).

CPC (213,301–305). Although leiomyosarcoma is among the most common of the sarcomas that arise in the uterus, it almost certainly does not evolve from "malignant degeneration" of a leiomyoma. Leiomyosarcomas are rarely associated with prior irradiation (306). Stage is the most important predictor of relapse-free survival, but there has been debate as to whether the histologic features of Stage I leiomyosarcomas provide additional prognostic insight. A recent study by Evans found that only size predicted outcome for Stage I leimyosarcoma and histologic features including the degree of cy-

tologic atypia and the level of mitotic activity provided no further insight into prognosis (305a). The only treatment known to be effective for leiomyosarcoma is surgical, and the value of postoperative adjuvant therapy has not been established (307–309). The mean age of patients with uterine leiomyosarcoma is around 50 years; they may be found in women in the fourth decade, but leiomyosarcoma is very rare in women under 30 years of age. The overall survival is 10% to 30% at 5 years.

Epithelioid leiomyosarcoma (267)

When epithelioid-type cells predominate or are abundantly present within a uterine smooth muscle tumor, experience indicates that the mitotic counts for leio-

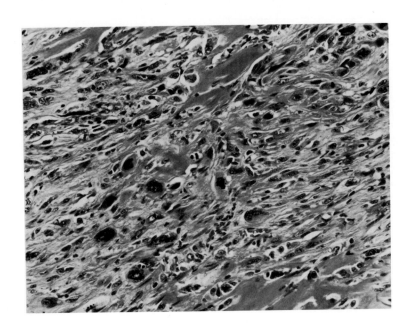

FIG. 50. Pleomorphic leiomyosarcoma. The pleomorphism and at least one abnormal mitotic figure can be appreciated. Most leiomyosarcomas have obvious malignant features similar to those in this photomicrograph, and only a minority will require careful mitotic counts in order to recognize aggressive potential.

myosarcoma should be lowered from 10 mf/10 hpf to 5 mf/10 hpf. Epithelioid leiomyosarcomas are rare in our experience and must be distinguished from infiltrating carcinoma. Electron microscopy and immunohistochemical techniques are potentially useful to make this distinction; however, normal smooth muscle cells may express keratin (312). Evolution of epithelioid areas into more characteristic spindled areas within the tumor is the most helpful finding in recognizing smooth muscle differentiation. Too few cases of epithelioid leiomyosarcoma have been reported to compare the prognosis to the usual type of leiomyosarcoma.

Myxoid leiomyosarcoma (297,310,311)

Description. This term denotes a malignant mesenchymal neoplasm of the uterus composed of hyperchromatic, pleomorphic smooth muscle cells suspended in a prominent myxoid matrix. The margin of this process is infiltrative, and mitotic figures may be very difficult to find.

CPC. These neoplasms have a tendency to recur over long periods of time, and they are potentially capable of metastasizing.

Differential Diagnosis

Other types of sarcoma versus high-grade leiomyosarcoma

Distinguishing leiomyosarcoma from other pure sarcomas, except low-grade endometrial sarcoma (see below), is not of great practical importance because the treatment and behavior of all high-grade uterine sarcomas will be the same. Accordingly, while it is certainly reasonable to attempt to properly classify uterine sarcomas using inexpensive traditional techniques, it is questionable whether other expensive techniques should be used for problematic cases. Malignant mixed müllerian tumors have a sarcomatous stroma, but they also contain carcinoma (see the section of mixed müllerian tumors). The stroma of müllerian adenosarcoma is fibroblastic rather than smooth muscle, and benign glands are present (see the section on adenosarcoma).

Well-differentiated leiomyosarcoma versus low-grade endometrial stromal sarcoma

Because the criteria for malignancy differ for smooth-muscle tumors and low-grade endometrial stromal sarcoma, an essential initial step is establishing the differentiation of a tumor. Low-grade endometrial stromal sarcoma is distinguished from the benign stromal nodule on the basis of the presence or absence of infiltrating margins independent of the number of mitotic figures.

On the other hand, smooth muscle neoplasms with fewer than 10 mf/10 hpf (and sometimes fewer than 5 mf/10 hpf; see Table 9) are considered benign or of uncertain malignant potential, even when they have infiltrating margins. As a result, the direction of differentiation is crucial for predicting outcome for neoplasms with fewer than 10 mf/10 hpf. Strategies for determining differentiation are presented in Table 4 and in the introduction to the section on smooth muscle lesions (page 1637). As noted above, when in doubt assign the case to the endometrial stromal group.

Spindle-cell epithelial proliferations versus leiomyosarcoma (Fig. 40)

Usually, reticulin is laid down around groups of cells in epithelial proliferations (carcinoma, morules, etc.), whereas it is often around individual cells in leiomyosarcoma. Immunohistochemical stains may be of use, but it should be remembered that normal smooth muscle cells express keratin (312).

Leiomyoma versus leiomyosarcoma

Almost all of the diagnostic problems that involve leiomyosarcoma center about distinguishing it from benign smooth muscle tumors. Careful attention to nuclear abnormalities, cellularity, cell size, tumor-cell necrosis, abnormal mitotic figures, and, most importantly, mitotic counts will allow accurate prediction of the behavior of almost all smooth muscle tumors. Tumor-cell necrosis and abnormal mitotic figures are histologic features that should never be ignored. The presence of either should trigger a compulsive search for more mitotic figures. Even when mitotic figures are found to be sparse, we never interpret tumors with tumor-cell necrosis or abnormal division figures as being completely benign. The criteria we use to define leiomyosarcoma, leiomyoma, and smooth-muscle tumor of uncertain malignant potential are presented in Table 9 and Fig. 43.

Pure Differentiated Sarcoma Other than Leiomyosarcoma and Low-Grade Endometrial Stromal Sarcoma

For references, see list of unusual neoplasms given in Table 6.

Description. Pure uterine sarcomas in which at least some of the tumor cells demonstrate either homologous or heterologous differentiation are classified on the basis of this differentiation, e.g., chondrosarcoma, osteosarcoma, rhabdomyosarcoma, etc. Rarely, two types of mesenchymal differentiation will be found in the same tumor; we classify such neoplasms as pure mixed uterine sarcomas. When the cells of a pure sarcoma do not demonstrate appreciable differentiation, we place the sarcoma in the undifferentiated category. Pure undifferentiated uterine sarcoma encompasses many of the neoplasms formerly classified as high-grade endometrial stromal sarcomas (see the discussion on this subject in the section on endometrial stromal tumors). Sarcomas containing multinucleated giant cells but no other evidence of differentiation are labeled "giant-cell sarcoma" of the uterus.

CPC. Setting aside low-grade endometrial stromal sarcoma, once a neoplasm has been classified as a pure uterine sarcoma, the direction of differentiation makes little difference; the treatment and outcome will be much the same for all pure uterine sarcomas.

Differential Diagnosis

Malignant mixed müllerian tumor versus pure sarcoma

Both carcinoma and high-grade sarcoma must be present in malignant mixed müllerian tumors; however, the carcinoma may be only focally present and not present in curettings or poorly sampled neoplasms. Misclassifying a malignant mixed müllerian tumor as a pure sarcoma is of little importance to the patient since both tumors have the same prognosis and both will be treated in essentially the same way.

Adenosarcoma versus pure differentiated sarcoma

The stroma of most adenosarcomas is low grade; however, even when the sarcoma is high grade, bland, often cystically dilated, glands are distributed throughout the tumor. These are not present in pure sarcomas. In addition, the sarcomatous stromal cells in adenosarcomas often condense circumferentially around the dilated glands. The diffusely distributed dilated glands and the stromal condensation help to distinguish adenosarcoma from pure sarcoma infiltrating among preexisting endometrial glands.

Mesenchymal metaplasia versus pure heterologous sarcoma

Rarely, benign bone or cartilage can be found in the uterus, and, at times, leiomyomas may contain benign metaplastic bone. Mesenchymal metaplasias are distinguished from sarcoma by their fully mature and bland constituent cells; i.e., the cells do not have the malignant cytologic features found in osteosarcoma and chondrosarcoma.

Anaplastic carcinoma versus lymphoma/leukemia versus pure sarcoma (see pattern 4 at the beginning of this chapter, page 1594)

Reticulin and chloracetate stains, as well as immunohistochemical stains for keratins and leukocyte common antigen, are useful in solving this differential diagnostic problem if large numbers of H&E sections do not allow definitive diagnosis.

Miscellaneous Neoplasms

Adenomatoid Mesothelioma (313–316) (Fig. 51)

Description. Adenomatoid tumors identical to those occurring in the fallopian tube may, less commonly, arise primarily in the uterus, usually in a subserosal location near the cornua. Grossly, adenometroid mesothe-

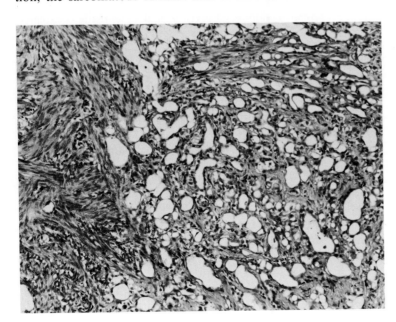

FIG. 51. Adenomatoid mesothelioma. These interesting neoplasms display spaces lined by bland cuboidal cells that appear to be infiltrating smooth muscle. The pattern is quite distinct.

liomas mimic leiomyomas, except the former often are yellow, and they are almost always under 2 cm in diameter. Microscopically, they feature irregular aggregates of cuboidal to flattened cells arranged in clumps, columns, or gland-like spaces interdigitating between bands of smooth muscle. Cellular atypia is minimal or absent, and mitotic figures are usually sparse, but rarely they may be numerous. The evidence to date suggests these neoplasms are differentiating along mesothelial lines. As would be expected, alcian blue stains may be positive while mucicarmine stains are negative.

CPC. Adenomatoid mesotheliomas occur chiefly during the reproductive years, and they are benign.

Lymphoma and Leukemia
(see pattern 4 above, page 1594)

Lymphoma and leukemia rarely involve endometrial biopsy specimens or a uterus which has been removed as a surgical specimen. Even when this rare event occurs, the knowledge that the patient has lymphoma or leukemia usually has been established. Thus, if history is provided, the pathologist is almost never faced with recognizing lymphoma or leukemia *de novo* in a surgical specimen. However, this possibility must always be kept in mind whenever an unusual neoplasm is encountered in the uterus. Moreover, large-cell lymphoma and granulocytic leukemia can resemble endometrial stromal sarcoma so that the former two are always in the differential diagnosis of the latter.

Rare and Unusual Neoplasms

For a listing of these with reference citations see Table 6.

GENERAL REFERENCES

Blaustein S, Kurman R, eds. *Pathology of the female genital tract,* 3rd edition. New York: Springer-Verlag, 1987.

Dallenbach-Hellweg G. *Histopathology of the endometrium,* 3rd edition. New York: Springer-Verlag, 1981.

DiSaia PJ, Creasman WT. *Clinical gynecologic oncology,* 3rd edition. St. Louis: CV Mosby, 1989.

Hendrickson MR, Kempson RL. *Surgical pathology of the uterine corpus.* Major problems in pathology series, vol. 12, James L. Bennington, consulting editor. Philadelphia: WB Saunders, 1980 (2nd edition in press, 1991).

Morrow CP, Townsend DE. *Synopsis of gynecologic oncology,* 3rd edition. New York: John Wiley & Sons, 1987.

Sherman RP, ed. *Clinical reproductive endocrinology.* Edinburgh: Churchill Livingstone, 1985.

Speroff L, Glass RH, Kase NG. *Clinical gynecologic endocrinology and infertility,* 4th edition. Baltimore: Williams & Wilkins, 1989.

REFERENCES

1. Nickelsen C. Diagnostic and curative value of uterine curettage. *Acta Obstet Gynecol Scand* 1980;65:693–697.
2. Daichman I, Mackles A. Diagnostic curettage: a 13 year study of 585 patients. *Am J Obstet Gynecol* 1966;95:212–218.
3. McElin TW, Bird CC, Reeves BD, Scott RC. Diagnostic dilatation and curettage: a 20 year survey. *Obstet Gynecol* 1969;33:807–812.
4. Carmichael DE. Asherman's syndrome. *Obstet Gynecol* 1970;36:922–928.
5. Sanfilippo JS, Fitzgerald MR, Badawy SZA, et al. Asherman's syndrome. A comparison of therapeutic methods. *J Reprod Med* 1982;27:328–330.
6. Baitlon D, Hadley JO. Endometrial biopsy. Pathologic findings in 3,600 biopsies from selected patients. *Am J Clin Pathol* 1975;63:9–15.
7. Dewhurst J. Postmenopausal bleeding from benign causes. *Clin Obstet Gynecol* 1982;26:769–776.
8. Rubin, SC. Postmenopausal bleeding: etiology, evaluation, and management. *Med Clin North Am* 1987;71:59–69.
9. Pacheco JC, Kempers RD. Etiology of postmenopausal bleeding. *Obstet Gynecol* 1968;32:40–46.
10. Schindler AE, Schmidt G. Post-menopausal bleeding: a study of more than 1000 cases. *Maturitas* 1980;2:269–274.
11. Van Bogaert L-J, Maldague P, Staquet J-P. Endometrial biopsy interpretation. Shortcomings and problems in current gynecologic practice. *Obstet Gynecol* 1978;51:25–28.
12. Noyes RW. Normal phases of the endometrium. In: Hertig AT, Norris HJ, eds. *The uterus.* IAP monograph no. 14, Baltimore, Williams & Wilkins, 1973: pp. 110–135.
13. Buxton DCL, Olson LE. Endometrial biopsy inadvertently taken during conception cycle. *Am J Obstet Gynecol* 1979;101:702.
13a. Ferenczy A. Endometrial cycles. In: Sciarra JJ, ed. *Gynecology and Obstetrics,* vol. 5. New York: Harper & Row, 1981:1–14.
14. Hendrickson MR, Kempson RL. *Surgical pathology of the uterine corpus.* Major problems in surgical pathology series, vol. 12. Philadelphia: WB Saunders, 1980 (2nd edition in preparation, 1988).
15. Allenby PA, Chowdhury LN. Histiocytic appearance of metastatic lobular breast carcinoma. *Arch Pathol Lab Med* 1986;110:759–760.
16. Kumar NB, Hart WR. Metastases to the uterine corpus from extragenital cancers. A clinicopathologic study of 63 cases. *Cancer* 1982;50:2163–2169.
17. Kumar A, Schneider V. Metastases to the uterus from extrapelvic primary tumors. *Int J Gynecol Pathol* 1983;2:134–140.
18. Johannisson E, Parker RA, Landgren B-M, Diczfalusy E. Morphometric analysis of the human endometrium in relation to peripheral hormone levels. *Fertil Steril* 1982;38:564–571.
19. Ferenczy A, Bertrand G, Gelfand MM. Proliferation kinetics of human endometrium during the normal menstrual cycle. *Am J Obstet Gynecol* 1979;133:859–867.
20. Noyes RW, Hertig AT, Rock J. Dating the endometrial biopsy. *Fertil Steril* 1950;1:3–25.
21. Robertson WB. A reappraisal of the endometrium in infertility. *Clin Obstet Gynaecol* 1984;11:209–226.
22. Dallenbach-Hellweg G. *Histopathology of the endometrium,* 3rd edition. New York: Springer-Verlag, 1981.
23. Dallenbach-Hellweg G. The endometrium of infertility. A review. *Pathol Res Pract* 1984;178:527–537.
24. Speroff L, Glass RH, Kase NG. *Clinical gynecologic endocrinology and infertility,* 3rd edition, Baltimore: Williams & Wilkins, 1983.
25. Koninckx PR, Goddeeris PG, Lauweryns JM, et al. Accuracy of endometrial biopsy dating in relation to the midcycle luteinizing hormone peak. *Fertil Steril* 1977;28:443.
26. Jansen RPRS, Johannisson E. Endocrine response in the female genital tract. In: Shearman R, ed. *Clinical reproductive endocrinology.* Edinburgh: Churchill Livingstone, 1985.
27. Radwanska E, Hammond MJ, Smith P. Single midluteal progesterone assay in the management of ovulatory infertility. *J Reprod Med* 1981;26:85.
28. Cumming DC, Honore LH, Scott JZ, Williams KP. The late luteal phase in infertile women: comparison of simultaneous endometrial biopsy and progesterone levels. *Fertil Steril* 1985;43:715–719.
29. Daly DC, Tohan N, Doney TJ, et al. The significance of lym-

phocyticleukocytic infiltrates interpreting late luteal phase endo-metrial biopsies. *Fertil Steril* 1982;37:786–791.

30. Daly DC, Walters CA, Soto-Albors CE, Riddick DH. Endome-trial biopsy during treatment of luteal phase defects is predictive of therapeutic outcome. *Fertil Steril* 1983;40:305–310.

31. Smith STK, Lenton EA, Landgren BM, Cooke ID. The short luteal phase and infertility. *Br J Obstet Gynaecol* 91:1120.

32. Zorn JR, Cedard L, Nessman C, Savale M. Delayed endometrial maturation in women with normal progesterone levels. The dy-shargmonic luteal phase syndrome. *Gynecol Obstet Invest* 1984;37:157–162.

33. Wentz AC. Diagnosing luteal phase inadequacy [Editorial]. *Fer-til Steril* 1982;37:334–335.

34. Annos T, Thompson IE, Taymor ML. Luteal phase deficiency and infertility: difficulties encountered in diagnosis and treat-ment. *Obstet Gynecol* 1980;55:705.

35. Huang K-E. The primary treatment of luteal phase inadaquacy: progesterone versus clomiphene citrate. *Am J Obstet Gynecol* 1986;155:824.

36. Jones GRS. Luteal phase insufficiency. *Clin Obstet Gynecol* 1973;16:255–273.

37. Ludwig H. The morphologic response of the human endome-trium to long-term treatment with progestational agents. *Am J Obstet Gynecol* 1982;142:796–808.

38. Ober WB. Effects of oral and intrauterine administration of con-traceptives on the uterus. *Hum Pathol* 1977;8:513–527.

39. Cruz-Aquino M, Shenker L, Blaustein A. Pseudosarcoma of the endometrium. *Obstet Gynecol* 1967;29:93–96.

40. Hertig AT. Gestational hyperplasia of endometrium: a morpho-logic correlation of ova, endometrium, and corpora lutea during early pregnancy. *Lab Invest* 1964;13:1153–1191.

41. Kjer JJ, Eldon K. The diagnostic value of the Arias-Stella phe-nomenon. *Zentralbl Gynakol* 1982;104:753–756.

42. Arias-Stella J. Atypical endometrial changes produced by chori-onic tissue. *Hum Pathol* 1972;3:450–453.

43. Arias-Stella J. Gestational endometrium. In: Hertig AT, Norris HJ, eds. *The uterus.* IAP monograph no. 14, Baltimore: Williams & Wilkins, 1973:185–212.

44. Silverberg SG. Arias-Stella phenomenon in spontaneous and therapeutic abortion. *Am J Obstet Gynecol* 1972;112:777–780.

45. Silverberg SG, Bolin MG, DeGiorgi LRS. Adenoacanthoma and mixed adenosquamous carcinoma of the endometrium: a clini-copathologic study. *Cancer* 1972;30:1307–1314.

46. Fienberg R, Lloyd HED. The Arias-Stella reaction in early nor-mal pregnancy—an involutional phenomenon. The ovary-pla-centa changeover as a possible cause. *Hum Pathol* 1974;5:183–190.

47. Johannisson E, Fournier K, Riotton G. Regeneration of the human endometrium and presence of inflammatory cells follow-ing diagnostic curettage. *Acta Obstet Gynecol Scand* 1981;60:451–457.

48. Winkler B, Reumann W, Mitao M, et al. Chlamydial endome-tritis. A histological and immunohistochemical analysis. *Am J Surg Pathol* 1984;8:771–778.

49. Jones RB, Mammal JB, Shephard MK, Fisher RR. Recovery of chlamydia trachomatis from the endometrium of women at risk for chlamydial infection. *Am J Obstet Gynecol* 1986;155:35.

50. Moyer DL, Mishell DR Jr. Reactions of human endometrium to the intrauterine foreign body. II. Long-term effects on the endo-metrial histology and cytology. *Am J Obstet Gynecol* 1971;111:66–80.

51. Moyer DL, Mishell DR Jr, Bell J. Reactions of human endome-trium to the intrauterine device. I. Correlation of endometrial histology and bacterial environment of the uterus following short-term insertion of the IUD. *Am J Obstet Gynecol* 1970;106:799–809.

52. Cadena D, Cavanzo FJ, Leone CL, Taylor HB. Chronic endo-metritis: a comparative clinicopathologic study. *Obstet Gynecol* 1973;41:733–738.

53. Greenwood SM, Moran JJ. Chronic endometritis: morphologic and clinical observations. *Obstet Gynecol* 1981;58:176–184.

54. Rotterdam H. Chronic endometritis: a clinicopathologic study. *Pathol Annu* 1978;13:209–231.

55. Platt LD, Yonekura ML, Ledger WJ. The role of anaerobic bac-teria in postpartum endometritis. *Am J Obstet Gynecol* 1979;135:814–817.

56. Barua R, Kirkland JA, Petrucco OM. Xanthogranulomatous endometritis: case report. *Pathology* 1978;10:161–164.

57. Dawagne MP, Silverberg SG. Foam cells in endometrial carci-noma—a clinicopathologic study. *Gynecol Oncol* 1982;13:67–75.

58. Nogales-Ortiz F, Tarancon I, Nogales FF. The pathology of fe-male genital tuberculosis. *Obstet Gynecol* 1979;53:422.

59. Bazaz-Malik G, Maheshwari B, Lal N. Tuberculous endome-tritis: a clinicopathological study of 1000 cases. *Br J Obstet Gyn-aecol* 1983;90:84–86.

60. Pepperell RJ. A rational approach to ovulation induction. *Fertil Steril* 1983;40:1.

61. Goldfarb JM, Little AB. Abnormal vaginal bleeding. *N Engl J Med* 1980;302:666–669.

62. Meyer WC, Malkasian GD, Dockerty MB, Decker DG. Post-menopausal bleeding from atrophic endometrium. *Obstet Gyne-col* 1971;38:731–738.

63. Daly JJ, Balogh K Jr. Hemorrhagic necrosis of the senile endo-metrium ("apoplexia uteri"): relation to superficial hemorrhagic necrosis of the bowel. *N Engl J Med* 1968;279:709–711.

64. Nedoss BR. Dysfunctional uterine bleeding: relation of endome-trial histology to outcome. *Am J Obstet Gynecol* 1971;109:103–107.

65. Coney P. Polycystic ovarian disease: current concepts of patho-physiology and therapy. *Fertil Steril* 1984;42:667.

66. Whitehead MRI, Townsend PT, Pryse-Davies J, et al. Effects of estrogens and progestins on the biochemistry and morphology of the postmenopausal endometrium. *N Engl J Med* 1981;305:1599–1605.

67. Fox H, Buckley CH. The endometrial hyperplasias and their relationship to endometrial neoplasia. *Histopathology* 1982;6:493–510.

68. Chamlian DL, Taylor HB. Endometrial hyperplasia in young women. *Obstet Gynecol* 1970;36:659–666.

69. Fraser IRS, Baird DT. Endometrial cystic hyperplasia in adoles-cent girls. *J Obstet Gynaecol Br Commonw.* 1972;79:1009–1015.

70. Scully RE. Definition of precursors in gynecologic cancer. *Cancer* 1981;48:531–537.

71. Scully RE. Definition of endometrial carcinoma precursors. *Clin Obstet Gynecol* 1982;25:39–48.

72. Hendrickson MR, Kempson RL. Endometrial hyperplasia and carcinoma. In: Fox H, ed. *Haines and Taylor: Obstetrical and gynecologic pathology.* Edinburgh: Churchill Livingstone, 1987.

73. Kurman RJ, Kaminski PF, Norris HJ. The behavior of endome-trial hyperplasia. A long term study of "untreated" hyperplasia in 170 patients. *Cancer* 1985;56:403–412.

74. Welch WR, Scully RE. Precancerous lesions of the endome-trium. *Hum Pathol* 1977;8:503–512.

75. Fenoglio CM, Crum CP, Ferenczy A. Endometrial hyperplasia and carcinoma: are ultrastructural, biochemical, and immuno-cytochemical studies useful in distinguishing between them? *Pathol Res Pract* 1982;174:257–284.

76. Hendrickson MR, Kempson RL. Invited review: the differential diagnosis of endometrial adenocarcinoma. Some viewpoints concerning a common diagnostic problem. *Pathology* 1980;12:35–61.

77. Hendrickson MR, Ross J, Kempson RL. Toward the develop-ment of morphologic criteria for well-differentiated adenocarci-noma of the endometrium. *Am J Surg Pathol* 1983;7:819–838.

78. Huang SJ, Amparo EG, Fu YS. Histologic classification and behavior of endometrial hyperplasia [Abstract]. *Lab Invest* 1988;58:40.

79. Kistner RW. Treatment of hyperplasia and carcinoma *in situ* of the endometrium. *Clin Obstet Gynecol* 1982;25:63–74.

80. Beutler HK, Dockerty MB, Randall LM. Precancerous lesions of the endometrium. *Am J Obstet Gynecol* 1963;86:433–443.

81. Sherman ARI, Brown S. The precursors of endometrial carci-noma. *Am J Obstet Gynecol* 1979;135:947–956.

82. Tavassoli F, Kraus FT. Endometrial lesions in uteri resected for atypical endometrial hyperplasia. *Am J Clin Pathol* 1978;70:770–779.

83. Campbell PE, Barter RA. The significance of atypical endome-trial hyperplasia. *J Obstet Gynecol* 1961;68:668–672.

84. Wolfe SA, Mackles A. Malignant lesions arising from benign endometrial polyps. *Obstet Gynecol* 1960;20:542–550.

85. Barwick KW, LiVolsi VA. Heterologous mixed mullerian tumor confined to an endometrial polyp. *Obstet Gynecol* 1979;53:512–514.

86. Atypical polypoid adenomyomas of the endometrium. *Am J Surg Pathol* 1981;5:473–482.

87. Young RH, Treger T, Scully RE. Atypical polypoid adenomyoma of the uterus. A report of 27 cases. *Am J Clin Pathol* 1986;86:139–145.

88. Gusberg SB. Current concepts in cancer: the changing nature of endometrial cancer. *N Engl J Med* 1980;302:729–731.

89. Silverberg SG. New aspects of endometrial carcinoma. *Clin Obstet Gynaecol* 1984;11:189–208.

90. Hendrickson M, Ross J, Eifel PJ, Cox RRS, et al. Adenocarcinoma of the endometrium: analysis of 256 cases with carcinoma limited to the uterine corpus. Pathology review and analysis of prognostic variables. *Gynecol Oncol* 1982;13:373–392.

91. Anderson B, Louis F, Watring WG, Edinger DD. Growth patterns in endometrial carcinoma. *Gynecol Oncol* 1980;10:134–145.

92. Aalders J, Abeler V, Kolstad P, Onsrud M. Postoperative external irradiation and prognostic parameters in stage I endometrial carcinoma: clinical and histopathologic study of 540 patients. *Obstet Gynecol* 1980;56:419–426.

93. Eifel P, Ross J, Hendrickson M, Cox RRS, et al. Adenocarcinoma of the endometrium: analysis of 256 cases with disease limited to the uterine corpus: Treatment Comparisons. *Cancer* 1983;52:1026–1031.

94. Quinn MA, Kneale BJ, Fortune DW. Endometrial carcinoma in premenopausal women: a clinicopathological study. *Gynecol Oncol* 1985;20:298–306.

95. Kempson RL, Pokorny, GE. Adenocarcinoma of the endometrium in women aged forty and younger. *Cancer* 1968;21:650–662.

96. Crissman JD, Azoury RRS, Barnes AE, Schellhas HF. Endometrial carcinoma in women 40 years of age or younger. *Obstet Gynecol* 1981;57:699–704.

97. Ostor AG, Adam R, Gutteridge BH, Fortune DW. Endometrial carcinoma in young women. *Aust NZ J Obstet Gynaecol* 1982;22:38–42.

98. Silverberg SG, Makowski EL, Roche WD. Endometrial carcinoma in women under 40 years of age: comparison of cases in oral contraceptive users and non-users. *Cancer* 1977;39:592–598.

99. Wilkinson EJ, Friedrich EG, Mattingly RF, Regali JA, et al. Turner's syndrome with endometrial adenocarcinoma and stilbestrol therapy. *Obstet Gynecol* 1973;42(2):193–200.

100. McCarroll AM, Montgomery DA, Harley JM, McKeown EF, et al. Endometrial carcinoma after cyclical oestrogen-progestogen therapy for Turner's syndrome. *Br J Obstet Gynaecol* 1975;82:421–423.

101. Fechner RE, Kaufman RH. Endometrial adenocarcinoma in Stein-Leventhal syndrome. *Cancer* 1974;34:444–452.

102. McDonald TW, Malkasian GD, Gaffey TA. Endometrial cancer associated with feminizing ovarian tumor and polycystic ovarian disease. *Obstet Gynecol* 1977;49:654–658.

103. Wood GP, Boronow RC. Endometrial adenocarcinoma and the polycystic ovary syndrome. *Am J Obstet Gynecol* 1976;124:140–142.

104. Robboy SJ, Miller AWR III, Kurman RJ. The pathologic features and behavior of endometrial carcinoma associated with exogenous estrogen administration. *Pathol Res Pract* 1982;174:237–256.

105. Robboy SJ, Bradley R. Changing trends and prognostic features in endometrial cancer associated with exogenous estrogen therapy. *Obstet Gynecol* 1979;54:269–277.

106. Scully RE. Estrogens and endometrial carcinoma. *Hum Pathol* 1977;8:481–483.

107. Silverberg SG, Mullen D, Faraci JA, Makowski EL, et al. Endometrial carcinoma: clinical-pathologic comparison of cases in postmenopausal women receiving and not receiving exogenous estrogens. *Cancer* 1980;45:3018–3026.

108. British Gynaecological Cancer Group. Oestrogen replacement and endometrial cancer: a statement by the British Gynaecological Cancer Group. *Lancet* 1981;June 20:1359–1360.

109. Collins J, Allen LH, Donner A, Adams O. Oestrogen use and survival in endometrial cancer. *Lancet* 1980;November 1:961–963.

110. Lipsett MB. Hormones, medication and cancer. *Cancer* 1983;51:2426–2429.

111. Smith DC, Prentice RL, Bauermeister, DE. Endometrial carcinoma: histopathology survival, and exogenous estrogens. *Gynecol Obstet Invest* 1981;12:169–179.

112. Mahboubi E, Eyler N, Wynder EL. Epidemiology of cancer of the endometrium. *Clin Obstet Gynecol* 1982;25:5–17.

113. Davies JL, Rosenshein NB, Antunes CM, Stolley PD. A review of the risk factors for endometrial carcinoma. *Obstet Gynecol Surv* 1981;36:107–115.

114. Bhagavan BRS, Parmley TH, Rosenshein NB, et al. Comparison of estrogen-induced hyperplasia to endometrial carcinoma. *Obstet Gynecol* 1984;64:12–15.

115. Horwitz RRI, Feinstein AR, Vidone RA, et al. Histopathologic distributions in the relationship of estrogens and endometrial cancer. *J Am Med Assoc* 1981;246:1425–1427.

116. Christopherson WM, Connelly PRS, Alberhasky RC. Carcinoma of the endometrium. V. An analysis of prognosticators in patients with favorable subtypes and Stage I disease. *Cancer* 1983;51:1705–1709.

117. Ng ABP, Reagan JW. Incidence and prognosis of endometrial carcinoma by histologic grade and extent. *Obstet Gynecol* 1970;35:437–443.

118. Piver MRS, Barlow JJ, Lele SB. Para-aortic lymph node metastasis in FIGO Stage I endometrial carcinoma: value of surgical staging and results of treatment. *NY State J Med* 1982;82:1321–1324.

119. DeVita VT, Hellman S, Rosenberg SA. *Cancer: principles and practice of oncology,* 2nd edition. Philadelphia: JB Lippincott, 1985.

120. Boronow RC. Staging of endometrial cancer. *Int J Radiat Oncol Biol Phys* 1980;6:355–359.

121. DiSaia PJ, Creasman WT. *Clinical gynecologic oncology,* 2nd edition. St. Louis: CV Mosby, 1984.

122. Hanson MB, van Nagell JR Jr, Powell DE, et al. The prognostic significance of lymph-vascular space invasion in stage I endometrial cancer. *Cancer* 1985;55:1753–1757.

123. Hall JB, Young RH, Nelson JH, Jr. The prognostic significance of adenomyosis in endometrial carcinoma. *Gynecol Oncol* 1984;17:32–40.

124. Hernandez E, Woodruff JD. Endometrial adenocarcinoma arising in adenomyosis. *Am J Obstet Gynecol* 1980;138:827–832.

125. Berman ML, Afridi MA, Kanbour AI, Ball HG. Risk factors and prognosis in stage II endometrial cancer. *Gynecol Oncol* 1982;14:49–61.

126. Kadar NRD, Kohorn ERI, LiVolsi VA, Kapp DRS. Histologic variants of cervical involvement by endometrial carcinoma. *Obstet Gynecol* 1982;59:85–92.

127. Choo YC, Naylor B. Multiple primary neoplasms of the ovary and uterus. *Int J Gynaecol Obstet* 1982;20:327–334.

128. Eifel P, Hendrickson M, Ross J, Ballon S, et al. Simultaneous presentation of carcinoma involving the ovary and the uterine corpus. *Cancer* 1982;50:163–170.

129. Ulbright TM, Roth LM. Metastatic and independent cancers of the endometrium and ovary: a clinicopathologic study of 34 cases. *Hum Pathol* 1985;16:28–34.

130. Kinsella TJ, Bloomer WD, Lavin PT, Knapp RC. Stage II endometrial carcinoma: a ten year follow-up of combined radiation and surgical treatment. *Gynecol Oncol* 1980;10:290–297.

131. Goplerud DR, Belgrad R. The importance of histologic grade in stage II endometrial carcinoma. *Surg Gynecol Obstet* 1979;148:406–408.

132. Burrell MO, Franklin EW III, Powell JL. Endometrial cancer: evaluation of spread and follow-up in one hundred eighty-nine patients with stage I or stage II disease. *Am J Obstet Gynecol* 1982;144:181–185.

133. Bruckman JE, Bloomer WD, March A, Ehrmann RL, et al. Stage III adenocarcinoma of the endometrium: two prognostic groups. *Gynecol Oncol* 1980;9:12–17.

134. Berman ML, Ballon SC, Lagasse LD, Watring WG. Prognosis

and treatment of endometrial cancer. *Am J Obstet Gynecol* 1980;136:679–688.

135. Figge DC, Otto PM, Tamimi HTK, Greer BE. Treatment variables in the management of endometrial cancer. *Am J Obstet Gynecol* 1983;146:495–500.

136. Morrow CP, Schlaerth JB. Surgical management of endometrial carcinoma. *Clin Obstet Gynecol* 1982;25:81–92.

137. Creasman WT, Soper JT, McCarty KRS Jr, McCarty KRS Sr, et al. Influence of cytoplasmic steroid receptor content on prognosis of early stage endometrial carcinoma. *Am J Obstet Gynecol* 1985;151:922–932.

138. Billiet G, DeHertogh R, Bonte J, Ide P, et al. Estrogen receptors in human uterine adenocarcinoma: correlation with tissue differentiation, vaginal karyopycnotic index, and effect of progestogen or anti-estrogen treatment. *Gynecol Oncol* 1982;14:33–39.

139. Ehrlich CE, Young PCM, Cleary RE. Cytoplasmic progesterone and estradiol receptors in normal, hyperplastic, and carcinomatous endometria: therapeutic implications. *Am J Obstet Gynecol* 1981;141:539–546.

140. Liao BRS, Twiggs LB, Leung BRS, et al. Cytoplasmic estrogen and progesterone receptors as prognostic parameters in primary endometrial carcinoma. *Obstet Gynecol* 1986;67:463–467.

141. Kurman RJ, Norris HJ. Evaluation of criteria for distinguishing atypical endometrial hyperplasia from well differentiated carcinoma. *Cancer* 1982;49:2547–2559.

142. Norris HJ, Tavassoli FA, Kurman RJ. Endometrial hyperplasia and carcinoma: diagnostic considerations. *Am J Surg Pathol* 1983;7:839–847.

143. Feichter GE, Hoffken H, Heep J, Haag D, et al. DNA-flow-cytometric measurements on the normal, atrophic, hyperplastic and neoplastic human endometrium. *Virchows Arch [A]* 1982;398:53–65.

144. Gray LA, Robertson RW, Christopherson WM. Atypical endometrial changes associated with carcinoma. *Gynecol Oncol* 1974;2:93–100.

145. Colgan TJ, Norris HRS, Foster W, Kurman RJ, et al. Predicting the outcome of endometrial hyperplasia by quantitative analysis of nuclear features using a linear discriminant function. *Int J Gynecol Pathol* 1983;15:1347–1352.

146. Hendrickson MR, Kempson RL. Endometrial epithelial metaplasias: proliferations frequently misdiagnosed as adenocarcinoma. Report of 89 cases and proposed classification. *Am J Surg Pathol* 1980;4:525–542.

147. Liu CT. A study of endometrial adenocarcinoma with emphasis on morphologically variant types. *Am J Clin Pathol* 1972;57:562–573.

148. Anderson WA, Taylor PT, Fechner RE, Pinkerton JAV. Endometrial metaplasia associated with endometrial carcinoma. *Am J Obstet Gynecol* 1987;157:597–604.

149. Dutra FR. Intraglandular morules of the endometrium. *Am J Clin Pathol* 1959;31:60–65.

150. Crum CP, Richart RM, Fenoglio CM. Adenoacanthosis of the endometrium: a clinicopathologic study in premenopausal women. *Am J Surg Pathol* 1981;5:15–20.

151. Lane ME, Dacalos E, Sobrero AJ, Ober WB. Squamous metaplasia of the endometrium in women with an intrauterine contraceptive device: follow-up study. *Am J Obstet Gynecol* 1974;119:693–697.

152. Ng ABP, Reagan JW, Storaasli JP, Wentz WB. Mixed adenosquamous carcinoma of the endometrium. *Am J Clin Pathol* 1973;59:765–781.

153. Alberhasky RC, Connelly PJ, Christopherson WM. Carcinoma of the endometrium. IV. Mixed adenosquamous carcinoma: a clinical-pathological study of 68 cases with long-term follow-up. *Am J Clin Pathol* 1982;77:655–664.

154. Haqqani MT, Fox H. Adenosquamous carcinoma of the endometrium. *J Clin Pathol* 1976;29:959–966.

155. Demopoulos RRI, Dubin N, Noumoff J, Blaustein A, Sommers GM. Prognostic significance of squamous differentiation in stage I endometrial adenocarcinoma. *Obstet Gynecol* 1986;68:245–250.

156. Connelly PJ, Alberhasky RC, Christopherson WM. Carcinoma of the endometrium. III. Analysis of 865 cases of adenocarcinoma and adenoacanthoma. *Obstet Gynecol* 1982;59:569–575.

157. Warhol MJ, Rice RH, Pinkus GRS, Robboy SJ. Evaluation of squamous epithelium in adenoacanthoma and adenosquamous carcinoma of the endometrium: immunoperoxidase analysis of involucrin and keratin localization. *Int J Gynecol Pathol* 1984;3:82–91.

158. Silverberg SG. Significance of squamous elements in carcinoma of the endometrium: a review. In: Fenoglio CM, Wolff M, eds. *Progress in surgical pathology.* New York: Masson, 1982:115–136.

159. Salazar OM, DePapp EW, Bonfiglio TA, Feldstein ML, et al. Adenosquamous carcinoma of the endometrium: an entity with an inherent poor prognosis? *Cancer* 1977;40:119–130.

159a.Zaino RJ, Kurman RJ. Squamous differentiation in carcinoma of the endometrium: a critical appraisal of adenoacanthoma and adenosquamous carcinoma. *Seminars in Diagnostic Pathol* 1988;5:154–171.

160. Christopherson WM, Alberhasky RC, Connelly PJ. Glassy cell carcinoma of the endometrium. *Hum Pathol* 1982;13:418–421.

161. Chen KTK, Kostich ND, Rosai J. Peritoneal foreign body granulomas to keratin in uterine adenoacanthoma. *Arch Pathol Lab Med* 1978;102:174–177.

162. Bibro MC, Kapp DRS, LiVolsi VA, Schwartz PE. Case report: squamous carcinoma of the endometrium with ultrastructural observations and review of the literature. *Gynecol Oncol* 1980;10:217–223.

163. Lifshitz S, Schauberger CW, Platz CA, Roberts JA. Primary squamous cell carcinoma of the endometrium. *J Reprod Med* 1981;26:25–27.

164. Tiltman AJ, Atad J. Verrucous carcinoma of the cervix with endometrial involvement. *Int J Gynecol Pathol* 1982;1:221–226.

165. Ryder DE. Verrucous carcinoma of the endometrium: a unique neoplasm with long survival. *Obstet Gynecol* 1982;59(Suppl):78s–80s.

166. Salm R. Superficial intrauterine spread of intraepithelial cervical carcinoma. *J Pathol Bacteriol* 1969;97:261–268.

167. Kanbour ARI, Stock RJ. Squamous cell carcinoma *in situ* of the endometrium and fallopian tube as superficial extension of invasive cervical carcinoma. *Cancer* 1978;42:570–580.

168. Demopoulos RRI, Greco MA. Mucinous metaplasia of the endometrium: ultrastructural and histochemical characteristics. *Int J Gynecol Pathol* 1983;1:383–390.

169. Honore LH. Benign obstructive myxometra: report of a case. *Am J Obstet Gynecol* 1979;133:227–229.

170. Tiltman AJ. Mucinous carcinoma of the endometrium. *Obstet Gynecol* 1980;55:244–247.

171. Ross JC, Eifel PJ, Cox RRS, Kempson RL, Hendrickson, MR. Primary mucinous adenocarcinoma of the endometrium: a clinicopathologic and histochemical study. *Am J Surg Pathol* 1983;7:715–729.

172. Melham MF, Tobon H. Mucinous adenocarcinoma of the endometrium: a clinico-pathological review of 18 cases. *Int J Gynecol Pathol* 1987;6:347–355.

173. Cohen C, Shulman G, Budgeon LR. Endocervical and endometrial adenocarcinoma: an immunoperoxidase and histochemical study. *Am J Surg Pathol* 1982;6:151–157.

174. Czernobilsky B, Katz Z, Lancet M, Gaton E. Endocervical components in endometrial carcinoma: a report of ten cases with emphasis on histochemical methods for differential diagnosis. *Am J Surg Pathol* 1980;4:481–489.

175. Bannatyne P, Russell P, Wills EJ. Argyrophilia and endometrial carcinoma. *Int J Gynecol Pathol* 1983;2:235–254.

176. Prade M, Gadenne C, Duvillard P, Bognel C, et al. Endometrial carcinoma with argyrophilic cells. *Hum Pathol* 1982;13:870–871.

177. Ueda G, Yamasaki M, Inoue M, Kurachi K. A clinicopathologic study of endometrial carcinomas with argyrophil cells. *Gynecol Oncol* 1979;7:223–231.

178. Scully RE, Aguirre P, DeLellis RA. Argyrophilia serotonin, and peptide hormones in the female genital tract and its tumors. *Int J Gynecol Pathol* 1984;3:51–70.

179. Aguirre P, Scully RE, Wolfe HJ, DeLellis RA. Endometrial carcinoma with argyrophil cells: a histochemical and immunohistochemical analysis. *Hum Pathol* 1984;15:210–217.

180. Inoue M, DeLellis RA, Scully RE. Immunohistochemical dem-

onstration of chromagranin in endometrial carcinomas with argyrophil cells. *Hum Pathol* 1986;17:841–847.

181. Sivridis E, Buckley CH, Fox H. Argyrophil cells in normal, hyperplastic, and neoplastic endometrium. *J Clin Pathol* 1984;37:378–381.

182. Rorat E, Wallach RC. Papillary metaplasia of the endometrium: clinical and histopathologic considerations. *Obstet Gynecol* 1984;64:90S–92S.

183. Christopherson WM, Alberhasky RC, Connelly PJ. Carcinoma of the endometrium. II. Papillary adenocarcinoma: a clinical pathological study of 46 cases. *Am J Clin Pathol* 1982;77:534–540.

184. Hendrickson MR, Ross J, Eifel P, Martinez A, Kempson R. Uterine papillary serous carcinoma: a highly malignant form of endometrial adenocarcinoma. *Am J Surg Pathol* 1982;6:93–108.

185. Lauchlan SC. Tubal (serous) carcinoma of the endometrium. *Arch Pathol Lab Med* 1981;105:615–618.

186. LiVolsi VA. Adenocarcinoma of the endometrium with psammoma bodies. *Obstet Gynecol* 1977;50:725–728.

187. Walker AN, Mills SE. Serous papillary carcinoma of the endometrium. A clinicopathologic study of 11 cases. *Diagn Gynecol Obstet* 1982;4:261–267.

188. Factor SM. Papillary adenocarcinoma of the endometrium with psammoma bodies. *Arch Pathol* 1974;98:201–205.

189. Fruin AH, Tighe JR. Tubal metaplasia of the endometrium. *J Obstet Gynaecol Br Commonw* 1967;74:93–97.

190. Hendrickson MR, Kempson RL. Ciliated carcinoma—a variant of endometrial adenocarcinoma: a report of 10 cases. *Int J Gynecol Pathol* 1983;2:1–12.

191. Christopherson WM, Alberhasky RC, Connelly PJ. Carcinoma of the endometrium. I. A clinicopathologic study of clear cell carcinoma and secretory carcinoma. *Cancer* 1982;49:1511–1523.

192. Crum CP, Fechner RE. Clear cell adenocarcinoma of the endometrium: a clinicopathologic study of 11 cases. *Am J Diagn Gynecol Obstet* 1979;1:261–267.

193. Eastwood J. Mesonephroid (clear cell) carcinoma of the ovary and endometrium: a comparative prospective clinicopathological study and review of literature. *Cancer* 1978;41:1911–1928.

194. Kurman RJ, Scully RE. Clear cell carcinoma of the endometrium: an analysis of 21 cases. *Cancer* 1976;37:872–882.

195. Photopulos GJ, Carney CN, Edelman DA, Hughes RR, et al. Clear carcinoma of the endometrium. *Cancer* 1979;43:1448–1456.

196. Silverberg SG, DeGiorgi LRS. Clear cell carcinoma of the endometrium: clinical, pathologic, and ultrastructural findings. *Cancer* 1973;31:1127–1140.

197. Ober WB. Uterine sarcomas: histogenesis and taxonomy. *Ann NY Acad Sci* 1959;75:568–585.

198. Zaloudek CJ, Norris HJ. Mesenchymal tumors of the uterus. In: Fenoglio CM, Wolff M, eds. *Progress in surgical pathology,* vol. III. New York: Masson 1981:1–35.

199. Clement PB, Scully RE. Uterine tumors with mixed epithelial and mesenchymal elements. *Semin Diagn Pathol* 1988;5:199–222.

199a.Clement PB, Scully RE. Mullerian adenosarcoma of the uterus: a clinicopathologic analysis of 100 cases with a review of the literature. *Hum Pathol* 1990;21:363–381.

200. Grimalt M, Arguelles M, Ferenczy A. Papillary cystadenofibroma of endometrium: a histochemical and ultrastructural study. *Cancer* 1975;36:137–144.

201. Vellios F, Ng ABP, Reagan JW. Papillary adenofibroma of the uterus: a benign mesodermal mixed tumor of mullerian origin. *Am J Clin Pathol* 1973;60:543–551.

202. Zaloudek CJ, Norris HJ. Adenofibroma and adenosarcoma of the uterus: a clinicopathologic study of 35 cases. *Cancer* 1981;48:354–366.

203. Clement PB, Scully RE. Mullerian adenosarcoma of the uterus: a clinicopathologic analysis of ten cases of a distinctive type of mullerian mixed tumor. *Cancer* 1974;34:1138–1149.

204. Czernobilsky B, Hohlweg-Majert P, Dallenbach-Hellweg, G. Uterine adenosarcoma: a clinicopathologic study of 11 cases with a re-evaluation of histologic criteria. *Arch Gynecol* 1983;233:281–294.

205. Christopherson WM. Mullerian adenosarcoma of the uterus [Letter]. *Am J Surg Pathol* 1980;4:413–414.

206. Hirschfield L, Kahn LB, Chen S, et al. Mullerian adenosarcoma with ovarian sex cord-like differentiation: a light- and electron-microscopic study. *Cancer* 1986;57:1197–1200.

207. Mortel R, Koss LG, Lewis JL Jr, D'Urso JR. Mesodermal mixed tumors of the uterine corpus. *Obstet Gynecol* 1974;43:248–252.

208. Geisinger KR, Dabbs DJ, Marshall RB. Malignant mixed mullerian tumors. An ultrastructural and immunohistochemical analysis with histogenetic considerations. *Cancer* 1987;59:1781–1790.

209. Norris HJ, Roth E, Taylor HB. Mesenchymal tumors of the uterus. II. A clinical and pathologic study of 31 mixed mesodermal tumors. *Obstet Gynecol* 1966;28:57–63.

210. Williamson EO, Christopherson WM. Malignant mixed mullerian tumors of the uterus. *Cancer* 1972;29:585–592.

211. Barwick KW, LiVolsi VA. Malignant mixed mullerian tumors of the uterus. A clinicopathologic assessment of 34 cases. *Am J Surg Pathol* 1979;3:125–135.

212. King ME, Kramer EE. Malignant mullerian mixed tumors of the uterus: a study of 21 cases. *Cancer* 1980;45:188–190.

213. Marchese MJ, Liskow ARS, Crum CP, et al. Uterine sarcomas: a clinicopathologic study, 1965–1981. *Gynecol Oncol* 1984;18:299–312.

214. Silverberg SG, Major F, Morrow P, Blessing J, Creasman W, Curry J. Malignant mixed mesodermal tumor of the endometrium. A clinicopathological study [Abstract]. *Lab Invest* 1988;58:86.

215. Macasaet MA, Waxman M, Fruchter RG, et al. Prognostic factors in malignant mesodermal (mullerian) mixed tumors of the uterus. *Gynecol Oncol* 1985;20:32–42.

216. Spanos WJ Jr, Peters LJ, Oswald MJ. Patterns of recurrence in malignant mixed mullerian tumor of the uterus. *Cancer* 1986;57:155–159.

216a.Silverberg SG, Major FJ, Blessing JA, et al. Carcinosarcoma (malignant mixed mesodermal tumor) of the uterus. A gynecologic oncology group pathologic study of 203 cases. *Int J Gynecol Pathol* 1990;9:1–19.

217. Kempson RL, Hendrickson MR. Pure mesenchymal neoplasms of the uterus corpus. In: Fox H, ed. *Haines and Taylor: Obstetrics and gynecologic pathology.* Edinburgh: Churchill Livingstone, 1987:411–456.

218. Kempson RL, Hendrickson MR. Pure mesenchymal neoplasms of the uterine corpus: selected problems. *Semin Diagn Pathol* 1988;5:172–198.

219. Evans HL. Endometrial stromal sarcoma and poorly differentiated endometrial sarcoma. *Cancer* 1982;50:2170–2182.

220. Norris HJ, Taylor HB. Mesenchymal tumors of the uterus. I. A clinical and pathologic study of 53 endometrial stromal tumors. *Cancer* 1966;19:755–766.

221. Tavassoli FA, Norris HJ. Mesenchymal tumors of the uterus. VII. A clinicopathological study of 60 endometrial stromal nodules. *Histopathology* 1981;5:1–10.

222. Chang KL, Crabtree GS, Lim-Tan, et al. Primary uterine endometrial stromal neoplasms. A clinicopathologic study of 117 cases. *Am J Surg Pathol* 1990;14(5):415–438.

223. Koss LG, Spiro RH, Brunschwig A. Endometrial stromal sarcoma. *Surg Gynecol Obstet* 1970;121:531–537.

224. Krieger PD, Gusberg SB. Endolymphatic stromal myosis—a grade I endometrial sarcoma. *Gynecol Oncol* 1973;1:299–313.

225. Hart WR, Yoonessi M. Endometrial stromatosis of the uterus. *Obstet Gynecol* 1977;49:393–403.

226. Mazur MT, Askin FB. Endolymphatic stromal myosis: unique presentation and ultrastructural study. *Cancer* 1978;42:2661–2667.

227. Fekete PRS, Vellios F. The clinical and histologic spectrum of endometrial stromal neoplasms: a report of 41 cases. *Int J Gynecol Pathol* 1984;3:198–212.

228. Kempson RL, Bari W. Uterine sarcomas: classification, diagnosis, and prognosis. *Hum Pathol* 1970;1:331–349.

229. Gloor E, Schnyder P, Cikes M, Hofstetter J, et al. Endolymphatic stromal myosis: surgical and hormonal treatment of extensive abdominal recurrence 20 years after hysterectomy. *Cancer* 1982;50:1888–1893.

230. Pulmonary metastases of uterine stromal sarcomas: unique histologic appearance suggesting their source [Abstract]. *Lab Invest* 1980;42:110.

231. Baker VVV, Walton LA, Fowler WB, Currie JL. Steroid receptors in endolymphatic stromal myosis. *Obstet Gynecol* 1984;63(Suppl):725–745.

232. Jacobsen KB, Haram K. Endolymphatic stromal myosis: report of a case treated surgically and with hormones. *Virchows Arch [A]* 1975;369:173–179.

233. Krumholz BA, Lobovsky FY, Halitsky V. Endolymphatic stromal myosis with pulmonary metastases. Remission with progestin therapy: report of a case. *J Reprod Med* 1973;10:85–89.

234. Katz L, Merino MJ, Sakamoto H, Schwartz PE. Endometrial stromal sarcoma: A clinicopathological study of 11 cases with determination of estrogen and progestin receptor levels in three tumors. *Gynecol Oncol* 1987;26:87–97.

235. Gerber MA, Toker C. Primary extrauterine endometrial stromal sarcoma. *Arch Pathol* 1970;89:477–480.

236. Sutton GP, Stehman FB, Michael H, et al. Estrogen and progesterone receptors in uterine sarcomas. *Obstet Gynecol* 1986;68:709–714.

237. Young RH, Prat J, Scully RE. Endometroid stromal sarcomas of the ovary: a clinicopathological analysis of twenty-three cases. *Cancer* 1984;53:43–55.

238. Berkowitz RRS, Ehrmann RL, Knapp RC. Endometrial stromal sarcoma arising from vaginal endometriosis. *Obstet Gynecol* 1976;51(Suppl):34–37.

239. Persaud V, Anderson MF. Endometrial sarcoma of the broad ligament arising in an area of endometriosis in a paramesonephric cyst: case report. *Br J Obstet Gynaecol* 1977;84:149–152.

240. Ulbright TM, Kraus FT. Endometrial stromal tumors of extrauterine tissue. *Am J Clin Pathol* 1981;76:371–377.

241. Hughesdon PE. The endometrial identity of benign stromatosis of the ovary and its relation to other forms of endometriosis. *J Pathol* 1976;119:201–209.

242. Brooks JJ, Wheeler JE. Malignancy arising in extragonadal endometriosis. A case report and summary of the world literature. *Cancer* 1977;40:3065–3073.

243. Yoonessi M, Hart WR. Endometrial stromal sarcomas. *Cancer* 1977;40:898–906.

244. Clement PB, Scully RE. Uterine tumors resembling ovarian sex-cord tumors. *Am J Clin Pathol* 1976;66:512–525.

245. Tang C-K, Toker C, Ances IG. Stromomyoma of the uterus. *Cancer* 1979;43:308–316.

246. Brown DC, Theaker JM, Banks PM, Gatter KC, Mason DY. Cytokeratin expression in smooth muscle and smooth muscle tumours. *Histopathology* 1987;11:477–486.

247. Azumi N, Sheibani K, Battifora H. Keratin-like immunoreactivity in leiomyosarcomas, uterine leiomyomas, and normal myometrium by multiple antikeratin antibodies [Abstract]. *Lab Invest* 1988;58:6.

248. Emge LA. The elusive adenomyosis of the uterus. *Am J Obstet Gynecol* 1962;83:1541–1563.

249. Mathur BL, Shah BRS, Bhende YM. Adenomyosis uteri. *Am J Obstet Gynecol* 1962;84:1820–1829.

250. Moliter JJ. Adenomyosis: a clinical and pathologic appraisal. *Am J Obstet Gynecol* 1971;110:275–284.

251. Weseley AC. The preoperative diagnosis of adenomyosis. *Diagn Gynecol Obstet* 1982;4:105–106.

252. Kempson RL, Hendrickson MR. Non-neoplastic conditions of the myometrium and the uterine serosa. In: Fox, H, ed. *Haynes and Taylor: Obstetrics and gynecologic pathology.* Edinburgh: Churchill Livingstone, 1987;1:405–411.

253. Burns B, Curry RH, Bell MEA. Morphologic features of prognostic significance in uterine smooth muscle tumors: a review of 84 cases. *Am J Obstet Gynecol* 1979;135:109–114.

254. Lisschitz-Mercer B, Czernobilsky B, Dgani R, et al. Immunocytochemical study of an endometrial diffuse clear cell stromal sarcoma and other endometrial sarcomas. *Cancer* 1987;59:1494–1499.

255. Poggetto CB, Virtanen I, Lehto V-P, Wahlstrom T, Saksela E. Expression of intermediate filaments in ovarian and uterine tumors. *Int J Gynecol Pathol* 1983;1:359–366.

256. Kempson RL. Mitosis counting. II. *Hum Pathol* 1976;7:482–483.

257. Norris HJ. Mitosis counting. III. *Hum Pathol* 1976;7:483–484.

258. Scully RE. Mitosis counting. I. *Hum Pathol* 1976;7:481–482.

259. Silverberg SG. Reproducibility of the mitosis count in the histologic diagnosis of smooth muscle tumors of the uterus. *Hum Pathol* 1976;7:451–454.

260. Taylor HB, Norris HJ. Mesenchymal tumors of the uterus. IV. Diagnosis and prognosis of leiomyosarcomas. *Arch Pathol* 1966;82:40–44.

261. Buttram VC, Reiter RC. Uterine leiomyomata: etiology, symptomatology, and management. *Fertil Steril* 1981;36:433–445.

262. Myles JL, Hart WR. Apoplectic leiomyomas of the uterus: a clinicopathologic study of five distinctive hemorrhagic leiomyomas associated with oral contraceptive usage. *Am J Surg Pathol* 1985;9:798–805.

263. Persaud V, Arjoon PD. Uterine leiomyoma: incidence of degenerative change and a correlation of associated symptoms. *Obstet Gynecol* 1970;35:432–436.

264. Prakash S, Scully RE. Sarcoma-like pseudopregnancy changes in uterine leiomyomas: report of a case resulting from prolonged norethindrone therapy. *Obstet Gynecol* 1964;24:106–110.

265. Fechner RE. Atypical leiomyomas and synthetic progestin therapy. *Am J Clin Pathol* 1968;49:697–703.

266. Tiltman AJ. The effect of progestins on the mitotic activity of uterine fibromyomas. *Int J Gynecol Pathol* 1985;4:89–96.

267. Kurman RJ, Norris HJ. Mesenchymal tumors of the uterus. VI. Epithelioid smooth muscle tumors including leiomyoblastoma and clear cell leiomyoma: a clinical and pathologic analysis of 26 cases. *Cancer* 1976;36:1853–1865.

268. Rywlin AM, Recher L, Benson J. Clear cell leiomyoma of the uterus: report of two cases of a previously undescribed entity. *Cancer* 1964;17:100–104.

269. Mazur MT, Priest JB. Clear cell leiomyoma (leiomyoblastoma) of the uterus: ultrastructural observations. *Ultrastruct Pathol* 1986;10:249–255.

270. Kaminski PS, Tavassoli FA. Plexiform tumorlet: a clinical and pathological study of 15 cases with ultrastructural observations. *Int J Gynecol Pathol* 1984;3:124–134.

271. Larbig GG, Clemmer JJ, Koss LG, Foote FW Jr. Plexiform tumorlets of endometrial stromal origin. *Am J Clin Pathol* 1965;44:32–35.

272. Nunez-Alonso C, Battifora HA. Plexiform tumors of the uterus: ultrastructural study. *Cancer* 1979;44:1707–1714.

273. Fisher ER, Paulson JD, Gregorio RM. The myofibroblastic nature of the uterine plexiform tumor. *Arch Pathol Lab Med* 1978;102:477–480.

274. Goodhue WM, Susin M, Kramer EBE. Smooth muscle origin of uterine plexiform tumors: ultrastructural and histochemical evidence. *Arch Pathol Lab Med* 1974;97:263–268.

275. Mazur MT, Kraus FT. Histogenesis of morphologic variations in tumors of the uterine wall. *Am J Surg Pathol* 1980;4:59–74.

276. Dharkar DD, Kraft JR, Gangadharam D. Uterine lipomas. *Arch Pathol Lab Med* 1981;105:43–45.

277. Jacobs ERS, Cohen H, Johnson JRS. Lipoleiomyomas of the uterus. *Am J Clin Pathol* 1965;44:45–51.

278. Pounder DJ. Fatty tumours of the uterus. *J Clin Pathol* 1982;35:1380–1383.

279. Gisser SD, Young I. Neurilemmoma-like uterine myomas: an ultrastructural reaffirmation of their non-Schwannian nature. *Am J Obstet Gynecol* 1977;129:389–392.

280. Clement PB, Young RH. Diffuse leiomyomatosis of the uterus: a report of four cases. *Int J Gynecol Pathol* 1987;6:322–330.

281. Aterman K, Fraser GM, Lea RH. Disseminated peritoneal leiomyomatosis. *Virchows Arch [A]* 1977;374:13–26.

282. Tavassoli FA, Norris HJ. Peritoneal leiomyomatosis (leiomyomatosis peritonealis disseminata): a clinicopathologic study of 20 cases with ultrastructural observations. *Int J Gynecol Pathol* 1982;1:59–74.

283. Goldberg MF, Hurt WG, Frabel WJ. Leiomyomatosis peritonealis disseminata: report of a case and review of the literature. *Obstet Gynecol* 1977;49(Suppl):46s–52s.

284. Parmley TH, et al. Histogenesis of leiomyomatosis peritonealis disseminata (disseminated fibrosing deciduosis). *Obstet Gynecol* 1975;46:511–516.

285. Pieslor PC, Orenstein JM, Hogan DL, Breslow A. Ultrastructure

of myofibroblasts and decidualized cells in leiomyomatosis peritonealis disseminata. *Am J Clin Pathol* 1979;72:875–882.

286. Herr JC, Platz CBE, Heidger PM, Curet LB. Smooth muscle within ovarian decidual nodules: a link to leiomyomatosis peritonealis disseminata? *Obstet Gynecol* 1979;53:451–456.

287. Wolff M, Silva F, Kaye G. Pulmonary metastases (with admixed epithelial elements) from smooth muscle neoplasms: report of nine cases, including three males. *Am J Surg Pathol* 1979;3:325–342.

288. Abell MR, Littiler ER. Benign metastasizing uterine leiomyoma with multiple lymph nodal metastases. *Cancer* 1975;36:2206–2213.

289. Boyce CR, Buddhdev HN. Pregnancy complicated by metastasizing leiomyoma of the uterus. *Obstet Gynecol* 1973;42:252–258.

290. Tench WD, Dail D, Gmelich JT, Matani N. Benign metastasizing leiomyomas: a review of 21 cases [Abstract]. *Lab Invest* 1978;38:367.

291. Harper RRS, Scully RE. Intravenous leiomyomatosis of the uterus: a report of 4 cases. *Obstet Gynecol* 1961;18:519–529.

292. Norris HJ, Parmley TH. Mesenchymal tumors of the uterus. V. Intravenous leiomyomatosis: a clinical and pathologic study of 14 cases. *Cancer* 1975;36:2164–2178.

292a.Clement PB, Young RH, Scully RE. Intravenous leiomyomatosis of the uterus. A clinicopathologic analysis of 16 cases with unusual histologic features. *Am J Surg Pathol* 1988;12:932–945.

293. Evans AT III, Symmonds RE, Gaffey TA. Recurrent pelvic intravenous leiomyomatosis. *Obstet Gynecol* 1981;57:260–264.

294. Cameron AE, Graham JC, Cotton LT. Intracaval leiomyomatosis. *Br J Obstet Gynaecol* 1983;90:272–275.

295. Tierney WM, Ehrlich CBE, Bailey JC, et al. Intravenous leiomyomatosis of the uterus with extension into the heart. *Am J Med* 1980;69:471–475.

296. Timmis AD, Smallpiece C, Davies AC, MacArthur AM, et al. Intracardiac spread of intravenous leiomyomatosis with successful surgical excision. *N Engl J Med* 1980;303:1043–1044.

297. King MBE, Dickersin GR, Scully RE. Myxoid leiomyosarcoma of the uterus: a report of six cases. *Am J Surg Pathol* 1982;6:589–598.

298. Silverberg SG. Leiomyosarcoma of the uterus: a clinicopathologic study. *Obstet Gynecol* 1971;38:613–628.

299. Hart WR, Billman JTK Jr. A reassessment of uterine neoplasms originally diagnosed as leiomyosarcomas. *Cancer* 1978;41:1902–1910.

300. Christopherson WM, Williamson EO, Gray LA. Leiomyosarcoma of the uterus. *Cancer* 1972;29:1512–1517.

301. Wheelock JB, Krebs HB, Schneider V, Goplerud DR. Uterine sarcoma: analysis of prognostic variables in 71 cases. *Am J Obstet Gynecol* 1985;151:1016–1022.

302. Kahanpaa KV, Wahlstrom T, Groehn P, et al. Sarcomas of the uterus: a clinicopathologic study of 119 patients. *Obstet Gynecol* 1986;67:417–424.

303. Hannigan E, Gomez L. Uterine leiomyosarcoma: a review of prognostic clinical and pathologic features. *Am J Obstet Gynecol* 1979;134:557–564.

304. Vardi JR, Tovell HMM. Leiomyosarcoma of the uterus: clinicopathologic study. *Obstet Gynecol* 1980;56:428–434.

305. Barter JF, Smith EB, Szpak CA, et al. Leiomyosarcoma of the uterus: clinicopathologic study of 21 cases. *Gynecol Oncol* 1985;21:220–227.

305a.Evans HL, Chawla SP, Simpson C, et al. Smooth muscle neoplasms of the uterus other than ordinary leiomyoma. A study of 46 cases, with emphasis on diagnostic criteria and prognostic factors. *Cancer* 1988;62(10):2239–2247.

306. Norris HJ, Taylor HB. Postirradiation sarcomas of the uterus. *Obstet Gynecol* 1965;26:689–694.

307. Salazar OM, Bonfiglio TA, Patten SF, Keller BBE, et al. Uterine sarcomas: natural history, treatment and prognosis. *Cancer* 1978;42:1152–1160.

308. Salazar OM, Bonfiglio TA, Patten SF, Keller BBE, et al. Uterine sarcomas: analysis of failures with special emphasis on the use of adjuvant radiation therapy. *Cancer* 1978;42:1161–1170.

309. Fleming WP, Peters WA, Kumar NB, Morley GW. Autopsy findings in patients with uterine sarcoma. *Gynecol Oncol* 1984;19:168–172.

310. Chen KT. Myxoid leiomyosarcoma of the uterus. *Int J Gynecol Pathol* 1984;3:389–392.

311. Pounder DJ, Iyer PV. Uterine leiomyosarcoma with myxoid stroma. *Arch Pathol Lab Med* 1985;109:762–764.

312. Yamasina M, Kobara TY. Primary squamous cell carcinoma with its spindle cell variant in the endometrium. A case report and review of literature. *Cancer* 1986;57:340–345.

313. Ferenczy A, Fenoglio J, Richart RM. Observations on benign mesothelioma of the genital tract (adenomatoid tumor): a comparative ultrastructural study. *Cancer* 1972;30:244–260.

314. Taxy JB, Battifora H, Ayasu R. Adenomatoid tumors: a light microscopic, histochemical and ultrastructural study. *Cancer* 1974;34:306–316.

315. Youngs LA, Taylor HB. Adenomatoid tumors of the uterus and fallopian tube. *Am J Clin Pathol* 1967;48:537–545.

316. Tiltman AJ. Adenomatoid tumours of the uterus. *Histopathology* 1980;4:437–443.

317. Bhagavan BRS, Gupta PK. Genital actinomysis and intrauterine contraceptive devices. Cytopathologic diagnosis and clinical significance. *Hum Pathol* 1978;9:567–578.

318. Berry A. A cytopathological and histopathological study of bilharziasis of the female genital tract. *J Pathol Bacteriol* 1966;91:325–338.

319. Westrom L. Gynecological chlamydial infections. *Infection* 1982;10(Suppl):S40–S45.

320. Salgia K, Bhatia L, Rajashekaraiah KR, Zangan M, et al. Coccidiomycosis of the uterus. *South Med J* 1982;75:614–616.

321. Dehner LP, Askin FB. Cytomegalovirus endometritis: report of a case associated with spontaneous abortion. *Obstet Gynecol* 1975;45:211–214.

322. McCracken AW, D'Agostino AN, Brucks AB, Kingsly WB. Acquired cytomegalovirus infection presenting as viral endometritis. *Am J Clin Pathol* 1974;61:556.

323. Wenckelbach GFC, Curry B. Cytomegalovirus infection of the female genital tract. Histologic findings in three cases and review of the literature. *Arch Pathol Lab Med* 1976;100:1609.

324. Schenken JR, Tamisica J. Enterobium vermicularis (pinworm) infection of the endometrium. *Am J Obstet Gynecol* 1956;72:913–914.

325. Robb JA, Benirschke K, Barmeyer R. Intrauterine latent herpes simplex virus infection. I. Spontaneous abortion. *Hum Pathol* 1986;17:1196.

326. Schneider V, Behm FG, Mumaw VR. Ascending herpetic endometritis. *Obstet Gynecol* 1982;59:259–262.

327. Remington JRS, Melton ML, Jacobs L. Chronic toxoplasma infection in the uterus. *J Lab Clin Med* 1960;56:879–883.

328. Stray-Pedersen B, Lorentzen-Styr A-M. Uterine toxoplasma infections and repeated abortions. *Am J Obstet Gynecol* 1977;128:716–721.

329. Venkataseshan VS, Woo TH. Diffuse viral papillomatosis (condyloma) of the uterine cavity. *Int J Gynecol Pathol* 1985;4:370.

330. Sherrick JC, Vega JG. Congenital intramural cysts of the uterus. *Obstet Gynecol* 1962;19:486–493.

331. Pirozynski WJ. Giant cell arteritis of the uterus. *Am J Clin Pathol* 1976;65:308–313.

332. Gronroos M, Meurman L, Kahra K. Proliferating glia and other heterotopic tissues in the uterus: fetal homografts? *Obstet Gynecol* 1983;61:261–266.

333. Newton CW III, Abell MR. Iatrogenic fetal implants. *Obstet Gynecol* 1972;40:686–691.

334. Mazur MT, Hendrickson MR, Kempson RL. Optically clear nuclei: an alteration of endometrial epthelium in the presence of trophoblast. *Am J Surg Pathol* 1983;7:415–423.

335. Buckley CH, Fox H. Histiocytic endometritis. *Histopathology* 1980;4:105–110.

336. Thomas W Jr, Sadeghieh B, Fresco R, et al. Malacoplakia of the endometrium, a probable cause of postmenopausal bleeding. *Am J Clin Pathol* 1978;69:637–642.

337. Perkins MB. Pneumopolycystic endometritis. *Am J Obstet Gynecol* 1960;80:332–336.

338. Kraus FT. Irradiation changes in the uterus. In: Hertig AT, Norris HJ, eds. *The uterus.* IAP monograph no. 14, Baltimore: Williams & Wilkins, 1973:457–488.

339. Ho KL. Sarcoidosis of the uterus. *Hum Pathol* 1979;10:219–222.

340. Arhelger RB, Bocian JJ. Brenner tumor of the uterus. *Cancer* 1976;38:1741–1743.

341. Young RH, Kleinman GM, Scully RE. Glioma of the uterus. Report of a case with comments on histogenesis. *Am J Surg Pathol* 1981;5:695–699.

342. Liao SY, Choi BH. Expression of glial fibrillary acidic protein by neoplastic cells of mullerian origin. *Virchows Arch [Cell Pathol]* 1986;52:185–193.

343. Roth E, Taylor HB. Heterotopic cartilage in the uterus. *Obstet Gynecol* 1966;27:838–844.

344. Bhatia NN, Hoshiko MG. Uterine osseous metaplasia. *Obstet Gynecol* 1982;60:256–259.

345. Nicholson GW. Studies of tumour formation: polypoid teratoma of the uterus. *Guy's Hospital Reports* 1956;105:157.

346. Olson N, Twiggs L, Sibley R. Small-cell carcinoma of the endometrium: light microscopic and ultrastructural study of a case. *Cancer* 1982;50:760–765.

347. Kumar NB. Small cell carcinoma of the endometrium in a 23-year-old woman: light microscopic and ultrastructural study. *Am J Clin Pathol* 1984;81:98–101.

348. Manivel C, Wick MR, Sibley RTK. Neuroendocrine differentiation in mullerian neoplasms. An immunohistochemical study of a "pure" endometrial small-cell carcinoma and a mixed mullerian tumor containing small-cell carcinoma. *Am J Clin Pathol* 1986;86:438–443.

349. Paz RA, Frigerio B, Sundblad ARS, Eusebi V. Small-cell (oat cell) carcinoma of the endometrium. *Arch Pathol Lab Med* 1985;109:270–272.

350. Civantos F, Rywlin AM. Carcinomas with trophoblastic differentiation and secretion of chorionic gonadotrophins. *Cancer* 1972;29:789–798.

351. Tsoutsoplides GC. Ectopic production of human chorionic gonadotropin by a highly anaplastic adenocarcinoma of the endometrium. *Am J Obstet Gynecol* 1980;136:694–695.

352. Gray GF Jr, Glick AD, Kurtin PJ, Jones HW III. Alveolar soft part sarcoma of the uterus. *Hum Pathol* 1986;17:297–300.

353. Ongkasuwan C, Taylor JE, Tang CTK, Prempree T. Angiosarcomas of the uterus and ovary: clinicopathologic report. *Cancer* 1982;49:1469–1475.

354. Clement PB. Chondrosarcoma of the uterus. Report of a case and review of the literature. *Hum Pathol* 1978;9:726–732.

355. Kofinas AD, Suarez J, Calame RJ, Chipeco Z. Chondrosarcoma of the uterus. *Gynecol Oncol* 1984;19:231–237.

356. Vakiani M, Mawad J, Talerman A. Heterologous sarcomas of the uterus. *Int J Gynecol Pathol* 1982;1:211–219.

357. Chou S, Fortune D, Beischer NA, et al. Primary malignant fibrous histiocytoma of the uterus—ultrastructural and immunocytochemical studies of two cases. *Pathology* 1985;17:36–40.

358. Fujii S, Kanzaki H, Konishi I, et al. Malignant fibrous histiocytoma of the uterus. *Gynecol Oncol* 1987;26:319–330.

359. Darby AJ, Papadaki L, Beilby JOW. An unusual leiomyosarcoma of the uterus containing osteoclast-like giant cells. *Cancer* 1975;36:495–504.

360. Pilon VA, Parikh N, Maccera J. Malignant osteoclast-like giant cell tumor associated with a uterine leiomyosarcoma. *Gynecol Oncol* 1986;23:381–386.

361. Crum CP, Rogers BH, Andersen W. Osteosarcoma of the uterus. Case report and review of the literature. *Gynecol Oncol* 1980;9:256–268.

362. Piscioli F, Govoni E, Polla E, et al. Primary osteosarcoma of the uterine corpus. Report of a case and critical review of the literature. *Int J Gynaecol Obstet* 1985;23:377–385.

363. Donkers B, Kazzaz BA, Meijering JH. Rhabdomyosarcoma of the corpus uteri: report of two cases with review of the literature. *Am J Obstet Gynecol* 1972;114:1025–1030.

364. Hart WR, Craig JR. Rhabdomyosarcomas of the uterus. *Am J Clin Pathol* 1978;70:217–223.

365. Hays DM, Shimada H, Raney RB Jr, et al. Sarcomas of the vagina and uterus: the Intergroup Rhabdomyosarcoma Study. *J Pediatr Surg* 1985;20:718–724.

366. Montag TW, D'Ablaing G, Schlaerth JB, et al. Embryonal rhabdomyosarcoma of the uterine corpus and cervix. *Gynecol Oncol* 1986;25:171–194.

367. Chen KTK, Vergon JM. Carcinomesenchymoma of the uterus. *Am J Clin Pathol* 1981;75:746–748.

368. Harris NL, Scully RE. Malignant lymphoma and granulocytic sarcoma of the uterus and vagina. A clinicopathologic analysis of 27 cases. *Cancer* 1984;53:2530–2545.

369. Kapadia SB, Krause JR, Kanbour ARI, Hartsock RJ. Granulocytic sarcoma of the uterus. *Cancer* 1978;41:687–691.

370. Hendrickson MR, Sheithauer B. Primitive neurectodermal tumors of the endometrium—report of 2 cases, one with electron microscopic observations. *Int J Gyncol Pathol* 1986;5:249–259.

371. Bittencourt AL, Britto JF, Fonseca LE Jr. Wilm's tumor of the uterus: the first report of the literature. *Cancer* 1981;47:2496–2499.

*Surgical Pathology of the Female
Reproductive System and Peritoneum,*
edited by Stephen S. Sternberg
and Stacey E. Mills. Raven Press, Ltd,
New York © 1991.

CHAPTER 6

The Ovary

Robert H. Young, Philip B. Clement, and Robert E. Scully

NON-NEOPLASTIC DISORDERS

The first section of this chapter reviews non-neoplastic ovarian lesions, which may form pelvic masses or have hormonal manifestations. Because they may mimic ovarian neoplasms on clinical examination, at operation, and even pathologically, their recognition is important. Normal ovarian structures are occasionally misinterpreted as neoplasms on histologic examination; these have been reviewed in detail elsewhere (1) and will not be discussed in this chapter.

Inflammatory Disorders

Infectious Diseases

Common bacterial infections

Pelvic inflammatory disease (PID) of bacterial origin accounts for most ovarian infections in the western world. Ovarian involvement is almost always secondary to salpingitis, and it typically takes the form of a tubo-ovarian abscess, which is usually bilateral. With resolution, the only sequela may be tubo-ovarian fibrous adhesions, but occasionally a healed abscess is converted into a tubo-ovarian cyst. Ovarian changes similar to polycystic ovarian disease have been reported as well (2). A unilateral or bilateral ovarian abscess without tubal involvement is much rarer than a tubo-ovarian abscess. The former is secondary to direct or lymphatic spread from a nongynecologic pelvic inflammatory process (diverticulitis, appendicitis, inflammatory bowel disease, postoperative pelvic infection) or, rarely, from a blood-borne infection (3). The external ovarian surface in such cases is often unremarkable, and the process may not be apparent until the organ is sectioned. Uncommonly, rupture of an ovarian or tubo-ovarian abscess leads to secondary peritonitis (4), or, rarely, fistulas involve the colon (5), bladder (6), or vagina.

A chronic ovarian abscess may rarely form a solid, yellow, tumor-like xanthogranuloma composed of foamy histiocytes and multinucleated giant cells, exhibiting chronic inflammation (7). Pseudotumorous xanthogranulomatous inflammation with more diffuse involvement of the adnexa has also been described (8).

Uncommon bacterial infections

Pelvic actinomycosis is uncommon and usually a complication of an intrauterine device (IUD), although most cases of IUD-associated PID are nonactinomycotic (9–11). The adnexal involvement is typically unilateral, with large abscesses containing actinomycotic "sulfur" granules. The actinomyces colonies may be extremely scarce microscopically, necessitating extensive sampling; a fluorescent antibody stain may help in their demonstration (12). The associated nonspecific inflammatory response consists of neutrophils, foamy histiocytes, lymphocytes, and plasma cells.

Ovarian involvement is present in only 10% of cases of pelvic tuberculosis and is usually secondary to more frequent tubal disease (13). Microscopically, ovarian disease is typically confined to the cortex. Involvement of the peritoneum may mimic an ovarian neoplasm with peritoneal implants (13,14).

Bacterial infections rarely involving the ovary include syphilis, leprosy, and malacoplakia; the last one may be due to several species of bacteria (15,16).

Other rare infections

Ovarian schistosomiasis is relatively common in endemic areas (17). A granulomatous inflammatory infiltrate, often containing eosinophils, is seen in response to the Schistosoma ova; dense fibrosis is frequently present in later stages. Ovarian involvement by *Enterobius vermicularis* is usually an incidental operative finding on the ovarian surface (18). Granulomas frequently contain eosinophils and may exhibit caseous necrosis. They surround the adult female worms and ova. Rare cases of ovarian echinococcosis have been described (19).

Fungal infections of the ovary are extremely rare, even in patients with disseminated mycoses. Rare examples of ovarian involvement by blastomycosis, coccidioidomycosis, and aspergillosis have been described (16).

Oophoritis secondary to cytomegalovirus is a rare autopsy finding in immunosuppressed patients, typically as part of a more generalized infection (20).

Noninfectious Granulomas

Foreign material may evoke a granulomatous reaction on the ovarian and peritoneal surfaces mimicking metastatic carcinoma. Starch granules from surgical gloves (21) or, more rarely, from starch-containing douche fluid or lubricants, can evoke a foreign-body or tuberculoid granulomatous response (21). Foreign-body granulomas may also be due to talc (22), hysterosalpingographic contrast material (23), keratin from ruptured cystic teratomas or adenocarcinomas with squamous differentiation (24), and bowel contents (25).

Isolated noninfectious ovarian granulomas occur typically in patients who have had prior ovarian surgery (26). These granulomas are usually multiple and bilateral. They have hyalinized or necrotic cores surrounded by palisading histiocytes and a fibrous pseudocapsule.

Granulomatous oophoritis can be rarely due to sarcoidosis (27) and Crohn's disease. The latter is usually secondary to direct extension from the bowel and also commonly affects the ipsilateral fallopian tube (28).

So-called cortical granulomas are common, incidental, microscopic lesions of unknown cause within the ovarian cortex of women in the late reproductive and postmenopausal age groups. They consist of epithelioid cells, lymphocytes, and multinucleated giant cells and have no known clinical significance (Fig. 1) (16,29).

Surface Proliferative Lesions

Epithelial Inclusion Glands

Epithelial inclusion glands arise from cortical invaginations of covering epithelium that have lost their connection to the surface. Although most numerous in postmenopausal women, they have also been found in fetuses, infants, and adolescents (30,31). These cysts may measure up to 1 cm in diameter and may be visible grossly, but most are incidental microscopic findings in the superficial cortex; less commonly, they extend into the deeper cortical or medullary stroma. They are typi-

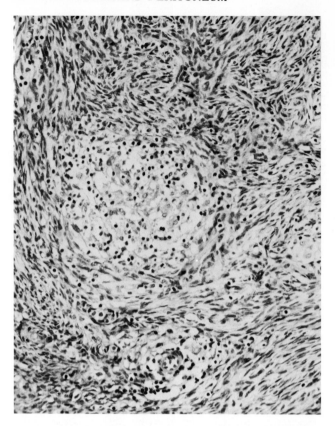

FIG. 1. Cortical granuloma of unknown cause composed of epithelioid cells and lymphocytes.

cally lined by a single layer of ciliated columnar epithelium; psammoma bodies may be present within cysts or in adjacent stroma (Fig. 2). Less commonly, their lining is a single layer of endometrioid or endocervical-type epithelium (32). An Arias-Stella-like reaction may occur in pregnant patients (31). The occasional finding of dysplastic epithelium lining the cysts supports the hypothesis that common epithelial carcinomas arise from them (33).

Surface Stromal Proliferations

Nodular or papillary stromal projections from the ovarian surface are common incidental histological findings in the late reproductive and postmenopausal age groups. They are composed of ovarian stroma exhibiting varying degrees of hyalinization covered by a single layer of surface epithelium.

Mesothelial Proliferations

Proliferations of mesothelial cells, which are occasionally atypical, may be encountered within periovarian adhesions. Similar proliferations are seen elsewhere on peritoneal surfaces (see Chapter 51).

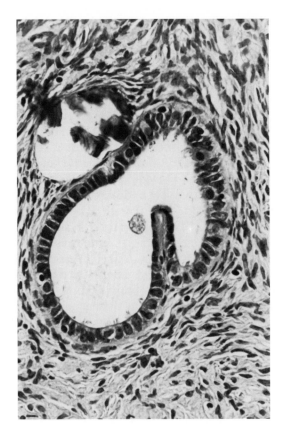

FIG. 2. Inclusion gland lined by tubal-type epithelium. Fragments of calcium are visible adjacent to the gland.

Solitary Cysts of Follicular Origin

Clinical Features

Solitary (one or occasionally a few) follicle cysts (FC) are common, particularly soon after menarche and around the time of menopause (Figs. 3 and 4). They may be encountered, however, at any age (34–38). Corpus luteum cysts (CLC) (Fig. 5) occur during the reproductive era but, exceptionally, may follow sporadic ovulation in a postmenopausal woman (39). Corpora lutea have been encountered very rarely in the ovaries of newborns. FC may be incidental findings, may result in palpable adnexal masses, or may manifest due to increased estrogen production with isosexual precocity (40), menstrual disturbances (36), or endometrial hyperplasia (37). An uncommon presentation of both FC and CLC is rupture with hemoperitoneum, a complication apt to occur in patients who are receiving anticoagulant therapy or who have a bleeding diathesis (41). A CLC arising in residual ovarian tissue is the most frequent finding in the ovarian remnant syndrome; complications have included ureteral and intestinal obstruction (42).

The great majority of FC result from gonadotropin stimulation. In some children, however, including those

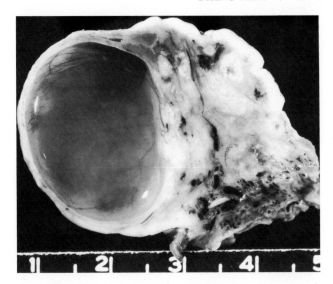

FIG. 3. Follicle cyst. The cyst is thin-walled and filled with clear fluid. (From ref. 39.)

with the McCune-Albright syndrome, the cysts are autonomous and the triggering mechanism is unknown. Isosexual pseudoprecocity caused by autonomous FC may regress spontaneously and may also be reversed by removal of the cyst (43). Autonomous cysts may be sin-

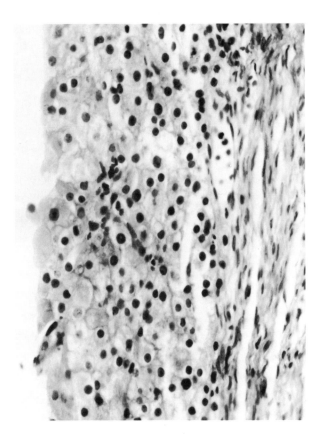

FIG. 4. Follicle cyst. The cyst is lined by luteinized cells. (From ref. 127.)

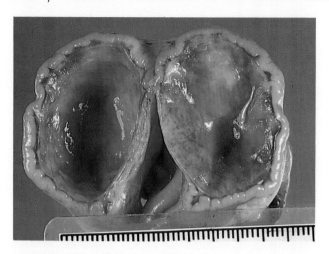

FIG. 5. Corpus luteum cyst. Note smooth lining of cyst and convoluted, yellow rim.

gle or multiple and, in the McCune-Albright syndrome, may be accompanied by corpora lutea and a potential for pregnancy. They may also recur after excision.

A rare type of solitary FC, the *large solitary luteinized follicle cyst of pregnancy and the puerperium* (LSLFCPP) is presumably related to hCG stimulation (45). The patients present with a palpable adnexal mass or with a unilateral ovarian cyst discovered during cesarean section. None of the cysts reported to date have been associated with clinical evidence of an endocrine disturbance.

Gross Features

FC and CLC are unilocular, smooth surfaced, thin walled, and rarely exceed 8 cm in diameter (Figs. 3 and 5). The reported examples of LSLFCPP, however, have had a median diameter of 25 cm. CLC are usually distinctive because all or part of their wall is typically yellow and sometimes convoluted. The contents of FC and CLC vary from serous or serosanguinous fluid to clotted blood.

Microscopic Features

FC are lined by an inner layer of granulosa cells and an outer layer of theca interna cells; either layer may be luteinized (Fig. 4). Distinction between the two is facilitated by a reticulin stain which reveals a dense network in the theca-cell layer but sparse or absent reticulin in the granulosa-cell layer. Either layer, but most often the granulosa-cell component, may be absent or present only focally. LSLFCPP has a distinctive appearance, being lined by one to several layers of large luteinized cells. It may be impossible to distinguish the granulosa-cell component from the theca-cell component. The luteinized cells typically vary markedly in size and shape and exhibit prominent nuclear pleomorphism and hyperchromatism (Fig. 6). CLC is lined by large luteinized granulosa cells interrupted externally by wedges of smaller theca lutein cells. A prominent innermost layer of connective tissue is typically present, and portions of the cyst wall may be lined predominantly by fibrous tissue. CLC associated with pregnancy may also contain hyaline bodies and calcification. Involution and fibrosis of a corpus luteum or CLC usually leads to a corpus albicans or, rarely, a small corpus albicans cyst.

Differential Diagnosis

Cysts otherwise identical to FC and CLC but measuring less than 2.5 cm in diameter are generally regarded as physiological and are designated cystic follicles and cystic corpora lutea, respectively. Differentiating large FC (including LSLFCPP) from unilocular cystic granulosa-cell tumors is discussed elsewhere (page 1690). Simple cysts have an absent lining, or they have a lining composed of nonspecific cuboidal or flattened cells; some are probably of follicular origin, whereas others are probably derived from surface epithelium.

Hyperreactio Luteinalis

Clinical Features

Hyperreactio luteinalis (HL) is characterized by multiple, bilateral, luteinized follicular cysts. It is most

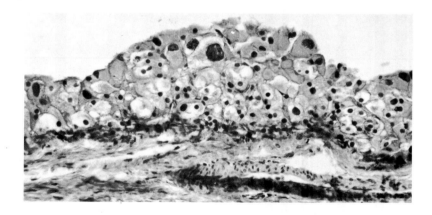

FIG. 6. Large luteinized solitary follicle cyst of pregnancy and puerperium. The lining cells are luteinized, and some have enlarged bizarre nuclei. (From ref. 235.)

commonly associated with disorders of pregnancy having high levels of serum chorionic gonadotropin (hCG), such as hydatidiform mole, choriocarcinoma, fetal hydrops, and multiple gestations (46–48). It also occurs during normal, singleton pregnancies (49). The disorder may become clinically apparent at any time during pregnancy or may be an incidental finding at cesarean section. Much less commonly, clinical manifestations occur within the first 10 days postpartum (46) or, exceptionally, late in the puerperium. The patients usually present with pain or palpable adnexal masses, or both. In patients with HL secondary to trophoblastic disease, cystic ovarian enlargement may be detected at the time of dilatation and curettage or during the postoperative follow-up period (50). In approximately 25% of cases unassociated with trophoblastic disease, the patient has been virilized (51). Complications include torsion, ascites, and rupture with intra-abdominal bleeding. HL typically regresses postpartum but may persist for up to 6 months. An iatrogenic form of HL, referred to as *ovarian hyperstimulation syndrome,* develops in women undergoing ovulation induction (52,53). Patients with this disorder may also have ascites and occasionally hydrothorax of acute onset (acute Meigs' syndrome).

Gross/Microscopic Features

Multiple, bilateral cysts result in moderate to massive ovarian enlargement up to 26 cm (Fig. 7). The cysts may be filled with clear or hemorrhagic fluid. One or more corpora lutea are present in patients with ovarian hyperstimulation syndrome. Microscopically, there are large follicle cysts with marked luteinization of the theca interna layer and, to a lesser extent, the granulosa-cell layer (Fig. 8). There is usually marked stromal edema, and stromal luteinization may be present as well.

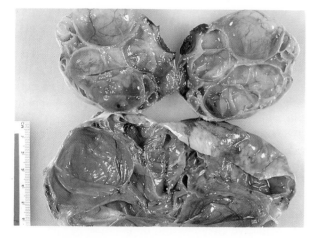

FIG. 7. Hyperreactio luteinalis. Both ovaries are replaced by multiple thin-walled cysts.

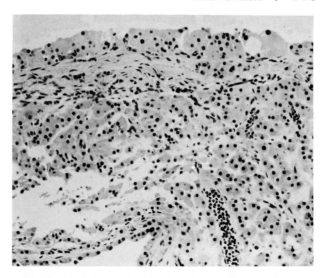

FIG. 8. Hyperreactio luteinalis. Two cysts are lined by luteinized granulosa cells, outside of which are thick layers of luteinized theca cells. (From ref. 127.)

Polycystic Ovarian Disease, Stromal Hyperthecosis and Stromal Hyperplasia

Morphologic and physiologic investigations have shown that these disorders are part of a continuum, and sharp distinctions cannot always be made. In spite of this overlap, it is appropriate to describe the typical clinical and pathologic features of each disorder separately, inasmuch as they differ in several aspects.

Polycystic Ovarian Disease (Stein-Leventhal Syndrome)

Clinical features

Polycystic ovarian disease (PCOD) has been estimated to affect 3.5% to 7.0% of the female population (54). The pathogenetic and endocrinologic features are complex and have been reviewed elsewhere (16,54). Patients typically present in their third decade with oligomenorrhea (rarely primary amenorrhea) or menometrorrhagia, infertility, and, in approximately half, hirsutism (54–56). Frank virilization is rare. The ovaries may be palpably enlarged. The endometrium may demonstrate a weakly proliferative appearance, cystic hyperplasia, atypical hyperplasia, or, uncommonly, adenocarcinoma that is almost always well-differentiated (57–60).

Gross features

Both ovaries are typically enlarged but may be of normal size. Cysts less than 1 cm in diameter may be visible just below the white surface. The central portion of the ovary is composed of stroma with few or no corpora lutea or albicantia (55,61).

Microscopic features

Hypocellular, fibrotic superficial cortex resembles a fibrous capsule (Figs. 9 and 10). Cystic follicles have an inner lining of granulosa cells and a prominent outer layer of luteinized theca interna cells ("follicular hyperthecosis") (Fig. 10). Maturing follicles (up to mid-antral stage) and atretic follicles, exhibiting prominent luteinization of the theca interna, may be twice as numerous as normal (54,62). Primordial follicles are normal in number and appearance (62). Although corpora lutea and albicantia are typically absent, the former occurs in up to 30% of otherwise typical PCOD (61,62). Distorted atretic follicles with persistence of granulosa cells have been described in rare cases (63). The deeper cortical and medullary stroma are often hyperplastic and may exhibit hyperthecosis; if the latter is more than minor in extent, stromal hyperthecosis is a more appropriate diagnosis.

The pathologic findings of PCOD may also be seen during or shortly after puberty, in childhood hypothyroidism, and in disorders disrupting cyclic gonadotropin release. These include late-onset congenital adrenal hyperplasia and primary hypothalamic-pituitary disorders, particularly those associated with hyperprolactinemia. Sclerocystic ovaries have also been described in patients ceasing long-term use of oral contraceptives (64,65), as well as in patients with periovarian adhesions (2). In the former group, PCOD may have been present in some cases before the initiation of oral contraceptives.

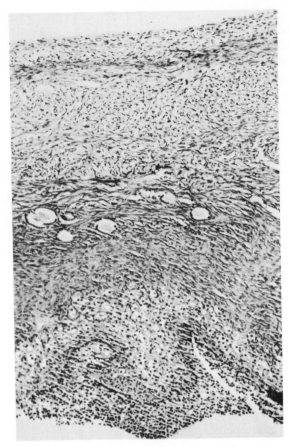

FIG. 10. Polycystic ovarian disease. Note collagenization of outermost cortex and thick band of luteinized theca cells around follicle in lower portion of illustration.

Stromal Hyperthecosis and Stromal Hyperplasia

Proliferation of ovarian stromal cells is common in perimenopausal and early postmenopausal age groups, and a sharp distinction cannot be made between normal stromal proliferation and so-called stromal hyperplasia. Nonetheless, the latter designation seems appropriate for cases in which stromal proliferation is of moderate to marked degree. Stromal hyperthecosis refers to the presence of luteinized cells in an almost invariably hyperplastic stroma.

Clinical features

Stromal hyperplasia is most common in the sixth and seventh decades of life (66). It is difficult to assess the endocrine effects of stromal hyperplasia because no investigators have analyzed simple hyperplasia separate from hyperplasia accompanied by hyperthecosis. There is evidence, however, that stromal hyperplasia may be associated with androgen hypersecretion, obesity, hypertension, and disorders of glucose metabolism. Such anomalies are not as common or obtrusive as in association with stromal hyperthecosis (66). Androgen production by nonluteinized stromal cells is consistent with their oxidative enzymes and designation as "enzymatically active stromal cells" (67).

Stromal hyperthecosis is usually encountered in the

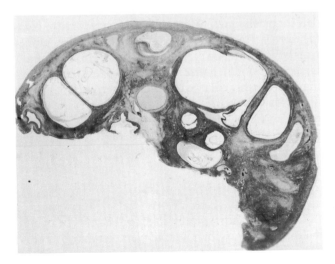

FIG. 9. Polycystic ovarian disease. Multiple follicular cysts are present; corpora lutea and albicantia are absent. (From ref. 460.)

sixth to ninth decades of life. It has been documented at autopsy in one-third of women over the age of 55 years (66). In this age group, it is usually mild and without obvious clinical manifestations (66). Younger patients may present with marked virilization, obesity, hypertension, and decreased glucose tolerance (68,69). In many patients, the clinical features of stromal hyperthecosis are similar to those of PCOD. As in cases of PCOD, estrogenic manifestations such as endometrial hyperplasia or carcinoma may be present (69,70). The disorder may be familial (71).

Gross features

Both stromal hyperplasia and hyperthecosis cause bilateral ovarian enlargement, with each gonad measuring up to 8 cm in diameter (39,66,69). The cut surface is homogeneous, firm, and white to yellow (Fig. 11) (66,72). In premenopausal patients with hyperthecosis, sclerocystic changes similar to those seen in PCOD may also be present (62,72).

Microscopic features

Both cortical and medullary stroma may be hyperplastic (66). In hyperthecosis, luteinized stromal cells appear singly, in small clusters (Fig. 12), or in nodules. They have abundant eosinophilic to vacuolated cytoplasm containing variable amounts of lipid, and they also have a round nucleus with a central small nucleolus (39,66). Associated ovarian findings include small foci of metaplastic smooth muscle (73), Leydig-cell hyperplasia (66,74), Leydig-cell tumors (74,75), and stromal luteomas (76).

Massive Edema and Fibromatosis

Tumor-like enlargement of one or both ovaries secondary to an accumulation of edema fluid within the ovarian stroma is referred to as "massive ovarian edema"; approximately 50 cases have been reported

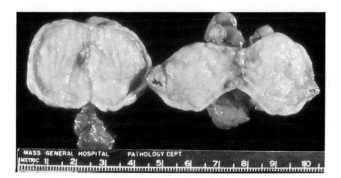

FIG. 11. Stromal hyperthecosis. Both ovaries are almost completely replaced by homogeneous yellow-white tissue.

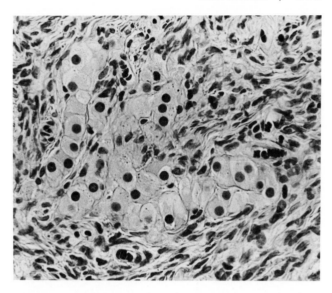

FIG. 12. Stromal hyperthecosis. A cluster of luteinized cells lies in the ovarian stroma.

(77–81). *Ovarian fibromatosis* has clinical and pathologic features that overlap with those of massive edema, suggesting a probable relationship between the two lesions (81).

Massive Edema

Clinical features

The patients range in age from 6 to 33 years (mean: 21 years). Three-quarters present with abdominal or pelvic pain, which may be acute and accompanied by abdominal swelling. In the remainder, the clinical manifestations include menstrual irregularities or evidence of androgen excess, or both. Serum testosterone may be elevated. Pelvic examination typically demonstrates a palpable adnexal mass. Ovarian enlargement is unilateral in about 90% of the cases. Partial or complete torsion of the involved ovary is present in at least 50% of the cases. Rare patients have Meigs' syndrome.

Gross features

The ovary is enlarged, soft, and fluctuant (Fig. 13), ranging in diameter from 5.5 to 35 cm (mean 11.5 cm). The cut surface is tan, homogeneous, and soft, exuding a watery fluid. The most superficial cortex appears white and fibrotic. Cystic follicles and corpora lutea within the edematous tissue strongly suggest the diagnosis of massive edema as opposed to an edematous fibroma.

Microscopic features

At low magnification, marked, diffuse, stromal edema surrounds follicles and their derivatives (Fig. 14) but

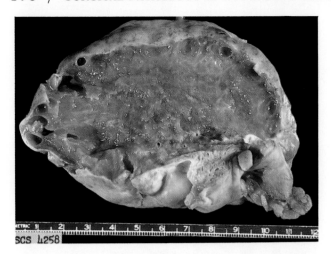

FIG. 13. Massive edema. The ovary is replaced by gelatinous tissue.

typically spares the thickened and fibrotic superficial cortex. Higher magnification demonstrates abundant, pale-staining fluid, which may have a microcystic appearance. In nonedematous areas, the stroma may appear normal or hyperplastic, or it may resemble the stroma of ovarian fibromatosis (81). Luteinized stromal cells are present in 40% of cases. Vascular and lymphatic dilatation may be seen within the ovary and, occasionally, the mesosalpinx. Foci of necrosis are rare (79). The contralateral ovary is typically normal but is occasionally enlarged and edematous, or, exceptionally, it is involved by stromal hyperthecosis or exhibits a sclerocystic appearance.

Differential diagnosis

Massive edema can be distinguished from ovarian neoplasms with an edematous or myxoid appearance. Included in the differential are an edematous fibroma, sclerosing stromal tumor, Krukenberg tumor, and the

rare ovarian myxoma. Distinction is based on the absence of characteristic features of these tumors, as well as the inclusion of follicular derivatives within massive ovarian edema.

Fibromatosis

Clinical features

The age of affected patients range from 13 to 39 years (mean: 25 years) (81). Clinical manifestations include menstrual abnormalities, abdominal pain, and, rarely, hirsutism or virilization. An adnexal mass is usually palpable. The process is usually unilateral; in 15% of the cases, the involved ovary has undergone torsion.

Gross/microscopic features

Involved ovaries are 6 to 12 cm in diameter with smooth, white external surfaces. Cut surfaces are firm, white, and solid, although residual cystic follicles are present within one-third of the cases (Fig. 15). Microscopically, a proliferation of spindle cells produces variable amounts of collagen. The appearance varies from cellular fascicles of spindle cells with a focal storiform pattern to acellular bands of dense collagen (Fig. 16) (81). The process typically surrounds normal follicular structures and produces collagenous thickening of the superficial cortex. Stromal edema is present in approximately half of the cases. Luteinized stromal cells and microscopic foci of sex-cord cells are seen occasionally.

Differential diagnosis

Ovarian fibromatosis should be distinguished from fibroma, which occurs in an older age group, is typically nonfunctioning, and rarely contains follicles or their derivatives. The small aggregates of sex-cord cells in fibro-

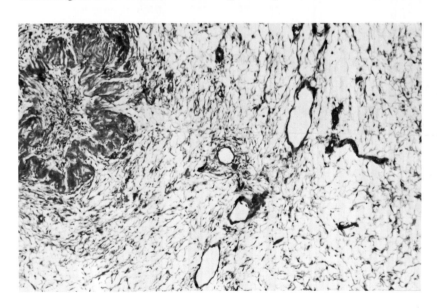

FIG. 14. Massive edema. Pale, edematous stroma partly surrounds a corpus fibrosum.

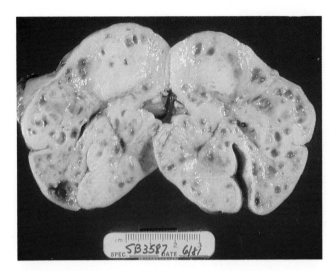

FIG. 15. Fibromatosis. The sectioned surfaces of the ovary reveal dense white tissue surrounding cystic follicles. (From ref. 81.)

matosis may lead to confusion with a sex-cord stromal tumor.

Pregnancy Luteoma

Pregnancy luteoma is characterized by tumor-like ovarian enlargement during pregnancy secondary to solid proliferations of luteinized cells derived from theca lutein cells or luteinized stromal cells (82–88). The disorder is likely related to hCG stimulation; however, its rarity in association with trophoblastic disease, along with almost exclusive occurrence during the third trimester when hCG levels are decreased, indicate that this hormone is not the only factor.

Clinical Features

The majority of patients are in their third or fourth decades, black, and multiparous. The lesion is usually discovered incidentally during cesarean section or postpartum tubal ligation. Rarely, a pelvic mass is palpable or obstructs delivery. In approximately 25% of the cases, there is hirsutism or virilization; two-thirds of female infants born to virilized mothers are also virilized (85,87,88). The ovarian enlargement begins to regress within days after delivery, and they return to normal size within several weeks.

Gross Features

The lesions range from small nodules to masses up to 20 cm in diameter. The cut surface of the nodules is soft, fleshy, circumscribed, and brown (Fig. 17) or gray; foci of hemorrhage are common. At least half of the cases have multiple nodules, and one-third are bilateral. Examination of ovaries days to weeks postpartum reveals focally infarcted lesions or brown puckered scars (39).

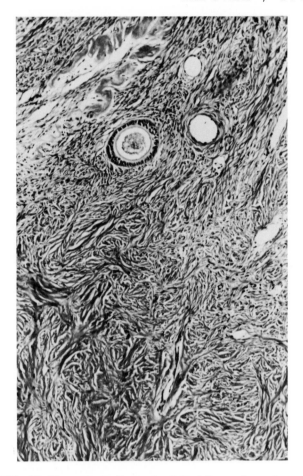

FIG. 16. Fibromatosis. Dense, hyalinized fibrous tissue has replaced the normal ovarian stroma and surrounds a primary follicle and a corpus fibrosum.

Microscopic Features

The sharply circumscribed nodules (Fig. 18) are composed of polygonal cells intermediate in size between

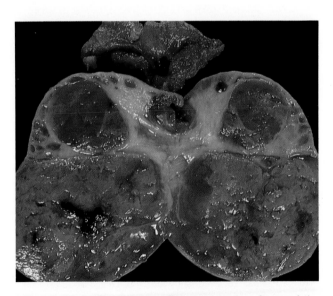

FIG. 17. Pregnancy luteoma. The sectioned surfaces of the ovary show several nodules of pale brown to red tissue.

luteinized granulosa and theca cells of adjacent follicles. Occasionally the cells form cords or small clusters, or they surround spaces (Fig. 18) containing colloid-like material. The cytoplasm is abundant, eosinophilic, and granular, and it contains little or no lipid. Less common features include cytoplasmic ballooning degeneration and intracellular colloid droplets similar to those seen in the corpus luteum of pregnancy. The nuclei may exhibit slight pleomorphism and hyperchromatism; mitotic figures range up to seven per 10 high-power fields, with an average of two or three, and occasional atypical forms may be seen (83). The stroma between the cells is scant, and reticulin fibrils surround groups of cells in an organoid pattern. Ultrastructural examination shows characteristic features of steroid-producing cells (89). Postpartum changes include intracytoplasmic lipid accumulation, round-cell infiltration, and fibrosis (39,86).

Differential Diagnosis

If multiple, bilateral nodules are present, confusion with metastatic carcinoma, especially a Krukenberg tumor, may be a major problem. As with pregnancy luteoma, the latter may also be virilizing. Frozen section of a biopsy specimen should establish the correct diagnosis. During pregnancy, other lesions composed of lu-

teinized cells may enter the differential diagnosis, microscopically, but the gross appearance of multiple, bilateral, solid nodules is distinctive. Neoplasms composed of luteinized cells (sex-cord–stromal and steroid(lipid)-cell tumors) are almost always unilateral and solitary. Sex-cord–stromal tumors typically contain nonluteinized foci, have denser reticulin, and contain more abundant intracellular lipid than do pregnancy luteomas. Tumors in the steroid-cell group, composed entirely of luteinized cells, may be indistinguishable from pregnancy luteomas. Features favoring a steroid-cell neoplasm include dense reticulin, intracellular lipid, lipochrome pigment, and, in Leydig-cell tumors, a hilar location with intracytoplasmic Reinke crystals.

Leydig-Cell Hyperplasia

Hilus-Cell Hyperplasia

Clinical features

Hilus-cell hyperplasia may be seen during pregnancy, following hCG administration, and in postmenopausal women where it is presumably related to elevated pituitary gonadotropins (66,90,91). Prominent hilus-cell hyperplasia was found in about 40% of women over 70 years of age in one autopsy study (66). The role of hilus-

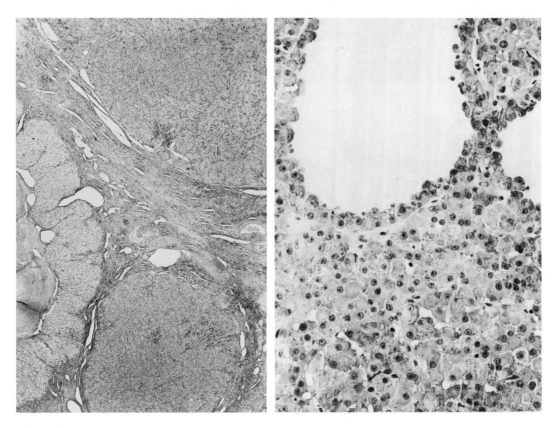

FIG. 18. Pregnancy luteoma. *Left:* Two large nodules of lutein cells lie to the right of a corpus luteum. *Right:* Follicle-like structures within luteoma. The luteoma cells have abundant dense cytoplasm. (From ref. 128.)

cell hyperplasia in endocrine disturbances is often complicated by coexisting stromal hyperthecosis or hilus-cell tumor, or both (90,92). In rare cases, however, isolated hilus-cell hyperplasia has been apparently responsible for androgenic and estrogenic manifestations. Elevated plasma testosterone also has been documented (93).

Gross/microscopic features

Hilus-cell hyperplasia may be grossly visible as multiple, yellow hilar nodules, usually less than 2 mm in diameter. On microscopic examination, the hilus cells are arranged in nodular (Fig. 19) or diffuse patterns; multinucleated cells and occasional mitotic figures may be seen (90,91). In older women, hyperplastic hilus cells may be enlarged with bizarre shapes and hyperchromatic nuclei (Fig. 19) (39).

Stromal Leydig-Cell Hyperplasia

Leydig cells containing Reinke crystals have been encountered rarely within ovarian stroma away from the hilus, typically as a microscopic finding in otherwise typical stromal hyperthecosis, hilus-cell hyperplasia, or hilus-cell tumor (74). Leydig cells have also been described rarely within the non-neoplastic stroma of a variety of ovarian neoplasms, most commonly those of surface epithelial or germ-cell origin (94,95).

Stromal Metaplasias Including Decidual Reaction

Decidual Reaction

Clinical features

An ectopic decidual reaction may be confined to the ovarian stroma or may be part of a widespread decidual transformation involving subperitoneal pelvic mesenchyme (see Chapter 51) (96–99). Ovarian decidual reaction is usually a response to high circulating or local levels of estrogen and progesterone (66). The process is seen most commonly during pregnancy, occurring as early as the ninth week of gestation, and is present in almost all ovaries at term (96–99). Less often it occurs in association with trophoblastic disease, in patients treated with progestins, in the vicinity of a corpus luteum, adjacent to a metastatic tumor, or in association with steroid-secreting lesions of the ovary and adrenal gland (39,66,100). Ovarian radiation may be a predisposing factor, increasing stromal cell sensitivity to hormonal stimulation (100). Occasionally, ectopic decidua may occur in the ovaries of premenopausal and postmenopausal women without obvious cause.

Gross/microscopic features

The decidual foci may be grossly visible as soft, red, subserosal nodules, ridges, or patches (97,99). More frequently they are incidental microscopic findings. The decidual cells are typically in the superficial cortex or in surface adhesions. They occur singly, as small nodules, in confluent sheets, or as small polypoid projections from the ovarian surface (97,101). Most cells are indistinguishable from eutopic decidua; cells transitional between spindle-shaped stromal cells and fully decidualized cells are also usually present. Ultrastructurally, some cells may exhibit smooth-muscle differentiation (102). A rich network of distended capillaries and a sprinkling of lymphocytes are typically found within decidual foci. Florid examples can simulate metastatic carcinoma, particularly if the decidual cells show focal cytologic atypia. Degenerative changes within the decidua are typically seen postpartum.

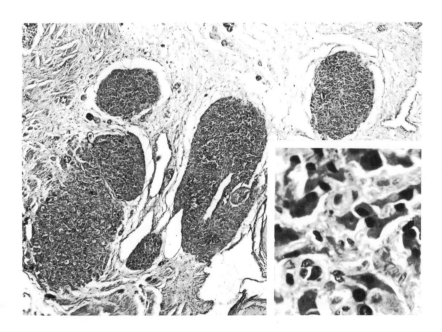

FIG. 19. Hilus-cell hyperplasia. Several nodules of hilus cells are prominent in the ovarian hilus. Inset shows hilus cells of bizarre shapes with hyperchromatic nuclei. (From ref. 39.)

Other Stromal Metaplasias

Small nodules of metaplastic smooth muscle are encountered occasionally in otherwise unremarkable ovarian stroma, in stromal hyperthecosis or PCOD, and in stroma surrounding non-neoplastic or neoplastic cysts (62,73). Mature fat may be an incidental finding in the superficial stroma (103). Heterotopic bone in the absence of an ovarian neoplasm is rare, typically occurring in adhesions, in the walls of endometriotic cysts, or, rarely, in otherwise normal ovaries (104).

Disorders of Ovarian Failure

Premature ovarian failure results from disorders causing secondary amenorrhea and infertility before the age of 35 years. If one excludes chromosomal abnormalities, as well as surgical, radiation-induced, or drug-induced ovarian ablation, at least three distinctive disorders are seen in patients with premature ovarian failure: premature follicle depletion (true premature menopause); resistant ovary; and autoimmune oophoritis. It is not known with certainty, however, whether each of these disorders includes several subtypes of diverse pathogenesis (105).

True Premature Menopause

True premature menopause is characterized by small ovaries that contain few or no primordial and developing follicles—an appearance resembling normal perimenopausal or postmenopausal ovary (105–108). If the gonads are streaks and the karyotype is 46XX, a diagnosis of 46XX pure gonadal dysgenesis is warranted.

Resistant Ovary Syndrome

Clinical features

Approximately 20% of patients with premature ovarian failure have resistant ovary syndrome characterized by primary or secondary amenorrhea, high gonadotropin levels, and resistance to both endogenous and even massive doses of exogenous gonadotropins (105,106,108–112). The pathogenesis is unknown, but a deficiency of follicular FSH and LH receptors, antibodies to these receptors, and a postreceptor defect have all been implicated (109,111).

Gross/microscopic features

The ovaries typically have a normal prepubertal or adult appearance on gross inspection. Primordial follicles are normal in number and appearance, but developing follicles beyond the antral stage are virtually absent.

Atretic follicles and stigmata of prior ovulation may be seen. Unusual histological findings include focal or diffuse follicular hyalinization in the preantral stage (112), as well as calcification of atretic follicles in the space normally occupied by the ovum (110). Stromal luteinization and hilus-cell hyperplasia may result from elevated LH, with associated virilization (92). A histologic pattern similar to resistant ovary syndrome may occur in morbid obesity, Cushing's syndrome, and hypogonadotropic ovarian failure secondary to hypothalamic-pituitary dysfunction (16).

Autoimmune Oophoritis

Clinical features

Less than a dozen cases of autoimmune oophoritis have been verified histologically (105,113–115). In most of these cases, as well as others in which ovarian biopsy was not performed, serum antibodies to steroid-producing cells have been present (116–122). The ovarian failure in such cases is often accompanied by one or more of the following predominantly autoimmune disorders: Addison's disease, idiopathic hypoparathyroidism, hyperthyroidism, Hashimoto's disease, hypothyroidism, myasthenia gravis, juvenile-onset diabetes mellitus, juvenile rheumatoid arthritis, sicca syndrome, vitiligo, pernicious anemia, alopecia, autoimmune hemolytic anemia, idiopathic thrombocytopenia purpura, and mucocutaneous candidiasis (108,118–121,123).

Microscopic features

Inflammatory cells infiltrate the theca-cell layer as it differentiates at the edge of maturing follicles (Fig. 20). Lymphocytes and plasma cells predominate, but eosinophils, histiocytes, and sarcoid-like granulomas have also been described. The intensity of the infiltrate increases with follicular maturation, and, as the follicles become cystic, inflammatory and degenerating granulosa cells fill the lumen. Primordial follicles appear normal.

Ovarian Changes Secondary to Cytotoxic Drugs and Radiation

Cytotoxic Drug Effects

Cytotoxic drugs may be associated with a variety of histologic changes in the ovary. These include reduction or depletion of follicles, impaired follicular maturation, and cortical fibrosis (16). These findings are consistent with the diminished ovarian function or failure in some patients. In occasional cases, the ovarian failure is reversible after cessation of therapy.

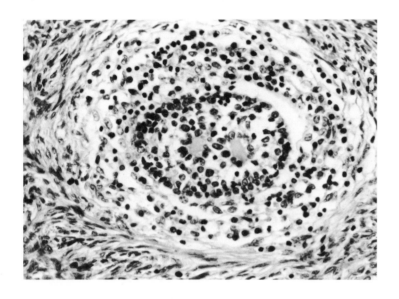

FIG. 20. Autoimmune oophoritis. Lymphocytes and plasma cells have infiltrated the theca interna layer of a preantral follicle. (From ref. 127.)

Radiation Effects

The ovary is among the most radiosensitive of organs, and ovarian failure occurs in the majority of patients who receive pelvic radiation (16). Low doses of radiation (500–600 R) to the ovaries are associated with complete or nearly complete disappearance of primordial and developing follicles, as well as stromal fibrosis and vascular sclerosis, in over 90% of patients. The ovarian stroma appears to be more radioresistant than the follicles and may continue to secrete androgens after radiation.

Congenital Lesions

Congenital lesions of the ovary are very rare and include (a) absent, lobulated, accessory, and supernumerary ovary, (b) splenic-gonadal fusion, (c) adrenal cortical rests, and (d) uterus-like ovarian masses (16).

TUMORS

Introduction

Most ovarian tumors cannot be distinguished on the basis of clinical or gross characteristics, but these features provide important diagnostic clues when considering a differential diagnosis. One of the most important clinical features is the patient's age. Less than one in 15 ovarian tumors in patients under 45 years of age is malignant, whereas in older women the corresponding figure is close to one in three. Some ovarian neoplasms are largely restricted to certain ages. For example, primitive germ-cell tumors are almost never encountered in women over 50 years of age. In the important common epithelial category, borderline tumors are often seen in women in their fourth decade, whereas invasive carcinomas are rare under 40 years of age.

The stage and laterality of ovarian tumors are also important clues. For example, sex-cord–stromal tumors are almost always confined to a single ovary. Therefore, when a tumor is bilateral, or has spread beyond the ovary, a diagnosis in this category should be made cautiously. On the other hand, the approximately 65% bilaterality of metastatic tumors indicates that a metastasis should always be considered when encountering a bilateral tumor. Nevertheless, diagnosis of ovarian tumors depends primarily on knowledge of the wide range of microscopic features they exhibit. In the following discussion, emphasis is placed on gross and microscopic features that are important in diagnosis. Clinical features are discussed only briefly, and histogenetic or therapeutic aspects, which are covered in detail elsewhere (39,124–127), receive little comment. Immunohistochemical and ultrastructural findings are included when they play an important diagnostic role. The World Health Organization (WHO) (128) classification is used with modifications (Table 1) due to the addition of recently described entities.

Common Epithelial Tumors

Common epithelial tumors account for approximately two-thirds of all ovarian neoplasms. Their malignant forms represent almost 90% of ovarian cancers in the western world (39). Most of these tumors are derived from surface ovarian epithelium, which develops from the coelomic epithelium (mesothelium) of the embryonic gonad. This surface epithelium often extends into the ovarian stroma to form surface epithelial inclusion glands and cysts. It may exhibit a variety of müllerian-type differentiations in its neoplastic transformations, including fallopian tube epithelium in serous neoplasms, endometrial epithelium in endometrioid tumors, and endocervical epithelium in mucinous neoplasms.

TABLE 1. *Modified WHO classification of ovarian tumors*

I. Common epithelial tumors

A. Serous tumors
  1. Benign
    a. Cystadenoma and papillary cystadenoma
    b. Surface papilloma
    c. Adenofibroma and cystadenofibroma
  2. Of borderline malignancy (carcinomas of low malignant potential)
    a. Cystadenoma and papillary cystadenoma
    b. Surface papilloma
    c. Adenofibroma and cystadenofibroma
  3. Malignant
    a. Adenocarcinoma, papillary adenocarcinoma, and papillary cystadenocarcinoma
    b. Surface papillary carcinoma
    c. Malignant adenofibroma and cystadenofibroma
B. Mucinous tumors
  1. Benign
    a. Cystadenoma
    b. Adenofibroma and cystadenofibroma
  2. Of borderline malignancy (carcinomas of low malignant potential)
    a. Cystadenoma
    b. Adenofibroma and cystadenofibroma
  3. Malignant
    a. Adenocarcinoma and cystadenocarcinoma
    b. Malignant adenofibroma and cystadenofibroma
C. Endometrioid tumors
  1. Benign
    a. Adenoma and cystadenoma
    b. Adenofibroma and cystadenofibroma
  2. Of borderline malignancy (carcinomas of low malignant potential)
    a. Adenoma and cystadenoma
    b. Adenofibroma and cystadenofibroma
  3. Malignant
    a. Carcinoma
      i. Adenocarcinoma
      ii. Adenocarcinoma with squamous differentiation
      iii. Malignant adenofibroma and cystadenofibroma
    b. Endometrioid stromal sarcomas
    c. Mesodermal (müllerian) mixed tumors (homologous and heterologous)
D. Clear-cell tumors
  1. Benign
  2. Of borderline malignancy (carcinomas of low malignant potential)
  3. Malignant: carcinoma and adenocarcinoma
E. Brenner tumors
  1. Benign
  2. Proliferating (of borderline malignancy)
  3. Malignant[a]
F. Undifferentiated carcinoma
G. Mixed epithelial tumors
  1. Benign
  2. Of borderline malignancy
  3. Malignant
H. Unclassified epithelial tumors

II. Sex-cord–stromal tumors

A. Granulosa-stromal cell tumor
  1. Granulosa-cell tumor
    a. Adult type
    b. Juvenile type
  2. Tumors in the thecoma–fibroma group
    a. Thecoma
      i. Typical
      ii. Luteinized[b]
    b. Fibroma-fibrosarcoma
      i. Fibroma
      ii. Cellular fibroma
      iii. Fibrosarcoma
    c. Stromal tumors with minor sex-cord elements
    d. Sclerosing stromal tumor
    e. Unclassified
B. Sertoli-stromal cell tumors (androblastomas)
  1. Sertoli-cell tumor
  2. Sertoli-Leydig cell tumor
    a. Well-differentiated
    b. Of intermediate differentiation
    c. Poorly differentiated
    d. With heterologous elements
    e. Retiform
    f. Mixed
  3. Leydig-cell tumors[c]
C. Gynandroblastoma
D. Sex-cord tumor with annular tubules
E. Unclassified

III. Steroid (lipid-lipoid)-cell tumors

A. Stromal luteoma
B. Leydig-cell tumor
  1. Hilus-cell tumor
  2. Leydig-cell tumor, nonhilar type
C. Steroid-cell tumor, NOS

IV. Tumors of the rete ovarii

V. Germ-cell tumors

A. Dysgerminoma
B. Yolk sac tumor (endodermal sinus tumor)
C. Embryonal carcinoma
D. Choriocarcinoma
E. Polyembryoma
F. Teratomas
  1. Immature
  2. Mature
    a. Solid
    b. Cystic
      i. Dermoid cyst (mature cystic teratoma)
      ii. Dermoid cyst with malignant transformation
      iii. Other
  3. Monodermal and highly specialized
    a. Struma ovarii
    b. Carcinoid
    c. Strumal carcinoid
    d. Mucinous carcinoid
    e. Neuroectodermal tumors
    f. Others
G. Mixed forms

VI. Germ-cell–sex-cord–stromal tumors

A. Gonadoblastoma
  1. Pure
  2. Mixed with dysgerminoma or other form of germ-cell tumor
B. Unclassified

TABLE 1. *Continued*

VII. Tumors of uncertain cell type

A. Ovarian tumor of probable wolffian origin
B. Small-cell carcinoma
C. Hepatoid carcinoma

VIII. Soft-tissue tumors not specific to ovary and miscellaneous other tumors

IX. Unclassified tumors

X. Secondary (metastatic) tumors

XI. Tumor-like lesions

A. Pregnancy luteoma
B. Hyperplasia of ovarian stroma and hyperthecosis

C. Massive edema
D. Fibromatosis
E. Solitary follicle cyst (including large solitary follicle cyst of pregnancy and the puerperium) and corpus luteum cyst
F. Multiple follicle cysts (polycystic ovaries)
G. Multiple luteinized follicle cysts (hyperreactio luteinalis) and/or corpora lutea
H. Endometriosis
I. Surface-epithelial inclusion cysts
J. Simple cysts
K. Inflammatory lesions
L. Parovarian cysts

[a] Tumors composed entirely of malignant transitional epithelium resembling that of the urinary tract are appropriately designated "transitional-cell carcinoma."

[b] Tumors that resemble luteinized thecomas but in which crystals of Reinke are identified in the steroid cells are designated "stromal–Leydig-cell tumors."

[c] Leydig-cell tumors are generally considered in the category of steroid-cell tumors because of their close resemblance to other tumors in that category.

Although common epithelial tumors may arise directly from the ovarian surface, more commonly they originate from inclusion glands, accounting for their cystic, endophytic nature.

Careful study of common epithelial tumors often demonstrates two or even three cell types. When less than 10% of a second cell type is present, the neoplasm is classified based on its predominant cellular element. Common epithelial tumors also are subclassified according to three other criteria. Some tumors, particularly serous neoplasms, may be exophytic or endophytic, or both. When exophytic growth is present, the word *surface* is added to the designation, as in, for example, serous surface papillary carcinoma. Except for benign Brenner tumors, most common epithelial neoplasms are primarily epithelial. When such tumors have a predominant stromal component, the terms *adenofibroma* and *cystadenofibroma* (if grossly visible cysts are present) are used (129).

Some common epithelial tumors have histologic and clinical features that are intermediate between benign and obviously malignant. The International Federation of Gynecology and Obstetrics (FIGO) adopted the designation *carcinoma of low malignant potential* for such tumors (130), but *tumor of borderline malignancy* is preferred by the WHO (128). Tumors in this category are characterized by epithelial proliferation exceeding that of benign tumors but have an absence of "destructive" stromal invasion (131–143). Borderline tumors are capable of implanting on peritoneal surfaces, and the implants are occasionally invasive. In a small number of cases, these tumors metastasize to lymph nodes; rarely, they metastasize distantly. The diagnosis of borderline malignancy is based on the ovarian tumor without re-

gard for the presence or absence of extraovarian extension. This approach is justified, because survival is typically long, even in cases with implants.

Serous Tumors

Clinical features

Serous neoplasms account for 20% to 50% of all ovarian tumors and for a similar proportion of benign ovarian neoplasms. Approximately 70% are benign, 5% to 10% are borderline, and 20% to 25% are carcinomas. Borderline and invasive serous tumors together account for 35% to 40% of all ovarian cancers. Benign serous tumors may occur at any age, but they are most common during the fifth decade. Borderline tumors are encountered most frequently between the ages of 30 and 60 years, and most carcinomas are encountered between the ages of 40 and 70 years.

Gross features

Benign serous tumors may be endophytic (cystadenomas) or exophytic (surface papillomas), or both. The serous cystadenoma is typically unilocular and is characterized by thin-walled cysts filled with watery, mucinous, or hemorrhagic fluid. The cysts may contain polypoid excrescences, which vary from firm to soft. Serous cystadenomas are bilateral in 10% of the cases, can be large, and occasionally attain the huge dimensions associated with mucinous cystadenomas.

Serous surface papillomas are polypoid excrescences on the ovarian surface. They are often associated with an underlying cystic neoplasm. Serous adenofibromas and cystadenofibromas are hard, white, fibromatous tumors, within which are microscopic or grossly visible cysts containing clear fluid and, sometimes, polypoid excrescences.

Serous cystadenomas (Fig. 21) and surface papillomas of borderline malignancy (Fig. 22) have gross features similar to those of benign serous papillary tumors, except that their papillae are finer and more extensive; microscopic examination is necessary to distinguish these lesions. Borderline tumors often secrete a thick, mucinous fluid, which should not lead to the erroneous diagnosis of a mucinous neoplasm. Serous borderline tumors are bilateral in approximately 25% of Stage I cases (144); an additional 10% microscopically involve the opposite ovary.

Serous carcinomas may be cystic and papillary, entirely solid and firm, or both cystic and solid. The poorly differentiated forms cannot be grossly distinguished from other ovarian carcinomas, sharing with them non-specific characteristics of malignancy such as friability, necrosis, and hemorrhage. Rarely, the tumor forms surface papillary or granular deposits (Fig. 23), which may be grossly inconspicuous (serous surface carcinoma) (145,146) or even undetectable (147). Serous carcinomas are bilateral in about two-thirds of all cases, but among Stage I and IIa tumors, only about one-third are bilateral (39).

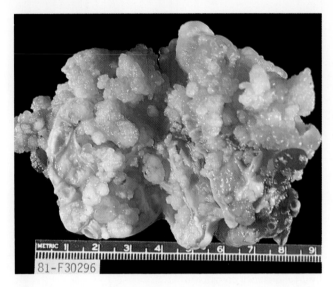

FIG. 22. Serous surface papilloma of borderline malignancy. Papillae and polypoid fronds cover most of the outer surface of the ovary.

Microscopic features

The cysts and papillae of benign serous tumors are typically lined by epithelium resembling that of fallopian tube. Tumors lined by nonciliated cuboidal or columnar cells resembling normal ovarian surface epithelium are also classified as serous, despite their indifferent appearance. If a cyst is lined entirely by flattened cells, the designation *simple cystadenoma* may be used. Benign serous tumor cells may secrete mucin, but it is confined to their surface and the apical portion of their cytoplasm. Psammoma bodies are absent or inconspicuous. Papillae, when present, are composed almost en-

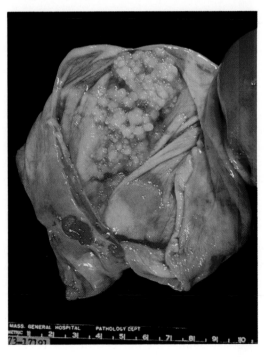

FIG. 21. Serous papillary cystadenoma of borderline malignancy. White, soft polypoid excrescences arise from the lining of the cyst.

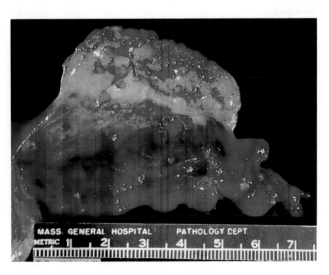

FIG. 23. Serous surface carcinoma. Small nodules with associated hemorrhage are visible on the external surface of the ovary; the normal ovarian shape is retained.

tirely of dense collagenous or markedly edematous stroma. In adenofibromas and cystadenofibromas, glands and cysts are scattered within a prominent fibrous stroma. Occasional, otherwise typical benign serous tumors exhibit minor degrees of focal nuclear stratification and atypia.

Serous borderline tumors are characterized by moderate to marked epithelial proliferation, as evidenced by cellular stratification, and solid cellular buds that often appear to be detached from the lining epithelium (Fig. 24) (134–143). A cribriform pattern may be seen. Tumor cells typically have scanty cytoplasm, but occasionally the cytoplasm is abundant and eosinophilic. Varying degrees of nuclear atypicality may be present; mitotic figures vary from rare to numerous. Ciliated cells are characteristically present, and psammoma bodies are found in approximately 25% of the cases. Some borderline tumors secrete thick mucin, which, as in benign serous tumors, is largely confined to the surface and apical portion of the cells. A minority of the tumors fall into the category of an adenofibroma or cystadenofibroma of borderline malignancy.

The absence of destructive stromal invasion distinguishes a serous borderline tumor from a low-grade carcinoma (Fig. 25). Tangential sectioning may mimic stromal invasion; however, the stroma in these areas of pseudoinfiltration does not differ from that elsewhere in the specimen, and the glands maintain an orderly arrangement. In contrast, destructive stromal invasion is characterized by a disorderly disposition of neoplastic glands. On rare occasions, focal microinvasion or lymphatic invasion is encountered in otherwise typical serous borderline tumors (Fig. 26). The prognosis of these tumors appears to be similar to that of borderline tumors without these findings (147a,147b). Serous tumors, whether benign, borderline, or malignant, tend to be uniform throughout a given specimen. They generally lack the mixtures of benign, borderline, and malignant foci that are often seen in mucinous, endometrioid, and clear-cell tumors.

Serous borderline tumors are associated with peritoneal serous cellular proliferations in 16% to 59% of the cases (148,148a). Some of these foci are composed of benign tubal-type cells, which are not considered to be ovarian implants and are designated *endosalpingiosis.* When peritoneal lesions contain moderately to severely atypical cells, they are regarded by some as primary peritoneal tumors. It is impossible to be certain whether these peritoneal lesions are true implants or independent proliferations, except when the ovarian surface is uninvolved or minimally affected. In the following discussion, for purposes of staging they will be referred to as *implants* when they accompany a borderline ovarian tumor. Peritoneal implants vary widely in their appearance. They have been classified into noninvasive and invasive categories (148–151), with the former subdivided into epithelial and desmoplastic subtypes (Figs. 27 and 28) (148). In the epithelial type of noninvasive implant, papillary proliferations of atypical serous cells are present on the peritoneal surface (Fig. 27), in smoothly contoured subperitoneal invaginations or between lobules of omental fat. The cytologic atypia in these cases approximates the parent ovarian tumor, and there is little or no stromal reaction. In contrast, the desmoplastic noninvasive implant is characterized by a prominent stromal reaction (Fig. 28) that is layered upon the peritoneal serosal surfaces, including those between omental fat lobules. Single cells, small glands, and papillae composed of atypical serous cells are entrapped and compressed by proliferating fibroblastic tissue (Fig. 28). Acute and chronic inflammation, as well as psammoma bodies, may also be present in the desmoplastic reaction.

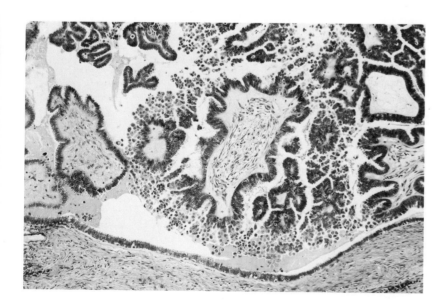

FIG. 24. Serous papillary cystadenoma of borderline malignancy. Papillae lined by stratified epithelial cells project into the lumen. Note the small cellular clusters off the larger papillae and the absence of stromal invasion. (From ref. 128.)

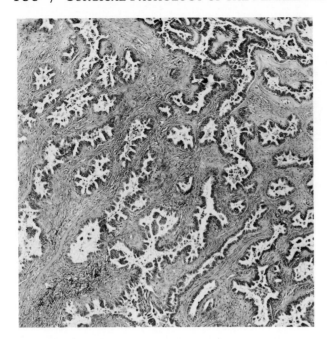

FIG. 25. Serous papillary cystadenoma of borderline malignancy. There is extensive, orderly invagination of glands into the unaltered stroma.

Necrosis, fibrin, and hemorrhage are frequent. Invasive implants are characterized by an irregular infiltration of the underlying tissue (Fig. 29). They histologically resemble grade 2 serous adenocarcinoma, but it should be emphasized that tumors with invasive implants are still classified according to the appearance of the primary neoplasm. Marked cytologic atypia may be present. In a large study of serous borderline tumors associated with peritoneal implants (148), separation of the implants into invasive and noninvasive categories had important prognostic implications. When followed for at least four years or until death, 90% of patients with noninvasive implants had no progression of disease, in contrast to only 17% of those with invasive implants. Severe nu-

clear atypicality in the implants was independently correlated with a poor prognosis.

Serous carcinomas exhibit obvious stromal invasion and are characterized by one or more of the following: fine papillae (Fig. 30); irregular, often slit-like, glandular lumens (Fig. 31); small tight nests of tumor cells; single tumor cells growing in a dense fibrous or hyalinized stroma; glomeruloid formations; and psammoma bodies (152–156). A serous carcinoma may grow as sheets of nonspecific cells lacking the tubular glands or squamous differentiation of endometrioid carcinoma, the intracellular mucin of mucinous carcinoma, or specific features of other ovarian carcinomas. When a solid pattern is exclusive, however, the tumor should be classified as an undifferentiated carcinoma.

Differential diagnosis

Although serous carcinoma is the common epithelial malignancy most typically associated with papillae, other tumors in this category, particularly endometrioid and clear-cell carcinomas, may be papillary. The papillae in endometrioid carcinoma tend to be larger, more regular, broader, and more villous than those of serous carcinoma. Those in clear-cell carcinoma are lined by hobnail or clear cells and frequently have hyalinized cores. These tumors, in addition, almost always exhibit other distinctive patterns of clear-cell carcinoma.

Mucinous Tumors

Clinical features

These neoplasms account for 15% to 25% of all ovarian tumors (39,157–160). The cystadenomas make up a higher proportion of benign ovarian neoplasms and account for approximately 85% of mucinous tumors (152,157). The remaining mucinous tumors are border-

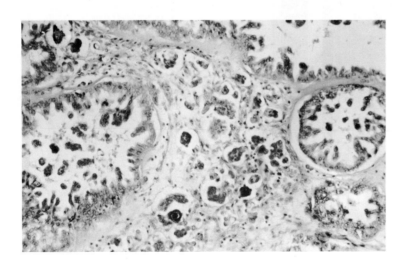

FIG. 26. Serous papillary cystadenoma of borderline malignancy with "microinvasion." Invasive carcinoma cells are present at the center.

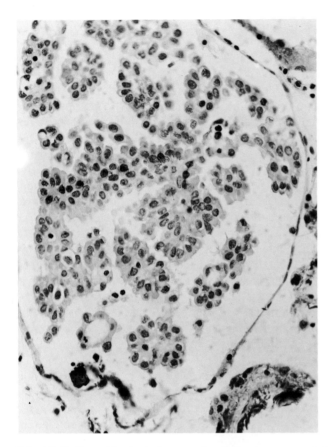

FIG. 27. Peritoneal implant of serous borderline tumor—noninvasive, epithelial.

line malignancies and carcinomas. Mucinous cystadenomas are most frequent during the third through fifth decades; borderline and invasive tumors usually occur during the fourth through seventh decades, with the mean age for the former being 5 to 10 years younger in most series. There is evidence that mucinous ovarian tumors occur with increased frequency in patients with Peutz-Jeghers syndrome (161). Some patients, both with and without this syndrome, have an associated mucinous adenocarcinoma of the cervix (161–163).

Gross features

Mucinous neoplasms tend to be the largest ovarian tumors. Many are 15 to 30 cm in diameter and weigh 4,000 g or more. Less than 5% of benign mucinous tumors are bilateral, whereas borderline and invasive forms involve both ovaries in 5% to 10% of cases. Borderline tumors of müllerian type (see below) are bilateral five or six times more often than those of intestinal type. Mucinous cystadenoma is often multilocular (Fig. 32); the cysts have thin walls and are filled with thick or watery mucinous fluid. Borderline and invasive tumors commonly contain papillae and solid areas, which may be soft and mucoid or firm. Necrosis and hemorrhage

are common in carcinomas, but their occasional presence in benign and borderline tumors may create a deceptively worrisome appearance. Because benign, borderline, and invasive mucinous components are frequently admixed, it is important to thoroughly sample mucinous tumors. Mucinous ovarian tumors associated with pseudomyxoma peritonei (166) usually have gross characteristics of mucinous neoplasms lacking this complication. They may, however, form very thin-walled sacs filled with jelly-like material, and they are more frequently bilateral (167).

Microscopic features

The usual mucinous cystadenoma is lined by epithelium resembling endocervix. Less often, the lining mimics intestinal epithelium, with goblet cells scattered among mucin-free cells, argyrophil cells, argentaffin cells, or, occasionally, Paneth cells. Intestinal type cells are more common in borderline (Figs. 33 and 34) and invasive mucinous tumors. Small papillae may project into the lumens of mucinous cystadenomas, but prominent papillarity is uncommon. Very rarely, squamous metaplasia is encountered. The stromal element is often conspicuous but rarely predominates (mucinous adeno-

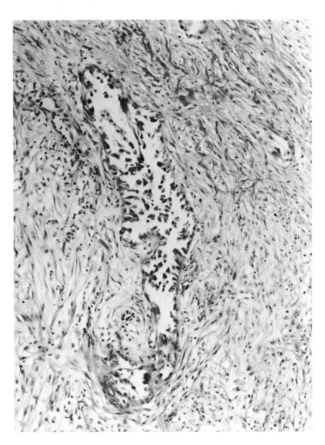

FIG. 28. Peritoneal implant of serous borderline tumor—noninvasive, desmoplastic.

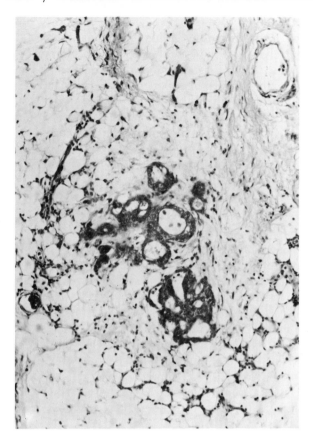

FIG. 29. Peritoneal implant of serous borderline tumor—invasive of omentum.

fibroma); occasionally, bands of smooth muscle and plaques of calcium or bone are present. Minor epithelial atypia is compatible with a mucinous cystadenoma, but significant degrees of epithelial stratification, budding and bridging, and nuclear atypia indicate borderline or invasive malignancy (132,164,165).

Borderline mucinous tumors may be of intestinal or müllerian type. Intestinal mucinous borderline tumors (IMBT) account for approximately 85% of cases and have been studied most extensively. They differ from mucinous cystadenomas by exhibiting significant nuclear atypia and cellular stratification (Figs. 33 and 34). Distinction between borderline and low-grade carcinoma may be difficult. Both borderline and invasive mucinous neoplasms contain glands in a normal, nondesmoplastic stroma, making detection of stromal invasion more difficult than in analogous serous tumors. To address this problem, Hart and Norris (164) suggested that, lacking clear-cut evidence of invasion, a carcinoma should be diagnosed when neoplastic cells are stratified to four layers or greater. Later, Hart proposed that a cribriform pattern also constituted carcinoma (132). These criteria are useful, but in our experience, the height of the epithelium is rarely used as the sole criterion of malignancy. When cells are stratified to four layers or more, it is usually obvious on conventional histologic grounds that the tumor is a carcinoma. Additionally, the glands in a borderline mucinous tumor may rarely have a cribriform appearance. Also, when a mucinous cystic tumor is lined by highly malignant cells, even if only a single layer in thickness, the tumor should be considered a carcinoma. It should be emphasized that an occasional high-power field showing carcinomatous features is acceptable in a borderline tumor but indicates the need for thorough sampling and merits comment in a microscopic description or note.

Mucinous tumors associated with pseudomyxoma peritonei (less than 5% of all mucinous tumors) are al-

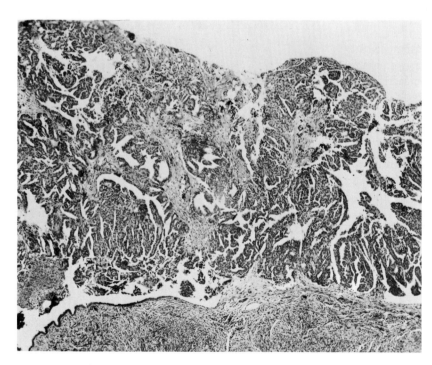

FIG. 30. Serous surface carcinoma. Note origin of the lesion from the ovarian surface in the lower portion. The neoplasm is characterized by many fine papillae and slit-like lumens.

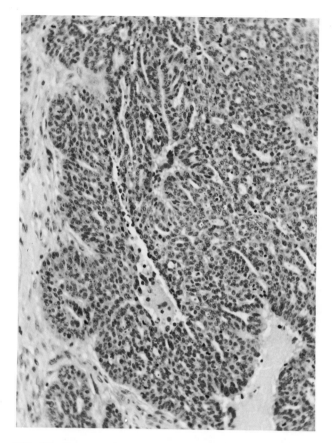

FIG. 31. Serous adenocarcinoma. Small, slit-like glandular lumens are prominent.

most always of borderline type, if adequately sampled (166). Acellular mucin pools in the ovarian stroma (pseudomyxoma ovarii) are a common finding in pseudomyxoma peritonei. In most cases that are associated with ovarian tumors, a "mucocele" of the appendix is also present (167). Its lining, as well as that of the peritoneal deposits, also typically has a borderline appearance. In most cases of appendiceal and ovarian borderline tumors, the former is probably primary and the latter is probably metastatic.

Müllerian mucinous borderline tumors (MMBT) (168) have only recently been delineated from IMBT. Their two major microscopic differences from IMBT are (i) papillae that resemble, architecturally, those of serous borderline tumors and (ii) a lining of endocervical-type epithelium (Fig. 35). Other differences include a prominent and typically extensive acute inflammatory infiltrate in MMBT, in contrast to only minimal inflammation in IMBT. Approximately 30% of MMBT are associated with endometriosis, which is rare in cases of IMBT. MMBT also differs from IMBT in its manner of spread as discrete peritoneal implants or lymph-node metastases, or both; pseudomyxoma peritonei has not been encountered. Even with peritoneal implants, MMBT has an excellent prognosis. The criteria of Hart

and Norris (164) for IMBT are not reliable in the distinction of MMBT from carcinoma. For example, MMBT may exhibit marked cellular stratification (up to 20 layers).

Otherwise typical mucinous cystic tumors, whether benign, borderline or malignant, may contain solid mural nodules. In some cases, the nodule is an anaplastic carcinoma with large cells having abundant, amphophilic cytoplasm (Fig. 36) (169). Rarely, the nodule is a high-grade sarcoma such as fibrosarcoma (170). In a third group, the nodule is composed of giant cells that are cytologically benign (171). A fourth category, which is most challenging diagnostically, includes sarcoma-like proliferations (171) with pleomorphic spindle-shaped cells, giant cells (commonly of epulis type), inflammatory cells, and histiocytes. Mitotic figures, including highly atypical forms, are usually present. Although their nature has not been fully elucidated, uneventful follow-up of patients with these sarcoma-like nodules suggests a histologically bizarre, but reactive, process.

Differential diagnosis

Mucinous adenocarcinomas and endometrioid carcinomas may be difficult to distinguish. Although it occasionally produces abundant mucin, endometrioid carcinoma has only minor quantities of intracellular mucin. Very small foci of endocervical-type cells may be encountered in endometrioid carcinoma, but their presence alone does not warrant a diagnosis of mucinous carcinoma. Squamous differentiation strongly favors endometrioid carcinoma over mucinous carcinoma. Metastatic mucinous tumors to the ovary, usually from the gastrointestinal tract, are also in the differential diagnosis. The best microscopic criterion for primary mucinous cystadenocarcinoma is its usual mixture with benign and borderline components. In one series, however, 11% of metastatic intestinal carcinomas had foci

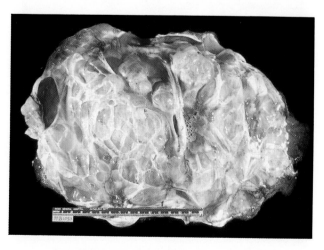

FIG. 32. Multilocular mucinous cystadenoma.

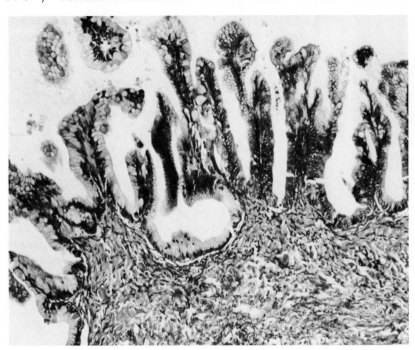

FIG. 33. Mucinous cystadenoma of borderline malignancy—intestinal type. Note filiform papillae, nuclear stratification, and goblet cells.

that were deceptively benign in appearance (172). Goblet cells are generally more common in an ovarian mucinous carcinoma, but they may be encountered in metastatic adenocarcinomas as well. Clinical and operative findings favoring metastasis, such as prior or synchronous bowel carcinoma, mesenteric lymph-node and liver metastases, and bilaterality and multinodularity of the ovarian tumor, may be more helpful diagnostic clues than the microscopic features.

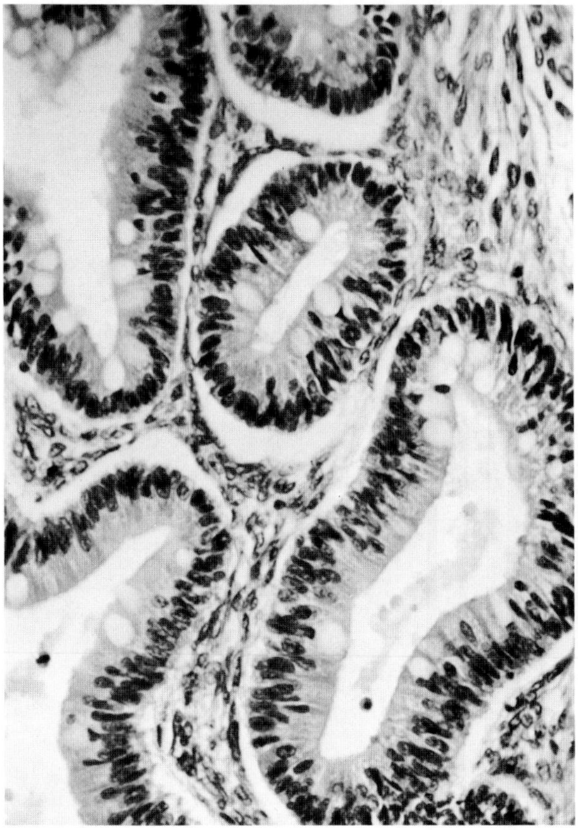

Endometrioid Tumors

Clinical features

Less than 5% of all ovarian tumors are endometrioid, but up to 15% of ovarian cancers are of this type. An origin from endometriosis, which can be demonstrated in 5% to 10% of cases, is not required for diagnosis. Endometriosis is not classified as a neoplasm; and benign endometrioid tumors, with the exception of adenofibromas (Fig. 37) (173–176), are exceedingly rare. Endometrioid tumors of borderline malignancy are also infrequent (175–177); and criteria for their diagnosis, except for those in the adenofibroma category, have not yet been clearly defined. Endometrioid carcinomas occur primarily from the fifth decade and involve an older age group than do serous carcinomas (178–183).

Gross features

Endometrioid carcinomas may be predominantly cystic or solid and do not have gross features that distinguish them from serous carcinomas, except for the minority that arise from the lining of an endometriotic cyst (184–187). In such cases, a chocolate cyst contains a papillary, or cauliflower-like growth, within its lumen,

FIG. 34. Mucinous cystadenoma of borderline malignancy—intestinal type. Note nuclear stratification and goblet cells.

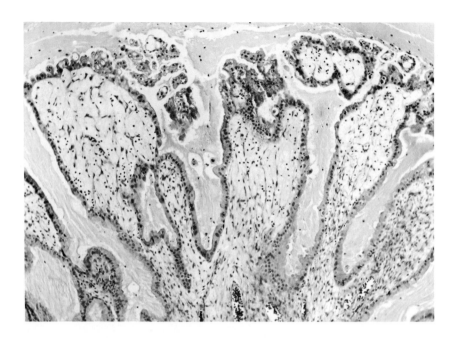

FIG. 35. Mucinous cystadenoma of borderline malignancy—müllerian type. Cellular clusters bud from edematous papillae.

usually accompanied by invasion of its wall. Up to one-third of endometrioid ovarian carcinomas are accompanied by carcinomas of the uterine corpus, which are usually independent primary tumors (see pages 1713 and 1724).

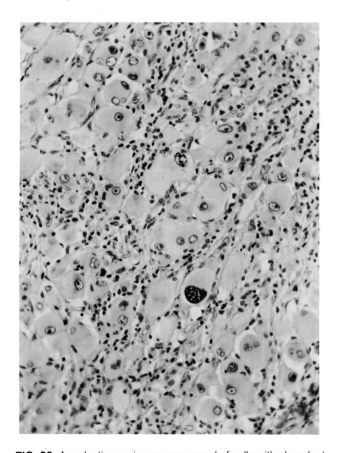

FIG. 36. Anaplastic carcinoma composed of cells with abundant cytoplasm in wall of mucinous cystic tumor.

Microscopic features

Endometrioid tumors are characterized by tubular glands similar to those of a proliferative or hyperplastic endometrium or of endometrial adenocarcinoma. Benign endometrioid tumors include rare lesions resembling endometrial polyps, which may arise in endometriotic cysts, and endometrioid adenofibromas, some of which show focal squamous differentiation (adeno-acanthofibromas) (Fig. 38). Endometrioid tumors of borderline malignancy include (a) rare, highly atypical polyps in endometriotic cysts and (b) endometrioid adenofibromas with epithelium resembling low-grade

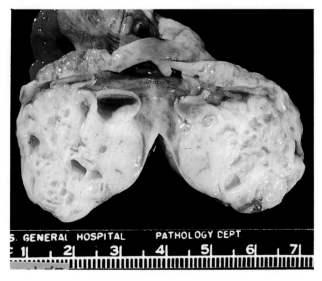

FIG. 37. Endometrioid adenofibroma. The sectioned surfaces show predominantly solid white tissue containing cysts. (From ref. 39.)

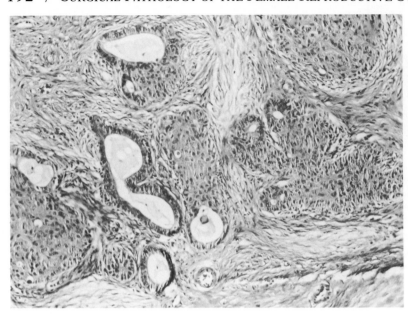

FIG. 38. Endometrioid adenoacanthofibroma. Endometrioid glands, with focal squamous differentiation, lie within a fibromatous stroma.

carcinoma but lacking stromal invasion. Atypical hyperplasia within endometriosis should be classified according to terminology used for endometrial lesions and not as a neoplasm.

Endometrioid adenocarcinomas are characterized by the presence of distinctive tubular glands lined by a pseudostratified, mucin-free epithelium (Fig. 39). The

glands may be cystically dilated and villiform papillae are also occasionally seen (Fig. 40). In one-fourth to one-half of cases, glandular cells differentiate focally into squamous cells, which have an appearance ranging from the benign-appearing cells of squamous morules to malignant-appearing squamous cells. Basal vacuolation similar to that seen in the 16- to 17-day secretory endo-

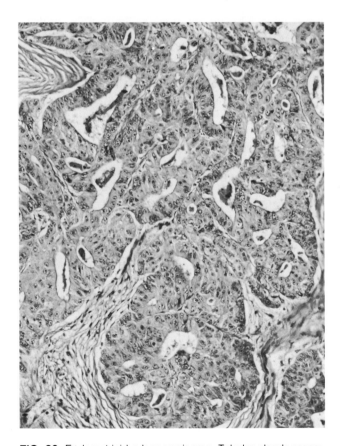

FIG. 39. Endometrioid adenocarcinoma. Tubular glands resemble those of endometrial adenocarcinoma.

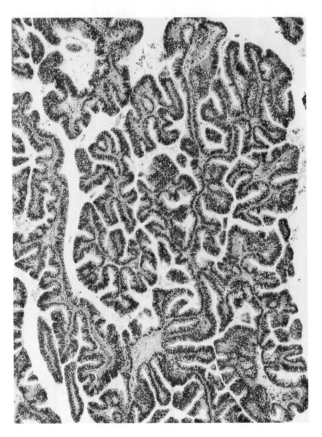

FIG. 40. Endometrioid adenocarcinoma. This neoplasm has a prominent villiform architecture.

metrium may be observed rarely, just as it is in an occasional endometrial adenocarcinoma. These "secretory carcinomas" may be related to progesterone production by the corpus luteum, but they are also encountered in postmenopausal women without an obvious source of excess progesterone. The secretion of abundant mucin is often a feature of endometrioid carcinomas, but typically the mucin appears to be secreted from the surfaces of the cells or appears to accumulate only in the upper portion of their cytoplasm. Occasionally, small foci resembling the lining of the endocervix or that of a mucinous cystadenoma are encountered.

Endometrioid carcinomas have a variety of additional, unusual patterns that may cause them to resemble sex-cord–stromal tumors (188,189). Small glands (Fig. 41) and solid tubules may be indistinguishable from the hollow or solid tubules of a Sertoli-Leydig cell tumor. Solid islands, trabeculae, and small cavities may mimic the insular, trabecular, and microfollicular (Fig. 42) patterns of a granulosa-cell tumor. Endometrioid carcinomas, like any ovarian tumor, may contain luteinized stromal cells; and when these are dispersed between small glands, the resemblance to a Sertoli-Leydig cell tumor may be striking. The variety of unusual patterns that occur in endometrioid carcinomas highlights the importance of thorough sampling of ovarian tumors.

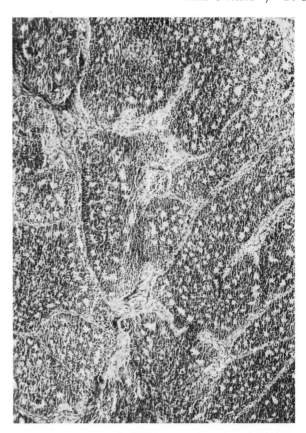

FIG. 42. Endometrioid carcinoma resembling granulosa-cell tumor. Numerous small cavities simulate Call-Exner bodies. (From ref. 188.)

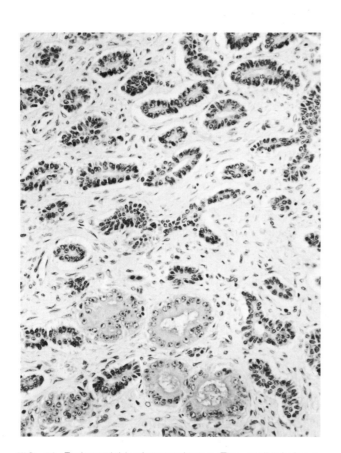

FIG. 41. Endometrioid adenocarcinoma. The small tubules resemble those of a Sertoli-cell tumor.

Differential diagnosis

A major difficulty in the recognition of endometrioid carcinoma arises because certain poorly differentiated forms merge almost imperceptibly with poorly differentiated serous carcinomas. This fact probably accounts, in large part, for the wide differences in the reported frequencies of these tumors. In questionable cases, the diagnosis of endometrioid carcinoma should be avoided. The differential diagnosis of endometrioid carcinoma and mucinous carcinoma is discussed in the section on the latter tumor.

Metastatic adenocarcinoma from the large intestine is occasionally difficult to distinguish from endometrioid carcinoma (190). The glandular lumens in the former are filled with eosinophilic debris containing nuclear fragments, which is usually absent in the latter. Also, the glands in metastatic intestinal carcinomas are typically lined by more poorly differentiated cells. Endometrioid carcinomas resembling sex-cord–stromal tumors contain at least some glands that are larger and more irregular in shape than the tubules of a Sertoli-Leydig cell tumor and are lined by epithelium that is less well differentiated. The presence of either (a) more than small amounts of intraluminal mucin, (b) squamous differentiation, or (c) an adenofibromatous component excludes a diagnosis of sex-cord–stromal tumor. In addition, Sertoli-Leydig cell tumors, in contrast to endometrioid tumors, typically occur in young women. The differential diagnosis of endometrioid carcinoma and endometrioid-like yolk sac tumor is discussed in the section on the latter tumor (see page 1707).

Malignant mesodermal (müllerian) mixed tumors

Malignant mesodermal mixed tumors (MMMTs) (carcinosarcomas) (191,192) are classified within the endometrioid category because they most often simulate tumors that arise in the endometrium and they contain epithelial and mesenchymal elements, both of which are malignant. The mesenchymal component may be homologous; or it may be heterologous, containing cartilage, striated muscle, osteoid, bone, fat, or a combination of these elements. Most of these tumors occur in postmenopausal women. At operation there is evidence of spread beyond the ovary in more than half of the cases.

Gross features. These tumors appear malignant with soft to firm, yellow to brown, solid areas exhibiting hemorrhage, necrosis, and cystic degeneration. They may be predominantly cystic. Occasionally, bone or cartilage is evident.

Microscopic features. The epithelial component most often resembles endometrioid or serous carcinoma, but malignant mucinous, squamous, or clear-cell elements are encountered. The mesenchymal component may resemble a fibrosarcoma, leiomyosarcoma, nonspecific sarcoma or, in heterologous tumors, may resemble rhabdomyosarcoma, chondrosarcoma, or osteosarcoma. Intracellular and extracellular PAS-positive hyaline droplets that stain for alpha-1-antitrypsin may be present in both the sarcomatous and the carcinomatous elements. Rare tumors are predominantly carcinomas with only minor foci of sarcoma.

Differential diagnosis. The neoplasm that is most often confused with the heterologous MMMT is the immature teratoma. In contrast to MMMTs, immature teratomas are extremely rare over the age of 50 years, contain elements derived from all three germ layers, generally lack a highly malignant epithelial component, and almost always contain prominent neuroepithelial components. Finally, the cartilage in immature teratomas has an embryonal or fetal appearance, whereas in MMMTs it resembles that seen in chondrosarcoma. Heterologous Sertoli-Leydig cell tumors with islands of cartilage or rhabdomyoblasts may cause difficulty, but the finding of Leydig cells, sex-cord formations, tubules, or elements of endodermal derivation should facilitate the latter diagnosis.

Mesodermal (müllerian) adenosarcomas

Mesodermal (müllerian) adenosarcomas, characterized by a malignant stromal component that is typically homologous and a proliferating endometrial glandular component, occur rarely in the ovary (193,194). The glandular component may show mucinous or squamous differentiation and may be atypical, occasionally having the appearance of adenocarcinoma *in situ*. These tumors should be distinguished from adenofibromas and endometriotic polypoid lesions. In contrast to the latter, the stroma of adenosarcomas is cellular and atypical with characteristic stromal collaring of the glands. In addition, large polypoid fronds may extend into the lumens of cystically dilated glands.

Endometrioid stromal sarcomas

Clinical features. These tumors occur in women with an average age of 54 years. Many are bilateral and have extended beyond the ovary (195,196). Some patients with an apparent ovarian primary have a history of endometrial stromal sarcoma of the uterus. In some of these instances the ovarian tumor may be metastatic, whereas others represent independent primary tumors of both organs (196).

Gross features. The appearance of these tumors is nonspecific. They are often large and may be solid, solid and cystic, or, rarely, predominantly cystic. The sectioned surface of the solid areas usually shows tan to yellow tissue, which may be soft or firm. Foci of hemorrhage and necrosis occur in approximately one-third of the cases.

Microscopic features. A diffuse pattern of small cells is most common. The tongue-like extravascular and intravascular growth seen in uterine tumors of the same type occurs most often when the tumor extends beyond the ovary. In most cases, small arteries resembling the spiral arteries of the uterus are distributed regularly throughout the tumor. The cells are typically small and oval to spindle-shaped, usually with scanty cytoplasm. Occasional tumors have cells containing small to moderate amounts of pale cytoplasm. Sometimes the neoplasms have focal epithelial patterns (Fig. 43) similar to those encountered in uterine endometrial stromal tumors (197). Large areas indistinguishable from ovarian fibroma, as well as collections of foam cells and hyaline plaques, may be present (196). In almost half of the cases, endometriosis is identified adjacent to the tumor, or glands of endometrial type are present focally within it.

Differential diagnosis. These tumors are frequently misinterpreted as sex-cord–stromal tumors—usually granulosa-cell tumors, thecomas, or fibromas. However, the frequent high stage and bilaterality militates against a diagnosis in the sex-cord–stromal category. In addition, sex-cord–stromal tumors lack the characteristic cell type, the numerous small arteries, and the frequent association with endometriosis of endometrioid stromal sarcomas. Granulosa-cell tumors lack the individual cellular investment by reticulin fibrils that is character-

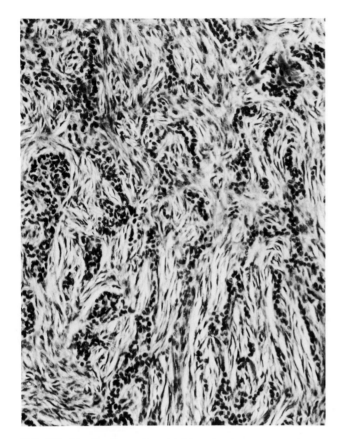

FIG. 43. Low-grade endometrioid stromal sarcoma with sex-cord-like differentiation. (From ref. 196.)

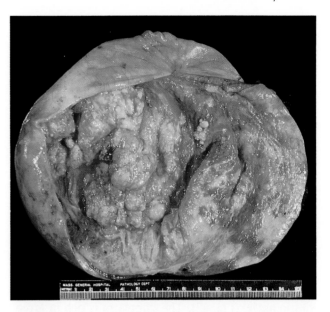

FIG. 44. Clear-cell adenocarcinoma arising in endometriotic cyst. A cauliflower-like mass of carcinoma protrudes into the cyst, the lining of which shows brown patches. (From ref. 200.)

istic of endometrial stromal sarcoma. The presence of epithelial foci may cause further confusion with a sex-cord–stromal tumor (Fig. 43). Endometrioid stromal sarcomas are distinguished from other pure ovarian sarcomas because of their characteristic cell type, vascular pattern, and frequent association with endometriosis.

Clear-Cell Tumors

Clinical features

Benign and borderline clear-cell tumors are uncommon, and almost all of them are in the adenofibroma category (173,198,199). Clear-cell carcinomas account for over 5% of all ovarian cancers; they occur most frequently between the ages of 40 and 70 years (200–208a).

Gross features

Clear-cell adenofibromas are indistinguishable, grossly, from other forms of adenofibroma except that the presence of closely packed, tiny cysts is suggestive of the diagnosis. Clear-cell carcinomas are often predominantly cystic masses, most commonly a unilocular cyst with one or more solid nodules protruding into its lumen (Fig. 44). The clear-cell carcinoma is the ovarian tumor that is most often associated with ovarian and

pelvic endometriosis and occasionally arises within an endometriotic cyst (187). Multilocular cysts are less common, and occasional tumors are predominantly solid. The neoplastic tissue may have a white, yellow, or light brown color with varying amounts of hemorrhage and necrosis (Fig. 45). Clear-cell carcinomas are rarely bilateral.

Microscopic features

Clear-cell adenofibromas are characterized by glands and cysts separated by varying amounts of fibromatous

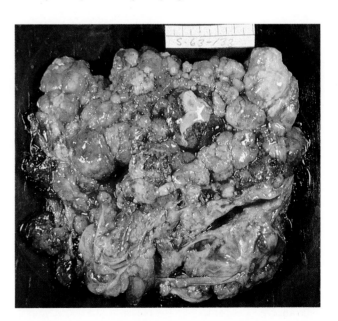

FIG. 45. Clear-cell carcinoma forms a solid tumor with cysts and necrosis.

stroma. The glands and cysts are lined by flat cells, slightly hobnail cells, typical hobnail cells, or clear cells. Clear-cell adenofibromas are subdivided into benign, borderline, and malignant categories according to criteria similar to those for endometrioid tumors (199). Before diagnosing clear-cell adenofibroma, one should sample the specimen carefully because foci of clear-cell carcinoma often coexist with the benign or borderline elements.

The clear-cell carcinoma is characterized by diffuse (Figs. 46 and 47), tubulocystic (Figs. 48 and 49), papillary (Figs. 50 and 51), and, rarely, trabecular (Fig. 52) patterns. The most common cell types are clear (Fig. 47), hobnail (Fig. 49), and flattened (Fig. 49). Clear cells can be found in almost all cases and are the most frequent cell type in tumors with a diffuse pattern. They are typically polyhedral, have distinct cell membranes, and contain abundant clear cytoplasm, often with eccentric nuclei (Fig. 47). The cytoplasm is rich in glycogen and may also contain lipid. Hobnail cells, found in most of the tumors, are characterized by prominent bulbous nuclei that protrude into the lumens of tubules and cysts (Fig. 49). Sometimes, the linings of dilated cysts become markedly flattened, producing a deceptively benign appearance (Fig. 49). The papillae of clear-cell carcinoma may be complex and often contain hyalinized cores (Fig. 51), a helpful diagnostic feature. The lumens of the tubules and cysts commonly contain mucin, but, as in the serous and endometrioid tumors,

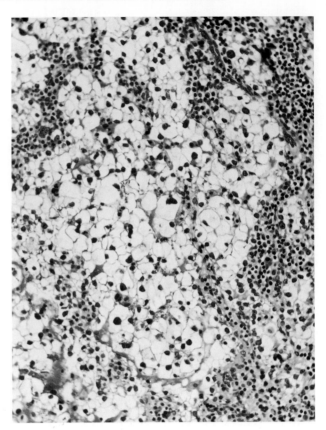

FIG. 47. Clear-cell carcinoma with eccentric nuclei and abundant clear cytoplasm. There is a chronic inflammatory-cell infiltrate.

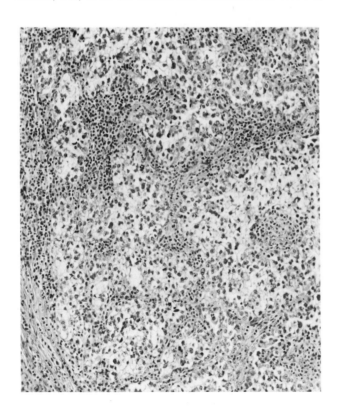

FIG. 46. Clear-cell carcinoma. The presence of a dense lymphocytic and plasmacytic infiltrate imparts a superficial resemblance to dysgerminoma on low-power examination.

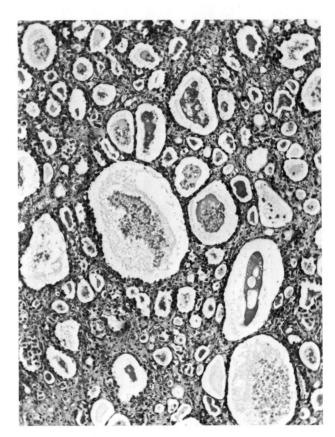

FIG. 48. Clear-cell carcinoma with tubulocystic pattern.

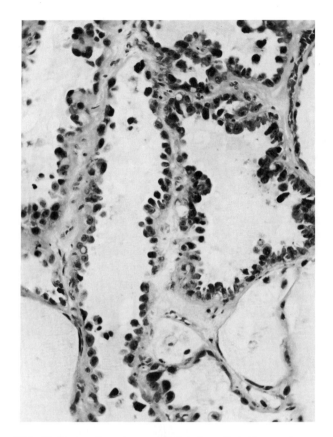

FIG. 49. Clear-cell carcinoma with tubulocystic pattern and prominent hobnail cells.

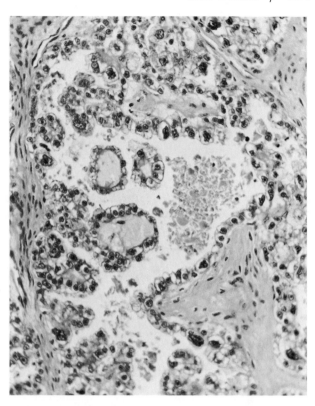

FIG. 51. Clear-cell carcinoma. Note two central papillae with hyalinized, eosinophilic cores.

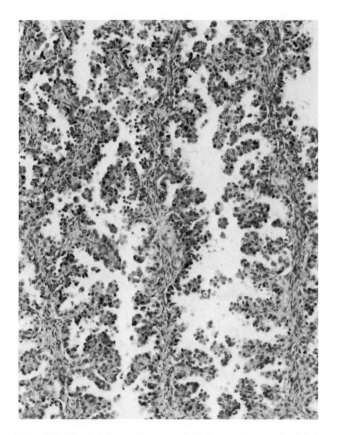

FIG. 50. Clear-cell carcinoma. Multiple papillae project into lumens of tubular glands.

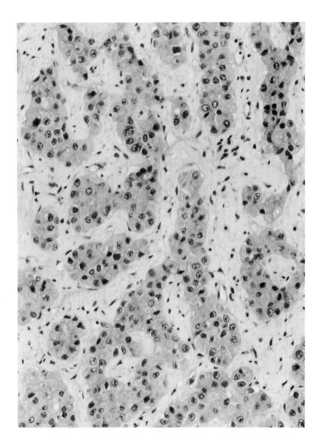

FIG. 52. Oxyphilic clear-cell carcinoma with trabecular pattern.

intracellular mucin is usually confined to the luminal tips of the cells. In some cells, mucin may displace the nucleus, creating a signet-ring cell appearance; in others it may form a central eosinophilic globule within an intracytoplasmic vacuole, producing a bull's-eye configuration. Occasional clear-cell carcinomas contain sheets, cords, or nests of cells with abundant eosinophilic cytoplasm (oxyphil cells) (Fig. 52). Rarely, this cell type predominates (208). Rarely, extensive amounts of basement membrane material occupy the stroma. When clear-cell carcinoma is poorly differentiated, many of its characteristic features are absent and a distinction from other carcinomas is difficult or impossible. Clear-cell carcinoma is often admixed with endometrioid carcinoma, with which it is closely related (200).

Differential diagnosis

Clear-cell carcinoma is most often confused with a germ-cell tumor, usually a dysgerminoma or yolk sac tumor (207), even though the usually older age of patients is strong evidence against a diagnosis of a primitive germ-cell tumor. Confusion with dysgerminoma occurs when the carcinoma has a diffuse pattern composed of clear cells. A mucin stain may show small foci of mucin that are absent in a dysgerminoma. The dysgerminoma cell is rounded with flattened edges, in contrast to the polyhedral cell of clear-cell carcinoma; and the nuclei of dysgerminomas are central, unlike those of the clear-cell carcinoma. Finally, at least a sprinkling of lymphocytes is almost always seen in dysgerminomas; occasional clear-cell carcinomas have a marked diffuse inflammatory-cell reaction (Fig. 46), but the infiltrate typically contains plasma cells and other inflammatory cells, as well as lymphocytes.

Clear-cell carcinomas may have a loose, edematous appearance simulating the reticular pattern of a yolk sac tumor (207), and both tumors may be papillary and contain hyaline bodies. The nuclei in yolk sac tumors, however, are almost always more primitive in appearance than those of a clear-cell carcinoma, and their papillae typically contain a central vessel and lack a hyalinized, eosinophilic core. Other typical patterns of clear-cell carcinoma or endometrioid foci help exclude a yolk sac tumor. Conversely, the presence of other types of germ-cell neoplasia exclude a diagnosis of clear-cell carcinoma. Finally, the immunohistochemical demonstration of alpha-fetoprotein strongly favors yolk sac tumor.

Rarely, metastatic renal-cell carcinoma may be indistinguishable from primary carcinoma of the ovary composed exclusively of clear cells. In most cases of ovarian clear-cell carcinoma, however, the presence of other patterns and cell types, as well as conspicuous extracellular luminal mucin, permits microscopic differentiation. Clinical data, including radiologic studies, may be necessary in some cases to exclude metastatic renal-cell carcinoma.

The rare clear-cell carcinoma composed predominantly of oxyphil cells may closely resemble a steroid-cell tumor, hepatoid yolk sac tumor (209), or hepatoid carcinoma (210). However, typical foci of clear-cell carcinoma are usually present in the oxyphilic variant. In addition, the nuclei in oxyphilic clear-cell carcinomas are typically eccentric, in contrast to the central nuclei of steroid-cell tumors. The degree of cytologic atypia in clear-cell carcinomas generally exceeds that of steroid-cell tumors, although occasional examples of the latter are highly pleomorphic. The hepatoid yolk sac tumor generally occurs in young females and, in addition, often contains foci of more typical yolk sac neoplasia. The hepatoid carcinoma occurs in an age group similar to that of clear-cell carcinoma but lacks the typical foci of clear-cell carcinoma usually present in the oxyphilic variant. Finally, in contrast to oxyphilic clear-cell carcinoma, hepatoid yolk sac tumor and hepatoid carcinoma stain immunohistochemically for alpha-fetoprotein.

Brenner Tumors

Clinical features

These tumors account for 2% to 3% of all ovarian neoplasms (211–217); less than 2% have been borderline (proliferative) or malignant (217–223), but the frequency of borderline or malignant change in palpable Brenner tumors is greater than 5% (218). Most of the benign neoplasms have been encountered in the fourth through eighth decades of life, with a peak in the late forties and early fifties. Borderline and malignant Brenner tumors occur in women who are, on the average, 5 to 10 years older than those with benign tumors.

Gross features

Benign Brenner tumors are typically less than 2 cm in diameter and incidental findings at operation or on pathological examination (Fig. 53); approximately 6% are bilateral. Most are solid; 10% to 25% appear as small, firm nodules in the wall of a mucinous cystadenoma. The benign tumors are well circumscribed with a hard, fibromatous, gray, white, or slightly yellow cut surface. Occasionally, the tissue has a gritty sensation due to calcific deposits, and, rarely, it is massively calcified. Sometimes tiny cysts are visible with a hand lens, and, occasionally, grossly visible cysts are conspicuous. Borderline tumors are characteristically cystic and unilocular or multilocular with cauliflower-like papillomatous masses protruding into one or more of the locules (Fig. 54). Rare borderline tumors are solid. Malignant Bren-

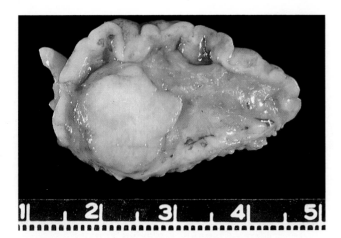

FIG. 53. Brenner tumor. A sharply demarcated, yellow-white fibrous tumor occupies a portion of the sectioned ovary.

ner tumors may be solid or cystic with mural nodules; they have no distinctive features.

Microscopic features

The typical, benign tumor is composed of round to oval, sharply demarcated nests of epithelial cells lying within an abundant fibrous stroma (Fig. 55). The tumor aggregates may be solid or may have a central lumen that contains dense eosinophilic material or mucin. Most of the neoplastic cells are polygonal or ovoid and have clear cytoplasm and oval, grooved nuclei. The cells lining the lumens range from flat to columnar and often contain mucin. Cysts of varying sizes lined entirely by mucinous or transitional epithelium are sometimes en-

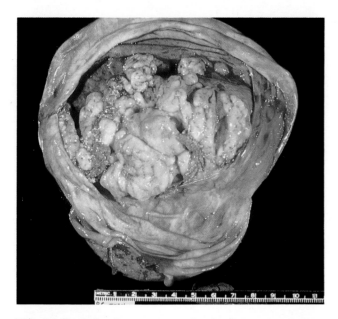

FIG. 54. Borderline Brenner tumor. A unilocular cyst contains a large polypoid mass of white tumor tissue arising from its lining.

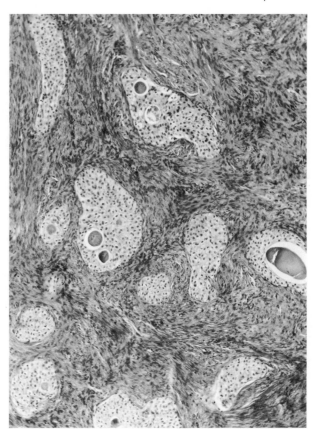

FIG. 55. Brenner tumor. Nests of transitional cells, some containing cysts, lie in a fibrous stroma.

countered. The stromal component may be focally hyalinized, and calcification is common.

Borderline tumors are characterized by cysts into which protrude papillae lined by proliferating cells of transitional type (Fig. 56). The lining cells resemble those of a Grade I papillary transitional-cell carcinoma. Mucin-containing cells may also be encountered, typically in the innermost layer. No invasion of the stroma is demonstrable, and typical Brenner tumor is also present in almost all cases. In a malignant Brenner tumor, the epithelium has the features of higher-grade transitional-cell carcinoma or squamous-cell carcinoma (Fig. 57). Scattered mucinous cells may be identified, but mucinous adenocarcinoma occurring in association with Brenner tumor should be diagnosed as such.

Agreement has not been reached concerning the criteria for malignant Brenner tumor. The diagnosis is clear when benign Brenner nests are associated with cytologically malignant nests that invade the stroma. Lacking invasion, we diagnose malignant Brenner tumor when the degree of atypia exceeds that of Grade I transitional-cell carcinoma, whereas others designate such cases as borderline malignancy. When malignant Brenner tumor is suspected the lesion should be sampled extensively in an attempt to demonstrate a benign

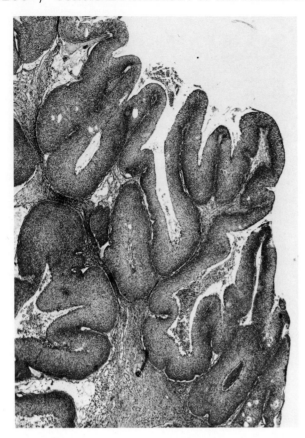

FIG. 56. Borderline Brenner tumor. Papillae lined by proliferating transitional epithelium protrude into a cyst. (From ref. 128.)

Brenner component. Tumors without the latter have been designated as transitional-cell carcinoma and have been associated with a worse prognosis than malignant Brenner tumor (223). The workers at the M. D. Anderson Hospital however, have shown that high–stage ovarian carcinomas with transitional cell carcinoma in extra-ovarian tumor have a very favorable prognosis compared to patients whose tumors do not have this component (223a).

Differential diagnosis

Metastatic transitional-cell carcinoma, which very rarely spreads to the ovary from the urinary bladder or ureter, may mimic a borderline or malignant Brenner tumor. In such cases, the presence of benign Brenner nests and mucinous elements, as well as the extent of invasion of the bladder tumor and the clinical history, may be of help in the differential diagnosis (224).

Squamous-Cell Tumors

Although squamous elements are often seen in endometrioid tumors and rarely in mucinous and Brenner tumors, very few pure squamous-cell neoplasms have been reported. Ten of them have been pure epidermoid cysts (225,226), which may not be true neoplasms. Nests of transitional epithelium were present in the walls of several of these cases, suggesting an origin from Walth-

ard nests or small Brenner tumors.

Four apparently pure squamous-cell carcinomas of the ovary have been described (227–229). In two, the tumor had the appearance of an *in situ* carcinoma lining a cyst, whereas the third case had both *in situ* and invasive components. There was a history of squamous-cell carcinoma *in situ* of the cervix in two of the cases. Because squamous-cell carcinomas may develop in a dermoid cyst (see page 1711), endometriotic cyst, or Brenner tumor, additional sections should be taken in an attempt to demonstrate such components before a diagnosis of pure squamous-cell carcinoma is rendered.

Mixed Common Epithelial Tumors

When only a small quantity of a second or third cell type is present in a common epithelial tumor it should be classified according to its predominant component. Tumors containing at least 10% of a second or third type, however, belong in the category of a mixed common epithelial tumor. Although one-third of Brenner tumors contain mucinous neoplastic elements and a much smaller proportion contain cells of serous type, it is excluded from the mixed-cell category. Mixed epithelial tumors can be benign, borderline, or malignant. Only one subtype, namely, mixed-epithelial papillary

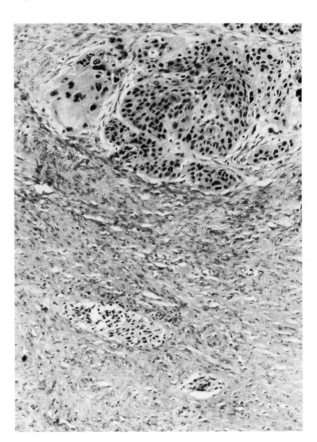

FIG. 57. Malignant Brenner tumor with squamous-cell carcinoma (*top*) and benign Brenner tumor (*bottom*).

THE OVARY / 201

cystadenoma of borderline malignancy, has been the subject of detailed investigation (231). Major findings in a recent study included the young age of the patients (average age: 35 years), a 22% frequency of bilateral ovarian involvement, and an association with endometriosis in 53% of the cases. On microscopic examination, the most striking feature is the presence of papillae reminiscent of those seen in serous borderline tumors but lined by combinations of endocervical-like mucinous cells, ciliated serous cells, endometrioid cells, and squamous cells. Many of the tumors had a heavy acute inflammatory infiltrate in the stroma and cyst lumens. These tumors are similar in their clinical and pathological features to the mucinous papillary cystadenomas of borderline malignancy of müllerian type that are discussed above.

Undifferentiated Carcinoma

The clinical features resemble those of serous carcinoma. Spread beyond the pelvis at presentation is common, and approximately 50% are bilateral. Undifferentiated carcinomas are predominantly solid and often show areas of hemorrhage, necrosis, and cyst formation.

A variety of patterns can be encountered, including diffuse masses, irregular nests (Fig. 58), and cords of epithelial cells separated by a desmoplastic stroma (39). Psammoma bodies, glands, papillae, and mucinous pools or droplets may be present in small numbers. The

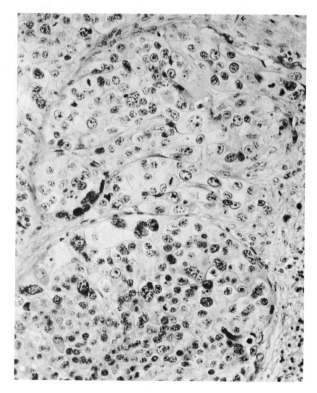

FIG. 58. Undifferentiated carcinoma. Note nuclear pleomorphism.

tumor cells vary greatly in size; tumor giant cells are often present. Occasional tumors resemble poorly differentiated transitional-cell or squamous-cell carcinoma; others have a superficial resemblance to a diffuse granulosa-cell tumor. The important distinction from the latter tumor is discussed in the section on granulosa-cell tumors. Before a diagnosis of undifferentiated carcinoma is rendered, numerous sections should be studied in an attempt to find better differentiated foci. The distinctive variant of undifferentiated carcinoma designated as small-cell carcinoma will be discussed below.

Sex-Cord–Stromal Tumors

These tumors account for approximately 6% of ovarian neoplasms and for most clinically functioning tumors (232); the most common form, however, is the endocrinologically inactive fibroma. The remainder most commonly exhibit differentiation toward ovarian-type cells (granulosa cells, theca cells, or both). Differentiation toward testicular-type cells (Sertoli cells, Leydig cells, or both) also occurs, and occasional tumors appear intermediate or indifferent or contain cells of both ovarian and testicular type. The stromal component of these tumors may resemble a spindle-cell sarcoma or a cellular fibromatous tumor; occasionally it is densely collagenized or markedly edematous. The tumors in this category contain sex-cord and stromal elements in varying combinations, with varying degrees of cytologic atypia and mitotic activity. The World Health Organization (WHO) classification used here (128) has been expanded to include several recently recognized subtypes (Table 1).

Granulosa-Cell Tumors

Clinical features

These tumors account for about 1.5% of all ovarian neoplasms (233) and for 6% of ovarian cancers (157). Approximately three-quarters are estrogenic, but rare examples, including a disproportionate number of large, thin-walled cystic tumors, are androgenic (234,235). Patients without endocrine symptoms usually present because of abdominal swelling or pain; the latter may be acute due to rupture and hemoperitoneum in up to 10% of cases (236). A mass is usually palpable on pelvic or abdominal examination. In about 10% of cases, the tumor is discovered during surgery for abnormal uterine bleeding or at the time of pathologic examination (237). Two-thirds of patients are postmenopausal (236–244); less than 5% are pre-pubertal. Most of the tumors in the latter patients differ pathologically from the usual granulosa-cell tumor encountered in older women, and the designations *adult granulosa-cell tumor* (AGCT) and *ju-*

venile granulosa-cell tumor (JGCT) (245) have been introduced to distinguish the two morphologic types. Occasional JGCTs are seen in older women, and, conversely, some AGCTs occur in children and young women. When GCTs of either type arise in prepubertal girls they are associated with isosexual pseudoprecocity in about 75% of cases. Both forms of GCT are almost always Stage I and are bilateral in less than 5% of the cases.

Adult granulosa-cell tumor

Gross features. These tumors vary greatly in size, with an average diameter of 12.5 cm (243). Their appearance ranges from uniformly solid to large, cystic tumors. Most characteristically, there is a yellow to white solid component and a hemorrhagic component that is solid or cystic (Fig. 59). Necrosis is uncommon. The cystic tumors are often thin-walled (Fig. 60), sometimes resembling serous cystadenomas (234,235).

Microscopic features. Examination reveals granulosa cells, usually accompanied by a stromal component of fibroblasts, theca cells, or lutein cells in varying combinations. Several patterns are encountered, with two or more commonly present in the same specimen. The microfollicular pattern (Fig. 61) is characterized by small follicles (Call-Exner bodies) that may contain eosinophilic material with nuclear debris, hyalinized basement-membrane-like material, or, rarely, basophilic mucinous secretion. A macrofollicular pattern of large, uniform follicles resembling follicle cysts is occasionally seen. Insular and trabecular patterns consist of islands and anastomosing bands of granulosa cells. The diffuse

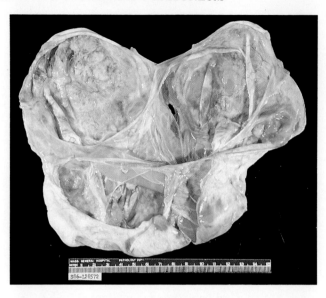

FIG. 60. Granulosa-cell tumor—adult type. This multiloculated neoplasm has small foci of pink-yellow tumor tissue adherent to its lining. (From ref. 461.)

pattern (Fig. 62) is characterized by sheets of round, oval, or slightly spindle-shaped cells imparting a "sarcomatoid" appearance. Uncommon patterns include "watered-silk" and gyriform variants. The former is characterized by a mosaic of thin winding cords, and the

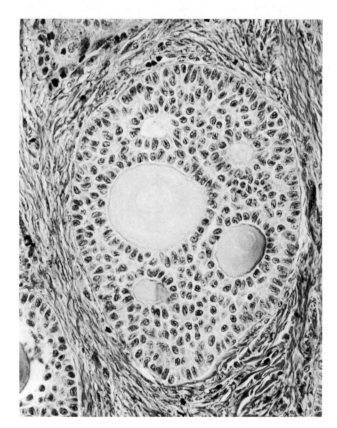

FIG. 61. Granulosa-cell tumor—follicular with Call-Exner bodies and larger follicles.

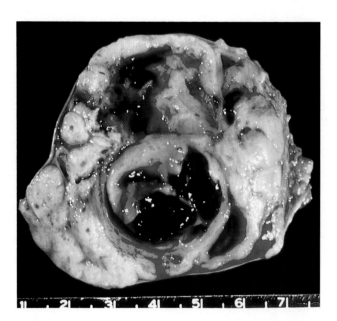

FIG. 59. Granulosa-cell tumor—adult type. The neoplasm is composed of yellow-white tissue with hemorrhage, some of which is intracystic. (From ref. 232.)

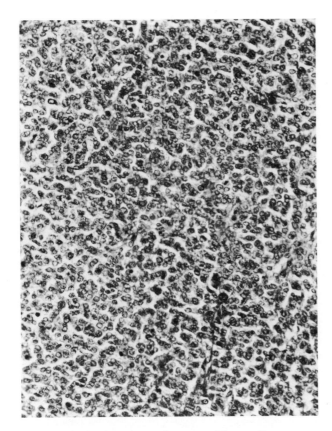

FIG. 62. Granulosa-cell tumor—diffuse pattern.

and poorly differentiated adenocarcinomas are often misinterpreted as diffuse and microfollicular AGCTs, respectively. In contrast to AGCTs, carcinomas are bilateral in over 25% of the cases, have often spread beyond the ovary, and may be extensively necrotic on gross examination. Microscopically, carcinomas, unlike AGCTs, have hyperchromatic, often pleomorphic, nuclei with frequent mitotic figures (Fig. 58) and may also contain rare glands, psammoma bodies, and intracellular mucin. The stroma of an undifferentiated carcinoma is typically composed of fibrous, often desmoplastic, tissue, in contrast to the fibrothecomatous stroma of an AGCT.

AGCTs may be difficult to distinguish from pure stromal tumors such as cellular thecomas, fibromas, and fibrosarcomas. Reticulin stains may show abundant intercellular fibrils in these tumors, unlike the scant reticulin of AGCTs. In some cases, the pattern of fibrils is intermediate between an AGCT and a typical thecoma, and, in such instances, the differential diagnosis may be difficult or impossible. The almost exclusively spindle-cell nature of fibromas and fibrosarcomas is rarely seen in AGCT. The differential diagnosis of the AGCT and endometrioid tumors, carcinoid tumors, endometrial stromal sarcomas, and small-cell carcinoma is discussed in the sections on those neoplasms.

latter by thin undulating cords. Rarely, true tubules with lumens and solid tubules are present in small numbers.

The nuclei of the granulosa cells are typically pale and round, oval, or angular and are often haphazardly oriented. They are commonly grooved (Fig. 63), but grooves may be inconspicuous, particularly in tumors with a diffuse pattern. Significant pleomorphism is typically absent, but approximately 2% contain cells with large, bizarre, hyperchromatic nuclei, resembling the bizarre nuclei occasionally seen in uterine leiomyomas (246). Mitotic activity is usually not conspicuous, and a mitotic rate of two or fewer per 10 high-power fields is seen in approximately three-quarters of the cases (236). The cytoplasm of granulosa cells is typically scanty, although occasional tumors contain cells with abundant, eosinophilic, luteinized cytoplasm or pale and vacuolated cytoplasm. Extensive luteinization is uncommon. A variable thecomatous or fibromatous component is usually present and may predominate. The designation of fibroma or thecoma with minor sex-cord elements (see below) should be reserved for tumors whose sex-cord element accounts for less than 5% of the tumor on any slide (247). Very rarely, the stroma of an AGCT has the appearance of a high-grade sarcoma (248) or exhibits adipose or osseous metaplasia (232).

Differential diagnosis. Undifferentiated carcinomas

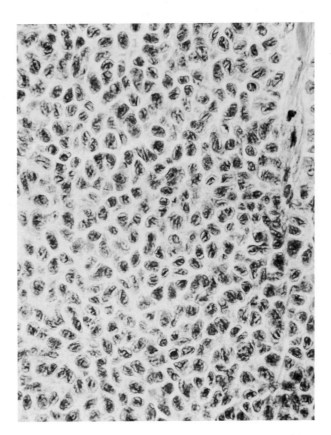

FIG. 63. Granulosa-cell tumor—diffuse pattern, with prominent nuclear grooves. (From ref. 462.)

Occasionally the distinction of a macrofollicular AGCT from one or more follicular cysts may be troublesome. This is particularly likely in gravid or recently gravid patients, because the large solitary luteinized follicle cyst of pregnancy and the puerperium (45) may be indistinguishable grossly from a unilocular cystic AGCT. The luteinized cells of the former, some of which contain large, bizarre nuclei, differ from those of a unilocular AGCT, which are rarely uniformly luteinized and rarely contain bizarre nuclei. In addition, the focal presence of neoplastic granulosa cells within the walls of most cystic AGCTs contrasts with their absence from follicle cysts.

Microscopic proliferations of granulosa cells mimicking small AGCTs are encountered rarely, usually within atretic follicles. These foci may be multiple and are seen most commonly in pregnant women, suggesting that they reflect a physiologic response to the elevated hCG level of pregnancy (249).

Juvenile granulosa-cell tumor

Gross features. The JGCT, like the AGCT, is typically partly solid, containing cysts that may be filled with blood (Fig. 64); uniformly solid or cystic tumors also occur. The neoplastic tissue may be gray, cream-colored, or yellow; occasionally, large areas of necrosis or hemorrhage are present (245).

Microscopic features. Sheets or nodular aggregates of neoplastic granulosa cells are usually punctuated by irregular or round to oval follicles (Fig. 65) (245,250–252). The follicles rarely attain the size of those in macrofollicular AGCT but are larger than Call-Exner bodies; typically they contain eosinophilic or basophilic, mucicarminophilic secretion. In the diffuse areas there

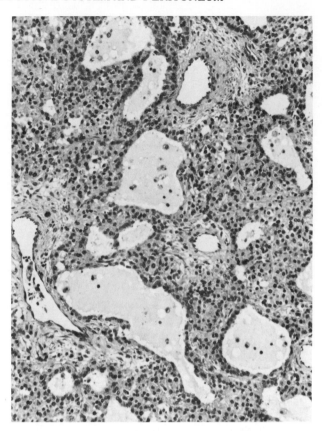

FIG. 65. Juvenile granulosa-cell tumor. Follicles of varying sizes and shapes are separated by cellular areas. (From ref. 463.)

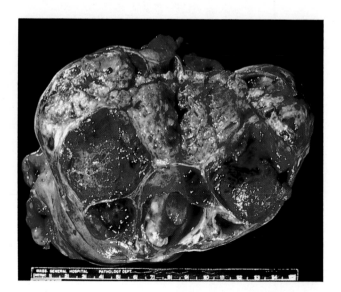

FIG. 64. Juvenile granulosa-cell tumor. The sectioned surface reveals solid, lobulated tissue, hemorrhage, necrosis, and cyst formation. (From ref. 245.)

maybe a background of basophilic, mucinous fluid. Theca cells are often present between nodules of granulosa cells; occasionally both cell types are arranged in a disorderly fashion and are difficult to distinguish. Both the granulosa and theca cells usually have abundant eosinophilic cytoplasm (Fig. 66) or are heavily vacuolated, i.e., are luteinized. The neoplastic cells have hyperchromatic, round nuclei that are only rarely grooved; mitotic figures, which may be atypical, are often numerous. In 10% to 15% of the cases, there is severe nuclear atypicality (245); in occasional tumors, hobnail-like cells line the follicles. Tumors from pregnant patient may exhibit prominent intercellular edema (253).

Differential diagnosis. The differential diagnosis of JGCT includes AGCT and a wide variety of other neoplasms. The follicles of JGCT are more irregular in size and shape than those of AGCT, and its cells are more extensively luteinized with nuclei that are typically round and hyperchromatic and that lack nuclear grooves. The mucicarminophilic, often basophilic, follicular content in JGCT also differs from the eosinophilic basement-membrane material and degenerating nuclei that often are present in the microfollicles of AGCT.

JGCT is often misdiagnosed as a malignant germ-cell tumor. The latter are more common in young females and may be associated with hCG-induced isosexual

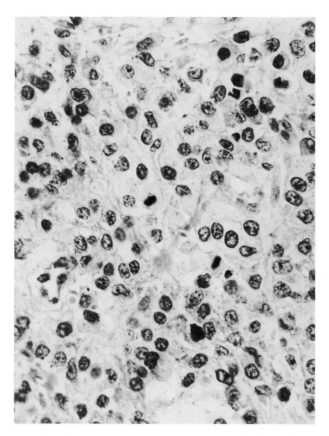

FIG. 66. Juvenile granulosa-cell tumor. Note abundant cytoplasm, mitotic activity, and absence of nuclear grooves. (From ref. 232.)

pseudoprecocity. The nuclei of JGCT are not as primitive-appearing as those of either yolk sac tumor or embryonal carcinoma, and the follicular pattern of JGCT is not a feature of either germ-cell tumor. Immunohistochemical demonstration of hCG in embryonal carcinomas and choriocarcinomas and of alpha-fetoprotein in yolk sac tumors may be helpful in difficult cases.

JGCT is sometimes misinterpreted as a thecoma because of the occasional absence or rarity of follicles, the typically abundant cytoplasm of the neoplastic cells, and the occasional predominance of theca cells. Thorough sampling to demonstrate follicles, as well as reticulin stains to establish the granulosa-cell nature of at least some of the tumor cells, is important diagnostically. Also, thecomas rarely exhibit significant mitotic activity, rarely occur before 30 years of age, and almost never develop in children. A focally diffuse pattern in a luteinized JGCT may suggest the diagnosis of a steroid(lipid)-cell tumor. The uniformity of the pattern, as well as the cytological features of the latter tumor, would be unusual for a JGCT, which almost always contains more diagnostic areas. Pregnancy luteoma rarely contains rounded, follicle-like spaces and may suggest a luteinized JGCT. As with the steroid-cell tumor, however, its cells are uniform and it is multiple and bilateral in one-half and one-third of the cases, respectively.

The only common epithelial tumors with which JGCT might be confused are clear-cell and undifferentiated carcinomas. The tubulocystic variant of clear-cell carcinoma is rarely suggested when follicles in JGCT are lined by hobnail-like cells. JGCT with high-grade nuclear atypia may suggest undifferentiated carcinoma. The absence of other patterns of clear-cell carcinoma, the young age of the patient, and the presence of follicles and of focal areas typical of JGCT provide evidence for its diagnosis. Finally, possible confusion between a JGCT and a small-cell carcinoma is discussed in the section on the latter tumor.

Tumors in the Thecoma-Fibroma Group

Fibroma

Clinical features. Fibromas typically occur in patients over 40 years of age with an average age of 48 years (254). They are rare in young patients, except for those with basal-cell nevus syndrome, in whom the tumors are almost always bilateral, multinodular, and calcified (255). Fibromas over 10 cm in diameter are associated with (a) ascites in up to 40% of cases and (b) Meigs' syndrome (ascites and pleural effusion) in about 1% of cases (256,257).

Gross features. Fibromas average 6 cm in diameter (254) and are typically solid, firm, white neoplasms; occasional specimens are soft and edematous. Rare specimens have yellow foci. Hemorrhage, necrosis, calcification, and cyst formation may be seen. The cellular fibroma is apt to be larger and softer with a much higher frequency of hemorrhage and necrosis (258).

Microscopic features. Spindle cells resembling fibroblasts and producing collagen, often in a storiform pattern, are typical. The cellularity is usually not pronounced. Hyaline plaques may be seen, and occasional tumors are diffusely edematous. Cytologic atypia and mitotic activity are absent or minor in extent. Fibromatous tumors that contain lutein cells belong in the category of luteinized thecoma (see below).

Differential diagnosis. Both fibromas and thecomas are derived from the ovarian stroma and, because a spectrum exists between the two, distinction may be arbitrary. We place tumors in the fibroma category unless the predominant cells are large and rounded and contain abundant vacuolated cytoplasm filled with lipid; such tumors are usually associated with estrogenic manifestations. Fat stains are not diagnostic, because slight to moderate amounts may be present in fibromas as well as in many other tumors. The term *fibrothecoma* has been used for tumors in the intermediate zone between fibroma and thecoma.

Fibromatosis of the ovary may closely resemble a fibroma (81). The former, however, enlarges the ovary diffusely and often envelops small follicle cysts. Microscopic examination discloses residual follicles entrapped within the lesion, in contrast to fibroma, which typically displaces them. Tiny aggregates of sex-cord cells, as well as foci of lutein cells, are occasionally seen in fibromatosis and should not lead to the misdiagnosis of a sex-cord–stromal tumor. Similar differences help to distinguish an edematous fibroma from an ovary involved by massive edema. Occasional Krukenberg tumors, Brenner tumors, and carcinoid tumors may closely resemble fibromas on gross examination, but their diagnostic epithelial components allow easy recognition, microscopically (259).

The most difficult and clinically important distinction is between a cellular fibroma and a fibrosarcoma. Cellular fibromatous tumors with three or fewer mitotic figures per 10 high-power fields and little or no nuclear atypia are almost always benign (cellular fibromas), whereas those with greater mitotic activity and moderate to marked nuclear atypia are almost always malignant (fibrosarcomas) (258). Neither mitotic activity nor nuclear atypia considered alone, however, is a valid predictor of behavior, and some tumors must be placed in the category "fibroma of uncertain malignant potential." Cellular fibromas and, less often, more innocuous-appearing fibromas rarely implant on the peritoneum.

Fibromas should be differentiated from rare leiomyomas and very rare schwannomas of the ovary using criteria and special techniques applied to these tumors at other sites. It must be emphasized that a storiform pattern in a fibromatous tumor of the ovary does not warrant a diagnosis of fibrous histiocytoma.

Thecoma (typical form)

Clinical features. Typical thecomas are about one-third as frequent as granulosa-cell tumors, if one uses stringent diagnostic criteria. The great majority are associated with estrogenic manifestations (260–263). In one large study (263), 84% of the patients were postmenopausal; only 10% of the women were under 30 years of age. Because thecomas are, in general, smaller than granulosa-cell tumors, they are less likely to be palpable on pelvic examination (237). Only 3% are bilateral (263).

Gross features. Thecomas are typically solid yellow masses (Fig. 67) but may be white and only focally yellow; they average about 7 cm in diameter. Cystic degeneration occasionally occurs but is rarely conspicuous.

Microscopic features. Large rounded cells with vacuolated cytoplasm containing lipid are typical (Fig. 68). The nuclei are round without significant atypia in most cases. Hyaline plaques are occasionally conspicuous (Fig. 68), and the stroma often contains a fibrous component separating sheets and nests of theca cells. In some cases there are large, confluent zones of hyaliniza-

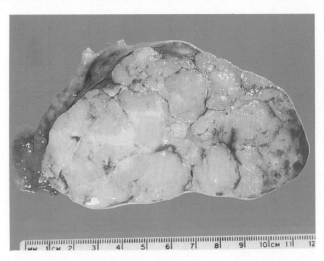

FIG. 67. Thecoma. The sectioned surface is solid, lobulated, and yellow. (From ref. 461.)

tion with focal calcification. Extensive calcification has been seen in rare cases, typically in young women (264). Occasional thecomas exhibit mild cytologic atypia, and, rarely, bizarre nuclei are seen in otherwise typical tumors (246). Prominent atypia and mitotic activity, accompanied by clinically malignant behavior, are very rare (265).

Luteinized thecoma

These tumors resemble fibromas or typical thecomas, but they contain lutein cells occurring singly, in clusters, or in masses (Fig. 69) (95,266,267). Patients are usually younger than those with typical thecomas. About half of luteinized thecomas are estrogenic, and about 10% are androgenic (95).

Differential diagnosis. Tumors that appear initially to be luteinized thecomas may rarely contain crystals of Reinke (268); such lesions have been designated "stromal Leydig-cell tumors" (74). When the lutein cells in a luteinized thecoma are extensive, the diagnosis of a steroid-cell tumor, not otherwise specified, or a stromal luteoma may be suggested. Because some steroid-cell tumors have minor fibromatous components, lesions intermediate between heavily luteinized thecomas and steroid-cell tumors are encountered rarely (269,270). By definition, however, the steroid-cell tumor is composed almost entirely of steroid cells with not more than a minimal component of thecoma or fibroma. Luteinized thecomas must also be distinguished from stromal hyperthecosis. The latter, may diffusely enlarge the ovaries up to 8 cm in diameter but in contrast to luteinized thecoma, is almost always bilateral. Microscopic examination of stromal hyperthecosis reveals lutein cells in a background of small stromal cells with minimal collagen production. In luteinized thecomas the background

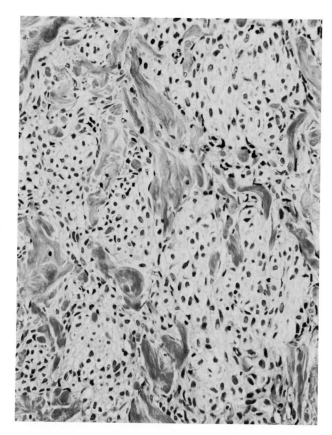

FIG. 68. Thecoma. Aggregates of rounded cells with abundant pale cytoplasm are traversed by bands of hyalinized collagen. (From ref. 232.)

consists of plump theca cells or of larger spindle cells producing collagen.

The extensive luteinization of thecomas that occurs in pregnancy may lead to confusion with pregnancy luteoma. The latter, however, are multiple in half of the cases, contain little or no lipid, and do not have a background of fibroma or thecoma. In addition, pregnancy luteomas usually exhibit more mitotic activity than luteinized thecomas.

Stromal tumors with minor sex-cord elements

Fibromas or thecomas rarely contain scattered sex-cord elements. Nests of indifferent cells, cells resembling granulosa cells, or tubules of Sertoli-like cells may be seen. The overall appearance and behavior of these tumors is more like that of fibroma or thecoma than a sex-cord–stromal tumor (247). The designation *fibroma* or *thecoma with minor sex-cord elements* should only be used when the sex-cord component accounts for less than 5% of the tumor on any slide (247).

Sclerosing stromal tumor

Clinical features. The sclerosing stromal tumor (SST) (271–275) occurs at a younger average age than typical

thecoma or fibroma, with over 80% of the patients being less than 30 years old (231). Most patients present with nonspecific symptoms related to an ovarian mass; estrogenic manifestations have been present only occasionally, and evidence of androgen secretion is rare. All reported tumors have been unilateral and benign.

Gross features. A well-demarcated, predominantly solid mass that is white with yellow flecks is typical; areas of edema and cyst formation are common (Fig. 70). Rare specimens are predominantly cystic (273–275). The average diameter is 10 cm; the largest reported tumor was 17 cm (271).

Microscopic features. Ill-defined cellular pseudolobules (Fig. 71) separated by densely hyalinized to markedly edematous stroma are characteristic. Two cell types are intermingled within the nodules: (i) spindle cells producing collagen and (ii) round to oval cells with small dark nuclei. The latter have vacuolated cytoplasm containing lipid and resemble degenerated luteinized stromal cells (Fig. 72). In an occasional tumor, the round or oval cells have dense eosinophilic cytoplasm and large nuclei containing prominent nucleoli and resemble typical lutein cells. Mitotic figures are absent or rare. Another distinctive feature is the presence of a network of thin-walled, often ectatic, blood vessels within the nodules.

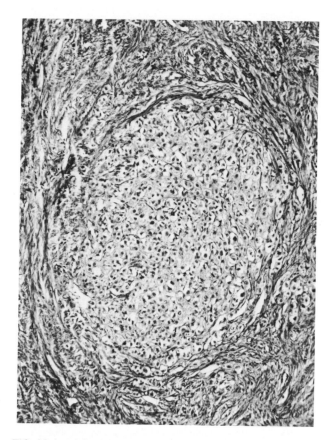

FIG. 69. Luteinized thecoma. A nodule of luteinized cells lies on a fibromatous background. (From ref. 463.)

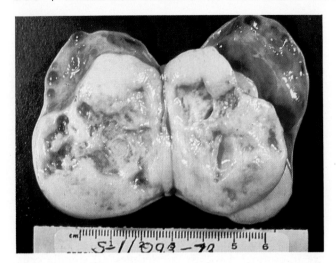

FIG. 70. Sclerosing stromal tumor forms a white mass with small cysts. (From ref. 39.)

Differential diagnosis. The heterogeneous appearance of SST contrasts with the homogeneity of fibromas and thecomas. Although fibromas may exhibit edema, it is generally diffuse rather than focal. Hyaline plaques, a conspicuous feature of many fibromas and thecomas, are rare in SST. The lutein cells in SST are typically

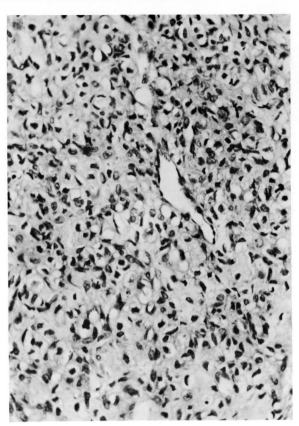

FIG. 72. Sclerosing stromal tumor is composed of rounded cells with clear cytoplasm. Some spindle-shaped cells are also present.

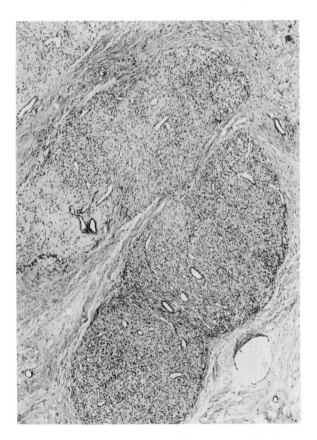

FIG. 71. Sclerosing stromal tumor. Cellular pseudolobules containing ectatic blood vessels are separated by hyalinized connective tissue.

vacuolated with dark nuclei, whereas in luteinized thecoma they usually have dense, eosinophilic cytoplasm and prominent nucleoli.

Rarely, the vacuolated lutein cells in SST have eccentric, compressed nuclei and simulate the signet-ring cells of Krukenberg tumor. The vacuoles in SST, however, contain lipid rather than mucin. The prominent vascularity in SST may suggest the diagnosis of hemangiopericytoma; no well documented ovarian case of the latter has been reported.

Ramzy (276) described an unusual signet-ring stromal tumor from a 28-year-old woman. The signet-ring cells failed to stain for lipid or mucin. Reticulin stains suggested that the neoplastic cells were mesenchymal.

Sertoli and Sertoli-Leydig Cell Tumors

Sertoli-cell tumors

Clinical features. These uncommon tumors occur at an average age of 27 years (277). Estrogenic effects are present in two-thirds of the cases; and occasional tumors, typically the lipid-rich type (278), cause isosexual pseudoprecocity (277–280). Two such tumors occurred in sisters with the Peutz-Jeghers syndrome (280).

Almost all the tumors have been confined to the ovary and have been unilateral; very rarely, they have malignant histologic features and metastasize distantly.

Gross features. Sertoli-cell tumors average 9 cm in diameter and are typically uniform, solid, yellow neoplasms.

Microscopic features. Hollow tubules or solid tubules (Fig. 73), or both, separated by a fibrous stroma, are characteristic. The hollow tubules are lined by columnar to cuboidal cells with moderate amounts of pale or slightly eosinophilic cytoplasm. The solid tubules are filled with cells having moderate to abundant, pale, lipid-rich cytoplasm (Fig. 73), the so-called lipid-rich Sertoli-cell tumor (folliculome lipidique) (278).

Differential diagnosis. Sertoli-cell tumors should be distinguished from rare, large Sertoli-cell adenomas composed of uniform, solid tubules filled with immature Sertoli cells. Such adenomas occur in the testes of patients with androgen insensitivity syndrome (testicular feminization). Sertoli-Leydig cell tumors are distinguished from Sertoli-cell tumors by the presence, in the former, of more than rare Leydig cells or their spindle-cell precursors. The distinctions from low-grade endometrioid carcinoma and Krukenberg tumor are discussed in the sections on those neoplasms. Ovarian tumors of probable wolffian origin (281) may have prominent solid tubules but typically contain other patterns, including sieve-like and solid areas composed of small, oval or spindle cells. Rare carcinoid tumors with a solid tubular pattern are distinguished from Sertoli-cell tumors (231) by argentaffin-argyrophil staining, electron microscopy, or immunohistochemical studies for neuroendocrine markers.

Sertoli-Leydig cell tumors

Sertoli-Leydig cell tumors (SLCT) account for less than 0.2% of ovarian neoplasms (282–286). They peak in incidence during early reproductive years (285). Approximately half of the patients develop hirsutism or virilization, but occasionally there are estrogen-related manifestations. Patients with no endocrine manifestations have symptoms attributable to a pelvic or abdominal mass.

Gross features. The diameter of SLCT varies greatly, averaging 10 cm. Typically, they form a firm, lobulated, yellow or tan mass (Fig. 74) with a smooth external surface. Cysts may be conspicuous, particularly if the tumor contains heterologous elements or has a retiform component. Tumors with a prominent mucinous component may simulate a mucinous epithelial neoplasm, and those with a retiform component are often soft, "spongy," or cystic with edematous intraluminal polypoid excrescences. Areas of hemorrhage and necrosis are uncommon, except in poorly differentiated subtypes. Only 2% of SLCT are bilateral (285).

Microscopic features. SLCT has been divided into four subtypes according to the WHO classification (Table 1). In our opinion, however, the clinical and pathologic features of SLCT that have a 10% or greater retiform pattern are sufficiently distinctive that a fifth subtype, the retiform SLCT, should be added. Mixtures of subtypes are frequently encountered.

Well-differentiated SLCT (286) is composed of hollow or solid tubules similar to those of pure Sertoli-cell tumor, but the surrounding fibrous stroma contains cells resembling Leydig cells. Crystals of Reinke have been identified within the latter in only a minority of cases. The tubules are usually small and round to oval but are occasionally large, varying in size and shape. They may be lined by stratified cells and, rarely, resemble the glands of low-grade endometrioid adenocarcinoma (287).

Tumors of intermediate differentiation often have a lobulated appearance with densely cellular areas intersected by acellular fibrous or edematous connective tissue. The latter often contains nests, small clusters (Fig. 75), and cords (Fig. 76) of cells compatible with immature Sertoli cells, as well as single cells or nests of cells consistent with Leydig cells (Figs. 75 and 76). Leydig cells are often most conspicuous at the periphery of the lobules, as well as at the periphery of the tumor as a

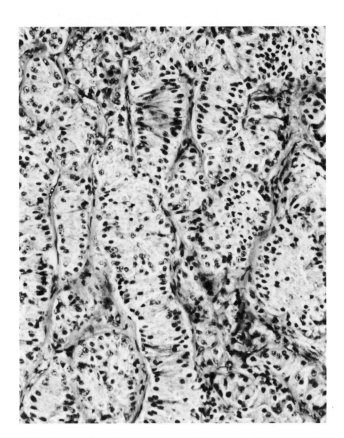

FIG. 73. Sertoli-cell tumor has a solid tubular architecture and is composed of cells with moderate to large amounts of pale cytoplasm.

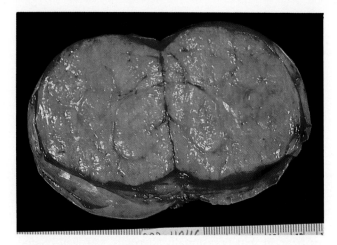

FIG. 74. Sertoli-Leydig-cell tumor of intermediate differentiation. The sectioned surface is lobulated and yellow.

whole. The cells resembling immature Sertoli cells have small, round to oval nuclei and, typically, scanty cytoplasm. Occasionally they contain abundant, pale or vacuolated cytoplasm and, in rare cases, eosinophilic cytoplasm. Sertoli cells are separated by variable numbers of Leydig cells and indifferent stromal cells. Some tumors

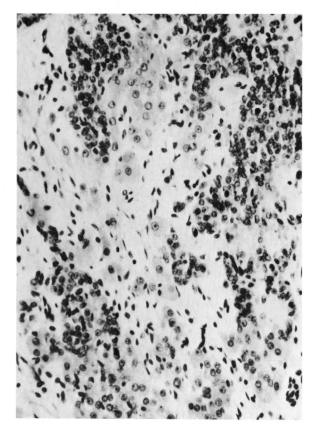

FIG. 75. Sertoli-Leydig cell tumor of intermediate differentiation. Note clusters of immature Sertoli cells with darkly staining nuclei. Pale Leydig cells have abundant cytoplasm, round nuclei, and prominent nucleoli.

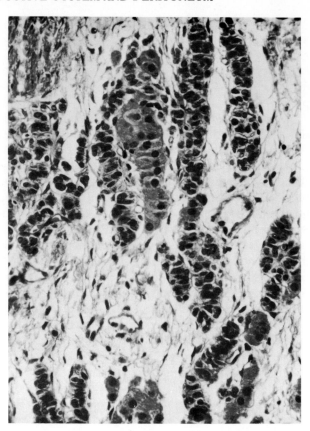

FIG. 76. Sertoli-Leydig cell tumor of intermediate differentiation. Cords of immature Sertoli cells reminiscent of the sex cords of the developing testis, accompanied by clumps of larger Leydig cells, are visible. (From ref. 288.)

contain foci of small, spindle-shaped cells with appreciable mitotic activity. Cysts of varying size, sometimes containing eosinophilic secretion, may be present; in addition, spaces reminiscent of thyroid follicles are occasionally seen. Rarely, SLCT, like granulosa-cell tumor and thecoma, contains cells with bizarre nuclei (246). SLCT from pregnant patients in the third trimester, as with other sex-cord–stromal tumors at this time, typically shows distinctive changes, particularly edema; large sheet-like aggregates of Leydig cells may also be seen (253).

Poorly differentiated SLCT is characterized by a diffuse growth of highly mitotically active cells that are usually spindle shaped, suggesting a fibrosarcoma. They may, however, be rounded and simulate an undifferentiated carcinoma. Tubules, sex-cord-like formations, and Leydig cells, as well as other, more distinctive patterns of Sertoli-Leydig cell neoplasia, are necessary to establish the diagnosis but may be minor in extent.

Patterns simulating the rete testis and characterized by irregular, slit-like tubules and cysts are found in approximately 10% of SLCT (288). They typically occur in children and women who are, on the average, younger than patients with other types of SLCT. The tubules are commonly lined by one or several layers of cells with round, usually regular nuclei and scanty cytoplasm. Papillae commonly project into the lumens of tubules and cysts. The papillae have cores that are small and hyalinized, large and edematous, or complex and branching with a lining of stratified atypical cells (Fig. 77). The retiform tubules are often continuous with solid columns of immature Sertoli cells. The stroma in the retiform areas varies from densely cellular to hyalinized or edematous. Occasional tumors are purely retiform, but most exhibit other patterns of Sertoli-Leydig cell tumor.

Heterologous elements occur in about 20% of SLCT (289–291). The most common component, present in almost 90% of the cases, is gastrointestinal-type epithelium (Fig. 78). The latter contains goblet cells in over half of the cases, argentaffin cells in one-third, and argyrophil cells in virtually all instances. The mucinous epithelium is usually benign but is occasionally borderline or a low-grade carcinoma (289,290). In over half of the cases with argentaffin cells, microscopic foci of carcinoid are also present (289,290). Approximately one-quarter of heterologous tumors contain cartilage or immature skeletal muscle, or both (291). Mesenchymal heterologous elements are usually found in tumors with a sarcomatoid background. Very rarely, cells resembling

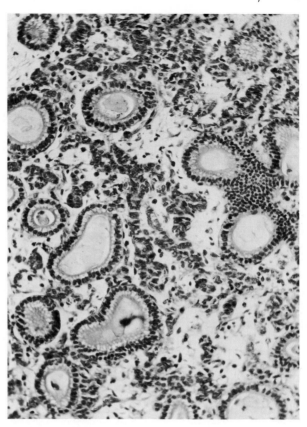

FIG. 78. Sertoli-Leydig cell tumor with heterologous elements. Mucinous glands are separated by cords and clusters of Sertoli cells.

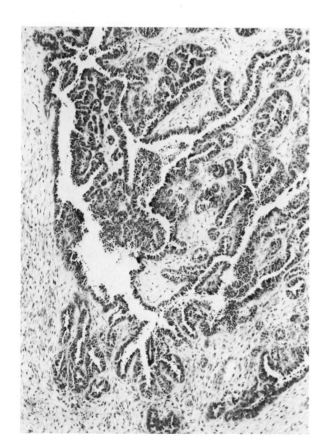

FIG. 77. Retiform Sertoli-Leydig cell tumor. Elongated tubules, papillae, and cellular stratification impart a resemblance to a malignant common epithelial neoplasm.

hepatocytes or neuroectodermal elements may be seen (292,293).

Differential diagnosis. SLCT is impossible to distinguish from granulosa-cell tumor (GCT) on gross inspection. However, SLCT, unlike GCT, almost never forms a unilocular thin-walled cyst and rarely forms multilocular thin-walled cysts. Microscopically, typical GCT and SLCT are quite different, but characteristic features of one are often seen focally in the other. The prominent tubules and discrete clusters of Leydig cells in well-differentiated SLCT readily distinguish it from GCT, although rare SCLT contain granulosa cells and rare GCT contain small numbers of well-formed tubules. Islands of well-differentiated granulosa cells are common in GCT but are infrequent in SLCT. The cells of GCT are typically more mature than those of SLCT, and, although nuclear grooves may be seen in Sertoli cells, they are seldom conspicuous. The stromal component of SLCT often has a sarcomatous appearance, which is rare in GCT. The presence of heterologous elements is almost specific for SLCT as opposed to GCT, and a retiform pattern is seen only in the former. Thecomatous stroma is unusual but is rarely present in SLCT. Finally, the Leydig cells of SLCT tend to cluster in small groups, whereas in GCT, luteinized theca cells are usually not prominent and tend to cluster less often than Leydig cells.

The retiform variant of SLCT is most commonly misdiagnosed as yolk sac tumor because of the young age of the patient, but the two tumors have little in common microscopically. Pure or almost pure retiform tumors, however, may bear a strong resemblance to common epithelial tumors and, indeed, have occasionally been reported as such. The papillae of retiform SLCT may simulate those of a serous borderline tumor. In addition, if nuclear stratification and papillarity are pronounced, SLCT may resemble a serous or endometrioid carcinoma. Juxtaposition of epithelium and immature mesenchyme in retiform SLCT has also caused confusion with malignant mesodermal mixed tumor. A variety of clinicopathologic features, including the young age of the patients, the presence of androgenic manifestations in 20% of the cases, and the finding of more typical SLCT in almost all cases, provide clues to the correct diagnosis.

Nonretiform SLCT are rarely misinterpreted as primitive germ-cell tumors, particularly during pregnancy, because the stromal edema in such cases (253) imparts a loose reticular appearance similar to that of yolk sac tumor. The nuclei of SLCT are not as primitive as those of yolk sac tumor, and the frequent presence of Sertoli-like tubules exclude the latter diagnosis.

Heterologous SLCT are most often misdiagnosed as teratomas, but, in contrast to the latter, almost never contain neuroectodermal tissues. Moreover, common constituents of teratoma, such as squamous epithelium, skin appendages, and respiratory epithelium, have not been reported in SLCT. Heterologous SLCT-containing glands and cysts lined by gastrointestinal-type epithelium may be confused with pure mucinous cystic tumors on gross examination. Although a history of virilization is much more suggestive of SLCT, occasional mucinous tumors containing luteinized stromal cells are masculinizing. The diagnosis of heterologous SLCT rests on finding a Sertoli-Leydig cell component, which is almost always of intermediate differentiation, between glands and cysts or at the periphery of the tumor. A carcinoid component in SLCT is usually a minor microscopic component and is unlikely to cause confusion. Heterologous tumors with mesenchymal elements may be confused with sarcoma when recognizable Sertoli-Leydig cells are scarce. Before a pure ovarian sarcoma is diagnosed, particularly in a young woman, heterologous SLCT should be excluded by adequate sampling. Criteria for the differentiation of SLCT from endometrioid carcinoma, tubular Krukenberg tumor, and carcinoid tumors are discussed elsewhere.

Gynandroblastoma

Tumors containing Sertoli-Leydig cell and granulosa-stromal cell elements in varying proportions have been reported as "gynandroblastoma." Because minor elements of one tumor type frequently occur in otherwise typical tumors of the other type, the diagnosis of gynandroblastoma should be reserved for neoplasms containing at least 10% of the minor component in a typical, easily recognizable form. If this strict definition is used, gynandroblastoma is exceedingly rare (294,295).

Unclassified Sex-Cord–Stromal Tumors

Approximately 5% to 10% of sex-cord–stromal tumors have microscopic features intermediate between SLCT and GCT, or they have unusual patterns not permitting reproducible placement in either category. In some cases, assignment as Sertoli-Leydig or granulosa cell is arbitrary. For example, Talerman et al. (296) have designated as *diffuse nonlobular androblastoma* tumors having a diffuse fibrothecomatous or granulosa-cell proliferation with focal Sertoli-tubular differentiation in almost all cases. Tumors of this type that we have seen have differed in appearance from the usual forms of SLCT, and it may be preferable to label them as unclassified sex-cord–stromal tumor.

Sex-cord–stromal tumors from pregnant patients are particularly likely to cause problems in diagnosis (253). In one study, 17% were unclassified, and others diagnosed as GCT or SLCT had large areas with an indifferent appearance (253). A major problem in classification was prominent intratumoral edema during the third trimester of pregnancy; increased luteinization in GCT, combined with extensive Leydig-cell maturation in SLCT, added to the diagnostic difficulty.

Sex-Cord Tumor with Annular Tubules (SCTAT)

This tumor is associated in one-third of cases with Peutz-Jeghers syndrome (PJS)—gastrointestinal polyposis, oral and cutaneous melanin pigmentation, and, rarely, minimal deviation adenocarcinoma of the cervix (297–299). In PJS patients, SCTAT is typically an incidental finding, whereas in patients without this syndrome it is typically detected clinically. In approximately 40% of SCTAT with or without the PJS, there are manifestations of hyperestrinism (including menstrual disturbances) and isosexual precocity when the tumor arises in a child (299); occasional SCTAT produce progesterone.

Gross features

Features differ depending on whether the patient has PJS. In patients with the syndrome, tumors are typically multifocal, bilateral, focally calcified, and no more than 3 cm in diameter (299). Those from patients without PJS are almost always unilateral, usually large, and rarely calcified. A large SCTAT is typically solid, but cysts are occasionally present, and, rarely, SCTAT is predominantly cystic (299).

Microscopic features

PJS-associated SCTAT form sharply circumscribed, rounded, ring-shaped tubules encircling nodules of hyalinized basement-membrane-like material (Fig. 79). Simple tubules encircle single hyaline nodules, whereas more common complex tubules surround multiple nodules. The centers of the tubules are filled with pale, lipid-rich cytoplasm, and the nuclei are located in an antipodal arrangement at the periphery; in some areas they proliferate toward the centers of the tubules. Rare tubules are elongated. Occasional nests are composed of cells containing large lipid-laden vacuoles. Focal calcification is observed in most of the cases.

Lesions unassociated with PJS are similar, but multifocality and calcification are rare, whereas areas of typical granulosa-cell tumor (300) or Sertoli-cell tumor (279), or both, are common. Because Charcot-Böttcher filaments have been demonstrated ultrastructurally in occasional cases, some regard SCTAT as a type of Sertoli-cell tumor (279); on the other hand, others consider it a variant of granulosa-cell tumor because of a prominent GCT component in many cases (300). Because of

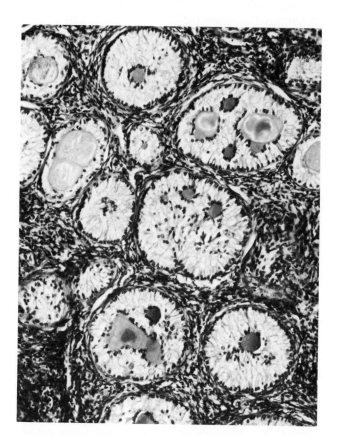

FIG. 79. Sex-cord tumor with annular tubules from a patient with Peutz-Jeghers syndrome. Simple and complex annular tubules encircle hyaline masses. (From ref. 464.)

its characteristic clinicopathologic features, it is preferable to consider the SCTAT as a distinct sex-cord–stromal tumor, with potential for bidirectional differentiation.

Another rare sex-cord–stromal tumor has been reported in two young girls with PJS and isosexual pseudoprecocity (301). The unusual microscopic features included diffuse areas, tubular differentiation, microcysts, and papillae formed by at least two distinctive cell types.

Steroid-Cell Tumors

The terms *lipoid-cell tumor* or *lipid-cell tumor* (10,30) have been used to describe neoplasms composed of large, rounded or polyhedral cells that resemble lutein, Leydig, and adrenocortical cells. Although most tumors in this category contain abundant intracellular fat, approximately 40% do not, leading to the paradox of lipid-free "lipid-cell" tumors. To avoid this incongruity, the designation *steroid-cell tumor* has been proposed (39,302). These tumors are divided into three major categories: stromal luteoma; Leydig-cell tumor; and steroid-cell tumor, not otherwise specified (NOS).

Stromal Luteoma

This designation (76) has been applied to small steroid-cell tumors that lie within the ovarian stroma and presumably arise from it. The capacity of ovarian stroma to form lutein cells is exemplified by the nonneoplastic disorder stromal hyperthecosis, a finding also present adjacent to over 90% of stromal luteomas (303). Microscopic nodules of lutein cells may develop in stromal hyperthecosis (nodular hyperthecosis), but the designation *stromal luteoma* should be reserved for grossly visible lesions. Some large steroid-cell tumors, NOS, are undoubtedly of stromal origin, but a specific diagnosis cannot be made when the tumor is no longer confined to the ovarian stroma.

Clinical/gross features

Approximately 20% of steroid-cell tumors belong in the stromal-luteoma category (303). These tumors occur over a wide age range but usually develop after menopause (average age: 58 years) (303). Approximately 60% are estrogenic and 12% are androgenic. Underlying stromal hyperthecosis may contribute to the associated endocrine abnormality, which is sometimes long-standing. Tumors rarely exceed 3 cm and are well circumscribed (303).

Microscopic features

A mass of luteinized cells, arranged diffusely or in nests and cords is characteristic. The cytoplasm is typically eosinophilic and contains relatively little lipid; lipochrome granules are present in over half of the cases; mitotic figures are rare. Approximately 20% of stromal luteomas exhibit a degenerative change seen only rarely in other steroid-cell tumors and characterized by irregular spaces simulating glands or vessels (Fig. 80) (76). The stroma is typically sparse but, in about 20% of cases, is focally fibrotic and hyalinized (303).

Leydig(Hilus)-Cell Tumors

Leydig-cell differentiation can be proven only when Reinke crystals are identified in the neoplastic cells by light microscopy or electron microscopy (304–306). Because only 35% to 40% of testicular Leydig-cell tumors contain these crystals light microscopically, some unclassified ovarian steroid-cell tumors are almost certainly Leydig-cell tumors that cannot be specifically identified.

Ovarian Leydig-cell tumors may originate in the hilus or within the ovarian stroma (74,75). Hilus-cell tumors, which are much more common, arise from hilus cells, which are present, usually in association with nonmyelinated nerve fibers, in 80% to 85% of normal ovaries. Only four stromal Leydig-cell tumors arising directly

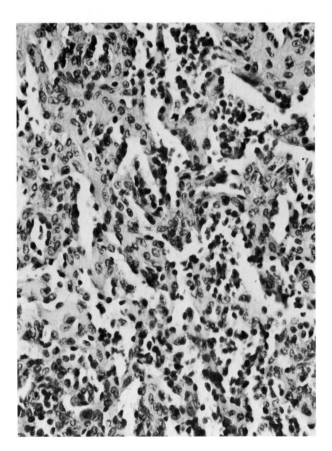

FIG. 80. Stromal luteoma. Degenerative changes have produced irregular spaces. (From ref. 464.)

from ovarian stromal cells have been reported (74). An ovarian stromal-cell derivation for these tumors is tenable because crystals of Reinke may be seen in otherwise typical cases of stromal hyperthecosis (74).

Clinical features

Hilus-cell tumors are diagnosed at an average age of 58 years; 75% cause hirsutism or virilization (306). The androgenic manifestations are typically milder and of longer duration than those associated with Sertoli-Leydig cell tumors. Occasionally, there are estrogenic manifestations.

Gross features

Hilus-cell tumors range from 1 to 15 cm in diameter, but the great majority measure less than 5 cm. Almost all are unilateral (89,304). They are well circumscribed, fleshy, and brown, orange, or yellow; hemorrhagic mottling is common.

Microscopic features

Sheets, cords, or nests of uniform, rounded or polyhedral cells with large, central nuclei and one or more prominent nucleoli are characteristic. In some areas, the nuclei may be aggregated or "pooled," usually in relation to blood vessels. The cytoplasm is eosinophilic and finely granular; small cytoplasmic lipid vacuoles may be present. Lipochrome pigment is seen in varying numbers of cells. Reinke crystals (Fig. 81) are present, by definition, but their detection may require prolonged search. Fibrinoid degeneration of large blood-vessel walls within the tumor is a frequent and seemingly distinctive feature. Except for their location, the pathologic features of Leydig-cell tumor, nonhilar type, are similar to those of hilus-cell tumor. The diagnosis of probable hilus-cell tumor is made if a steroid-cell tumor lacking Reinke crystals is located in the hilus, has a background of hilus-cell hyperplasia, is closely associated with nonmyelinated nerve fibers, exhibits nuclear pooling, or has fibrinoid degeneration of its vessels.

Steroid-Cell Tumor, Not Otherwise Specified

Clinical features

Steroid-cell tumors, which cannot be diagnosed as stromal-luteoma or Leydig-cell tumor, are the most common subtype, accounting for 56% of cases in one series (307). They may occur at any age (mean age: 43 years) (307). They are most often virilizing (41% of the cases) (307) but occasionally are estrogenic or unassociated with endocrine manifestations (307,308). Rare

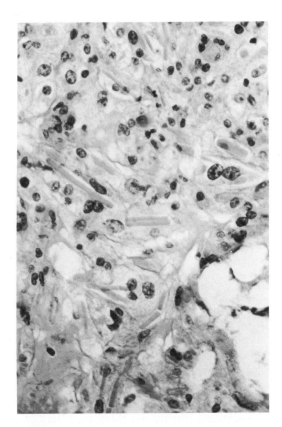

FIG. 81. Crystals of Reinke in Leydig-cell tumor.

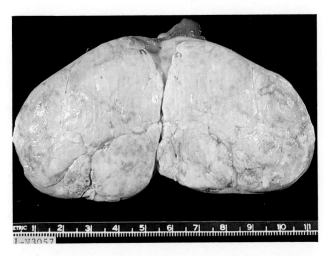

FIG. 82. Steroid-cell tumor, not otherwise specified. The neoplasm has a lobulated, yellow, sectioned surface. (From ref. 307.)

plasm (Fig. 84); transitions between the two cell types are usually seen (Fig. 84). Both have distinct cell borders and central nuclei, often with a prominent nucleolus. Intracytoplasmic lipochrome pigment is present in about one-third of the cases (307). In most cases, nuclear atypia is absent or slight, but it is moderate or marked in approximately 25%. The mitotic rate varies and does not clearly correlate with nuclear atypia.

examples in children have caused isosexual pseudoprecocity (308). Four tumors in this category have caused Cushing's syndrome (309,310). Neoplasms in this group are almost always unilateral and Stage I, but approximately 40% are clinically malignant (307).

Gross features

Examination typically discloses well-circumscribed masses that vary greatly in size, ranging up to 45 cm, with an average diameter of 8.5 cm (307). Most are yellow (Fig. 82) or orange because of abundant intracytoplasmic lipid. They may be red to brown if they are lipid-poor, or they may be dark brown to black if they contain abundant lipochrome pigment. Necrosis, hemorrhage, and cystic degeneration are occasionally observed.

Microscopic features

Cells arranged diffusely, in nests, or in columns separated by a rich vascular network are characteristic. A minor fibromatous component and areas of hyalinization are rarely seen. The more common steroid cell is polygonal and of medium to large size, and it contains slightly granular, eosinophilic cytoplasm (Fig. 83). A second cell type is larger with abundant spongy cyto-

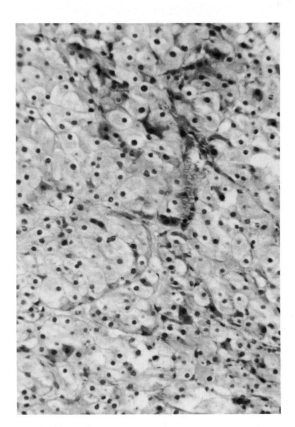

FIG. 83. Steroid-cell tumor. The cells have abundant dense cytoplasm. [From Case Records of the Massachusetts General Hospital (Case 8, 1969).]

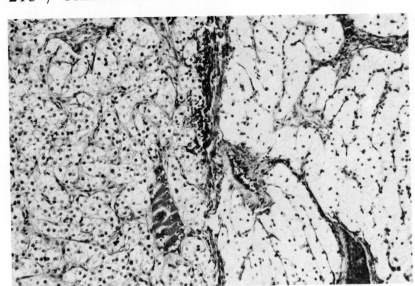

FIG. 84. Steroid-cell tumor. The cells have moderate to large amounts of vacuolated cytoplasm. (From ref. 462.)

Although the only absolute evidence of malignancy is metastasis, a variety of clinicopathologic features correlate with malignant behavior. In a recent large study (307), the clinically malignant tumors occurred in patients who were, on average, 16 years older than those with a favorable outcome. Approximately 78% of tumors over 7 cm in diameter were malignant, whereas smaller tumors have been invariably benign (307). Approximately two-thirds of tumors with high nuclear atypia, as well as 80% of those with two or more mitotic figures per 10 high-power fields, proved to have a malignant course (307).

Differential diagnosis

Steroid-cell tumors may be confused with other neoplasms, including extensively luteinized granulosa-cell tumors and thecomas, clear-cell carcinomas, metastatic renal-cell carcinomas, and lipid-rich Sertoli-cell tumors. Rare, extensively luteinized granulosa-cell tumors and thecomas can be identified by the presence of (a) nonluteinized granulosa-cell tumor in the former and (b) fibrothecomatous areas with abundant reticulin in the latter. Clear-cell carcinoma and metastatic renal-cell carcinoma have glycogen-rich cytoplasm and typically eccentric nuclei, in contrast to the characteristic lipid-filled cytoplasm and central nuclei of lipid-rich steroid-cell tumors. Oxyphilic clear-cell carcinomas (208) exhibit, at least focally, architectural patterns characteristic of typical clear-cell carcinoma. The differentiation between a steroid-cell tumor and a lipid-rich Sertoli-cell tumor with a prominent diffuse pattern depends on identifying focal tubules in the latter.

Pregnancy luteomas may be difficult to differentiate from lipid-free or lipid-poor steroid-cell tumors occurring during pregnancy, and both may be virilizing. Unlike steroid-cell tumors, however, approximately one-third of pregnancy luteomas are bilateral and one-half are multiple. The latter may also contain numerous mitotic figures. In contrast, a steroid-cell tumor with minimal cytologic atypia usually contains only rare mitotic figures. Although it may be impossible to be certain given a solitary lesion, a nodule of lipid-poor steroid cells encountered during the third trimester of pregnancy is presumed to be a pregnancy luteoma, unless clear-cut evidence indicates otherwise.

Tumors of the Rete Ovarii

These lesions are uncommon; most are cysts (cystadenomas) (311). Rete cysts are found most often in postmenopausal women, who have nonspecific symptoms. Occasional patients with a rete cyst have androgenic manifestations.

Gross Features

The cysts range up to 24 cm in diameter (mean: 8.7 cm), have a hilar location, and are usually unilocular. They typically contain clear or yellow fluid and have thin walls with smooth linings. Adenomas have usually been incidental microscopic findings, and the only rete carcinoma reported had nonspecific gross features.

Microscopic Features

The walls of rete cysts are composed of fibrovascular tissue, which typically contains fascicles of smooth muscle. The luminal surfaces characteristically have thin crevices (Fig. 85) and are usually lined by cuboidal or flat cells, which are only rarely ciliated. Hyperplasia of hilus cells, frequently seen in the cyst wall (Fig. 85), accounts for the virilization that may accompany the

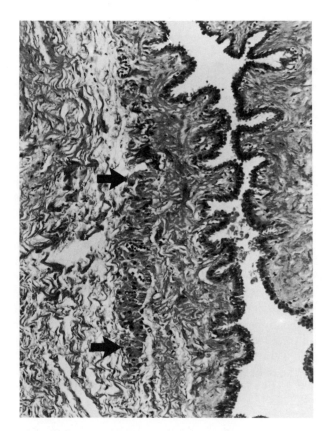

FIG. 85. Rete cyst. Note the nonciliated, columnar epithelial lining, the formation of crevices, and the fibrous wall. A thin band of hilus cells is present (*arrows*). (From ref. 94.)

lesion. Adenomas are composed of closely packed small tubules, some of which may be dilated and contain simple papillae. A single rete adenocarcinoma was characterized by an irregular network of branching tubules and cysts that contained papillae with fibrovascular or hyalinized cores. The tubules, cysts, and papillae were lined by obviously malignant, nonciliated cuboidal cells. There were also areas with a solid growth pattern and extensive transitional-cell metaplasia.

Differential Diagnosis

Rete cysts are often misdiagnosed as serous cystadenomas but are distinguished by their location, characteristic crevices in their linings, the resemblance of their lining cells to the normal rete, and the frequent presence of smooth-muscle bundles and hilus cells in their walls. Rete adenomas may be confused with female adnexal tumors of probable wolffian origin, but the latter typically have patterns other than tubular or papillary that are incompatible with a rete nature. The rete carcinoma was distinguished from a pure retiform Sertoli-Leydig cell tumor, primarily by its focal solid pattern and transitional-cell metaplasia which we have not seen in the latter. It also occurred in an elderly woman.

Germ-Cell Tumors

Germ-cell tumors account for approximately 30% of ovarian neoplasms. Ninety-five percent are dermoid cysts (mature cystic teratomas), and most of the remainder are malignant. Dermoid cysts account for one-third of benign ovarian neoplasms, and malignant germ-cell tumors account for approximately 3% of all ovarian cancers in western countries. The latter figure, however, is as high as 15% in native Oriental and black populations, in which common epithelial carcinomas are infrequent. Germ-cell tumors account for two-thirds of ovarian cancers during the first two decades of life.

Most malignant germ-cell tumors occur in pure form (Table 1), but each may be mixed with other types. It is essential, therefore, to examine every germ-cell tumor carefully and sample all areas that differ in gross appearance. If the tumor proves to be mixed on microscopic examination, the relative amount of each component should be reported.

Dysgerminoma

Clinical features

Dysgerminomas account for nearly 50% of malignant germ-cell tumors, for 1% of all ovarian cancers, and for 5% to 10% of ovarian cancers in the first two decades. Eighty percent occur before the age of 30 years (mean: 21 years); they are extremely rare over the age of 50 and under the age of 5 years. Most of the patients present with signs or symptoms related to an abdominal mass. In patients with an associated gonadoblastoma, an underlying abnormality in gonadal development may dominate the clinical presentation. Dysgerminomas rarely elaborate hCG, leading to hormonal manifestations that are typically estrogenic (isosexual pseudoprecocity, menstrual irregularities) but occasionally androgenic (virilization) (312). The clinical picture may mimic that of an ectopic or intrauterine pregnancy or of a hydatidiform mole (313,314).

About 65% of dysgerminomas are Stage IA; in higher stages, the contralateral ovary, pelvic and para-aortic lymph nodes, or peritoneum, or combinations thereof, are typically involved. The 5-year survival rates approach 100% for Stage I tumors (315,316). Because of the sensitivity of dysgerminomas to radiation therapy and chemotherapy, the 5-year survival rate for patients with higher stage or recurrent tumors is currently over 80% (315–317).

Gross features

Dysgerminomas are typically solid tumors with a median diameter of 15 cm. The serosal surface is smooth or bosselated. The cut surface is typically soft, fleshy, and lobulated and may be cream-colored, gray, pink, or tan (Fig. 86). Areas of cystic degeneration, necrosis, and hemorrhage occasionally occur and should be sampled to exclude other germ-cell elements. Calcification suggests an underlying gonadoblastoma. The tumor is grossly bilateral in about 10% of the cases; in another 10%, microscopic foci of tumor are present in a grossly negative contralateral ovary.

Microscopic features

The appearance is monotonous (Fig. 87), with primordial germ cells in diffuse, insular, or trabecular patterns. The uniform, rounded tumor cells have eosinophilic to clear cytoplasm (which is almost always glycogen-rich), discrete cell membranes, and a central, large, rounded or flattened nucleus (Fig. 88). The nucleus contains coarsely clumped chromatin and one or a few prominent nucleoli. Mitotic figures are usually numerous. The characteristic stroma consists of thin to broad fibrous bands infiltrated by mature lymphocytes with occasional lymphoid follicles. Sarcoid-like granulomas are present in 20% of the cases and very rarely are numerous, obscuring the underlying tumor (314). Less than 5% of dysgerminomas are of the so-called "anaplastic" type, characterized by a high mitotic rate (30 or more mitotic figures per 10 high-power fields) and marked nuclear pleomorphism (314). The prognostic and therapeutic implications, if any, of this subtype have not been established.

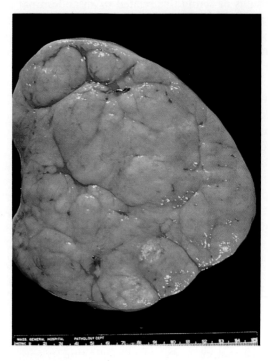

FIG. 86. Dysgerminoma. The neoplasm has a lobulated, tan-white, sectioned surface.

Approximately 3% of dysgerminomas contain syncytiotrophoblastic giant cells (SGC) that are immunoreactive for hCG; serum hCG is frequently elevated in such cases (314). The SGC may be intimately associated with blood-filled sinusoids (312), but the biphasic growth pattern of choriocarcinoma with accompanying cytotrophoblasts is absent. Exhaustive sampling of tumors producing hCG is important to exclude foci of choriocarcinoma or embryonal carcinoma. In contrast to SGC, the presence of the last two components warrants a diagnosis of mixed germ-cell tumor. Rare patients with pure dysgerminoma have elevated hCG but no demonstrable SGC; in such cases, the dysgerminoma cells may be immunoreactive for hCG (318).

Luteinized stromal cells, which may be admixed with the neoplasm or confined to the periphery of the tumor (94), are occasionally present, especially in the tumors producing hCG; they may be the source of the excessive estrogens or androgens found in some cases. Foci of calcification suggest origin in a focally obliterated or completely obliterated gonadoblastoma. Extensive sampling is warranted to identify residual gonadoblastoma, and the patient's karyotype should be determined.

Differential diagnosis

Dysgerminoma should be distinguished from other malignant germ-cell tumors in which a diffuse pattern may occur, specifically yolk sac tumor and embryonal carcinoma. Yolk sac tumor has greater nuclear variation, hyaline bodies, immunoreactivity for AFP, and, almost always, characteristic patterns lacking in dysgerminoma. The extremely rare embryonal carcinoma has nuclei that are more hyperchromatic and variable than those of the dysgerminoma and almost always contains SGC. The distinction of dysgerminoma from clear-cell carcinoma has been discussed earlier. Large-cell lymphomas may simulate dysgerminoma both grossly and microscopically, and the frequent stromal lymphocytes of the latter enhance their microscopic similarity. The differing nuclear features, the almost invariable absence of glycogen in lymphomas, and a variety of distinctive immunohistochemical reactions facilitate differential diagnosis. Other tumors with solid growth patterns of round cells, such as granulosa-cell tumor and primary or metastatic poorly differentiated carcinoma, belong in the differential diagnosis but differ from dysgerminoma histologically to the extent that they rarely present a diagnostic problem.

Yolk Sac Tumor

Clinical features

Yolk sac tumor (YST; endodermal sinus tumor) accounts for approximately 20% of malignant primitive germ-cell tumors. It is almost as common as dysgermi-

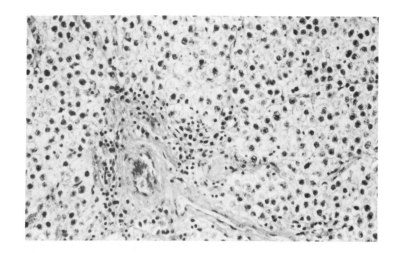

FIG. 87. Dysgerminoma. The tumor cells have clear cytoplasm and predominantly central nuclei. Note lymphocytes in vicinity of vessels.

noma in females under the age of 20 years. YST is most common in childhood and adolescence (mean age: 19 years) and is very rare over the age of 40 years. Patients typically present with abdominal pain, frequently of sudden onset, and a large abdominal or pelvic mass (319–322). Serum alpha-fetoprotein is almost invariably elevated preoperatively; its measurement is also useful in monitoring therapy and detecting recurrent tumor.

YST is a rapidly growing tumor, with evidence of extraovarian spread to the peritoneum or retroperitoneal lymph nodes, or both, in approximately one-third of patients. Before the use of combination chemotherapy, survival was poor; more recently, however, such treatment has achieved survivals of over 80% with Stage I YST and over 50% with higher-stage tumors (323).

Gross features

The tumors are typically large, with a median diameter of 15 cm. About 25% have capsular tears as a result of preoperative or intraoperative rupture (320). The sectioned surfaces are typically solid and cystic (Fig. 89) and composed of soft, friable, yellow to gray tissue; very rare tumors are entirely cystic (324). Extensive areas of hemorrhage and necrosis are common. A honeycomb appearance due to many small cysts may indicate a polyvesicular-vitelline pattern (Fig. 90) (see below). Gross evidence of other germ-cell elements, most commonly benign cystic teratoma, may be seen. YST is virtually never bilateral, unless the opposite ovary is involved as part of generalized peritoneal spread.

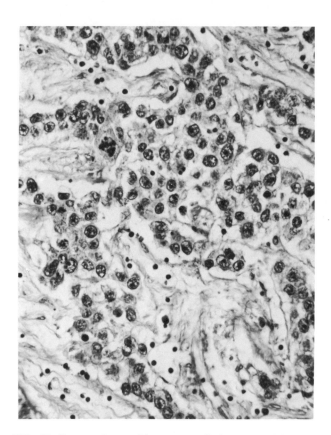

FIG. 88. Dysgerminoma. The tumor cells have rounded nuclei with prominent nucleoli. Note sprinkling of lymphocytes.

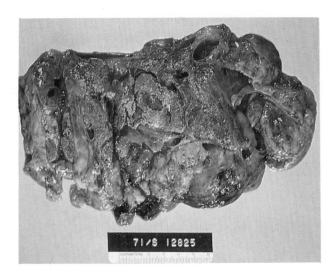

FIG. 89. Yolk sac (endodermal sinus) tumor. The neoplasm is solid and cystic with focal necrosis. (From ref. 209.)

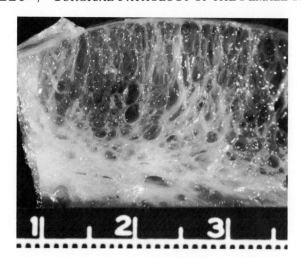

FIG. 90. Yolk sac tumor with polyvesicular vitelline pattern. Numerous small cysts with thin walls are visible.

Microscopic features

Almost all YST have at least one of three cardinal histologic features: a reticular pattern, Schiller-Duval bodies, and hyaline droplets (320). The reticular pattern (Fig. 91) consists of a loose meshwork of communicating spaces lined by primitive tumor cells with typically clear cytoplasm containing glycogen and, occasionally, lipid. The hyperchromatic, irregular, large nuclei contain prominent nucleoli; mitotic figures are numerous. Schiller-Duval (S-D) bodies, which are present in up to 75% of YST (320), consist of single papillae with a connective tissue core containing a single central vessel (Fig. 92). These structures typically are covered by primitive columnar cells and lie in a space lined by cuboidal, flattened, or hobnail cells. S-D bodies are usually sparsely distributed, but when they are closely packed, a distinctive papillary pattern is created (320). Variably sized, eosinophilic, PAS-positive, diastase resistant, hyaline droplets are present in most YST and are numerous in areas with a reticular or hepatoid pattern (see below).

Other less common, but characteristic, patterns also occur in YST. These are usually admixed with reticular foci but may predominate or occur in pure form (Table 2). The polyvesicular-vitelline pattern (Fig. 93) is characterized by cysts that are lined by columnar, cuboidal, or flattened cells and that are usually separated by a dense spindle-cell stroma (320,325). The cysts may exhibit eccentric constrictions. The hepatoid pattern (Fig. 94) resembles hepatocellular carcinoma. It is characterized by large, polygonal cells with abundant eosinophilic cytoplasm growing in compact masses separated by thin fibrous bands (209,326). In some cases, glandular spaces filled with mucin impart a honeycomb pattern (209). YST may contain glands lined by nonspecific or vacuo-

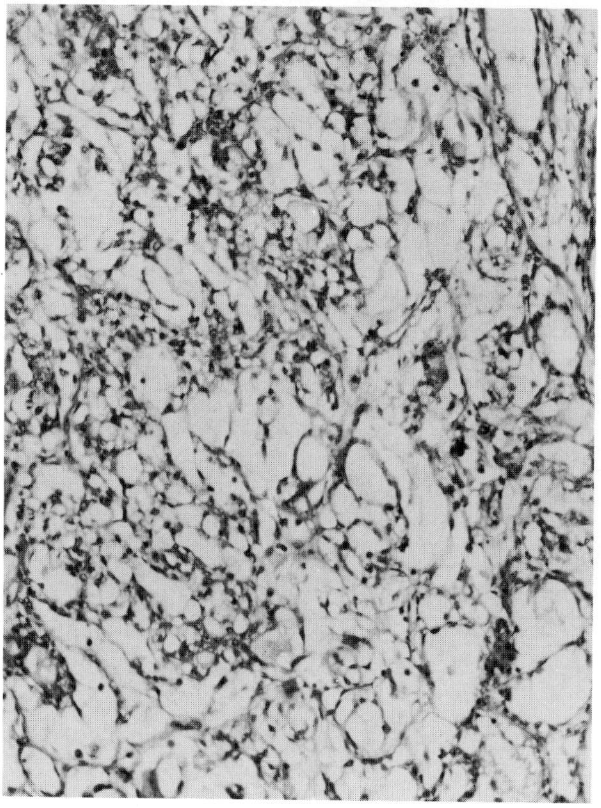

FIG. 91. Yolk sac tumor, reticular pattern.

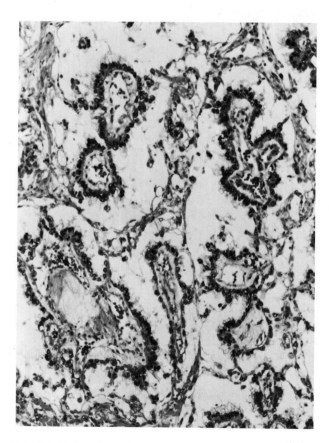

FIG. 92. Yolk sac tumor. Numerous Schiller-Duval bodies are present.

TABLE 2. *Histological classification of yolk sac tumors*

Typical
    Reticular (often with Schiller-Duval bodies)
    Papillary
    Solid
    Parietal
Polyvesicular-vitelline
Hepatoid
Endometrioid-like
Mixed[a]

[a] At least 10% of second pattern present.

lated cells, and, in rare tumors, a predominant glandular pattern resembling typical or secretory endometrioid carcinoma is seen (Fig. 95). Tumors of the latter type have been designated as *endometrioid-like* YST (324). "Parietal" differentiation is characterized by small, extracellular accumulations of basement-membrane material, typically within reticular foci (322).

Nonspecific patterns in YST include solid, papillary, and adenofibromatous. Occasional YST contain cells with large, intracellular vacuoles that displace the nucleus, creating an appearance resembling liposarcoma. Enteric-type glands occur up to 50% of YST; they are lined by bland mucinous columnar cells, goblet cells, and, rarely, Paneth cells (320,322). Rare YST contain small numbers of syncytiotrophoblastic giant cells. Luteinized stromal cells, granulomatous inflammation, and erythropoietic foci are occasionally found in YST.

Immunohistochemical findings are useful in diagnosing YST, particularly when confronted with unusual or nonspecific histologic patterns. YST is almost always immunoreactive for alpha-fetoprotein (AFP) and alpha-1-antitrypsin (AAT), although the staining may be focal. The contents of glands and cysts in YST with polyvesicular-vitelline, hepatoid, and endometrioid-like patterns

are also positive for these antigens. Most hyaline droplets are immunoreactive for AAT but stain for AFP only occasionally.

Differential diagnosis

Clear-cell carcinoma is most commonly confused with YST. The differential diagnosis is discussed in the section on the former tumor.

Embryonal Carcinoma

Clinical features

Embryonal carcinoma of testicular type is very rare in the ovary, accounting for only about 3% of primitive ovarian germ-cell tumors (327,328). Patients are typically children or young adults (median age: 15 years). In over half of the cases, there is isosexual pseudoprecocity, abnormal uterine bleeding, or amenorrhea. Serum hCG and AFP are typically elevated. Laparotomy reveals extraovarian spread in 40% of the cases. Five-year survival with Stage I disease in the only reported series was 50%, but most patients did not receive chemotherapy (327).

Gross features

The tumors are typically large (median diameter: 17 cm). The cut surface is predominantly solid and variegated, with white, tan-gray, and yellow soft tissue alternating with cysts containing mucoid material; hemorrhage and necrosis are common (327).

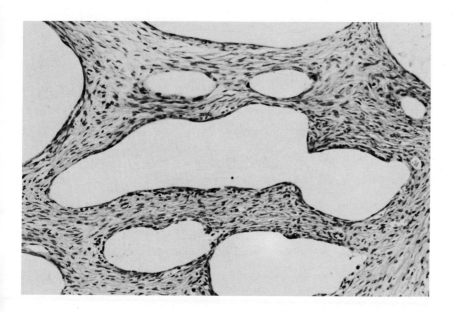

FIG. 93. Yolk sac tumor, polyvesicular vitelline pattern. The cysts are lined by flattened cells, imparting a deceptively bland appearance.

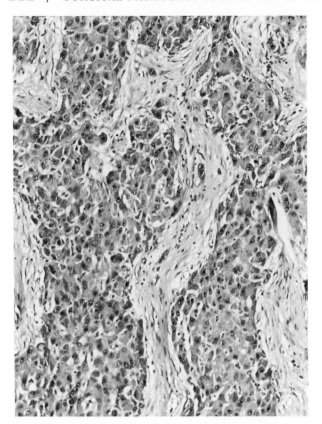

FIG. 94. Yolk sac tumor, hepatoid pattern. Trabeculae of cells with abundant eosinophilic cytoplasm impart a resemblance to hepatocellular carcinoma.

Microscopic features

The tumors are characterized by solid masses, glands, and papillae composed of, or lined by, large anaplastic cells with amphophilic, slightly vacuolated cytoplasm and well-defined cell membranes. The nuclei are round and vesicular with one or more prominent nucleoli; mitotic figures are numerous. Isolated syncytiotrophoblastic giant cells (SGC) are found in almost all the cases (327). Some tumor cells are typically immunoreactive for AFP; whether they are AFP-reactive embryonal carcinoma or foci of yolk sac differentiation is controversial. Both SGC and occasional mononucleate cells stain for hCG. Enteric glands and minor foci of mature teratomatous elements may be encountered.

Differential diagnosis

The distinction from dysgerminoma is discussed above. Differentiation from YST is based primarily on the absence of characteristic patterns of that tumor. Although embryonal carcinoma typically contains isolated SGC, it lacks the biphasic pattern of choriocarcinoma.

Polyembryoma

This very rare primitive germ-cell tumor is characterized by a preponderant content of embryoid bodies mimicking normal early embryos. Teratomatous elements are seen in most cases. Because these tumors contain trophoblasts, they may be associated with high levels of hCG and related endocrine manifestations; serum AFP may also be elevated (329).

Choriocarcinoma

Ovarian choriocarcinoma is rarely encountered as a pure form and is present in less than 1% of primitive ovarian germ-cell tumors (330,331). The occurrence of choriocarcinoma prepubertally or the presence of other germ-cell elements establishes a germ-cell origin and excludes a gestational-type tumor. Choriocarcinoma typically occurs in patients under the age of 20 years who present with abdominal enlargement and pain. Serum hCG is elevated, leading to isosexual pseudoprecocity in children, and menstrual abnormalities, and occasionally, androgenic changes in adults. The tumors are typically fatal, although improved prognosis has been reported with aggressive chemotherapy (331).

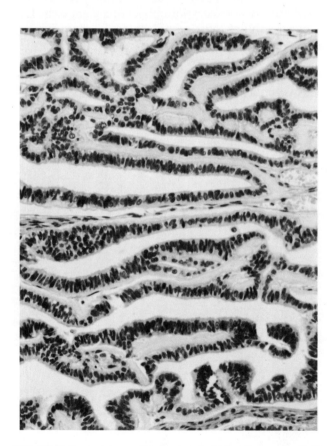

FIG. 95. Yolk sac tumor with glands resembling those of well-differentiated endometrioid carcinoma.

On gross examination, the pure choriocarcinoma is typically solid, hemorrhagic, and friable. A biphasic pattern consisting of an intimate admixture of cytotrophoblast and syncytiotrophoblast, accompanied by hemorrhage, is seen microscopically. In areas, however, the tumor may have a nonspecific appearance. The syncytiotrophoblastic elements are intensely immunoreactive for hCG. Choriocarcinoma should be distinguished from malignant germ-cell tumors containing isolated syncytiotrophoblastic cells, such as embryonal carcinoma, dysgerminoma, and YST. In addition, poorly differentiated carcinomas in older women may somewhat resemble choriocarcinoma and even secrete hCG (332).

Teratomas

Almost all teratomas are composed of tissues representing at least two, but usually all three, embryonic layers. If the neoplastic tissue is completely mature, the tumor is designated as a *mature teratoma* (almost always a dermoid cyst), whereas the presence of any immature tissue warrants a designation of *immature teratoma.* Occasionally a teratoma has a large component of a single endodermal or ectodermal tissue type or is composed exclusively of such tissue. Tumors of this type are referred to as *monodermal teratomas.*

Immature teratomas

Clinical features. Immature teratomas are the third most common among the primitive germ-cell tumors, accounting for almost 20% of them, 1% of ovarian cancers in general, and 10% to 20% of those encountered in the first two decades. They are most common in children and young adults (median age: 18 years), who typically have a palpable abdominal or pelvic mass, frequently accompanied by pain (333). Rarely, an immature teratoma is preceded by an ipsilateral dermoid cyst that was removed months to years previously (334). An occasional patient has an elevated serum AFP or hCG (335).

Approximately one-third of immature teratomas have spread beyond the ovary at the time of operation, typically as peritoneal implants and less commonly as lymphatic or hematogenous metastases. The frequency of extraovarian spread increases with the histologic grade of the primary tumor (see below) (333). Prior to combination chemotherapy, survival with high-grade tumors, particularly those with high-grade implants, was poor (333). In contrast, 90% of patients in a recent study who received combination chemotherapy achieved a sustained remission (336). Chemotherapy typically transforms high-grade implants into mature tissue, necrotic tumor, or fibrous tissue, or combinations of the

above. Patients with exclusively mature, typically glial implants (see below) almost always have a benign clinical course even without postoperative treatment (337,338).

Gross features. The tumors are usually large (median diameter: 18 cm), encapsulated masses. The cut surface is predominantly solid, but small cysts containing hair or mucinous, serous, or bloody fluid are frequently present (Fig. 96). Grossly evident dermoid cysts can be identified in approximately 25% of cases (334). The solid areas, which are usually composed of neural tissue, are typically soft, fleshy, and gray to pink, with focal hemorrhage and necrosis. Bone and cartilage may be visible or palpable. Bilateral involvement is very rare in the absence of extraovarian spread, but the opposite ovary harbors a dermoid cyst or, less often, another benign tumor in approximately 10% of cases (334).

Microscopic features. Immature tissue varies from rare foci to a predominant component. It is composed mainly of immature neuroectodermal elements (Figs. 97 and 98) in the form of neuroepithelial rosettes and tubules, cellular foci of mitotically active glia, and, in occasional cases, areas resembling glioblastoma or neuroblastoma. Immature or embryonal epithelium of ectodermal and endodermal types, as well as immature cartilage (Fig. 97) and skeletal muscle, are frequently encountered. Uncommon findings include isolated syncytiotrophoblastic giant cells, endodermal elements (yolk sac tissue, enteric glands, hepatic tissue) (335), and immature renal tissue.

Immature teratomas have been graded 1 to 3, based on increasing amounts of immature, usually neural tissue (333,339,340). Grade 1 tumors have rare foci of immature neural tissue occupying less than one low-power-field (LPF) per slide, grade 2 tumors have moderate quantities of immature neural tissue occupying more than one, but three or fewer, LPF per slide, and grade 3 tumors have large quantities of immature neural tissue

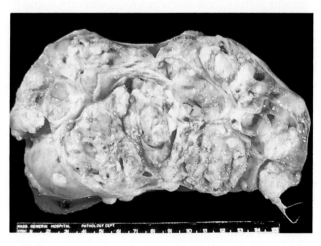

FIG. 96. Immature teratoma. The neoplasm has a solid and cystic sectioned surface.

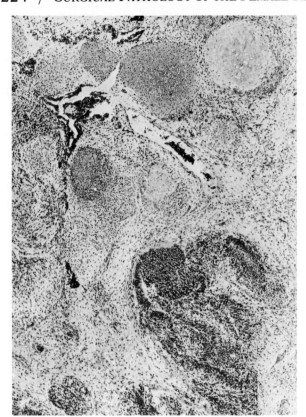

FIG. 97. Immature teratoma with immature neural tissue and nodules of cartilage.

occupying four or more LPF per slide. A similar grading system can be applied to extraovarian tumor. Rarely, immature or mature solid teratomas are associated with peritoneal implants composed of mature, predominantly glial tissue, so-called peritoneal gliomatosis (Fig. 99) (337,338,341,342). Occasionally, mature epithelial elements are also present. Pelvic and para-aortic lymph nodes in such cases may contain similar tumor (342).

Differential diagnosis. Distinction between immature and mature teratoma is clinically important and is based on finding even rare foci of immature tissue. Predominantly solid teratomas should therefore be extensively sampled to exclude immaturity. Distinction from heterologous malignant mixed mesodermal tumors and primitive neuroectodermal tumors is discussed in the sections dealing with those neoplasms.

Mature teratomas

Clinical features. Mature teratomas account for almost 30% of all ovarian tumors, 30% of benign ovarian tumors, and over two-thirds of ovarian tumors in patients under the age of 15 years. These tumors usually develop in young females but are sometimes not detected until years after menopause. Patients typically present with manifestations related to a pelvic mass. The

tumors may undergo torsion or rupture, leading to acute abdominal symptoms. Rupture into an adjacent organ may lead to passage of cyst contents into the urinary bladder, vagina, or rectum (343). Slow leakage of a dermoid cyst may result in peritoneal foreign-body granulomas that mimic tumor implants or tuberculosis. Rare complications include Coombs' + hemolytic anemia cured by removal of the tumor (344), infection, and peritoneal melanosis (see Chapter 51).

Mature teratomas are benign, except for the 1% to 2% that harbor an adult-type cancer, most commonly squamous-cell carcinoma. This complication should be suspected when the tumor is adherent to surrounding structures or has areas of surface nodularity, hemorrhage, or necrosis. Squamous-cell carcinoma that has penetrated the capsule, as well as rarer forms of malignant change, typically have a poor prognosis. In contrast, the survival with squamous-cell carcinoma confined to the ovary is over 90% (345).

Gross features. Mature teratomas are almost always dermoid cysts but are rarely predominantly solid. In the latter, the gross appearance is similar to that of immature teratoma except that areas of softening, hemorrhage, and necrosis are much less common. Dermoid cysts are globular or ovoid with a white to gray external surface; most are less than 15 cm in diameter. Yellow to

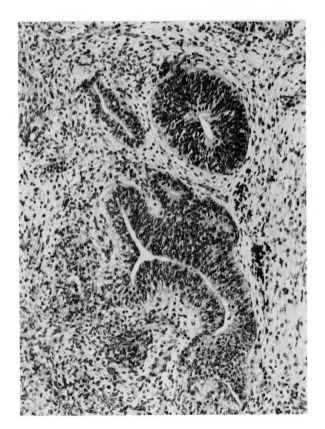

FIG. 98. Immature teratoma with immature neuroepithelial tubules.

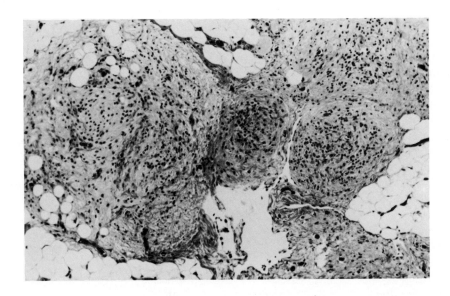

FIG. 99. Glial implants in omentum in patient with ovarian teratoma.

brown sebaceous material and hair fill the cysts, which are typically lined by skin-like tissue. One or more rounded, polypoid masses designated mamillae or Rokitansky's protuberances typically protrude into the lumen. Teeth are present in one-third of the cases; occasionally they are embedded in a rudimentary mandible or maxilla. Bone, cartilage, mucinous cysts, fat, thyroid, and brain tissue may be seen grossly. Rarely, partially developed organs (bowel, appendix, skull, vertebrae, limb buds, external genitalia, eyes) or a fetiform structure (homunculus) may be present (346,347). Approximately 12% of dermoid cysts are bilateral and occasionally there are multiple tumors in one ovary (334). A malignant tumor arising within a dermoid cyst may appear as a polypoid intracystic mass, a mural nodule, or a plaque. If extensive, the malignant component may almost obliterate the dermoid cyst. Hemorrhage and necrosis are common within the malignant component.

Microscopic features. The tumors are composed exclusively of adult-type tissues, usually from all three germ layers. Ectodermal derivatives almost always predominate; these include keratinized epidermis, pilosebaceous structures, sweat glands, and neural tissue. The last component is most commonly glial, but organized structures such as cerebrum, cerebellum, and choroid plexus may be present. Mesodermal derivatives take the form of smooth muscle, bone, cartilage, and fat. Endodermal elements include respiratory and gastrointestinal epithelium as well as thyroid. Rare tissues include retina, pancreas, thymus, adrenal gland, pituitary gland, kidney, lung, breast, and prostate (39,348–350). Mitotic figures are virtually absent.

The above tissues are often arranged in an organoid fashion; e.g., cartilage and mucinous glands underlie respiratory epithelium, and layers of smooth muscle surround intestinal mucosa. Respiratory and glial tissue may partially line cysts. Lipogranulomatous and fibros-

ing inflammation may be seen in surrounding tissue in response to the escape of cyst contents.

Approximately 75% of malignant tumors arising in dermoid cysts are squamous-cell carcinomas that are invasive or rarely, *in situ.* The remainder have been carcinoids (see below), undifferentiated carcinomas, adenocarcinomas, sarcomas, malignant melanoma, or, rarely, lymphoma or basal-cell carcinoma (351–356). Rarely, sebaceous gland tumors with varying degrees of cellular atypicality are found. Exceptionally, benign tumors may arise within dermoid cysts, including ACTH or prolactin-secreting pituitary adenomas (350) and hemangiomas (357).

Monodermal teratomas

Struma ovarii

Clinical features. This is the most common monodermal teratoma. Thyroid tissue can be identified microscopically in up to 20% of dermoid cysts, and *struma ovarii* is an appropriate term only when such tissue is grossly recognizable or when it is the predominant or sole component, microscopically. The peak incidence is in the fifth decade; occasional cases have been reported in both prepubertal and postmenopausal females. Ascites occurs in approximately one-third of the cases, and, rarely, a Meigs'-type syndrome is present. Very rare cases are associated with hyperthyroidism.

Although 5% to 10% of cases have been considered malignant, only 40% of this group developed extraovarian spread (358–361). In the remainder, the diagnosis of malignancy was based on microscopic criteria alone. Many of the latter cases are now known to be strumal carcinoids. Occasionally, benign nodules of thyroid tissue implant on the peritoneum (peritoneal strumosis), a condition that is compatible with longevity (362).

Gross features. Thyroid elements are usually brown or green-brown, predominantly solid, gelatinous tissue. Some strumas appear as uni- or multilocular cysts containing brown to green, mucoid or gelatinous fluid (Fig. 100). Strumas may be pure, or, less often, they are associated with a dermoid cyst or mixed with carcinoid (strumal carcinoid). Rarely, struma is found within the wall of a mucinous or serous cystadenoma or is admixed with a Brenner tumor (39,363). Occasionally, the opposite ovary contains a dermoid cyst and, rarely, another struma.

Microscopic features. The struma may resemble normal thyroid tissue or a thyroid adenoma of any type. Oxyphil cells and areas of "thyroiditis" may be seen (364). Follicular colloid often contains birefringent calcium oxalate crystals and is immunoreactive for thyroglobulin. Accepted microscopic criteria for malignant change have not been established. As in the thyroid gland, a papillary pattern with typical nuclear characteristics, or a follicular pattern with vascular or capsular invasion, provides evidence of malignancy.

Differential diagnosis. Cystic strumas can be mistaken grossly for mucinous tumors; the green to brown color of the former helps in the differential diagnosis. Clear-cell carcinomas, endometrioid carcinomas, Sertoli-Leydig cell tumors, and pregnancy luteomas may contain thyroid-like areas, but other features almost always permit correct identification. In problematic cases, the demonstration of calcium oxalate crystals and immunoreactivity for thyroblobulin are helpful in confirming struma.

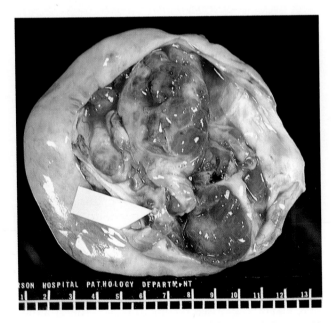

FIG. 100. Struma ovarii. A large cystic neoplasm contains multiple locules that have a brown-green color.

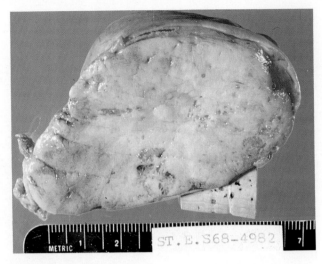

FIG. 101. Primary carcinoid tumor. The neoplasm has a tan sectioned surface.

Carcinoid

Clinical features. Carcinoids are the second most common type of monodermal ovarian teratoma. They are divided into insular and trabecular pure carcinoids, strumal carcinoids, and mucinous carcinoids. The patients range in age from early reproductive to postmenopausal, although the latter age group predominates. A pelvic mass is typically evident. Approximately one-third of insular carcinoids are accompanied by the carcinoid syndrome, which disappears after removal of the tumor (365); one case of strumal carcinoid was also associated with the syndrome (366). Patients with carcinoid syndrome are usually over 50 years of age and have large tumors (over 7 cm in diameter). Androgenic or estrogenic manifestations may also occur as a result of stromal luteinization within, or adjacent to, the tumor (94,367). In addition, probable thyroid hyperfunction has been associated with strumal carcinoid, as has Cushing's syndrome (368).

Fewer than 5% of ovarian carcinoids metastasize and cause death. Malignant tumors are most commonly of insular or mucinous type (365,367,369–371). Rare patients have died of carcinoid heart disease despite eradication of their tumor (365).

Gross features. All recorded primary carcinoid tumors have been unilateral, although in 15% the opposite ovary contains a cystic teratoma, mucinous tumor, or Brenner tumor. Ovarian carcinoid is typically firm, tan to yellow, predominantly solid, and variably fibrous (Fig. 101). Cysts filled with clear fluid are occasionally present; rarely, the tumor is predominantly cystic. Approximately 75% are mixed with other teratomatous elements. In such cases, the carcinoid may form a nodule that protrudes into the lumen or thickens the wall of a dermoid cyst or mucinous tumor. Alternately, it may lie within a solid teratoma, be admixed with a Brenner tumor, or be associated with struma (strumal carcinoid) (365,367,372). In strumal carcinoid, the two elements may each be grossly identifiable or they may form a homogenous mass (367,373,374). A dermoid cyst or mucinous tumor is associated with 60% of strumal carcinoids.

Microscopic features. Insular carcinoid resembles midgut carcinoid and is characterized by discrete cellular masses and nests (Fig. 102) separated by scant to abundant fibrous stroma (365). Small acini lined by columnar cells with copious cytoplasm commonly punctuate the cellular islands, particularly at their periphery. Eosinophilic secretion, which may be concentrically calcified, is typically present within the lumens. The tumor cells have round, uniform nuclei containing coarse chromatin and rare mitotic figures. The peripheral cells of the islands and the acinar cells typically contain red-brown, argentaffin-positive granules, which are often visible on routine staining. An intimate relation of the tumor to respiratory or gastrointestinal epithelium is sometimes evident (365). Pleomorphic, reniform, or dumbbell-shaped dense-core granules are present, ultrastructurally (365).

Trabecular carcinoid resembles foregut and hindgut carcinoid and is characterized by long, wavy, parallel ribbons of cells separated by a scant to abundant fibrous stroma (371,375). The ribbons are composed of columnar cells, usually one or two cells thick, with oblong nuclei oriented perpendicular to the axis of the ribbon. The moderately abundant eosinophilic cytoplasm typically contains argyrophilic granules. The nuclei contain finely dispersed chromatin and occasional mitotic figures. An insular pattern is observed as a minor feature in about 20% of cases. Associated teratomatous elements are almost always present. Dense-core granules, in contrast to those of insular carcinoids, are small, round, and uniform (371,376).

Strumal carcinoid is characterized by the presence of both struma and carcinoid. The components typically are intimately admixed (Fig. 103), and either one may predominate (367,373,374). The carcinoid component is trabecular in half of the cases, mixed trabecular-insular in most of the remainder, and pure insular occasionally. The thyroid component resembles normal tissue or a follicular adenoma, including the presence of calcium oxalate crystals. Argyrophilic granules are typically present within cells forming trabeculae and lining thyroid follicles (374,377). Almost half of the tumors also contain argentaffin granules (367). Occasionally, there is stromal amyloid (377). Ultrastructurally, trabecular cells contain neuroendocrine-type granules; the follicles are lined by similar neuroendocrine-type cells or thyroid epithelial-type cells, or a mixture of the two (373,374).

Mucinous carcinoid (goblet-cell carcinoid) resembles analogous tumors of appendiceal origin (369,370). They are usually pure but may be associated with mature teratoma or epidermoid cyst. They consist of small nests or glands composed of goblet cells and argyrophil cells, some of which may also be argentaffinic. Nuclei are uniform, small, and round to oval. Small pools of mucin may lie within cystically dilated glands or in the stroma. More poorly differentiated cells, often of signet-ring type, may invade the stroma. Irregular dense-core granules have been identified on ultrastructural examination (369).

Rare ovarian carcinoids include a spindle-cell type, resembling its pulmonary counterpart, and nonspecific, sometimes poorly differentiated tumors (378).

Immunohistochemical findings. Serotonin has been demonstrated in insular (370), strumal (373,374), and mucinous subtypes (370). In addition, approximately

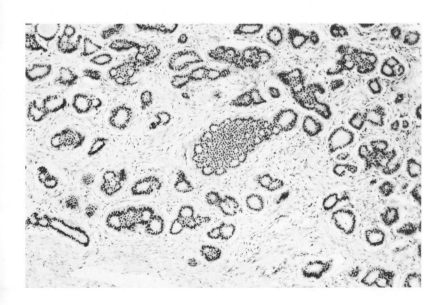

FIG. 102. Carcinoid tumor, insular pattern. Note many small acini within the nests.

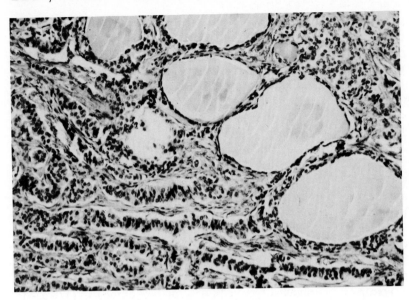

FIG. 103. Strumal carcinoid. Several trabeculae of carcinoid tumor are intimately associated with thyroid follicles.

25% of the tumors contain neurohormonal peptides, most commonly pancreatic polypeptide, glucagon, enkephalin, and somatostatin (379). Trabecular, strumal, and insular carcinoids were immunoreactive for at least one neurohormonal peptide in 53%, 42%, and 7% of cases, respectively (379). Other investigators have demonstrated the presence of (a) "neuron-specific" enolase in insular and strumal carcinoids (380) and (b) thyroglobulin within the follicular cells and, occasionally, the trabecular cells of strumal carcinoid (373,374).

Differential diagnosis. In the absence of teratomatous elements, primary carcinoid may be difficult to distinguish from a metastasis. Evidence favoring or establishing the diagnosis of metastasis includes the presence of a definite or probable carcinoid in the small bowel or elsewhere, extraovarian metastases, bilateral involvement, intraovarian growth as multiple nodules, and persistance of the carcinoid syndrome after ovarian removal. Most of the above features are equally useful in differentiating a signet-ring carcinoid from a metastatic signet-ring carcinoma.

Despite their distinctive microscopic characteristics, ovarian carcinoids can be confused with other primary tumors, especially granulosa-cell tumor, Sertoli-Leydig cell tumor (SLCT), and Brenner tumor. In contrast to the acini of carcinoid, Call-Exner bodies of granulosa-cell tumor have irregular margins and contain watery eosinophilic material as well as occasional shrunken nuclei. The granulosa cells surrounding a Call-Exner body lack the copious cytoplasm that separates the nucleus from the lumen of a carcinoid acinus and typically have pale, grooved, haphazardly oriented nuclei. The cords of Sertoli cells in SLCT of intermediate differentiation tend to be shorter, less uniform, and more sparsely distributed than the elongated trabeculae of a trabecular carcinoid. In addition, several other distinctive patterns

of SLCT may be present to facilitate the diagnosis. The epithelial cells of Brenner tumor, in contrast to those of carcinoid tumor, have a urothelial appearance with grooved nuclei. Additionally, the acini within Brenner nests are often lined by mucinous cells, unlike those of a carcinoid acinus.

Strumal carcinoid is most frequently misdiagnosed as thyroid carcinoma arising in struma. The latter exhibits the patterns of papillary or follicular thyroid carcinoma. It lacks the trabeculae and argyrophil/argentaffin granules of strumal carcinoid.

Rare monodermal teratomas

A distinctive monodermal ovarian teratoma is characterized by malignant neuroectodermal differentiation (381–384). The patients are usually in their second or third decades, and the tumors typically pursue a malignant course. In contrast to immature teratoma, malignant neuroectodermal tumors have pure, or almost pure, histologic patterns resembling analogous intracranial tumors in children (385). Patterns resembling glioblastoma, medulloblastoma, and neuroblastoma (or, occasionally, ependymoma) may be seen alone or in combination (382,384). Minor foci of mature teratoma may also be present. Primitive neuroectodermal tumor may be difficult to distinguish from other ovarian tumors occurring in young women and characterized by highly malignant small cells, such as small-cell carcinoma (see below). Thorough sampling and immunohistochemical staining for glial fibrillary acidic protein are often helpful. Ependymoma may be confused with sex-cord–stromal and common epithelial tumors, but the distinctive features of ependymoma, combined with immunohistochemical stains, should permit recognition.

Other rare monodermal teratomas of the ovary include sebaceous gland tumor (386), tumors resembling retinal anlage tumor (387), and cysts lined exclusively by mature glial tissue (388), ependyma (389), or respiratory epithelium (390). Epidermoid cysts, lined exclusively by mature squamous epithelium, may be monodermal teratomas but are more likely of surface epithelial origin (391,392).

Mixed Malignant Germ-Cell Tumors

Approximately 8% of malignant primitive germ-cell tumors of the ovary have a mixed histology (393). Their occurrence emphasizes the importance of careful gross examination and judicious sampling. The prognosis for mixed germ-cell neoplasia may depend on both the quantity and nature of the malignant elements (393). In one study, a highly malignant component did not adversely affect prognosis unless it accounted for more than one-third of the tumor volume. Such a correlation, however, was not confirmed in a later series (394).

A unique mixed germ-cell tumor consisted predominantly of immature pancreatic tissue, with foci of benign and malignant mucinous epithelium, dysgerminoma, YST, and immature teratoma (395).

Mixed Germ-Cell–Sex-Cord–Stromal Tumors

Gonadoblastoma

Clinical features

Gonadoblastoma is a rare tumor that occurs almost exclusively in patients with an underlying gonadal disorder. It accounts for two-thirds of gonadal tumors in women with abnormal gonadal development (396). Affected patients are typically children or young adults. The clinical picture includes a tumor mass, occasional hormonal secretion, and intrinsic abnormalities of involved gonads and secondary sex organs. Because at least a portion of one gonad is replaced by tumor, a diagnosis of the underlying gonadal abnormality may be impossible. When a sexual disorder is identifiable, it is almost always pure or mixed gonadal dysgenesis; a Y chromosome is detected in over 90% of cases. Patients with gonadoblastoma are typically phenotypic females who are usually virilized. A minority are phenotypic males with varying degrees of feminization. Gonadoblastoma without an invasive germ-cell tumor is clinically benign. Because of the high frequency with which it gives rise to a malignant germ-cell tumor, it should be regarded as an *in situ* malignancy.

Gross features

The gross appearance varies with size, the presence or absence of malignant germ cell tumor, and the degree of calcification. Tumors may be soft and fleshy, firm and cartilaginous, flecked with calcification, or totally calcified. Their color varies from brown to yellow to gray. Pure gonadoblastomas are typically less than 8 cm in diameter, and 25% are microscopic; those with germinomatous overgrowth may be much larger. Approximately one-third of gonadoblastomas are bilateral; less often the opposite ovary contains a malignant germ-cell tumor, usually a germinoma, with no trace of underlying gonadoblastoma. The gonad in which a gonadoblastoma develops is of unknown nature in 60%, an abdominal or inguinal testis in 20%, and a gonadal streak in 20%. Extremely rare tumors arise in apparently normal ovaries.

Microscopic features

Cellular aggregates composed of mixed germ cells and small epithelial cells of sex-cord type (Fig. 104) are the cardinal histologic feature (396). The germ cells are germinoma-like (dysgerminoma, seminoma) and usually exhibit mitotic activity. The smaller, round to oval epithelial cells have pale nuclei, are mitotically inactive, and resemble immature Sertoli or granulosa cells. These cells surround circular spaces filled with eosinophilic

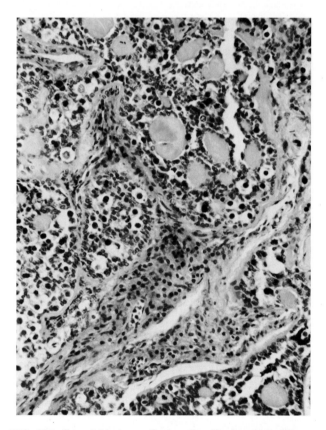

FIG. 104. Gonadoblastoma. Germ cells with abundant clear cytoplasm, accompanied by smaller cells of sex-cord type and hyaline bodies, are visible. Note lutein-Leydig cells in stroma.

basement membrane-like material, line the periphery of germ-cell nests, or surround individual germ cells. The epithelial nests are separated by a scanty to abundant fibrous stroma. Stromal Leydig cells or luteinized cells are present in two-thirds of the cases (Fig. 104). Rare, otherwise typical gonadoblastomas focally resemble the unclassified mixed germ-cell–sex-cord–stromal tumors discussed in the next section (397).

The appearance of gonadoblastoma can be altered or obliterated by extensive deposition of basement-membrane-like material, calcification, or overgrowth of a malignant component. Calcification, present in over 80% of the cases, occurs within the basement-membrane-like material in the form of laminated spheres and mulberry-like masses. Overgrowth by a malignant germ-cell tumor develops in approximately 60% of the cases. In over 80%, the associated malignant tumor is a germinoma (Fig. 105), which may vary in extent from microscopic stromal penetration to massive replacement of the entire gonad. Less commonly, a yolk sac tumor, embryonal carcinoma, choriocarcinoma, or immature teratoma overgrows the gonadoblastoma (398,399).

Differential diagnosis

Gonadoblastoma can be confused with pure dysgerminoma and sex-cord tumor with annular tubules (SCTAT). A dysgerminoma or seminoma in a patient with abnormal gonads should be suspected to arise in a gonadoblastoma; the only clue may be a tiny focus of calcification or a rare nest of typical gonadoblastoma. SCTAT resembles gonadoblastoma because of its similar growth pattern, basement-membrane-like material, and calcification. It contains no germ cells, however. Gonadoblastoma should also be distinguished from the unclassified germ-cell–sex-cord–stromal tumors discussed in the following section. Finally, it should be noted that microscopic gonadoblastoma-like structures have been found in 15% of normal fetuses and newborn infants (400).

Germ-Cell–Sex-Cord–Stromal Tumors—Unclassified

This category includes all tumors that contain germ cells, sex-cord elements, and, occasionally, lutein or Leydig-type cells but that lack the distinctive pattern of gonadoblastoma (39,401,402). Patients are usually infants or girls under the age of 10 years with normal gonadal development and a normal karyotype. All reported tumors have been benign.

The few such tumors in the ovary constitute a heterogenous group. The microscopic picture is that of an infiltrative growth of sex-cord and germ-cell elements, with both components varying widely in proportion. The combination of cells may grow in diffuse masses, broad cords likened to Pfluger's tubules (sex cords) of the developing ovary, or small solid tubules (Fig. 106) similar to those of Sertoli-cell adenoma of the androgen insensitivity syndrome. Rarely, the sex-cord cells form retiform patterns (403,404). The sex-cord element may be even less mature than in gonadoblastoma, and the germ cells may resemble dysgerminoma, but, in some cases, they have large round nuclei without prominent nucleoli. In such tumors, doubt exists as to whether the large clear cells are germ cells or cells of another type. Hyaline bodies and calcification, characteristic of gonadoblastoma, are very infrequent or absent. An associated dysgerminoma, or, rarely, a more malignant germ-cell tumor, may be seen.

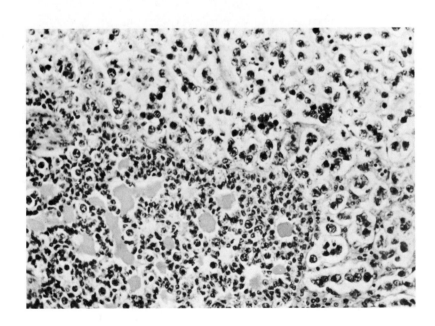

FIG. 105. Gonadoblastoma (*lower left*) associated with germinoma (*top* and *right*). (From ref. 128.)

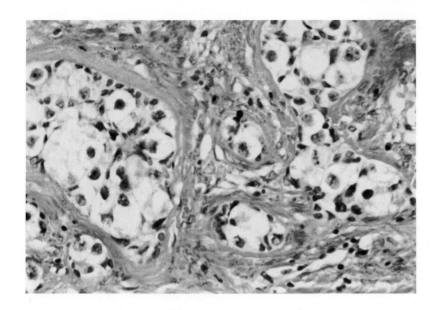

FIG. 106. Germ-cell–sex-cord–stromal tumor—unclassified. Nests composed of germ cells and sex-cord cells are separated by a hyaline stroma.

Nonspecific Mesenchymal and Miscellaneous Other Tumors

Benign

Fibromas, the most common mesenchymal tumors of the ovary, are discussed elsewhere in this chapter (page 1691). Leiomyomas account for almost 1% of benign ovarian neoplasms (39,405,406). They vary tremendously in size and are histologically similar to leiomyomas encountered elsewhere, including occasional tumors with epithelioid features (leiomyoblastoma). Leiomyomas may arise from frequently observed smooth-muscle metaplasia of stromal cells.

About 20 ovarian hemangiomas have been reported (39); a few have been associated with isolated hemangiomas elsewhere or generalized hemangiomatosis (407). Many have been incidental findings at autopsy. These tumors are usually of the cavernous type and are most commonly situated in the medulla and hilus. They must be distinguished from large vessels in the ovarian medulla present normally in older women. One or a few benign neural tumors, lipomas, lymphangiomas, myxomas, chondromas, osteomas, ganglioneuromas, and pheochromocytomas have been described in the ovary (408). In a recent review, Talerman (408) identified six ovarian adenomatoid tumors. These are typically small, round to oval, incidentally discovered lesions in the hilus. They are histologically similar to analogous tumors elsewhere in the female genital tract, but their rare occurrence in the ovary leads to potential misdiagnosis. We have seen an ovarian adenomatoid tumor misdiagnosed as yolk sac tumor because the clefts and spaces suggested the reticular pattern of the latter. However, the bland nuclear features of adenomatoid tumor contrast markedly with the primitive appearance of the nuclei in a yolk sac tumor.

Sarcomas

Rare pure, or apparently pure, sarcomas such as fibrosarcoma (258,408–412), leiomyosarcoma (413), malignant schwannoma (414), lymphangiosarcoma (408), and angiosarcoma (415) may arise from the nonspecific ovarian mesenchyme. Alternately, sarcomas including rhabdomyosarcoma (416), chondrosarcoma (417), and osteogenic sarcoma result from sarcomatous overgrowth of a complex tumor such as malignant mesodermal mixed tumor, mesodermal adenosarcoma, immature teratoma, dermoid cyst, or heterologous Sertoli-Leydig cell tumor. Some apparently pure sarcomas probably reflect incomplete sampling of more complex tumors. The microscopic features of ovarian sarcomas are analogous to their counterparts in other organs and tissues.

Malignant Lymphoma and Leukemic Involvement of the Ovary

Clinical features

Ovarian involvement is found in approximately 25% of non-Hodgkin's lymphomas at autopsy and in up to 50% of leukemias (39). Clinically detectable ovarian enlargement is much less common (418–420). With the exception of Burkitt's lymphoma, ovarian involvement as the initial manifestation of disease is very rare (0.3% of extranodal lymphomas).

Gross features

Lymphomas and leukemic tumors form smooth or nodular masses composed typically of homogeneous, fleshy, gray, pink, white, or yellow tissue. Areas of necrosis and cystic degeneration may be present. About half the cases are bilateral.

Microscopic features

The diffuse or nodular patterns seen in lymph nodes are reproduced within the ovary but may be distorted and compartmentalized by ovarian stroma. Stromal sclerosis may result in an insular or cord-like pattern. The cells of lymphoma and leukemia can infiltrate ovarian follicles without destroying them. Giemsa and chloroacetate esterase stains may facilitate the diagnosis of granulocytic sarcoma.

A study of 42 patients with lymphoma or leukemia presenting in the ovary subtyped the histologic variants (419). In 16 patients under the age of 20 years, there were 10 small noncleaved lymphomas (undifferentiated Burkitt's and non-Burkitt's lymphoma), four immunoblastic sarcomas, and two leukemias. In 26 adult patients, there were 10 diffuse large follicular-center-cell lymphomas, nine immunoblastic sarcomas, and seven nodular lymphomas.

In about two-thirds of ovarian lymphomas, extragenital involvement is found at laparotomy. Burkitt's lymphoma is almost invariably disseminated at the time of detection. Ovarian granulocytic leukemia (sarcoma) is also almost always accompanied by blood and marrow involvement. Exceptionally, ovarian disease may be the site of relapse in children with acute lymphoblastic leukemia.

Differential diagnosis

The gross appearance of ovarian malignant lymphoma may be indistinguishable from that of dysgerminoma. The former, however, is bilateral in approximately half of the cases, in contrast to the 10% frequency of grossly evident bilaterality for dysgerminoma. Although these tumors may resemble each other at low-power, high-power examination of their nuclei discloses striking differences. The single-file arrangement of lymphoma and leukemia cells within the ovary may simulate metastatic carcinoma, particularly of breast origin. Evaluation of cytologic features, combined with clinical information, is important in the differential diagnosis. A diffuse pattern of lymphoma may also simulate granulosa-cell tumor at low-power, but, again, the cytologic features of these two neoplasms are markedly dissimilar. Numerous immunohistochemical reactions (leukocyte common antigen, etc.) are available to distinguish difficult cases.

Tumors of Uncertain Cell Type

Small-Cell Carcinoma of the Ovary

Clinical features

This distinctive ovarian tumor (421) has occurred in females from 10 to 42 (mean: 22) years of age and is the most common undifferentiated ovarian carcinoma in this age group. Approximately two-thirds of patients have hypercalcemia, accounting for half of the ovarian tumors associated with this disorder. Small-cell carcinomas are almost always unilateral, but approximately one-third have spread beyond the ovary at laparotomy.

Gross features

The tumors are usually large and predominantly solid, tan to gray masses, often with areas of softening, necrosis, and hemorrhage. They may closely resemble ovarian lymphoma and dysgerminoma.

Microscopic features

A diffuse arrangement of small, closely packed epithelial cells with scanty cytoplasm, small nuclei, and single nucleoli is characteristic. Mitotic figures are frequent. The tumor cells also form small islands, cords (Fig. 107) and trabeculae. Follicle-like structures lined by tumor cells and filled with eosinophilic fluid are present in most cases (Fig. 108). In approximately one-quarter of the tumors, a variable proportion of cells have abundant, eosinophilic, sometimes hyaline-like cytoplasm. Mucinous epithelium is encountered in about 10% of the tumors. In most cases, electron microscopy demonstrates nonspecific epithelial features with abundant rough endoplastic reticulum as the most characteristic finding (421a). Occasionally, whorls of microfilaments are found. The cells stain variably for vimentin, cytokeratin, and epithelial membrane antigen (421b).

Differential diagnosis

Small-cell carcinoma is most commonly misinterpreted as an adult-type granulosa-cell tumor, but it may also be confused with the juvenile variant. Hypercalcemia or evidence of estrogen excess strongly favors small-cell carcinoma or granulosa-cell tumor, respectively. Approximately 30% of small-cell carcinomas have spread beyond the ovary; in contrast, a high proportion of granulosa-cell tumors are confined to the ovary. The nuclear features of the small-cell carcinoma are not compatible with granulosa-cell tumor. Mitotic figures are generally numerous, and nuclear grooves are absent. The rare presence of mucinous epithelium is also

spread beyond the ovary. Sheets, trabeculae, and cords of cells with moderate to large amounts of eosinophilic cytoplasm and round to oval, central nuclei are characteristic. Tumor cells stained immunohistochemically in varying numbers for alpha fetoprotein.

Differential diagnosis

Distinction from rare metastatic hepatocellular carcinomas and other ovarian tumors with abundant eosinophilic cytoplasm must be made. Two of five reported hepatoid carcinomas contained extracellular mucin, a rare feature of hepatocellular carcinoma. Hepatoid yolk sac tumor (309) occurs typically in younger women and usually contains foci of more typical yolk sac neoplasia. Nuclear pleomorphism is greater in hepatoid carcinoma than in hepatoid yolk sac tumor. Hepatoid carcinoma also must be distinguished from the oxyphil variant of clear-cell carcinoma and steroid-cell tumors. All of the oxyphil clear-cell carcinomas that we have seen have contained foci of typical clear-cell carcinoma (208). The cells of steroid-cell tumors resemble those of hepatoid carcinoma in their abundant eosinophilic cytoplasm. Steroid-cell tumors, unlike hepatoid carcinomas, are usually confined to the ovary and lack significant nuclear atypia in most cases. Steroid-cell tumors are also usually associated with endocrine manifestations and

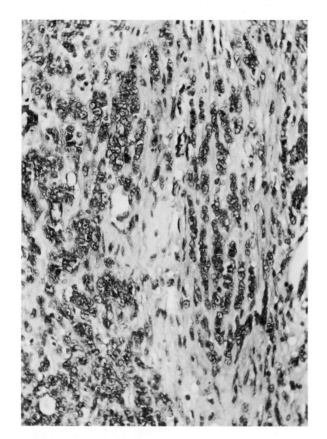

FIG. 107. Small-cell carcinoma associated with hypercalcemia. The tumor cells grow in small clusters and cords.

inconsistent with granulosa-cell tumor. The follicle-like structures of small-cell carcinoma, combined with the young age at which it occurs, may suggest a juvenile granulosa-cell tumor. Unlike the latter, the cells of the former have scanty cytoplasm in most cases; those containing cells with abundant eosinophilic cytoplasm usually have more typical areas that facilitate diagnosis. The follicular content of juvenile granulosa-cell tumor is typically mucicarminophilic, in contrast to that of small-cell carcinoma. Small-cell carcinoma can also be confused with malignant lymphoma. The usual presence of follicles in small-cell carcinoma, combined with the differing cytologic, immunohistochemical, and ultrastructural features, allows distinction. The differential diagnosis with other rare small cell tumors of the ovary is sometimes difficult (421c).

Hepatoid Carcinoma

Clinical and microscopic features

The designation *hepatoid carcinoma* has been proposed for a rare subtype of ovarian carcinoma resembling hepatocellular carcinoma and gastric hepatoid carcinoma (210). Four of the five reported patients were postmenopausal, and one was of reproductive age. The tumors were highly malignant; four of the five had

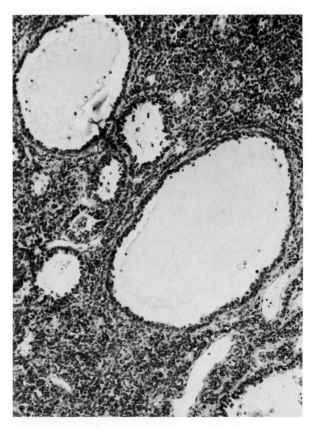

FIG. 108. Small-cell carcinoma associated with hypercalcemia. Follicle formation is striking. (From ref. 266.)

would not be expected to stain immunohistochemically for alpha fetoprotein.

Ovarian Tumors of Probable Wolffian Origin

Tumors of this type are rare (281,422) and are identical, microscopically, to their more common counterparts involving the broad ligament and fallopian tube (423) (see page 1745).

Gross features

The tumors average 12 cm in diameter, are solid or partially cystic, and are always Stage 1A at the time of presentation. The solid tissue varies from gray-white to tan or yellow and may be rubbery or firm.

Microscopic features

Solid areas consisting of diffuse sheets of cells or closely packed tubules are most typical on low-power examination. A variable fibrous stroma may produce lobulations. Cysts that focally impart a sieve-like pattern (Fig. 109) and typically contain eosinophilic secretion may be conspicuous. The tubules may be either solid or hollow. In apparently diffuse areas, a tubular pattern

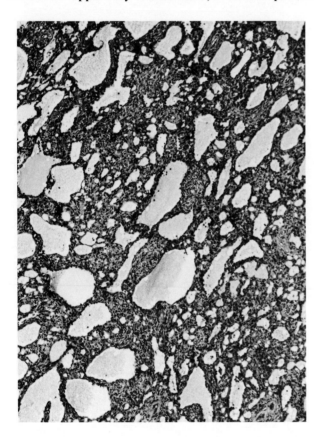

FIG. 109. Ovarian tumor of probable wolffian origin. The cysts impart a sieve-like pattern. (From ref. 266.)

may be unmasked by PAS or reticulin stains. The cells are oval or spindle-shaped and contain small amounts of eosinophilic cytoplasm. Rare tumors contain poorly differentiated cells and may behave in a malignant fashion (281).

Differential diagnosis

Misinterpretation as a sex-cord–stromal tumor, particularly a Sertoli-cell tumor, is common because the tubules of the two neoplasms may be indistinguishable. The other patterns typically present are incompatible, however, with a Sertoli-cell tumor. Rarely, large tubules in tumors of probable Wolffian origin resemble the glands of endometrioid adenocarcinoma. Again, other patterns of the neoplasm and the absence or scarcity of intraluminal mucin rule out the latter diagnosis. Wolffian-like tumors with a diffuse growth can be misinterpreted as undifferentiated carcinoma on low-power, but high-power evaluation generally demonstrates cells with bland cytologic features and few mitotic figures.

Metastatic Tumors

Certain clinical and operative findings should alert the pathologist to the probability of an ovarian metastasis. These include: (a) a prior or synchronous primary tumor elsewhere that is known to metastasize to the ovary, and (b) extraovarian spread of tumor that is highly atypical for ovarian cancer and more consistent with origin at another site. For example, the presence of hepatic or pulmonary metastases in the absence of extensive peritoneal spread would be unusual for an ovarian cancer. Because metastases to the ovary are bilateral in two-thirds to three-quarters of the cases, this possibility should be considered in the evaluation of bilateral tumors. Probably 15% to 20% of surgically encountered bilateral ovarian cancers are metastatic. Two other gross findings that are highly suggestive, but not pathognomonic, of metastasis are multiple nodules and location on the surface of the ovary without significant involvement of the underlying parenchyma. Single or multiple cysts, even when thin-walled, should not be regarded as establishing a primary ovarian tumor. Cysts that simulate follicules on microscopic examination may be encountered in many metastatic tumors, including gastric and intestinal carcinoma, carcinoid, small-cell carcinoma of pulmonary origin, and malignant melanoma.

Krukenberg Tumors

Clinical features

Krukenberg tumors are carcinomas with a prominent component of signet-ring cells (259,424–429). They usually arise from the stomach; the primary tumor may be very small, escaping detection at operation, or even for several years postoperatively. Rare Krukenberg tumors originate in breast, other portions of gastrointestinal tract, gallbladder, uterine cervix, or urinary bladder. Exceptionally rare Krukenberg tumors have been associated with disease-free survival for 10 years or more after removal, or an exhaustive autopsy has disclosed no extraovarian primary site. Such cases may represent true ovarian primaries (430).

Women with Krukenberg tumors tend to be unusually young for patients with metastatic carcinoma. The majority are between 40 and 50 years of age (mean age: 45 years) (425–429), but a sizable proportion are in their twenties. The symptoms are usually nonspecific, but endocrine manifestations may occur, particularly during pregnancy, as a result of stromal luteinization.

Gross features

Krukenberg tumor is bilateral in 60% to 80% of cases. They are typically solid with a smooth or bosselated contour (Fig. 110). Sectioning shows firm, solid, white or yellow tissue that is often lobulated. Focal gelatinous and cystic change may be seen; necrosis and hemorrhage are common.

Microscopic features

Rounded malignant epithelial cells, many of which have a signet-ring appearance, are embedded in a densely cellular stroma (Fig. 111). The cells occur singly or in clumps, or they form small acini; occasionally, they line tubules (tubular Krukenberg tumor) (Fig. 112) (431). Cysts lined by better-differentiated cells resembling those of mucinous cystadenoma may be seen.

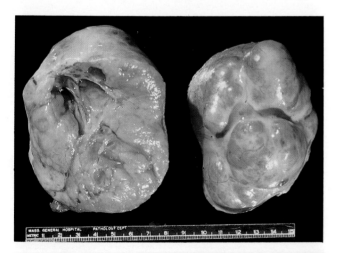

FIG. 110. Krukenberg tumor. The neoplasm has a bosselated external surface, and its sectioned surface shows lobulated, tan tissue.

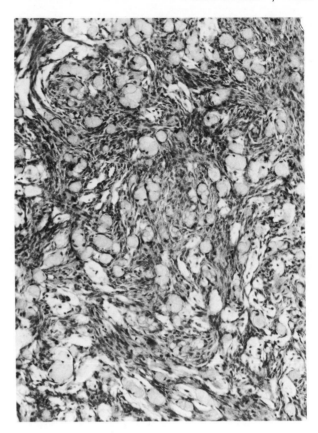

FIG. 111. Krukenberg tumor. Signet-ring cells lie within a cellular stroma. (From ref. 455.)

Often, pools of cell-free mucin are present in the stroma. The stromal cells are typically closely packed, plump, and spindle-shaped; occasionally the stroma is luteinized.

Differential diagnosis

In addition to their distinction from fibroma and sclerosing stromal tumor, discussed above, Krukenberg tumors must be distinguished from Sertoli-Leydig cell tumor and rare clear cell carcinomas having signet-ring cells. Confusion with Sertoli-Leydig cell tumor occurs in relation to tubular Krukenberg tumor. The latter are bilateral in a high proportion of cases and are usually associated with tumor outside the ovary (431). Microscopically, signet-ring cells are incompatible with Sertoli-Leydig cell tumor, with the very rare exception of heterologous tumors containing a component of mucinous carcinoid (289). In addition, the cells of tubular Krukenberg tumor are more atypical than those in Sertoli-Leydig cell tumor. Clear cell carcinomas that contain signet-ring cells typically have prominent components of conventional clear cell carcinoma.

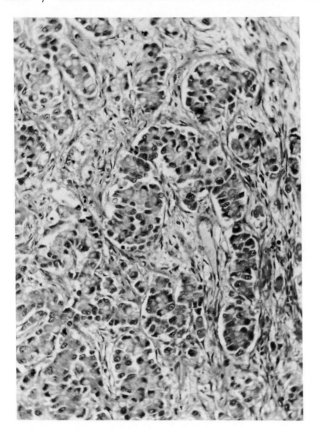

FIG. 112. Tubular Krukenberg tumor. Note signet-ring cells in many of the solid tubules.

Intestinal Carcinoma

Clinical features

From 2% to 10% of women with intestinal cancer have ovarian metastases during the course of their disease (172,432–437). Ovarian involvement is more common in women under 40 years of age. Patients fall into three categories: (i) those who present with an intestinal carcinoma and subsequently develop ovarian metastasis (50–75% of the cases); (ii) those with ovarian involvement found during resection of the intestinal carcinoma; and (iii) those who present with an "ovarian tumor" (3–20% of the cases) (435).

Gross features

Approximately two-thirds of the cases are bilateral. Sectioning of smaller tumors generally reveals firm or soft, solid tissue, whereas larger tumors are composed of friable yellow, red, or gray tissue with cysts that contain necrotic tumor, mucinous or clear fluid, or blood. Very rare examples are composed of multiple, thin-walled cysts resembling a mucinous cystadenoma (Fig. 113) (438).

Microscopic features

The tumors resemble primary intestinal carcinomas and typically form small or large glands lined by stratified epithelial cells, with scattered goblet cells. Necrosis is common and often extensive; glands may surround necrotic foci in a "garland arrangement" (190). Occasionally, cystic glands lined by well-differentiated, mucin-rich cells are prominent (438), or the tumor may be a colloid carcinoma. The stroma varies from negligible to abundant; it may be desmoplastic, edematous, or mucoid but often resembles ovarian stroma. Theca externa cells or lutein cells are present in about one-third of the cases (439). These tumors are among those most often associated with stromal luteinization (440).

Differential diagnosis

The most difficult tumors to exclude, microscopically, are primary mucinous and endometrioid carcinomas, the differential diagnoses of which have been discussed above.

Metastatic Carcinoid Tumors

Clinical features

Carcinoid tumors account for approximately 2% of ovarian metastases (440). Almost all patients are over 40 years of age (441); approximately half have features of the carcinoid syndrome. The ileum is usually the primary site, but cecum, jejunum, appendix, colon, stomach, pancreas, and lung are rarely sources (441).

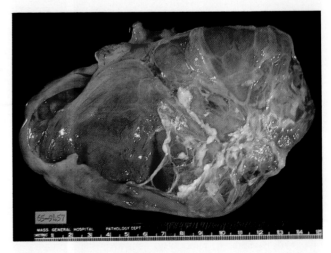

FIG. 113. Metastatic rectal carcinoma. This multicystic neoplasm simulates a mucinous cystadenoma. (From ref. 455.)

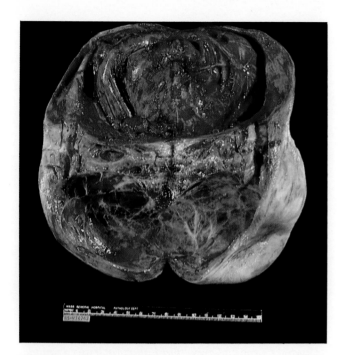

FIG. 114. Metastatic carcinoid tumor. The tumor is predominantly cystic with extensive hemorrhage. (From ref. 455.)

Gross features

Metastatic carcinoids are typically bilateral. They vary in size and are typically solid. Sectioning demonstrates single or confluent, firm, white or yellow nodules, which may resemble a fibroma, thecoma, or Brenner tumor. Cysts are present in some cases and are typically filled with clear, watery fluid, resembling a cystadenofibroma. Rare tumors are predominantly cystic (Fig. 114). Necrosis and hemorrhage may occur in solid tumors, and some of the cysts may contain blood.

Microscopic features

An insular pattern is most typical (Fig. 115), but trabecular and, rarely, solid tubular patterns are also encountered. Small, round acini are common; they often contain homogeneous eosinophilic secretion (Fig. 115), which may calcify, sometimes forming psammoma bodies. With rare exceptions, carcinoid is the only ovarian metastasis that elicits a fibroma-like stromal proliferation, which may become extensively hyalinized. Metastatic mucinous or goblet-cell carcinoid (adenocarcinoid) is composed of rounded nests containing goblet cells (Figs. 116 and 117). These tumors may also have foci resembling a Krukenberg tumor, as well as cystic glands filled with mucin (370). On high-power examination in all such cases, the characteristic features of carcinoid cells can be appreciated and confirmed by silver stains or immunocytochemical techniques.

Differential diagnosis

The acini of carcinoids are sometimes confused with Call-Exner bodies. Examination of the neoplastic cells is most important in the differential diagnosis. The sexcord-like formations of SLCT may resemble the ribbons of a trabecular carcinoid, but the latter are longer, thicker, and have a more orderly architecture. The acini of insular carcinoids may simulate the tubules of Sertoli or SLCT. Further confusion may be caused by the presence of a heterologous carcinoid component in a SLCT. Finally, a metastatic carcinoid tumor with solid tubules may resemble a solid tubular Sertoli-cell tumor. The presence of other distinctive patterns, the lack of cytologic features of carcinoid, and, if necessary, negative silver or immunohistochemical stains for neuroendocrine markers should facilitate the diagnosis of SLCT.

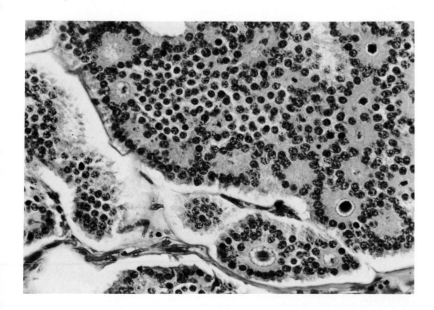

FIG. 115. Metastatic carcinoid tumor. Note round nuclei with coarse chromatin and acini containing inspissated secretion. (From ref. 128.)

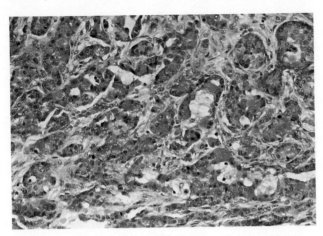

FIG. 116. Metastatic mucinous carcinoid. Note staining of goblet cells for mucin (mucicarmine stain).

Breast Carcinoma

Approximately one-third of patients with breast cancer have ovarian metastases during the course of their disease (442). The involvement is bilateral in 60% to 80% of cases (443). About two-thirds of affected ovaries are grossly normal (444). Only 2% to 11% of prophylactic oophorectomy specimens for breast cancer contain metastases (437,445). It is unusual for metastatic breast carcinoma to produce signs or symptoms of an ovarian tumor (446); stromal luteinization is uncommon, in contrast to metastatic intestinal carcinoma. Rarely, the features are those of a Krukenberg tumor (444). Lobular carcinomas, including those of the signet-ring cell subtype, spread to the ovary more frequently than ductal carcinomas (447), but metastases of the latter are more common because of its greater prevalence.

Tumors of the Appendix, Pancreas and Biliary Tract

Most metastatic appendiceal tumors are adenocarcinomas, including occasional signet-ring cell (448) and colloid subtypes, but approximately one-quarter are mucinous carcinoids (449). An unknown percentage of patients with low-grade mucinous cystadenocarcinomas of the appendix, which typically appear as mucoceles on gross examination, have similar tumors in one or both ovaries, accompanied by pseudomyxoma peritonei (167). As discussed elsewhere, the tumors at both sites characteristically resemble ovarian borderline mucinous tumors. It is probable that the ovarian tumors in such cases are metastatic from the appendix. Metastatic tumors from the pancreas (449a) and biliary tract (449b) may also closely simulate primary mucinous tumors.

Malignant Melanoma

At autopsy, 18% of patients with malignant melanoma have ovarian involvement; 95% of the tumors are bilateral (450,451). Metastatic melanoma must be distinguished from rare primary ovarian melanoma arising in the wall of a dermoid cyst. Recognition of teratomatous elements is therefore important in establishing the primary nature of a melanoma. Apparently pure ovarian melanomas may be metastases from regressed cutaneous primaries.

Metastatic melanoma may closely resemble a lipid-poor steroid-cell tumor or, if clinically appropriate, a pregnancy luteoma. In one report, three of 10 metastatic melanomas were initially misinterpreted as ovarian stromal tumors (451). Melanin can be misinterpreted as lipochrome pigment, the presence of which is a feature of steroid-cell tumors. As with other metastases, occasional metastatic melanomas contain follicle-like spaces (Fig. 118). The diagnosis of melanoma is supported in problem cases by the immunohistochemical demonstration of S-100 protein and negative staining for keratin and other antigens.

Uterine Corpus, Cervix, and Fallopian Tube Tumors

Endometrial carcinoma

Ovarian involvement accompanies endometrial carcinoma in 34% to 40% of autopsy cases (452,453), and in 5% to 15% of surgical specimens (39). When the uterine corpus and ovary are both involved by carcinoma, usually of endometrioid type, the great majority are probably independent primaries (454–456). This interpretation is supported by the high survival rates in these cases. If the endometrial carcinoma deeply invades the myometrium, permeates vascular spaces, is present in fallopian tube, involves the ovarian surface, or is present within ovarian vessels, it is probable that the ovarian involvement is secondary. Conversely, if (a) lymphatic or hematogenous spread is absent, (b) the corpus carci-

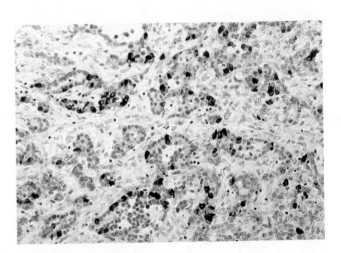

FIG. 117. Metastatic mucinous carcinoid. Note staining of argentaffin granules (Masson-Fontana stain).

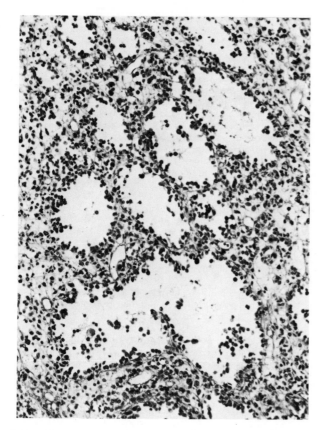

FIG. 118. Metastatic malignant melanoma. Note the follicle-like spaces.

noma is small and is limited to the superficial myometrium, (c) the carcinoma is accompanied by atypical hyperplasia, and (d) there is a centrally located ovarian tumor, sometimes accompanied by endometriosis, the tumors are probably independent primaries. In occasional cases of combined involvement it is impossible to establish the site of origin.

Uterine sarcomas

Endometrial stromal sarcomas are much more apt to spread to the ovary than leiomyosarcomas. As previously noted, when uterine endometrial stromal sarcoma is associated with a histologically similar ovarian tumor, it may be difficult to distinguish independent primaries from a metastasis to the ovary (196). The finding of endometriosis is continuity with an ovarian sarcoma indicates the primary nature of the tumor.

Carcinoma of the cervix

Mucinous adenocarcinomas of the cervix are associated with ovarian tumors of similar type (161,163). In one series, 10% of cervical mucinous adenocarcinomas were accompanied by similar ovarian tumors (163). As in other instances, it is difficult to distinguish metastases

from independent primaries (161–163). Consideration of criteria similar to those utilized for coexistent ovarian and corpus carcinomas may enable one to reach a conclusion, or it may be impossible to be certain. Less than 1% of cervical squamous cell carcinomas metastasize to the ovary (455). The rare association of ovarian squamous-cell carcinoma and cervical squamous-cell carcinoma *in situ* suggests that in exceptional cases the ovarian squamous-cell cancer may be a separate primary (227).

Trophoblastic tumors

Uterine choriocarcinoma involves the ovary in up to 22% of cases. It may be difficult or impossible to differentiate between (a) a primary ovarian tumor of either gestational or germ-cell origin and (b) a metastasis from a regressed uterine choriocarcinoma. The presence of teratomatous elements in the ovarian tumor establishes a primary, germ-cell origin. Invasive hydatidiform mole and placental site trophoblastic tumor may also spread to the ovary.

Fallopian tube

The ovary is involved in approximately 13% of tubal carcinomas, usually by direct extension (457). If involvement of the tube and ovary is extensive, the primary site may be uncertain; the term *tubo-ovarian carcinoma* has been suggested for such cases (458). Because most tubal carcinomas closely resemble serous or undifferentiated ovarian carcinomas, microscopic examination is seldom helpful in establishing the primary site. However, because tubal mucinous, endometrioid, and clear-cell carcinoma are rare, a tumor of these types involving both organs is probably an ovarian primary.

REFERENCES

1. Clement PB. Histology of the ovary. *Am J Surg Pathol* 1987;11:277–303.
2. Quan A, Charles D, Craig JM. Histologic and functional consequences of periovarian adhesions. *Obstet Gynecol* 1963;22:96–101.
3. Willson JB, Black JR III. Ovarian abscess. *Am J Obstet Gynecol* 1964;90:34–43.
4. Mickal A, Sellmann AH, Beebe JL. Ruptured tuboovarian abscess. *Am J Obstet Gynecol* 1968;100:432–436.
5. Simstein NL. Colo-tubo-ovarian fistula as complication of pelvic inflammatory disease. *South Med J* 1981;74:512–513.
6. London AM, Burkman RT. Tuboovarian abscess with associated rupture with fistula formation into the urinary bladder. *Am J Obstet Gynecol* 1979;135:1113–1114.
7. Pace EH, Voet EH, Melancon JT. Xanthogranulomatous oophoritis: an inflammatory pseudotumor of the ovary. *Int J Gynecol Pathol* 1984;3:398–402.
8. Shalev E, Zuckerman H, Rizescu I. Pelvic inflammatory pseudotumor (xanthogranuloma). *Acta Obstet Gynecol Scand* 1982;61:285–286.

9. Bhagavan BS, Gupta PK. Genital actinomycosis and intrauterine contraceptive devices. *Hum Pathol* 1978;9:567–578.

10. Schmidt WA, Bedrossian CWM, Ali V, et al. Actinomycosis and intrauterine contraceptive devices. *Diagn Gynecol Obstet* 1980;2:165–177.

11. Schmidt WA. IUDs, inflammation, and infection: assessment after two decades of IUD use. *Hum Pathol* 1982;13:878–881.

12. Pine L, Curtis EM, Brown JM. Actinomyces and the intrauterine contraceptive device: aspects of the fluorescent antibody stain. *Am J Obstet Gynecol* 1985;152:287–290.

13. Nogales-Ortiz F, Taracon I, Nogales FF. The pathology of female genital tract tuberculosis. *Obstet Gynecol* 1979;53:422–428.

14. Sutherland AM. Postmenopausal tuberculosis of the female genital tract. *Obstet Gynecol* 1982;59:54S–57S.

15. Chalvardjian A, Picard L, Shaw R, et al. Malacoplakia of the female genital tract. *Am J Obstet Gynecol* 1980;138:391–394.

16. Clement PB. Nonneoplastic lesions of the ovary. In: Kurman RJ, ed. *Blaustein's pathology of the female genital tract.* New York: Springer-Verlag, 1987:471–515.

17. Tiboldi T. Involvement of human and primate ovaries in schistosomiasis. A review of the literature. *Ann Soc Belg Med Trop* 1978;58:9–20.

18. McMahon JN, Connolly CE, Long SV, et al. Enterobius granulomas of the uterus, ovary and pelvic peritoneum. Two case reports. *Br J Obstet Gynaecol* 1984;91:289–290.

19. Hangval H, Habibi H, Moshref A, et al. Case report of an ovarian hydatid cyst. *J Trop Med Hyg* 1979;82:34–35.

20. Subietas A, Deppisch LM, Astarloa J. Cytomegalovirus oophoritis: ovarian cortical necrosis. *Hum Pathol* 1977;8:285–292.

21. Nissim F, Ashkenazy M, Borenstein R, et al. Tuberculoid cornstarch granulomas with caseous necrosis. A diagnostic challenge. *Arch Pathol Lab Med* 1981;105:86–88.

22. Mostofa SAM, Bargeron CB, Flower RW, et al. Foreign body granulomas in normal ovaries. *Obstet Gynecol* 1985;66:701–702.

23. Teilum G, Madsen V. Endometriosis ovarii et peritonaei caused by hysterosalpingography. *Br J Obstet Gynaecol* 1950;57:10–16.

24. Chen KTK, Kostich ND, Rosai J. Peritoneal foreign body granulomas to keratin in uterine adenoacanthoma. *Arch Pathol Lab Med* 1978;102:174–177.

25. Gilks CB, Clement PB. Colo-ovarian fistula. A report of two cases. *Obstet Gynecol* 1987;533–537.

26. Herbold DR, Frable WJ, Kraus FT. Isolated noninfectious granuloma of the ovary. *Int J Gynecol Pathol* 1984;2:380–391.

27. Chalvardjian A. Sarcoidosis of the female genital tract. *Am J Obstet Gynecol* 1978;132:78–80.

28. Honore LH. Combined suppurative and noncaseating granulomatous oophoritis combined with distal ileitis (Crohn's disease). *Eur J Obstet Gynecol Reprod Biol* 1981;12:91–94.

29. Hughesdon PE. The endometrial identity of benign stromatosis of the ovary and its relation to other forms of endometriosis. *J Pathol* 1976;119:201–209.

30. Blaustein A. Surface cells and inclusion cysts in fetal ovaries. *Gynecol Oncol* 1981;12:222–233.

31. Blaustein A, Kantius M, Kaganowicz A, et al. Inclusions in ovaries of females aged day 1 to 30 years. *Int J Gynecol Pathol* 1982;1:145–153.

32. Mulligan RM. A survey of epithelial inclusions in the ovarian cortex of 470 patients. *J Surg Oncol* 1976;8:61–66.

33. Scully RE. Ovary. In: Henson DE, Albores-Saavedra J, eds. *The pathology of incipient neoplasia.* Philadelphia: WB Saunders, 1986:279–293.

34. Brune WH, Pulaski EJ, Shuey HE. Giant ovarian cyst. Report of a case in a premature infant. *N Engl J Med* 1957;257:876–878.

35. Landrum B, Ogburn PL Jr, Feinberg S, et al. Intrauterine aspiration of a large fetal ovarian cyst. *Obstet Gynecol* 1986;68:11S–14S.

36. Piver MS, Williams LJ, Marcuse PM. Influence of luteal cysts on menstrual function. *Obstet Gynecol* 1970;35:740–751.

37. Stevens ML, Plotka ED. Functional lutein cyst in a postmenopausal woman. *Obstet Gynecol* 1977;50:27S–29S.

38. Strickler RC, Kelly RW, Askin FB. Postmenopausal ovarian follicle cyst: an unusual cause of estrogen excess. *Int J Gynecol Pathol* 1984;3:318–322.

39. Scully RE. Tumors of the ovary and maldeveloped gonads. *Atlas of tumor pathology,* second series, fascicle 16. Washington, DC: Armed Forces Institute of Pathology, 1979.

40. Kosloske AM, Goldthorn JF, Kaufman E, et al. Treatment of precocious pseudopuberty associated with follicular cysts of the ovary. *Am J Dis Child* 1984;138:147–149.

41. Hallatt JG, Steele CH Jr, Snyder M. Ruptured corpus luteum with hemoperitoneum: a study of 173 surgical cases. *Am J Obstet Gynecol* 1984;149:5–9.

42. Payan HM, Gilbert EF. Mesenteric cyst-ovarian implant syndrome. *Arch Pathol Lab Med* 1987;111:282–284.

43. Monteleone JA, Monteleone PL, Danis RK. Pseudoprecocious puberty associated with isolated follicle cyst of the ovary. *J Pediatr Surg* 1973;8:949–950.

44. Danon M, Robboy SJ, Kim S, et al. Cushing syndrome, sexual precocity and polyostotic fibrous dysplasia (Albright syndrome) in infancy. *J Pediatr* 1975;87:917–921.

45. Clement PB, Scully RE. Large solitary luteinized follicle cyst of pregnancy and puerperium. *Am J Surg Pathol* 1980;4:431–438.

46. Caspi E, Schreyer P, Bukovsky J. Ovarian lutein cysts in pregnancy. *Obstet Gynecol* 1973;42:388–398.

47. Girouard DP, Barclay DL, Collins CG. Hyperreactio luteinalis. Review of the literature and report of 2 cases. *Obstet Gynecol* 1964;23:513–525.

48. Samaan NA, Smith JP, Rutledge FN, et al. Plasma testosterone levels in trophoblastic disease and the effects of oophorectomy and chemotherapy. *J Clin Endocrinol Metab* 1972;34:558–561.

49. Barad DH, Gimovsky ML, Petrie RH, et al. Diagnosis and management of bilateral theca lutein cysts in a normal term pregnancy. *Diagn Gynecol Obstet* 1981;3:27–30.

50. Planner RS, Abell DA, Barbaro CA, et al. Massive enlargement of the ovaries after evacuation of hydatidiform moles. *Aust NZ J Obstet Gynaecol* 1982;22:96–100.

51. Berger NG, Repke JT, Woodruff JD. Markedly elevated serum testosterone in pregnancy without fetal virilization. *Obstet Gynecol* 1984;63:260–262.

52. Haning RV Jr, Strawn EY, Nolten WE. Pathophysiology of the ovarian hyperstimulation syndrome. *Obstet Gynecol* 1985;66:220–224.

53. Tulandi T, McInnes RA, Arronet GH. Ovarian hyperstimulation syndrome following ovulation induction with human menopausal gonadotropin. *Int J Fertil* 1984;29:113–117.

54. Futterweit W. Polycystic ovarian disease. In: *Clinical perspectives in obstetrics and gynecology.* New York: Springer-Verlag, 1985.

55. Biggs JSG. Polycystic ovarian disease—current concepts. *Aust NZ J Obstet Gynaecol* 1981;21:26–36.

56. Yen SSC. The polycystic ovary syndrome. *Clin Endocrinol* 1980;12:177–207.

57. Fechner RE, Kaufman RH. Endometrial adenocarcinoma in Stein-Leventhal syndrome. *Cancer* 1974;34:444–452.

58. Gallup DG, Stock RJ. Adenocarcinoma of the endometrium in women 40 years of age or younger. *Obstet Gynecol* 1984;64:417–419.

59. McDonald TW, Malkasian GD, Gaffey TA. Endometrial cancer associated with feminizing ovarian tumor and polycystic ovarian disease. *Obstet Gynecol* 1977;49:654–658.

60. Ramzy I, Nisker JA. Histologic study of ovaries from young women with endometrial adenocarcinoma. *Am J Clin Pathol* 1979;71:253–256.

61. Green JA, Goldzieher JW. The polycystic ovary. IV. Light and electron microscope studies. *Am J Obstet Gynecol* 1965;91:173–181.

62. Hughesdon PE. Morphology and morphogenesis of the Stein-Leventhal ovary and of so-called "hyperthecosis." *Obstet Gynecol Surv* 1982;37:59–77.

63. Hughesdon PE, Anderson MC. Giant nodular ovaries with aberrant follicles. *Histopathology* 1985;9:51–62.

64. Plate WP. Ovarian changes after long-term oral contraception. *Acta Endocrinol* 1967;55:71–77.

65. Ryan GM, Craig J, Reid DE. Histology of the uterus and ovaries after long-term cyclic norethynodrel therapy. *Am J Obstet Gynecol* 1964;90:715–725.

66. Boss JH, Scully RE, Wegner KH, et al. Structural variations in

the adult ovary—clinical significance. *Obstet Gynecol* 1965;25:747–763.

67. Scully RE, Cohen RB. Oxidative-enzyme activity in normal and pathologic human ovaries. *Obstet Gynecol* 1964;24:667–681.

68. Braithwaite SS, Erkman-Balis B, Avila TD. Postmenopausal virilization due to ovarian stromal hyperthecosis. *J Clin Endocrinol Metab* 1978;46:295–300.

69. Madeido G, Tieu TM, Aiman J. Atypical ovarian hyperthecosis in a virilized postmenopausal woman. *Am J Clin Pathol* 1985;83:101–107.

70. Stearns HC, Sneeden VD, Fearl JD. A clinical and pathologic review of ovarian stromal hyperplasia and its possible relationship to common diseases of the female reproductive system. *Am J Obstet Gynecol* 1974;119:375–381.

71. Judd HL, Scully RE, Herbst AL, et al. Familial hyperthecosis: comparison of endocrinologic and histologic findings with polycystic ovarian disease. *Am J Obstet Gynecol* 1973;117:976–982.

72. Nagamani M, Lingold JC, Gomez JR, et al. Clinical and hormonal studies in hyperthecosis of the ovaries. *Fertil Steril* 1981;36:326–332.

73. Scully RE. Smooth-muscle differentiation in genital tract disorders [Editorial]. *Arch Pathol Lab Med* 1981;105:505–507.

74. Sternberg WH, Roth LM. Ovarian stromal tumors containing Leydig cells. I. Stromal-Leydig cell tumor and non-neoplastic transformation of ovarian stroma to Leydig cells. *Cancer* 1973;32:940–951.

75. Roth LM, Sternberg WH. Ovarian stromal tumors containing Leydig cells. II. Pure Leydig cell tumor, non-hilar type. *Cancer* 1973;32:952–960.

76. Scully RE. Stromal luteoma of the ovary. *Cancer* 1964;17:769–778.

77. Kalstone CE, Jaffe RB, Abell MR. Massive edema of the ovary simulating fibroma. *Obstet Gynecol* 1969;34:564–571.

78. Kanbour AI, Salazar H, Tobon H. Massive ovarian edema. A nonneoplastic pelvic mass of young women. *Arch Pathol Lab Med* 1979;103:42–45.

79. Roth LM, Deaton RL, Sternberg WH. Massive ovarian edema. A clinicopathologic study of five cases including ultrastructural observations and review of the literature. *Am J Surg Pathol* 1979;3:11–21.

80. Chervenak FA, Castadot MJ, Wiederman J, et al. Massive ovarian edema: review of world literature and report of two cases. *Obstet Gynecol Surv* 1980;35:677–684.

81. Young RH, Scully RE. Fibromatosis and massive edema of the ovary, possibly related entities: a report of 14 cases of fibromatosis and 11 cases of massive edema. *Int J Gynecol Pathol* 1984;3:153–178.

82. Sternberg WH, Barclay DL. Luteoma of pregnancy. *Am J Obstet Gynecol* 1966;95:165–181.

83. Norris HJ, Taylor HB. Nodular theca-lutein hyperplasia of pregnancy (so-called "pregnancy luteoma"). A clinical and pathologic study of 15 cases. *Am J Clin Pathol* 1967;47:557–566.

84. Rice BF, Barclay DL, Sternberg WH. Luteoma of pregnancy. *Am J Obstet Gynecol* 1969;104:871–878.

85. Garcia-Bunuel R, Berek JS, Woodruff JD. Luteomas of pregnancy. *Obstet Gynecol* 1975;45:407–414.

86. Sternberg WH, Dhurandhar HN. Functional ovarian tumors of stromal and sex cord origin. *Hum Pathol* 1977;8:565–582.

87. Polansky S, dePapp EW, Ogden EB. Virilization associated with bilateral luteomas of pregnancy. *Obstet Gynecol* 1975;45:516–522.

88. Thomas E, Mestman J, Henneman C, et al. Bilateral luteomas of pregnancy with virilization. *Obstet Gynecol* 1972;39:577–584.

89. Garcia-Bunuel R, Brandes D. Luteoma of pregnancy: ultrastructural features. *Hum Pathol* 1976;7:205–214.

90. Sternberg WH. The morphology, androgenic function, hyperplasia, and tumours of the human ovarian hilus cells. *Am J Pathol* 1949;25:493–521.

91. Sternberg WH, Segaloff A, Gaskill CJ. Influence of chorionic gonadotropin on human ovarian hilus cells (Leydig-like cells). *J Clin Endocrinol Metab* 1953;13:139–153.

92. Davidson BJ, Waisman J, Judd HL. Longstanding virilism in a woman with hyperplasia and neoplasia of ovarian lipidic cells. *Obstet Gynecol* 1981;58:753–759.

93. Meldrum DR, Frumar AM, Shamonki IM, et al. Ovarian and adrenal steroidogenesis in a virilized patient with gonadotropin-resistant ovaries and hilus cell hyperplasia. *Obstet Gynecol* 1980;56:216–221.

94. Rutgers JL, Scully RE. Functioning ovarian tumors with peripheral steroid cell proliferation: a report of twenty-four cases. *Int J Gynecol Pathol* 1986;5:319–337.

95. Zhang J, Young RH, Arseneau J, et al. Ovarian stromal tumors containing lutein or Leydig cells (luteinized thecomas and stromal Leydig cell tumors)—a clinicopathological analysis of fifty cases. *Int J Gynecol Pathol* 1982;1:270–285.

96. Bersch W, Alexy E, Heuser HP, et al. Ectopic decidua formation in the ovary (so-called deciduoma). *Virchows Arch [A]* 1973;360:173–177.

97. Herr JC, Heidger PM Jr, Scott JR, et al. Decidual cells in the human ovary at term. I. Incidence, gross anatomy and ultrastructural features of merocrine secretion. *Am J Anat* 1978;152:7–28.

98. Rewell RE. Extra-uterine decidua. *J Pathol* 1972;105:219–222.

99. Starup J, Visfeldt J. Ovarian morphology in early and late human pregnancy. *Acta Obstet Gynecol Scand* 1974;53:211–218.

100. Ober WB, Grady HG, Schoenbucher AK. Ectopic ovarian decidua without pregnancy. *Am J Pathol* 1957;33:199–217.

101. Israel SL, Rubenstone A, Meranze DR. The ovary at term. I. Decidua-like reaction and surface cell proliferation. *Obstet Gynecol* 1954;3:399–407.

102. Herr JC, Platz CE, Heidger PM Jr, et al. Smooth muscle within ovarian decidual nodules: a link to leiomyomatosis peritonealis disseminata? *Obstet Gynecol* 1979;53:451–456.

103. Honore LH, O'Hara KE. Subcapsular adipocytic infiltration of the human ovary: a clinicopathological study of eight cases. *Eur J Obstet Gynaecol Reprod Biol* 1980;10:13–20.

104. Shipton EA, Meares SD. Heterotopic bone formation in the ovary. *Aust NZ J Obstet Gynaecol* 1965;5:100–102.

105. Russell P, Bannatyne P, Shearman RP, et al. Premature hypergonadotropic ovarian failure: clinicopathological study of 19 cases. *Int J Gynecol Pathol* 1982;1:185–201.

106. Starup J, Sele V. Premature ovarian failure. *Acta Obstet Gynecol Scand* 1973;52:259–268.

107. Board JA, Redwine FO, Moncure CW, et al. Identification of differing etiologies of clinically diagnosed premature menopause. *Am J Obstet Gynecol* 1979;134:936–944.

108. Aiman J, Smentek C. Premature ovarian failure. *Obstet Gynecol* 1985;66:9–14.

109. Koninckx PR, Brosens IA. The "gonadotropin-resistant ovary" syndrome as a cause of secondary amenorrhea and infertility. *Fertil Steril* 1977;28:926–931.

110. Gloor E, Juillard E, Curchod A, et al. Ovarian hypoplasia with follicular calcifications. *Am J Clin Pathol* 1982;78:857–860.

111. Talbert LM, Raj MHG, Hammond MG, et al. Endocrine and immunologic studies in a patient with resistant ovary syndrome. *Fertil Steril* 1984;42:741–744.

112. Massachusetts General Hospital Case Records. Case 46-1986. Resistant-ovary syndrome, with hyalinization of preantral follicles. *N Engl J Med* 1986;315:1336–1343.

113. Coulam CB, Kempers RD, Randall RV. Premature ovarian failure: evidence for autoimmune function. *Fertil Steril* 1981;36:238–240.

114. Gloor E, Hurlimann J. Autoimmune oophoritis. *Am J Clin Pathol* 1984;81:105–109.

115. Sedmak DD, Hart WR, Tubbs RR. Autoimmune oophoritis: a histopathologic study of involved ovaries with immunologic characterization of the mononuclear cell infiltrate. *Int J Gynecol Pathol* 1987;6:73–81.

116. Irvine WJ, Chan MMW, Scarth L, et al. Immunological aspects of premature ovarian failure associated with idiopathic Addison's disease. *Lancet* 1968;2:883–887.

117. Irvine WJ, Chan MMW, Scarth L. The further characterization of autoantibodies reactive with extra-adrenal steroid-producing cells in patients with adrenal disorders. *Clin Exp Immunol* 1969;4:489–503.

118. Ruehsen MDM, Blizzard RM, Garcia-Bunuel R, et al. Autoimmunity and ovarian failure. *Am J Obstet Gynecol* 1972;112:693–703.

119. Irvine WJ, Barnes EW. Addison's disease, ovarian failure and hypoparathyroidism. *Clin Endocrinol Metab* 1975;4:379–433.
120. Coulam CB, Ryan RJ. Premature menopause I. Etiology. *Am J Obstet Gynecol* 1979;133:639–643.
121. Coulam CB. The prevalence of autoimmune disorders among patients with primary ovarian failure. *Am J Reprod Immunol* 1983;4:63–66.
122. Damewood MD, Zacur HA, Hoffman GJ, et al. Circulating antiovarian antibodies in premature ovarian failure. *Obstet Gynecol* 1986;68:850–854.
123. Alper MM, Garner PR. Premature ovarian failure: its relationship to autoimmune disease. *Obstet Gynecol* 1985;66:27–30.
124. Kurman RJ, ed. *Blaustein's pathology of the female genital tract*, 3rd edition. New York: Springer-Verlag, 1987.
125. Fox H, Langley FA. *Tumours of the ovary*. Chicago: Year Book Medical Publishers, 1976.
126. Morrow CP, Townsend DE. *Synopsis of gynecologic oncology*, 2nd edition. New York: John Wiley & Sons, 1981.
127. Haines and Taylor *Obstetrical and Gynaecological Pathology*, Fox H, ed. New York: Churchill Livingstone, 1987.
128. Serov SF, Scully RE, Sobin LH. *International histological classification of tumors No. 9. Histological typing of ovarian tumors*. Geneva: World Health Organization, 1973.
129. Czernobilsky B. Cystadenofibroma, adenofibroma and malignant adenofibroma of the ovary. In: Sommers SC, Rosen PP, eds. *Pathology annual, vol. 12, part I*. New York: Appleton-Century-Crofts, 1977:201–216.
130. International Federation of Gynaecology and Obstetrics: Classification and staging of malignant tumors in the female pelvis. *Acta Obstet Gynaecol Scand* 1971;50:1–7.
131. Taylor HC Jr. Studies in the clinical and biological evolution of adenocarcinoma of the ovary. *J Obstet Gynecol Br Commonwealth* 1959;66:827–842.
132. Hart WR. Ovarian epithelial tumors of borderline malignancy (carcinomas of low malignant potential). *Hum Pathol* 1977;8:541–549.
133. Russell P. The pathological assessment of ovarian neoplasms. III: The malignant 'epithelial' tumors. *Pathology* 1979;11:493–532.
134. Scully RE. Common epithelial tumors of borderline malignancy (carcinomas of low malignant potential). *Bull Cancer (Paris)* 1982;69:228–238.
135. Colgan TJ, Norris HJ. Ovarian epithelial tumors of low malignant potential: a review. *Int J Gynecol Pathol* 1983;1:367–382.
136. Katzenstein A-L A, Mazur MT, Morgan TE, Kao MS. Proliferative serous tumors of the ovary. *Am J Surg Pathol* 1978;2:339–355.
137. Fox H. Ovarian tumors of borderline malignancy. In: Morrow CP, et al, eds. *Recent clinical developments in gynecologic oncology*. Progress in Cancer Research and Therapy, vol. 24. New York: Raven Press, 1983:137–150.
138. The Ovarian Tumour Panel of the Royal College of Obstetricians and Gynaecologists. Ovarian epithelial tumours of borderline malignancy: pathological features and current status. *Br J Obstet Gynecol* 1983;90:743–750.
139. Barnhill D, Heller P, Brzozowski P, Advani H, Gallup D, Park R. Epithelial ovarian carcinoma of low malignant potential. *Obstet Gynecol* 1985;65:53–59.
140. Tasker M, Langley FA. The outlook for women with borderline epithelial tumours of the ovary. *Br J Obstet Gynecol* 1985;92:969–973.
141. Ulbright TM, Roth LM. Common epithelial tumors of the ovary: proliferating and of low malignant potential. *Sem Diagn Pathol* 1985;2:2–15.
142. Bostwick DG, Tazelaar HD, Ballon SC, Hendrickson MR, Kempson RL. Ovarian epithelial tumors of borderline malignancy. A clinical and pathologic study of 109 cases. *Cancer* 1986;58:2052–2065.
143. Kliman L, Rome RM, Fortune DW. Low malignant potential tumors of the ovary: a study of 76 cases. *Obstet Gynecol* 1986;68:338–344.
144. Julian GC, Woodruff JD. The biological behavior of low-grade papillary serous carcinoma of the ovary. *Obstet Gynecol* 1972;40:860–868.
145. Gooneratne S, Sassone M, Blaustein A, Talerman A. Serous surface papillary carcinoma of the ovary; a clinicopathologic study of 16 cases. *Int J Gynecol Pathol* 1982;1:258–269.
146. White PF, Merino MJ, Barwick KW. Serous surface papillary carcinoma of the ovary: a clinical, pathologic, ultrastructural, and immunohistochemical study of 11 cases. In: Sommers SC, Rosen PP, Fechner RE, eds. *Path annual, vol. 20, part 1*. Norwalk, Connecticut: Appleton-Century-Crofts, 1985; 403–418.
147. Chen KTK, Schooley JL, Flam MS. Peritoneal carcinomatosis after prophylactic oophorectomy in familial ovarian cancer syndrome. *Obstet Gynecol* 1985;66:93s–94s.
147a. Tavassoli FA. Serous tumor of low malignant potential with early stromal invasion (serous LMP with microinvasion). *Modern Pathol* 1988;1:407–414.
147b. Bell DA, Scully RE. Ovarian serous borderline tumors with stromal microinvasion: A report of 21 cases. *Human Pathol* 1990;21:397–403.
148. Bell DA, Weinstock MA, Scully RE. Peritoneal implants of serous borderline tumors: histologic features and prognosis. *Cancer* 1988;62:2212–2222.
148a. Gershenson DM, Silva EG. Serous ovarian tumors of low malignant potential with peritoneal implants. *Cancer* 1990;65:578–585.
149. McCaughey WTE, Kirk ME, Lester W, Dardick I. Peritoneal epithelial lesions associated with proliferative serous tumours of the ovary. *Histopathology* 1984;8:195–208.
150. Russell P. Borderline epithelial tumours of the ovary: a conceptual dilemma. *Clin Obstet Gynecol* 1984;11:259–277.
151. Michael H, Roth LM. Invasive and noninvasive implants in ovarian serous tumors of low malignant potential. *Cancer* 1986;57:1240–1247.
152. Kent SW, McKay DG. Primary cancer of the ovary. An analysis of 349 cases. *Am J Obstet Gynecol* 1960;80:430–438.
153. Aure JC, Høeg K, Kolstad P. Clinical and histologic studies of ovarian carcinoma. Long-term follow-up of 990 cases. *Obstet Gynecol* 1971;37:1–9.
154. Bergman F. Carcinoma of the ovary. A clinicopathological study of 86 autopsied cases with special reference to mode of spread. *Acta Obstet Gynecol Scand* 1966;45:211–231.
155. Allan MS, Hertig AT. Carcinoma of the ovary. *Am J Obstet Gynecol* 1949;58:640–653.
156. Turner JC, ReMine WH, Dockerty MB. A clinicopathologic study of 172 patients with primary carcinoma of the ovary. *Surg Gynecol Obstet* 1959;105:198–206.
157. Bennington JL, Ferguson BR, Haber SL. Incidence and relative frequency of benign and malignant ovarian neoplasms. *Obstet Gynecol* 1968;32:627–632.
158. Cariker M, Dockerty M. Mucinous cystadenomas and mucinous cystadenocarcinomas of the ovary. A clinical and pathological study of 355 cases. *Cancer* 1954;7:302–310.
159. Reagan JW. Histopathology of ovarian pseudomucinous cystadenoma. *Am J Pathol* 1949;25:689–707.
160. Chaitin BA, Gershenson DM, Evans HL. Mucinous tumors of the ovary. A clinicopathologic study of 70 cases. *Cancer* 1985;55:1958–1962.
161. Young RH, Scully RE. Mucinous ovarian tumors associated with mucinous adenocarcinomas of the cervix. A clinicopathological analysis of 16 cases. *Int J Gynecol Pathol* 1988;7:99–111.
162. LiVolsi VA, Merino MJ, Schwartz PE. Coexistent endocervical adenocarcinoma and mucinous adenocarcinoma of ovary: a clinicopathologic study of four cases. *Int J Gynecol Pathol* 1983;1:391–402.
163. Kaminski PF, Norris HJ. Coexistence of ovarian neoplasms and endocervical adenocarcinoma. *Obstet Gynecol* 1984;64:553–556.
164. Hart WR, Norris HJ. Borderline and malignant mucinous tumors of the ovary. Histologic criteria and clinical behavior. *Cancer* 1973;31:1031–1045.
165. Agrofojo Blanco A, Gibbs ACC, Langley FA. Histological discrimination of malignancy in mucinous ovarian tumors. *Histopathology* 1977;1:431–443.
166. Limber GK, King RE, Silverberg SG. Pseudomyxoma peritonei: a report of ten cases. *Ann Surg* 1973;178:587–593.
167. Campbell JS, Lou P, Ferguson JP, Krongold I, Kemeny T, Mitton DM, Allam N. Pseudomyxoma peritonei et ovarii with occult neoplasm of appendix. *Obstet Gynecol* 1973;42:897–902.

168. Rutgers JL, Scully RE. Ovarian mullerian mucinous papillary cystadenomas of borderline malignancy. A clinicopathological analysis. *Cancer* 1988; 61:340–348.

169. Prat J, Young RH, Scully RE. Ovarian mucinous tumors with foci of anaplastic carcinoma. *Cancer* 1982;50:300–304.

170. Prat J, Scully RE. Sarcomas in ovarian mucinous tumors. A report of two cases. *Cancer* 1979;44:1327–1331.

171. Prat J, Scully RE. Ovarian mucinous tumors with sarcoma-like mural nodules. A report of seven cases. *Cancer* 1979;44:1333–1344.

172. Ulbright TM, Roth LM, Stehman FB. Secondary ovarian neoplasia. A clinicopathologic study of 35 cases. *Cancer* 1984;53:1164–1174.

173. Kao GF, Norris HJ. Unusual cystadenofibromas: endometrioid, mucinous, and clear cell types. *Obstet Gynecol* 1979;54:729–736.

174. Kao GF, Norris HJ. Cystadenofibromas of the ovary with epithelial atypia. *Am J Surg Pathol* 1978;2:357–363.

175. Hughesdon PE. Benign endometrioid tumours of the ovary and the Müllerian concept of ovarian epithelial tumours. *Histopathology* 1984;8:977–990.

176. Roth LM, Czernobilsky B, Langley FA. Ovarian endometrioid adenofibromatous and cystadenofibromatous tumors: benign, proliferating, and malignant. *Cancer* 1981;48:1838–1845.

177. Bell DA, Scully RE. Atypical and borderline endometroid adenofibromas of the ovary. *Am J Surg Pathol* 1985;9:205–214.

178. Malloy JJ, Dockerty MB, Welch JS, Hunt AB. Papillary ovarian tumors. II. Endometrioid cancers and mesonephroma ovarii. *Am J Obstet Gynecol* 1965;93:880–885.

179. Gray LA, Barnes ML. Endometrioid carcinoma of the ovary. *Obstet Gynecol* 1967;29:694–701.

180. Czernobilsky B, Silverman BB, Mikuta JJ. Endometrioid carcinoma of the ovary. A clinicopathologic study of 75 cases. *Cancer* 1970;26:1141–1152.

181. Kurman RJ, Craig JM. Endometrioid and clear cell carcinoma of the ovary. *Cancer* 1972;29:1653–1664.

182. Long ME, Taylor HC Jr. Endometrioid carcinoma of the ovary. *Am J Obstet Gynecol* 1964;90:936–950.

183. Fu YS, Stock RJ, Reagan JW, Storaasli JP, Wentz WB. Significance of squamous components in endometrioid carcinoma of the ovary. *Cancer* 1979;44:616–621.

184. Corner GW Jr, Hu YC, Hertig AT. Ovarian carcinoma arising in endometriosis. *Am J Obstet Gynecol* 1950;59:760–774.

185. Fathalla MF. Malignant transformation in ovarian endometriosis. *J Obstet Gynaecol Br Commonwealth* 1967;74:85–92.

186. Aure JC, Høeg K, Kolstad P. Carcinoma of the ovary and endometriosis. *Acta Obstet Gynecol Scand* 1971;50:63–67.

187. Mostoufizadeh M, Scully RE. Malignant tumors arising in endometriosis. *Clin Obstet Gynecol* 1980;23:951–963.

188. Young RH, Prat J, Scully RE. Ovarian endometrioid carcinomas resembling sex cord-stromal tumors. A clinicopathologic analysis of 13 cases. *Am J Surg Pathol* 1982;6:513–522.

189. Roth LM, Liban E, Czernobilsky B. Ovarian endometrioid tumors mimicking Sertoli and Sertoli-Leydig cell tumors. Sertoliform variant of endometrioid carcinoma. *Cancer* 1982;50:1322–1331.

190. Lash RH, Hart WR. Intestinal adenocarcinomas metastatic to the ovaries. A clinicopathological evaluation of 22 cases. *Am J Surg Pathol* 1987;11:114–121.

191. Dehner LP, Norris HJ, Taylor HB. Carcinosarcomas and mixed mesodermal tumors of the ovary. *Cancer* 1971;27:207–216.

192. Hernandez W, Di Saia PJ, Morrow CP, Townsend DE. Mixed mesodermal sarcoma of the ovary. *Obstet Gynecol* 1977;49:59s–63s.

193. Clement PB, Scully RE. Extrauterine mesodermal (mullerian) adenosarcoma. *Am J Clin Pathol* 1978;69:276–283.

194. Kao GF, Norris HJ. Benign and low grade variants of mixed mesodermal tumor (adenosarcoma) of the ovary and adnexal region. *Cancer* 1978;42:1314–1324.

195. Silverberg SG, Fernandez FN. Endolymphatic stromal myosis of the ovary: a report of three cases and literature review. *Gynecol Oncol* 1981;12:129–138.

196. Young RH, Prat J, Scully RE. Endometrioid stromal sarcomas of the ovary. A clinicopathologic analysis of 23 cases. *Cancer* 1984;53:1143–1155.

197. Clement PB, Scully RE. Uterine tumors resembling ovarian sex-cord tumors. *Am J Clin Pathol* 1976;66:512–525.

198. Roth LM, Langley FA, Fox H, Wheeler JE, Czernobilsky B. Ovarian clear cell adenofibromatous tumors: benign, of low malignant potential, and associated with invasive clear cell carcinoma. *Cancer* 1984;53:1156–1163.

199. Bell DA, Scully RE. Benign and borderline clear cell adenofibromas of the ovary. *Cancer* 1985;56:2922–2931.

200. Scully RE, Barlow JF. "Mesonephroma" of ovary. Tumor of mullerian nature related to the endometrioid carcinoma. *Cancer* 1967;20:1405–1417.

201. Anderson MC, Langley FA. Mesonephroid tumours of the ovary. *J Clin Pathol* 1970;23:210–218.

202. Aure JC. Mesonephroid tumors of the ovary. Clinical and histopathologic studies. *Obstet Gynecol* 1971;37:860–867.

203. Doshi N, Tobon H. Primary clear cell carcinoma of the ovary. An analysis of 15 cases with review of the literature. *Cancer* 1977;39:2658–2664.

204. Eastwood J. Mesonephroid (clear cell) carcinoma of the ovary and endometrium. A comparative prospective clinico-pathological study and review of the literature. *Cancer* 1978;41:1911–1928.

205. Norris HJ, Robinowitz M. Ovarian adenocarcinoma of mesonephric type. *Cancer* 1971;28:1074–1081.

206. Shevchuk MM, Winkler-Monsanto B, Fenoglio CM, Richart RM. Clear cell carcinoma of the ovary: a clinicopathologic study with review of the literature. *Cancer* 1981;47:1344–1351.

207. Klemi PJ, Meurmann L, Grönroos M, Talerman A. Clear cell (mesonephroid) tumor of the ovary with characteristics resembling endodermal sinus tumor. *Int J Gynecol Pathol* 1982;1:95–100.

208. Young RH, Scully RE. Oxyphilic clear cell carcinoma of the ovary. A report of nine cases. *Am J Surg Pathol* 1987;11:661–667.

208a. Kennedy AW, Biscotti CV, Hart WR, Webester KD. Ovarian clear cell adenocarcinoma. *Gynecol Oncol* 1989;32:342–349.

209. Prat J, Bhan AK, Dickersin GR, Robboy SJ, Scully RE. Hepatoid yolk sac tumor of the ovary (endodermal sinus tumor with hepatoid differentiation). A light microscopic, ultrastructural and immunohistochemical study of seven cases. *Cancer* 1982;50:2355–2368.

210. Ishikura H, Scully RE. Hepatoid carcinoma of the ovary: a report of five cases of newly described tumor. *Cancer* 1987;60:2775–2784.

211. Berge T, Borglin NE. Brenner tumors. Histogenetic and clinical studies. *Cancer* 1967;20:308–318.

212. Bransilver BR, Ferenczy A, Richart RM. Brenner tumors and Walthard cell nests. *Arch Pathol* 1974;98:76–86.

213. Ehrlich CE, Roth LM. The Brenner tumor. A clinicopathologic study of 57 cases. *Cancer* 1971;27:332–342.

214. Silverberg SG. Brenner tumor of the ovary. A clinicopathologic study of 60 tumors in 54 women. *Cancer* 1971;28:588–596.

215. Fox H, Agrawal K, Langley FA. The Brenner tumour of the ovary. A clinicopathological study of 54 cases. *J Obstet Gynecol Br Commonw* 1972;79:661–665.

216. Jorgensen EO, Dockerty MB, Wilson RB, Welch JS. Clinicopathologic study of 53 cases of Brenner's tumors of the ovary. *Am J Obstet Gynecol* 1970;108:122–127.

217. Trebeck CE, Friedlander ML, Russell P, Baird PJ. Brenner tumors of the ovary: a study of the histology, immunohistochemistry and cellular DNA content in benign, borderline and malignant ovarian tumours. *Pathology* 1987;19:241–246.

218. Hallgrimson J, Scully RE. Borderline and malignant Brenner tumours of the ovary. A report of 15 cases. *Acta Pathol Microbiol Scand [A]* 1972;80(suppl):233:56–66.

219. Miles PA, Norris HJ. Proliferative and malignant Brenner tumors of the ovary. *Cancer* 1972;30:174–186.

220. Roth LM, Sternberg WH. Proliferating Brenner tumors. *Cancer* 1971;27:687–693.

221. Roth LM, Dallenbach-Hellweg G, Czernobilsky B. Ovarian Brenner tumors. I. Metaplastic, proliferating, and of low malignant potential. *Cancer* 1985;56:582–591.

222. Roth LM, Czernobilsky B. Ovarian Brenner tumors. II. Malignant. *Cancer* 1985;56:592–601.

223. Austin RM, Norris HJ. Malignant Brenner tumor and transitional cell carcinoma of the ovary. A comparison. *Int J Gynecol Pathol* 1987;6:29–39.

223a. Robey SS, Silva EG, Gershenson DM, McLemore D, El-Naggar A, Ordonez NG. Transitional cell carcinoma in high-grade high-stage ovarian carcinoma. *Cancer* 1989;63:839–847.

224. Young RH, Scully RE. Urothelial and ovarian carcinomas of identical cell types. Problems in interpretation. A report of three cases and review of the literature. *Int J Gynecol Pathol* 1988;7:197–211.

225. Nogales FF, Silverberg SG. Epidermoid cysts of the ovary: a report of five cases with histogenetic considerations and ultrastructural findings. *Am J Obstet Gynecol* 1976;124:523–528.

226. Young RH, Prat J, Scully RE. Epidermoid cyst of the ovary. A report of three cases with comments on histogenesis. *Am J Clin Pathol* 1980;73:272–276.

227. Black WC, Benitez RE. Nonteratomatous squamous cell carcinoma in situ of the ovary. *Obstet Gynecol* 1964;24:865–868.

228. Lele SB, Piver S, Barlow JJ, Tsukada Y. Squamous cell carcinoma arising in ovarian endometriosis. *Gynecol Oncol* 1978;6:290–293.

229. Shingleton HM, Middleton FF, Gore H. Squamous cell carcinoma in the ovary. *Am J Obstet Gynecol* 1974;120:556–560.

230. Tetu B, Silva EG, Gershenson DM. Squamous cell carcinoma of the ovary. *Arch Pathol Lab Med* 1987;111:864–866.

231. Rutgers JL, Scully RE. Ovarian mixed-epithelial papillary cystadenomas of borderline malignancy. A clinicopathological analysis. *Cancer* 1988;61:546–554.

232. Young RH, Scully RE. Ovarian sex cord-stromal tumors. Recent advances and current status. *Clin Obstet Gynaecol* 1984;11:93–134.

233. Hodgson JE, Dockerty MB, Mussey RD. Granulosa cell tumor of the ovary. A clinical and pathologic review of sixty-two cases. *Surg Gynecol Obstet* 1945;81:631–642.

234. Norris HJ, Taylor HB. Virilization associated with cystic granulosa cell tumors. *Obstet Gynecol* 1969;34:629–635.

235. Nakashima N, Young RH, Scully RE. Androgenic granulosa cell tumors of the ovary. A clinicopathologic analysis of 17 cases and review of the literature. *Arch Pathol Lab Med* 1984;108:786–791.

236. Stenwig JT, Hazekamp JT, Beecham JB. Granulosa cell tumors of the ovary. A clinicopathological study of 118 cases with long term follow-up. *Gynecol Oncol* 1979;7:136–152.

237. Fathalla MF. The occurrence of granulosa and theca tumors in clinically normal ovaries. *J Obstet Gynaecol Br Commonwealth* 1967;74:279–282.

238. Burslem RW, Langley FA, Woodcock AS. A clinicopathological study of oestrogenic ovarian tumours. *Cancer* 1954;7:522–538.

239. Busby T, Anderson GW. Feminizing mesenchymomas of the ovary. Includes 107 cases of granulosa-cell, granulosa-theca-cell, and theca-cell tumors. *Am J Obstet Gynecol* 1954;68:1391–1420.

240. Diddle AW. Granulosa and theca cell ovarian tumors: Prognosis. *Cancer* 1952;5:215–228.

241. Sjöstedt S, Wahlén T. Prognosis of granulosa cell tumors. *Acta Obstet Gynecol Scand* 1961;40(suppl 6):3–26.

242. Norris HJ, Taylor HB. Prognosis of granulosa-theca tumors of the ovary. *Cancer* 1968;21:255–263.

243. Fox H, Agrawal K, Langley FA. A clinicopathologic study of 92 cases of granulosa cell tumor of the ovary with special reference to the factors influencing prognosis. *Cancer* 1975;35:231–241.

244. Björkholm E, Silferswürd C. Prognostic factors in granulosa cell tumors. *Gynecol Oncol* 1981;11:261–274.

245. Young RH, Dickersin GR, Scully RE. Juvenile granulosa cell tumor of the ovary. A clinicopathologic analysis of 125 cases. *Am J Surg Pathol* 1984;8:575–596.

246. Young RH, Scully RE. Ovarian sex cord-stromal tumors with bizarre nuclei. A clinicopathologic analysis of seventeen cases. *Int J Gynecol Pathol* 1983;1:325–335.

247. Young RH, Scully RE. Ovarian stromal tumors with minor sex cord elements: a report of seven cases. *Int J Gynecol Pathol* 1983;2:227–234.

248. Susil BJ, Sumithran E. Sarcomatous change in granulosa cell tumor. *Hum Pathol* 1987;18:397–399.

249. Clement PB, Young RH, Scully RE. Ovarian granulosa cell proliferations of pregnancy. A report of nine cases. *Hum Pathol* 1988;19:657–662.

250. Roth LM, Nicholas TR, Ehrlich CE. Juvenile granulosa cell tumor. A clinicopathologic study of three cases with ultrastructural observations. *Cancer* 1979;44:2194–2205.

251. Lack EE, Perez-Atayde AR, Murthy ASK, Goldstein DP, Crigler JF, Vawter GF. Granulosa theca cell tumors in premenarchal girls. A clinical and pathologic study of ten cases. *Cancer* 1981;48:1846–1854.

252. Zaloudek C, Norris HJ. Granulosa tumors of the ovary in children. A clinical and pathologic study of 32 cases. *Am J Surg Pathol* 1981;6:503–512.

252a. Biscotti CV, Hart WR. Juvenile granulosa cell tumors of the ovary. *Arch Pathol Lab Med* 1989;113:40–46.

253. Young RH, Dudley AG, Scully RE. Granulosa cell, Sertoli-Leydig cell and unclassified sex cord-stromal tumors associated with pregnancy. A clinicopathological analysis of thirty-six cases. *Gynecol Oncol* 1984;18:181–205.

254. Dockerty MB, Masson JC. Ovarian fibromas: A clinical and pathologic study of two hundred and eighty-three cases. *Am J Obstet Gynecol* 1944;47:741–752.

255. Gorlin RJ. Nevoid basal cell carcinoma syndrome. *Medicine (Baltimore)* 1987;66:98–113.

256. Meigs JV. Fibroma of the ovary with ascites and hydrothorax—Meigs' syndrome. *Am J Obstet Gynecol* 1954;67:962–987.

257. Samanth KK, Black WC. Benign ovarian stromal tumors associated with free peritoneal fluid. *Am J Obstet Gynecol* 1970;107:538–545.

258. Prat J, Scully RE. Cellular fibromas and fibrosarcomas of the ovary: a comparative clinicopathologic analysis of seventeen cases. *Cancer* 1981;47:2663–2670.

259. Holtz F, Hart WR. Krukenberg tumors of the ovary. A clinicopathological analysis of 27 cases. *Cancer* 1982;50:2438–2447.

260. Geist SH, Gaines JA. Theca cell tumors. *Am J Obstet Gynecol* 1928;35:39–51.

261. Banner EA, Dockerty MB. Theca cell tumors of the ovary. A clinical and pathologic study of twenty-three cases (including thirteen new cases) with a review. *Surg Gynecol Obstet* 1945;81:234–242.

262. Sternberg WH, Gaskill CJ. Theca-cell tumors. With a report of twelve new cases and observations on the possible etiologic role of ovarian stromal hyperplasia. *Am J Obstet Gynecol* 1950;59:575–587.

263. Björkholm E, Silfverswürd C. Theca-cell tumors. Clinical features and prognosis. *Acta Radiol Oncol Radiat Phys Biol* 1980;19:241–244.

264. Young RH, Clement PB, Scully RE. Calcified thecomas in young women: a report of four cases. *Int J Gynecol Pathol* 1988;7:343–350.

265. Waxman M, Vuletin JC, Urcuyo R, Belling CG. Ovarian low grade stromal sarcoma with thecomatous features. A critical reappraisal of the so-called "malignant thecoma." *Cancer* 1979;44:2206–2217.

266. Young RH, Scully RE. Ovarian sex-cord stromal tumors: recent progress. *Int J Gynecol Pathol* 1982;101–123.

267. Roth LM, Sternberg WH. Partly luteinized theca cell tumor of the ovary. *Cancer* 1983;51:1697–1704.

268. Scully RE. An unusual ovarian tumor containing Leydig cells but associated with endometrial hyperplasia in a postmenopausal woman. *J Clin Endocrinol Metab* 1953;13:1254–1263.

269. Hughesdon PE. Ovarian lipoid and theca cell tumors: their origins and interrelations. *Obstet Gynecol Surv* 1966;21:245–288.

270. Hughesdon PE. Lipid cell thecomas of the ovary. *Histopathology* 1983;7:681–692.

271. Chalvardjian A, Scully RE. Sclerosing stromal tumors of the ovary. *Cancer* 1973;31:664–670.

272. Gee DC, Russell P. Sclerosing stromal tumours of the ovary. *Histopathology* 1979;3:367–376.

273. Hsu C, Ma L, Mak L. Sclerosing stromal tumor of the ovary: case report and review of the literature. *Int J Gynecol Pathol* 1983;2:192–200.

274. Tiltman AJ. Sclerosing stromal tumor of the ovary: demonstration of Ligandin in three cases. *Int J Gynaecol Pathol* 1985;4:362–369.

275. Katayama I, Kimura Y, Hata T, Ikeda S. Sclerosing stromal tumor of the ovary. *Eur J Gynaecol Oncol* 1987;8:247–252.

276. Ramzy I. Signet-ring stromal tumor of ovary. Histochemical, light, and electron microscopic study. *Cancer* 1976;38:166–172.

277. Young RH, Scully RE. Ovarian Sertoli cell tumors. A report of ten cases. *Int J Gynecol Pathol* 1984;2:349–363.

278. Teilum G. Homologous ovarian and testicular tumors. III. Estrogen producing Sertoli cell tumors (androblastoma tubulare lipoides) of the human testis and ovary. *J Clin Endocrinol* 1949;9:301–318.

279. Tavassoli FA, Norris H. Sertoli tumors of the ovary. A clinicopathologic study of 28 cases with ultrastructural observations. *Cancer* 1980;46:2281–2297.

280. Solh HM, Azoury RS, Najjar SS. Peutz-Jeghers syndrome associated with precocious puberty. *J Pediatr* 1983;103:593–595.

281. Young RH, Scully RE. Ovarian tumors of probable wolffian origin. A report of 11 cases. *Am J Surg Pathol* 1983;7:125–135.

282. O'Hern TM, Neubecker RD. Arrhenoblastoma. *Obstet Gynecol* 1962;19:758–770.

283. Roth LM, Anderson MC, Govan ADT, Langley FA, Gowing NFC, Woodcock AS. Sertoli-Leydig cell tumors. A clinicopathologic study of 34 cases. *Cancer* 1981;48:187–197.

284. Zaloudek C, Norris HJ. Sertoli-Leydig tumors of the ovary. A clinicopathologic study of 64 intermediate and poorly differentiated neoplasms. *Am J Surg Pathol* 1984;8:405–418.

285. Young RH, Scully RE. Ovarian Sertoli-Leydig cell tumors: a clinicopathological analysis of 207 cases. *Am J Surg Pathol* 1985;9:543–569.

286. Young RH, Scully RE. Well-differentiated ovarian Sertoli-Leydig cell tumors: a clinicopathological analysis of 23 cases. *Int J Gynecol Pathol* 1984;3:277–290.

287. Dardi LE, Miller AW, Gould VE. Sertoli-Leydig cell tumor with endometrioid differentiation. *Diagn Gynecol Obstet* 1982;4:227–234.

288. Young RH, Scully RE. Ovarian Sertoli-Leydig cell tumors with a retiform pattern: A problem in histopathologic diagnosis. A report of 25 cases. *Am J Surg Pathol* 1983;7:755–771.

289. Young RH, Prat J, Scully RE. Ovarian Sertoli-Leydig cell tumors with heterologous elements (i). Gastrointestinal epithelium and carcinoid: a clinicopathologic analysis of thirty-six cases. *Cancer* 1982;50:2448–2456.

290. Waxman M, Damjanov I, Alpert L, Sardinsky T. Composite mucinous ovarian neoplasms associated with Sertoli-Leydig and carcinoid tumors. *Cancer* 1981;47:2044–2052.

291. Prat J, Young RH, Scully RE. Ovarian Sertoli-Leydig cell tumors with heterologous elements (ii). Cartilage and skeletal muscle: a clinicopathological analysis of twelve cases. *Cancer* 1982;50:2465–2475.

292. Young RH, Perez-Atayde AR, Scully RE. Ovarian Sertoli-Leydig cell tumor with retiform and heterologous components. Report of a case with hepatocytic differentiation and elevated serum alpha-fetoprotein. *Am J Surg Pathol* 1984;8:709–718.

293. Chadha S, Honnebier WJ, Schaberg A. Raised serum alpha-fetoprotein in Sertoli-Leydig cell tumor (androblastoma) of ovary: report of two cases. *Int J Gynecol Pathol* 1987;6:82–88.

294. Anderson MC, Rees DA. Gynandroblastoma of the ovary. *Br J Obstet Gynaecol* 1975;82:68–73.

295. Chalvardjian A, Derzko C. Gynandroblastoma. Its ultrastructure. *Cancer* 1982;50:710–721.

296. Talerman A, Hughesdon PE, Anderson MC. Diffuse nonlobular ovarian androblastoma usually associated with feminization. *Int J Gynecol Pathol* 1982;1:155–171.

297. Scully RE. Sex cord tumor with annular tubules. A distinctive ovarian tumor of the Peutz-Jeghers syndrome. *Cancer* 1970;25:1107–1121.

298. McGowan L, Young RH, Scully RE. Peutz-Jeghers syndrome with adenoma malignum of cervix. A report of two cases. *Gynecol Oncol* 1980;10:125–133.

299. Young RH, Welch WR, Dickersin GR, Scully RE. Ovarian sex cord tumor with annular tubules: review of 74 cases including 27 with Peutz-Jeghers syndrome and four with adenoma malignum of the cervix. *Cancer* 1982;50:1384–1402.

300. Hart WR, Kumar N, Crissman JD. Ovarian neoplasms resembling sex cord tumors with annular tubules. *Cancer* 1980;45:2352–2363.

301. Young RH, Dickersin GR, Scully RE. A distinctive ovarian sex cord-stromal tumor causing sexual precocity in the Peutz-Jeghers syndrome. *Am J Surg Pathol* 1985;7:233–243.

302. Scully RE. Ovarian tumors with endocrine manifestations. In: DeGroot LJ, ed. *Endocrinology*, 2nd edition. Orlando: Grune-Stratton Inc. 1988 (*in press*).

303. Hayes MC, Scully RE. Stromal luteoma of the ovary: a clinicopathological analysis of 25 cases. *Int J Gynecol Pathol* 1987;6:313–321.

304. Allander E, Wagermark J. Leydig cell tumors of the ovary. Report of three cases. *Acta Obstet Gynecol Scand* 1969;48:433–439.

305. Boivin Y, Richart RM. Hilus cell tumors of the ovary. A review with a report of 3 new cases. *Cancer* 1965;28:231.

306. Dunnihoo DR, Grieme DL, Woolf RB. Hilar-cell tumors of the ovary. Report of 2 new cases and a review of the world literature. *Obstet Gynecol* 1966;27:703.

307. Hayes MC, Scully RE. Ovarian steroid cell tumors, not otherwise specified (lipid cell tumors): a clinicopathological analysis of 63 cases. *Am J Surg Pathol* 1987;11:835–845.

308. Taylor HB, Norris HJ. Lipid cell tumors of the ovary. *Cancer* 1967;20:1953–1962.

309. Marieb HJ, Spangler S, Kashgarian M, Heiman A, Schwartz ML, Schwartz PE. Cushing's syndrome secondary to ectopic cortisol production by an ovarian carcinoma. *J Clin Endocrinol Metab* 1983;57:737–740.

310. Young RH, Scully RE. Ovarian steroid cell tumors associated with Cushing's syndrome: a report of three cases. *Int J Gynecol Pathol* 1987;6:40–48.

311. Rutgers JL, Scully RE. Cysts (cystadenomas) and tumors of the rete ovarii. *Int J Gynecol Pathol* 1988;7:330–342.

312. Case Records of the Massachusetts General Hospital. Case 11-1972. Dysgerminoma of left ovary, with syncytiotrophoblastic-like giant cells and minute focus of embryonal carcinoma and with luteinization of stroma. *N Engl J Med* 1972;286:594–600.

313. Brettell JR, Miles PA, Herrera G, et al. Dysgerminoma with syncytiotrophoblastic giant cells presenting as a hydatidiform mole. *Gynecol Oncol* 1984;18:393–401.

314. Zaloudek CJ, Tavassoli FA, Norris HJ. Dysgerminoma with syncytiotrophoblastic giant cells. A histologically and clinically distinctive subtype of dysgerminoma. *Am J Surg Pathol* 1981;5:361–367.

315. De Palo G, Lattuada A, Kenda R, et al. Germ cell tumors of the ovary: the experience of the national cancer institute of Milan. I. Dysgerminoma. *Int J Radiat Oncol Biol Phys* 1987;13:853–860.

316. Thomas GM, Dembo AJ, Hacker NF, et al. Current therapy for dysgerminoma of the ovary. *Obstet Gynecol* 1987;70:268–275.

317. LaPolla JP, Benda J, Vigliotti AP, et al. Dysgerminoma of the ovary. *Obstet Gynecol* 1987;69:859–867.

318. Mullin TJ, Lankerani MR. Ovarian dysgerminoma: immunocytochemical localization of human chorionic gonadotropin in the germinoma cell cytoplasm. *Obstet Gynecol* 1986;68:80S–83S.

319. Huntington RW, Bullock WK. Yolk sac tumors of the ovary. *Cancer* 1970;25:1357–1367.

320. Kurman RJ, Norris HJ. Endodermal sinus tumor of the ovary. A clinical and pathologic analysis of 71 cases. *Cancer* 1976;38:2404–2419.

321. Langley FA, Govan ADT, Anderson MC, et al. Yolk sac and allied tumours of the ovary. *Histopathology* 1981;5:389–401.

322. Ulbright TM, Roth LM, Brodhecker CA. Yolk sac differentiation in germ cell tumors. A morphologic study of 50 cases with emphasis on hepatic, enteric, and parietal yolk sac features. *Am J Surg Pathol* 1986;10:151–164.

323. Gershenson DM, Del Junco G, Herson J, et al. Endodermal sinus tumor of the ovary: the M.D. Anderson experience. *Obstet Gynecol* 1983;61:194–202.

324. Clement PB, Young RH, Scully RE. Endometrioid-like yolk sac tumor of the ovary. A clinicopathological analysis of eight cases. *Am J Surg Pathol* 1987;11:767–778.

325. Nogales FF Jr, Matilla A, Nogales-Ortiz F, et al. Yolk sac tumors with pure and mixed polyvesicular vitelline patterns. *Hum Pathol* 1978;9:553–566.

326. Nakashima N, Fukatsu T, Nagasaki T, et al. The frequency and

histology of hepatic tissue in germ cell tumors. *Am J Surg Pathol* 1987;11:682–692.

327. Kurman RJ, Norris HJ. Embryonal carcinoma of the ovary. A clinicopathologic entity distinct from endodermal sinus tumor resembling embryonal carcinoma of the adult testis. *Cancer* 1976;38:2420–2433.

328. Nakakuma K, Tashiro S, Uemura K, et al. Alpha-fetoprotein and human chorionic gonadotropin in embryonal carcinoma of the ovary. An 8-year survival case. *Cancer* 1983;52:1470–1472.

329. Takeda A, Ishizuka T, Goto T, et al. Polyembryoma of ovary producing alpha-fetoprotein and HCG: immunoperoxidase and electron microscopic study. *Cancer* 1982;14:1878–1889.

330. Vance RP, Geisinger KR. Pure nongestational choriocarcinoma of the ovary. Report of a case. *Cancer* 1985;56:2321–2325.

331. Jacobs AJ, Newland JR, Green RK. Pure choriocarcinoma of the ovary. *Obstet Gynecol Surv* 1982;37:603–609.

332. Civantos F, Rywlin A. Carcinomas with trophoblastic differentiation and secretion of chorionic gonadotrophins. *Cancer* 1972;29:789–798.

333. Norris HJ, Zirkin HJ, Benson WL. Immature (malignant) teratoma of the ovary. A clinical and pathologic study of 58 cases. *Cancer* 1976;37:2359–2372.

334. Yanai-Inbar I, Scully RE. Relation of ovarian dermoid cysts and immature teratomas: an analysis of 350 cases of immature teratoma and 10 cases of dermoid cyst with microscopic foci of immature tissue. *Int J Gynecol Pathol* 1987;6:203–212.

335. Perrone T, Steiner M, Dehner LP. Nodal gliomatosis and alpha-fetoprotein production. Two unusual facets of grade I ovarian teratoma. *Arch Pathol Lab Med* 1986;110:975–977.

336. Gershenson DM, Del Junco G, Silva EG, et al. Immature teratoma of the ovary. *Obstet Gynecol* 1986;68:624–629.

337. Robboy SJ, Scully RE. Ovarian teratoma with glial implants on the peritoneum. *Hum Pathol* 1970;1:643–653.

338. Nogales FF Jr, Favara BE, Major FJ, et al. Immature teratoma of the ovary with a neural component ("solid" teratoma). A clinicopathologic study of 20 cases. *Hum Pathol* 1976;7:625–642.

339. Thurlbeck WM, Scully RE. Solid teratoma of the ovary. A clinicopathological analysis of 9 cases. *Cancer* 1960;13:804–811.

340. Steeper TA, Mukai K. Solid ovarian teratomas: an immunocytochemical study of thirteen cases with clinicopathologic correlation. In: Sommers SC, Rosen PP, eds. *Pathology annual, part 1.* New York: Appleton-Century-Crofts, 1984:81–92.

341. Nielsen SNJ, Scheithauer BW, Gaffey TA. Gliomatosis peritonei. *Cancer* 1985;56:2499–2503.

342. Boehner JF, Gallup DG, Talledo OE, et al. Solid ovarian teratoma with neuroglial metastases to periaortic lymph nodes and omentum. *South Med J* 1987;80:649–652.

343. Pantoja E, Noy MA, Axtmayer RW, et al. I. Ovarian dermoids and their complications. Comprehensive historical review. *Obstet Gynecol Surv* 1975;30:1–20.

344. Payne D, Muss HB, Homesley HD, et al. Autoimmune hemolytic anemia and ovarian dermoid cysts. Case report and review of the literature. *Cancer* 1981;48:721–724.

345. Krumerman MS, Chung A. Squamous carcinoma arising in benign cystic teratoma of the ovary. A report of four cases and review of the literature. *Cancer* 1977;39:1237–1242.

346. Woodfield B, Katz DA, Cantrell CJ, et al. A benign cystic teratoma with gastrointestinal tract development. *Am J Clin Pathol* 1985;83:236–240.

347. Abbott TM, Hermann WJ, Scully RE. Ovarian fetiform teratoma (homunculus) in a 9-year-old girl. *Int J Gynecol Pathol* 1984;2:392–402.

348. Ulirsch RC, Goldman RL. An unusual teratoma of the ovary: neurogenic cyst with lactating breast tissue. *Obstet Gynecol* 1982;60:400–402.

349. Brumback RA, Brown BS, di Sant'Agnese A. Unique finding of prostatic tissue in a benign cystic ovarian teratoma. *Arch Pathol Lab Med* 1985;109:675–677.

350. Axiotis CA, Lippes HA, Merino MJ, et al. Corticotroph cell pituitary adenoma within an ovarian teratoma. A new cause of Cushing's syndrome. *Am J Surg Pathol* 1987;11:218–224.

351. Genadry R, Parmley T, Woodruff JD. Secondary malignancies in benign cystic teratomas. *Gynecol Oncol* 1979;8:246–251.

352. Tsukamoto N, Matsukuma K, Matsumura M, et al. Primary

malignant melanoma arising in cystic teratoma of the ovary. *Gynecol Oncol* 1986;23:395–400.

353. Peterson WF. Malignant degeneration of benign cystic teratomas of the ovary. A collective review of the literature. *Obstet Gynecol Surv* 1957;12:793–830.

354. Ueda G, Sato Y, Yamasaki M, et al. Malignant fibrous histiocytoma arising in a benign cystic teratoma of the ovary. *Gynecol Oncol* 1977;5:313–322.

355. Climie ARW, Heath LP. Malignant degeneration of benign cystic teratomas of the ovary. Review of the literature and report of a chondrosarcoma and carcinoid tumor. *Cancer* 1968;22:824–832.

356. Seifer DB, Weiss LM, Kempson KL. Malignant lymphoma arising within thyroid tissue in a mature cystic teratoma. *Cancer* 1986;58:2459–2461.

357. Feuerstein IM, Aronson BL, McCarthy EF. Bilateral ovarian cystic teratomata mimicking bilateral pure ovarian hemangiomata: case report. *Int J Gynecol Pathol* 1984;3:393–397.

358. Gonzalez-Angulo A, Kaufman RH, Braungart CD, et al. Adenocarcinoma of thyroid arising in struma ovarii (malignant struma ovarii). Report of two cases and review of the literature. *Obstet Gynecol* 1963;21:567–576.

359. Hasleton PS, Kelehan P, Whittaker JS, et al. Benign and malignant struma ovarii. *Arch Pathol Lab Med* 1978;102:180–184.

360. Pardo-Mindan FJ, Vazquez JJ. Malignant struma ovarii. Light and electron microscopic study. *Cancer* 1983;51:337–343.

361. Yannopoulos D, Yannopoulos K, Ossowski R. Malignant struma ovarii. In: Sommers SC, Rosen PP, eds. *Pathology annual.* New York: Appleton-Century-Crofts, 1976:403–413.

362. Willemse PHB, Oosterhuis JW, Aalders JG, et al. Malignant struma ovarii treated by ovariectomy, thyroidectomy, and ^{131}I administration. *Cancer* 1987;60:178–182.

363. Moon S, Waxman M. Mixed ovarian tumor composed of Brenner and thyroid elements. *Cancer* 1976;38:1997–2001.

364. Nieminen U, Von Numers C, Widholm O. Struma ovarii. *Acta Obstet Gynecol Scand* 1963;42:399–424.

365. Robboy SJ, Norris HJ, Scully RE. Insular carcinoid primary in the ovary. A clinicopathologic analysis of 48 cases. *Cancer* 1975;36:404–418.

366. Ulbright TM, Roth LM, Ehrlich CE. Ovarian strumal carcinoid. An immunocytochemical and ultrastructural study of two cases. *Am J Clin Pathol* 1982;77:622–631.

367. Robboy SJ, Scully RE. Strumal carcinoid of the ovary: an analysis of 50 cases of a distinctive tumor composed of thyroid tissue and carcinoid. *Cancer* 1980;46:2019–2034.

368. Brown H, Lane M. Cushing's and malignant carcinoid syndromes from ovarian neoplasm. *Arch Intern Med* 1965;115:490–494.

369. Alenghat E, Okagaki T, Talerman A. Primary mucinous carcinoid tumor of the ovary. *Cancer* 1986;58:777–783.

370. Talerman A. Carcinoid tumors of the ovary. *J Cancer Res Clin Oncol* 1984;107:125–135.

371. Robboy SJ, Scully RE, Norris HJ. Primary trabecular carcinoid of the ovary. *Obstet Gynecol* 1977;49:202–207.

372. Robboy SJ. Insular carcinoid of ovary associated with malignant mucinous tumors. *Cancer* 1984;54:2273–2276.

373. Stagno PA, Petras RE, Hart WR. Strumal carcinoids of the ovary. An immunohistologic and ultrastructural study. *Arch Pathol Lab Med* 1987;111:440–446.

374. Snyder RR, Tavassoli FA. Ovarian strumal carcinoid: immunohistochemical, ultrastructural, and clinicopathologic observations. *Int J Gynecol Pathol* 1986;5:187–201.

375. Talerman A, Evans MI. Primary trabecular carcinoid tumor of the ovary. *Cancer* 1982;50:1403–1407.

376. Talerman A, Okagaki T. Ultrastructural features of primary trabecular carcinoid tumor of the ovary. *Int J Gynecol Pathol* 1985;4:153–160.

377. Dayal Y, Tashjian AH Jr, Wolfe HJ. Immunocytochemical localization of calcitonin-producing cells in a strumal carcinoid with amyloid stroma. *Cancer* 1979;43:1331–1338.

378. Czernobilsky B, Segal M, Dgani R. Primary ovarian carcinoid with marked heterogeneity of microscopic features. *Cancer* 1984;54:585–589.

379. Sorrong B, Falkmer S, Robboy SJ, et al. Neurohormonal peptides in ovarian carcinoids: an immunohistochemical study of 81

primary carcinoids and of intraovarian metastases from six midgut carcinoids. *Cancer* 1982;49:68–74.

380. Inoue M, Ueda G, Nakajima T. Immunohistochemical demonstration of neuron-specific enolase in gynecologic malignant tumors. *Cancer* 1985;55:1686–1690.

381. Aguirre P, Scully RE. Malignant neuroectodermal tumor of the ovary, a distinctive form of monodermal teratoma. Report of five cases. *Am J Surg Pathol* 1982;6:283–292.

382. Dekmezian R, Sneige N, Ordonez NG. Ovarian and omental ependymomas in peritoneal washings: cytologic and immunocytochemical features. *Diagn Cytopathol* 1986;2:62–68.

383. Kleinman GM, Young RH, Scully RE. Neuroepithelial tumors arising in the female genital tract [Abstract]. *J Neuropathol Exp Neurol* 1980;39:367.

384. Kleinman GM, Young RH, Scully RE. Ependymoma of the ovary: report of three cases. *Hum Pathol* 1984;15:632–638.

385. Hart MN, Earle KM. Primitive neuroectodermal tumors of the brain in children. *Cancer* 1973;32:890–897.

386. Kaku T, Toyoshima S, Hachisuga T, et al. Sebaceous gland tumor of the ovary. *Gynecol Oncol* 1987;26:398–402.

387. King ME, Mouradian JA, Micha JP, et al. Immature teratoma of the ovary with predominant malignant retinal anlage component. A parthenogenically derived tumor. *Am J Surg Pathol* 1985;9:221–231.

388. Karten G, Sher JH, Marsh MR, et al. Neurogenic cyst of the ovary. A rare form of benign cystic teratoma. *Arch Pathol* 1968;86:563–567.

389. Tiltman AJ. Ependymal cyst of the ovary. *S Afr Med J* 1985;68:424–425.

390. Clement PB, Dimmick JE. Endodermal variant of mature cystic teratoma of the ovary. Report of a case. *Cancer* 1979;43:383–385.

391. Nogales FF Jr, Silverberg SG. Epidermoid cysts of the ovary. A report of five cases with histogenetic considerations and ultrastructural findings. *Am J Obstet Gynecol* 1976;124:523–528.

392. Young RH, Prat J, Scully RE. Epidermoid cyst of the ovary. A report of three cases with comments on histogenesis. *Am J Clin Pathol* 1980;73:272–276.

393. Kurman RJ, Norris HJ. Malignant mixed germ cell tumors of the ovary. A clinical and pathologic analysis of 30 cases. *Obstet Gynecol* 1976;48:579–589.

394. Gershenson DM, Del Junco G, Copeland LJ, et al. Mixed germ cell tumors of the ovary. *Obstet Gynecol* 1984;64:200–206.

395. Ueda G, Yamasaki M, Inoue M, et al. A rare malignant ovarian mixed germ cell tumor containing pancreatic tissue with islet cells. *Int J Gynecol Pathol* 1984;3:220–231.

396. Scully RE. Gonadoblastoma. A review of 74 cases. *Cancer* 1970;25:1340–1356.

397. Bhathena D, Haning RV Jr, Shapiro S. Coexistence of a gonadoblastoma and mixed germ cell-sex cord stroma tumor. *Pathol Res Pract* 1985;180:203–206.

398. Talerman A. Gonadoblastoma associated with embryonal carcinoma. *Obstet Gynecol* 1974;43:138–142.

399. Hart WR, Burkons DM. Germ cell neoplasms arising in gonadoblastomas. *Cancer* 1979;43:669–789.

400. Kedzia H. Gonadoblastoma: structures and background of development. *Am J Obstet Gynecol* 1983;147:81–85.

401. Talerman A, van der Harten JJ. A mixed germ cell-sex cord stroma tumor of the ovary associated with isosexual precocious puberty in a normal girl. *Cancer* 1977;40:889–894.

402. Talerman A. A distinctive gonadal neoplasm related to gonadoblastoma. *Cancer* 1972;30:1219–1224.

403. Tokuoka S, Aoki Y, Hayaski Y, et al. A mixed germ cell-sex cord-stromal tumor of the ovary with retiform tubular structure: a case report. *Int J Gynecol Pathol* 1985;4:161–170.

404. Talerman A. A combined germ cell-gonadal stromal-epithelial tumor of the ovary or a hamartoma [Letter]. *Am J Surg Pathol* 1984;8:638–639.

405. Fallahzadeh H, Dockerty MB, Lee RA. Leiomyoma of the ovary: report of five cases and review of the literature. *Am J Obstet Gynecol* 1972;113:394–398.

406. Tsalacopoulos G, Tiltman AJ. Leiomyoma of the ovary. A report of 3 cases. *S Afr Med J* 1981;59:574–575.

407. Miyauchi J, Mukai M, Yamazaki K, Kosi I, Higashi S, Hori S.

408. Talerman A. Nonspecific tumors of the ovary, including mesenchymal tumors and malignant lymphoma. In: Kurman RJ, ed. *Blaustein's pathology of the female genital tract,* 3rd edition. New York: Springer-Verlag, 1987:772–741.

409. Azoury RS, Woodruff JD. Primary ovarian sarcomas. Report of 43 cases from the Emil Novak Ovarian Tumor Registry. *Obstet Gynecol* 1971;37:920–941.

410. Nieminen V, von Numers C, Purola E. Primary sarcoma of the ovary. *Acta Obstet Gynecol Scand* 1969;48:423–432.

411. Kraemer BB, Silva EG, Sneige N. Fibrosarcoma of ovary. A new component in the nevoid basal-cell carcinoma syndrome. *Am J Surg Pathol* 1984;8:231–236.

412. Miles PA, Kiley KC, Mena H. Giant fibrosarcoma of the ovary. *Int J Gynecol Pathol* 1985;4:83–87.

413. Reddy SA, Poon TP, Ramaswamy G, Tchertkoff V. Leiomyosarcoma of the ovary. *NY State J Med* 1985;85:218–220.

414. Stone GC, Bell DA, Fuller A, Dickersin GR, Scully RE. Malignant Schwannoma of the ovary. Report of a case. *Cancer* 1986;58:1575–1582.

415. Ongkasuwan C, Taylor JE, Tang C-K, Prempree T. Angiosarcomas of the uterus and ovary: clinicopathologic report. *Cancer* 1982;49:1469–1475.

416. Guerard MJ, Arguelles MA, Ferenczy A. Rhabdomyosarcoma of the ovary: ultrastructural study of a case and review of the literature. *Gynecol Oncol* 1983;15:325–339.

417. Talerman A, Auerbach WM, Van Meurs AJ. Primary chondrosarcoma of the ovary. *Histopathology* 1981;5:319–324.

418. Chorlton I, Norris HJ, King FM. Malignant reticuloendothelial diseases involving the ovary as a primary manifestation. A series of 19 lymphomas and one granulocytic sarcoma. *Cancer* 1974;34:397–407.

419. Osborne BM, Robboy SJ. Lymphomas or leukemia presenting as ovarian tumors. An analysis of 42 cases. *Cancer* 1983;52:1933–1943.

420. Cecalupo AJ, Frankel LS, Sullivan P. Pelvic and ovarian extramedullary leukemic relapse in young girls. *Cancer* 1982;50:587–593.

421. Dickersin GR, Kline IW, Scully RE. Small cell carcinoma of the ovary with hypercalcemia. A report of eleven cases. *Cancer* 1982;49:188–197.

421a. McMahon JT, Hart WR. Ultrastructural analysis of small cell carcinomas of the ovary. *Am J Clin Pathol* 1988;90:523–529.

421b. Aguirre P, Thor AD, Scully RE. Ovarian small cell carcinoma: Histogenetic considerations based on immunohistochemical and other findings. *Am J Clin Pathol* 1989;92:140–149.

421c. Young RH, Scully RE. Alveolar rhabdomyosarcoma metastatic to the ovary. A report of two cases and a discussion of the differential diagnosis of small cell malignant tumors of the ovary. *Cancer* 1989;64:899–904.

422. Hughesdon PE. Ovarian tumours of wolffian or allied nature: their place in ovarian oncology. *J Clin Pathol* 1982;35:526–535.

423. Kariminejad MH, Scully RE. Female adnexal tumor of probable wolffian origin. A distinctive pathologic entity. *Cancer* 1973;31:671–677.

424. Novak E, Gray LA. Krukenberg tumors of the ovary. Clinical and pathological study of 21 cases. *Surg Gynecol Obstet* 1938;66:157–167.

425. Diddle AW. Krukenberg tumors: Diagnostic problem. *Cancer* 1955;8:1026–1034.

426. Hale RW. Krukenberg tumor of the ovaries. A review of 81 records. *Obstet Gynecol* 1968;32:221–225.

427. Karsh J. Secondary malignant disease of the ovaries. A study of 72 autopsies. *Am J Obstet Gynecol* 1951;61:154–160.

428. Leffel JM Jr, Masson JC, Dockerty MB. Krukenberg tumors. A survey of forty-four cases. *Ann Surg* 1942;115:102–113.

429. Yakusshiji M, Tazaki T, Nishimura H, Kato T. Krukenberg tumors of the ovary: a clinicopathological analysis of 112 cases. *Acta Obstet Gynaecol Jpn* 1987;39:479–485.

430. Joshi VV. Primary Krukenberg tumor of ovary. Review of literature and case report. *Cancer* 1968;22:1199–1207.

431. Bullon A, Arseneau J, Prat J, Young RH, Scully RE. Tubular

Krukenberg tumor. A problem in histopathologic diagnosis. *Am J Surg Pathol* 1981;5:225–232.

432. Burt CAV. Prophylactic oophorectomy with resection of the large bowel for cancer. *Am J Surg* 1951;82:571–577.

433. Cutait R, Lesser ML, Enker WE. Prophylactic oophorectomy in surgery for large-bowel cancer. *Dis Colon Rectum* 1983;26:6–11.

434. Graffner HOL, Alm POA, Oscarson JEA. Prophylactic oophorectomy in colorectal carcinoma. *Am J Surg* 1983;146:233–235.

435. Harcourt KF, Dennis DL. Laparotomy for "ovarian tumors" in unsuspected carcinoma of the colon. *Cancer* 1968;21:1244–1246.

436. O'Brien PH, Newton BB, Metcalf JS, Rittenbury MS. Oophorectomy in women with carcinoma of the colon and rectum. *Surg Gynecol Obstet* 1981;153:827–830.

437. Johansson H. Clinical aspects of metastatic ovarian cancer of extragenital origin. *Acta Obstet Gynecol Scand* 1960;39:681–697.

438. Ulbright TM, Roth LM. Secondary tumors of the ovary. In: Roth LM, Czernobilsky B, eds. *Tumors and tumor-like conditions of the ovary.* Contemporary Issues in Surgical Pathology, No. 6. New York: Churchill Livingstone, 1985:129–152.

439. Blamey SL, McDermott FT, Pihl E, Hughes SR. Resected ovarian recurrence from colorectal adenocarcinoma: A study of 13 cases. *Dis Colon Rectum* 1981;24:272–275.

440. Scully RE, Richardson GS. Luteinization of the stroma of metastatic cancer involving the ovary and its endocrine significance. *Cancer* 1961;14:827–840.

441. Robboy SJ, Scully RE, Norris HJ. Carcinoid metastatic to the ovary. A clinicopathologic analysis of 35 cases. *Cancer* 1974;33:798–811.

442. Lee YN, Hori JM. Significance of ovarian metastases in therapeutic oophorectomy for advanced breast cancer. *Cancer* 1971;27:1374–1378.

443. Puga FJ, Gibbs CP, Williams TJ. Castrating operations associated with metastatic lesions of the breast. *Obstet Gynecol* 1973;41:713–719.

444. Lumb G, Mackenzie DH. The incidence of metastases in adrenal glands and ovaries removed for carcinoma of the breast. *Cancer* 1959;12:521–526.

445. Brickman M, Ferreira B. Metastasis of breast carcinoma to the ovaries—incidence, significance, and relationship to survival. A preliminary study. *Grace Hosp Bull* 1967;45:44–49.

446. Young RH, Carey RW, Robboy SJ. Breast carcinoma masquerading as a primary ovarian neoplasm. *Cancer* 1981;48:210–212.

447. Harris M, Howell A, Chrissohou M, Swindell RIC, Hudson M, Sellwood RA. A comparison of the metastatic pattern of infiltrating lobular carcinoma and infiltrating duct carcinoma of the breast. *Br J Cancer* 1984;50:23–30.

448. Hirschfield LS, Kahn LB, Winkler B, Bochner RZ, Gibstein AA. Adenocarcinoid of the appendix presenting as bilateral Krukenberg tumor of the ovaries. *Arch Pathol Lab Med* 1985;109:930–933.

449. Merino MJ, Edmonds P, LiVolsi V. Appendiceal carcinoma metastatic to the ovaries and mimicking primary ovarian tumors. *Int J Gynecol Pathol* 1985;4:110–120.

449a. Young RH, Hart WR. Metastases from carcinomas of the pancreas simulating primary mucinous tumors of the ovary: A report of seven cases. *Am J Surg Pathol* 1989;13:748–756.

449b. Young RH, Scully RE. Ovarian metastases from carcinoma of the gallbladder and extrahepatic bile ducts simulating primary tumors of the ovary: A report of six cases. *Int J Gynecol Pathol* 1990;9:60–72.

450. Hameed K. Melanotic ovarian neoplasms. *Prog Clin Cancer* 1973;5:209–217.

451. Fitzgibbons PL, Martin SE, Simmons TJ. Malignant melanoma metastatic to the ovary. *Am J Surg Pathol* 1987;11:959–964.

452. Beck RP, Latour JPA. Necropsy reports on 36 cases of endometrial carcinoma. *Am J Obstet Gynecol* 1963;85:307–311.

453. Bunker ML. The terminal findings in endometrial carcinoma. *Am J Obstet Gynecol* 1959;77:530–538.

454. Eifel P, Hendrickson M, Ross J, Ballon S, Martinez A, Kempson R. Simultaneous presentation of carcinoma involving the ovary and the uterine corpus. *Cancer* 1982;50:163–170.

455. Ulbright TM, Roth LM. Metastatic and independent cancers of the endometrium and ovary: a clinicopathologic study of 34 cases. *Hum Pathol* 1985;16:28–34.

456. Zaino RJ, Unger ER, Whitney C. Synchronous carcinomas of the uterine corpus and ovary. *Gynecol Oncol* 1984;19:329–335; 1985;21:337–350.

457. Mazur MT, Hsueh S, Gersell DJ. Metastases to the female genital tract. Analysis of 325 cases. *Cancer* 1984;53:1978–1984.

458. Sedlis A. Primary carcinoma of the fallopian tube. *Obstet Gynecol Surv* 1961;16:209–226.

459. Green TH Jr, Scully RE. Tumors of the fallopian tube. *Clin Obstet Gynecol* 1962;5:886–906.

460. Scully RE. Androgenic lesions of the ovary. In: Grady HG, Smith DE, eds. *The Ovary.* International Academy of Pathology Monograph No. 3. Baltimore: Williams & Wilkins, 1962.

461. Young RH, Scully RE. *Ovarian sex cord–stromal tumors: problems in differential diagnosis.* Pathology Annual. Norwalk, CT: Appleton-Century-Crofts, 1988;23 (Part 1):237–296.

462. Young RH, Scully RE. Ovarian sex cord–stromal and steroid cell tumors. In: Roth LM, Czernobilsky B, eds. *Tumors and tumor-like conditions of the ovary.* New York: Churchill-Livingstone, 1985;43–73.

463. Young RH. *Update on ovarian sex cord–stromal tumors.* Pathology Update Series, vol. 27. Princeton, NJ: Continuing Professional Education Center, Inc., 1985.

464. Young RH, Scully RE. Sex cord stromal, steroid cell, and other ovarian tumors with endocrine, paraendocrine, and paraneoplastic manifestations. In: Kurman RJ, ed. *Blaustein's pathology of the female genital tract,* 3rd edition. New York: Springer-Verlag, 1987;607–658.

*Surgical Pathology of the Female
Reproductive System and Peritoneum,*
edited by Stephen S. Sternberg
and Stacey E. Mills. Raven Press, Ltd,
New York © 1991.

CHAPTER 7

The Fallopian Tube and Broad Ligament

Robert H. Young, Philip B. Clement, and Robert E. Scully

INFLAMMATORY DISEASES

Acute Salpingitis

Acute salpingitis may be secondary to sexually transmitted infection by *Neisseria gonorrhoeae, Chlamydia,* or *Mycoplasma.* Alternately, it may result from infection by streptococci, staphylococci, coliform bacilli, and anaerobic bacteria that reach the tubes by way of lymphatic or blood vessels, especially after an abortion or pregnancy (1–3). The tube is typically enlarged, edematous, and erythematous (Fig. 1), frequently with fibrinopurulent serosal and luminal exudate. It is often adherent to adjacent tissues, including the ovary, which may be involved as part of a tubo-ovarian abscess. Microscopic examination reveals a marked neutrophilic infiltration of the tubal plicae associated with congestion and edema. The mucosa may be ulcerated with purulent exudate in the lumen. The epithelium is often hyperplastic and may exhibit reactive atypia, occasionally simulating carcinoma (see below). In some cases of salpingitis, chlamydial antigens have been demonstrable with immunoperoxidase staining (4).

Acute inflammatory cells may be seen in the lumen and lamina propria of the tube during menstruation, during the puerperium (5,6), and, occasionally, to a lesser extent, throughout the menstrual cycle (7). In these cases of "physiologic salpingitis" (5–7), edema and lymphatic dilatation in the tubal plicae are usually present as well. The inflammation, which is maximal at mid-menstruation, only rarely involves the muscularis, is unaccompanied by necrosis or ulceration, and is not followed by chronic inflammatory-cell infiltration.

Chronic Salpingitis

In chronic salpingitis, the tube is usually enlarged, distorted, and adherent to the ovary and adjacent tissues (Fig. 2). If infection has obliterated the ostium, there may be a hydrosalpinx or a pyosalpinx. Hydrosalpinx is typically bilateral (Fig. 3). Resolution of a tubo-ovarian abscess may result in a tubo-ovarian cyst. Microscopic examination of the tube reveals shortened, blunted, and fibrotic plicae containing chronic inflammatory cells. Plical fusion produces pseudoglandular spaces [chronic follicular salpingitis (Fig. 4)]. In hydrosalpinx, only a few small plicae usually remain, and the lining epithelium is typically flattened or low cuboidal. Late stages of chronic salpingitis may result in fibrous obliteration of the lumen, typically in the cornual-isthmic region.

Granulomatous Salpingitis

Mycobacterial

The most common cause of granulomatous salpingitis is mycobacterium tuberculosis or mycobacterium bovis; 80% to 90% of women with genital tuberculosis have tubal involvement (8), and the process is bilateral in 90% of cases (8–10). Early or mild infection results in irregular thickening or nodularity of the wall; serosal tubercles are visible in about 20% of the cases (9). In more severe forms of tuberculous salpingitis, there may be dense tubo-ovarian adhesions, a thickened wall, ulcerated mucosa, and a caseous luminal exudate. The ostium of the tube generally remains open. On micro-

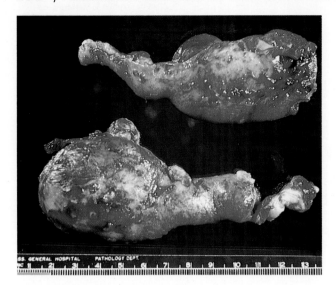

FIG. 1. Acute and chronic salpingitis. Both tubes are distended, and there is closure of the fimbriated ends, extensive congestion, and hemorrhage on the serosal surfaces.

scopic examination, tuberculous granulomas, which may be caseating, are characteristic (Figs. 5 and 6); a marked epithelial hyperplasia may simulate adenocarcinoma (Fig. 5) (see below), and Schaumann bodies may be conspicuous. The muscularis shows varying degrees of chronic inflammation and fibrosis. The diagnosis should be confirmed with special stains or culture. The differential diagnosis includes very rare cases of leprous salpingitis (11).

Actinomycosis

Actinomycosis of the fallopian tube is encountered most often in patients wearing an intrauterine contraceptive device (12,13). The disease is bilateral in almost

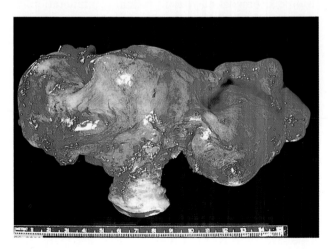

FIG. 2. Chronic salpingo-oophoritis. Both tubes and ovaries are bound down in hemorrhagic adhesions that largely obscure the tube on one side.

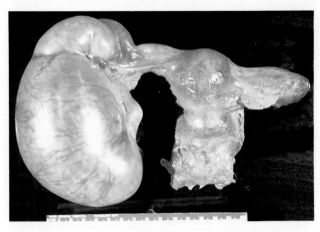

FIG. 3. Unilateral hydrosalpinx. The tube is markedly dilated and thin-walled.

half the cases (12) and frequently involves the ovaries. The only specific gross finding is small yellow flecks ("sulfur granules") within the luminal exudate. A fistulous communication with the bowel, urinary bladder, or skin may be present. Microscopically, the diagnostic granules are composed of gram-positive filamentous bacteria surrounded by a purulent exudate; a typical granulomatous response is rare.

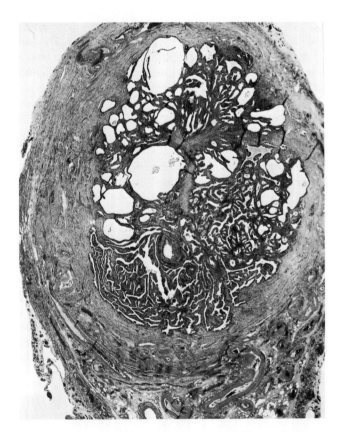

FIG. 4. Chronic follicular salpingitis. The tubal plicae are adherent to one another, and variably sized follicle-like spaces have resulted. (From ref. 10.)

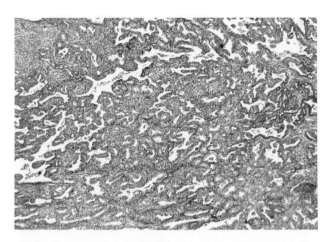

FIG. 5. Tuberculous salpingitis. The plicae contain tubercles (*upper left*) with marked epithelial hyperplasia simulating the appearance of adenocarcinoma.

Fungal Infections

Fungi rarely cause granulomatous salpingitis, with blastomycosis and, more commonly, coccidioidomycosis reported in the American literature (14–17). Typically, a tubo-ovarian abscess or inflammatory tubo-ovarian mass is associated with tubercle-like nodules on the peritoneal surfaces. The causative organisms are generally identifiable on microscopic examination.

Parasitic Infestations

Schistosomiasis of the tube is rare in the United States but common in areas of endemic disease (18,19). *Schistosoma haematobium* is the usual agent. Grossly, the tube may exhibit nodularity or scarring due to the fibrosis elicited by the deposition of ova. Microscopically, there is a granulomatous reaction to the characteristic ova (20).

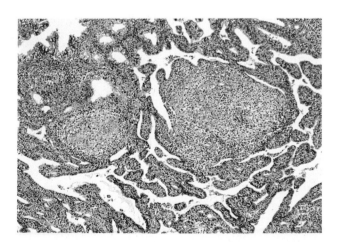

FIG. 6. Tuberculous salpingitis. Note granulomas within inflamed plicae.

Involvement of the tube by *Enterobius vermicularis* is probably secondary to migration of the pinworm from the lower female genital tract. Infestation may cause a nodular thickening of the wall (21); seeding of the pelvic peritoneum by ova with surrounding reaction may simulate tubercles. Fragments of worms or ova are surrounded by necrotic debris, an eosinophil-rich infiltrate, foreign-body giant cells, granulation tissue, and fibrous tissue. Cysticercosis of the tube has also been reported (22).

Foreign-Body Salpingitis

Granulomatous salpingitis may result when irritative agents such as lubricant jellies, mineral oil, powder containing talc or starch, and radiographic contrast media are introduced into the genital tract (Fig. 7) (23–25). Grossly, the tube may have a yellow or a chocolate-brown appearance suggesting endometriosis. When lipid material is causative, numerous foamy histiocytes in the mucosa are characteristic. Typically, a foreign-body giant-cell reaction is present and may extend to the serosa. Although so-called lipoid salpingitis usually results from the introduction of foreign material, occasional lipoid granulomas have been reported in gonococcal

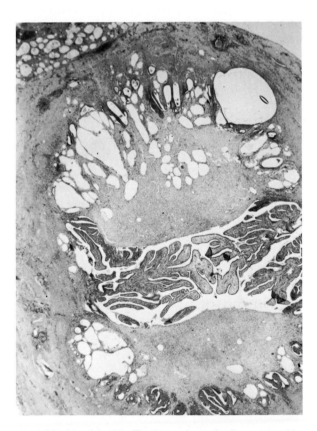

FIG. 7. Lipoid salpingitis. The lumen is markedly narrowed by a granulomatous reaction to oily contrast medium (clear spaces). (From ref. 10.)

and tuberculous salpingitis (24). Thus an infectious process should be excluded before attributing the lesion to foreign material.

Other Causes of Granulomatous Salpingitis

Other causes of granulomatous salpingitis include involvement by Crohn's disease (26) and sarcoidosis (27,28). With regard to the distinction between sarcoidosis and tuberculosis it should be remembered that Schaumann bodies may be seen in tuberculosis. Diffuse infiltration of the endosalpinx by histiocytes can be seen in chronic pelvic inflammatory disease (xanthogranulomatous salpingitis) (29–31) and malacoplakia (32,33). Numerous pigmented histiocytes (pseudoxanthoma cells) containing lipofuscin (ceroid) may be encountered in the tubal mucosa in pelvic endometriosis (34,35) and after pelvic irradiation (36). Tubal palisading granulomas with central necrosis have been described secondary to tubal diathermy (37). A granulomatous reaction may also be encountered in small to medium-sized arteries in cases of giant-cell arteritis (38).

Changes Secondary to Ligation

Following ligation the fallopian tube may develop proximal luminal dilatation, plical attenuation with pseudopolyp formation and chronic inflammation, and plical thickening in the distal tubal segment (39). These changes become more pronounced with increasing postoperative intervals.

TUMOR-LIKE LESIONS

Amyloidosis

Involvement of the fallopian tube by amyloidosis is rare. In one unusual case, a 47-year-old woman had heavy menstrual bleeding with extensive amyloidosis of the genital organs, appendix, and omentum (40).

Salpingitis Isthmica Nodosa (SIN)

This lesion is of uncertain pathogenesis and may cause infertility or predispose to ectopic pregnancy. It usually occurs in young women with a mean age of 26 years (41–44). SIN typically appears as one or more yellow-white nodular swellings up to 2 cm in diameter in the tubal isthmus, but it may be grossly inconspicuous. It is bilateral in approximately 85% (44). Microscopically, glands lined by tubal epithelium lie within hyperplastic smooth muscle (Fig. 8). Occasionally, glands are surrounded by endometrial-type stroma or are cystically dilated. Serial sectioning shows that the glands are diverticula that communicate with the tubal

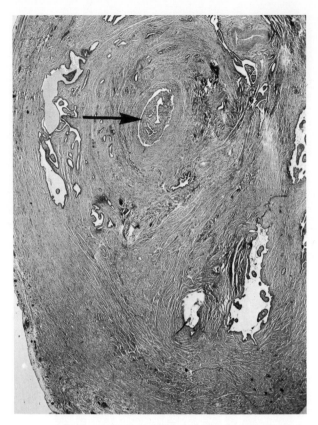

FIG. 8. Salpingitis isthmica nodosa. The tubal isthmic lumen (*arrow*) is surrounded by numerous small, gland-like diverticula that extend deeply into the muscularis. (From ref. 10.)

lumen. SIN should be easily distinguished from carcinoma by the regular distribution of its widely spaced glands, the lack of significant cellular atypia, and the absence of a stromal response (Fig. 9). SIN accompanied by severe tubal inflammation, however, may have a pseudocarcinomatous appearance, as described below.

Ectopic Pregnancy

In the usual tubal pregnancy there is distension of the ampullary segment (45), typically resulting in a sausage-shaped appearance with a thinned or ruptured wall and a dusky red serosa (Fig. 10). Microscopic examination may reveal fetal parts, villi which are frequently degenerative, trophoblast, and blood clot (46). The lamina propria shows decidual change in about one-third of the cases (45). Evidence of an underlying predisposing disorder such as chronic salpingitis, salpingitis isthmica nodosa, endometriosis, or a small tumor may be present. Rarely, the hemorrhagic mass resulting from ectopic pregnancy dissects into the broad ligament and may even extend to the contralateral adnexa (47). Tubal trophoblastic tumors (48) should be diagnosed with criteria used for analogous uterine tumors.

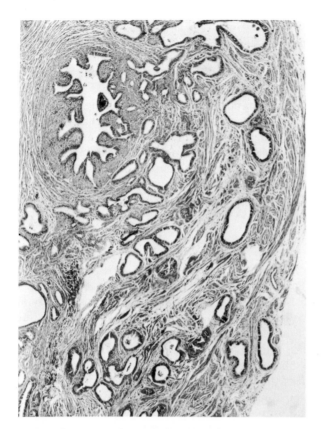

FIG. 9. Salpingitis isthmica nodosa. Gland-like structures have extended to the serosa. Note lack of any stromal reaction around the glands.

Torsion

Isolated torsion of the tube is rare (49), but tubal torsion often accompanies torsion of the adjacent ovary. The disorder occurs in women of all ages (50,51). Most often the patient is a young woman whose ovary is the seat of a neoplasm or cyst, usually of only moderate size. In 18% of cases, however, both the tube and ovary are otherwise normal (50). On gross inspection, the involved tube, which is right-sided in two-thirds of cases (50), is swollen and typically dusky blue.

A rare complication of torsion is tubo-ovarian autoamputation (52–54). Such patients are found at operation to have no tube or ovary on one side. In some cases, a calcified nodule is present in the vicinity or lying free in the peritoneal cavity; microscopic examination may disclose features compatible with calcified ovarian or tubal tissue.

Prolapse

Prolapse of the fallopian tube occasionally occurs after a prior hysterectomy, which has been performed by the vaginal route in approximately 80% of cases (55–58). On clinical examination a lesion simulating granulation tissue is visible at the vaginal apex (see page 1544). In a unique case, the fallopian tube prolapsed into the urinary bladder, clinically mimicking a carcinoma (59).

Endometriosis

The term "endometriosis" has been applied to three distinct lesions in the fallopian tube. Most commonly, it refers to serosal or subserosal endometriotic foci associated with endometriosis elsewhere in the pelvis; the myosalpinx is not involved in most cases (60).

Endometrial tissue may extend directly from the uterine cornu, replacing the interstitial and isthmic mucosa of the tube in 25% and 10% of women, respectively (Fig. 11). This finding is considered a normal morphologic variation, although the ectopic endometrial tissue may give rise to intratubal polyps. The latter have been found in from 1% of hysterosalpingographic studies to 11% of hysterectomy and salpingo-oophorectomy specimens (61). The polyps may be associated with ectopic pregnancy, and, particularly if bilateral, infertility. They are typically unilateral, pink to red lesions, 0.1 to 1.3 cm in diameter, with a smooth surface and a broad-based mucosal attachment. Microscopically, they consist of nonfunctioning endometrium (62–66). When ectopic endometrial tissue causes luminal occlusion, the term "endometrial colonization" has been arbitrarily applied (67–70). The process may represent only an exaggeration of the normal variation described above. This lesion accounts for 15% to 20% of cases of infertility and may be associated with tubal pregnancy.

The third type of tubal endometriosis has been designated "postsalpingectomy endometriosis" (71–73). It occurs at the tip of the proximal tubal stump, typically 1 to 4 years after tubal ligation. It is closely related to, and may be associated with, salpingitis isthmica nodosa. The lesion is analogous to uterine adenomyosis, consisting of endometrial glands and stroma extending from the endosalpinx into the muscularis; the lesion frequently extends to the serosal surface. Hysterosalpingography or India ink injection may show tuboperitoneal fistulous tracts (74) through which postligation pregnancies may result. Postsalpingectomy endometriosis has been documented in 20% to 50% of tubes examined after ligation.

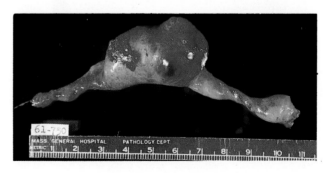

FIG. 10. Tubal pregnancy.

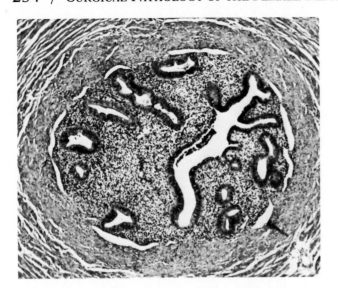

FIG. 11. Endometriosis (colonization) of the fallopian tube. The tubal lumen is occluded by endometrial glands and stroma.

The frequency of this complication is increased if electrocautery is used, if the proximal stumps are short, and if the postligation interval is long.

Walthard Nests

Nests of transitional (urothelial) epithelium referred to as "Walthard nests" are commonly found on the serosal surfaces of the fallopian tubes (Fig. 12), mesosal-

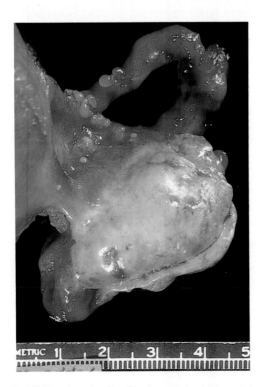

FIG. 12. Walthard nests. Small yellow cysts are present on the tubal serosa.

pinx, and mesovarium. They are often visible grossly as white to yellow nodules or cysts a few millimeters in diameter and have been mistaken for granulomas. Histologically, they are well-circumscribed, small solid nests, cysts, or, less commonly, surface plaques. The nests are composed of cytologically benign, mitotically inactive, transitional-type cells; their nuclei have fine chromatin, a prominent nuclear groove, and one or two small nucleoli. Less commonly, the cells have a nonkeratinized squamous appearance. The cysts are also lined by transitional cells, which may be flattened; inspissated eosinophilic secretion and mucin may be seen within the lumens.

Cysts

Paratubal cysts are common incidental findings (Fig. 13) that are rarely of clinical significance. They are usually of müllerian (paramesonephric) origin and lined by a single layer of tubal-type, ciliated epithelium (so-called hydatids of Morgagni) (75–78). Some cysts have a few plicae. They are generally attached to the fimbriated end of the tube by a pedicle. Mesonephric remnants lie in the broad ligament (79); they may be cystic but more often form small tubules lined by low columnar to cuboidal, nonciliated cells surrounded by a prominent layer of smooth muscle. Some paratubal cysts are of mesothelial origin and lined by flattened cells with surrounding fibrous or fatty tissue.

Ectopic Tissue in Fallopian Tube and Broad Ligament

Ectopic hilus cell nests may occur in the fallopian tube and paratubal tissue (80–82). In a thorough examination of over 2,000 fallopian tubes, Honoré and O'Hara (82) found hilus cells in 0.5%. The cells were found only in the endosalpinx and paratubal connective tissue, being most common in the fimbriae. Encapsu-

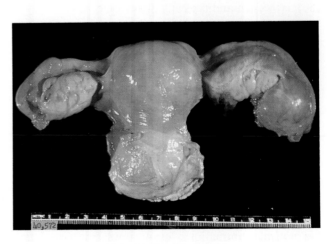

FIG. 13. Paratubal cyst.

lated adrenal cortical nests have been found in the broad ligament in 23% of hysterectomy specimens (83). They typically form small yellow nodules in the infundibulo-pelvic ligament, just beneath the peritoneum. Microscopically, all three layers of the adrenal cortex are present, but the medulla is absent. A single case of ectopic pancreas in the fallopian tube has been reported (84).

Metaplastic Lesions

The tubal epithelium rarely undergoes mucinous or squamous metaplasia. Mucinous metaplasia may be associated with mucinous tumors of the cervix, ovary, or both, most commonly in patients with the Peutz-Jeghers syndrome (85–89). Serotonin and somatostatin have been detected immunohistochemically in the metaplastic mucinous cells, as well as within adjacent normal-appearing epithelial cells in cases of Peutz-Jeghers syndrome (90).

A rare lesion designated "metaplastic papillary tumor of the fallopian tube" occurs as an incidental microscopic finding in pregnant and postpartum women (91). The lesion involves only part of the circumference of the mucosa; small, rounded cysts may be present within the papillae. The epithelial cells are large with abundant, eosinophilic cytoplasm (Fig. 14), which occasionally contains mucin and large, oval vesicular nuclei; mitotic figures are rare. The lesion is distinguishable from primary tubal carcinoma by its microscopic size, lack of invasion, and bland-appearing or only slightly atypical nuclei. Whether this lesion is metaplastic or neoplastic is unclear, but it has been associated with an uneventful course in the small number of cases encountered to date.

Decidual transformation of tubal stromal cells in the lamina propria may occur in pregnant patients (6) as well as in women on progestin therapy (92).

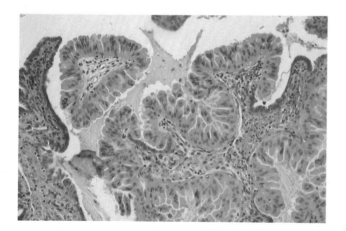

FIG. 14. Metaplastic papillary tumor. The papillae are lined by stratified cells with abundant eosinophilic cytoplasm.

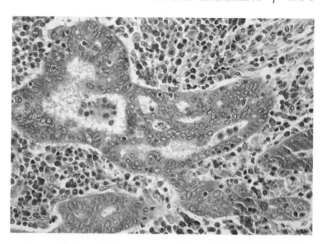

FIG. 15. Atypical epithelial hyperplasia with intraglandular bridging associated with severe chronic salpingitis.

Hyperplastic and Pseudocarcinomatous Lesions

In patients with functioning ovarian tumors and excess estrogen production, epithelial hyperplasia associated with occasional mitotic figures but unaccompanied by cytologic atypia is common and may be the only pathologic evidence of estrogen excess, if the endometrium is not available for microscopic examination. More commonly, epithelial hyperplasia is an incidental microscopic finding or is present in a tube that is the site of acute or chronic inflammation (93–98).

In one study, 18.5% of unselected fallopian tubes removed surgically showed epithelial proliferative changes such as nuclear stratification and atypia (95). In half of these cases there was an associated salpingitis. Some authors have designated examples of atypical hyperplasia unassociated with inflammation as carcinoma *in situ,* but no evidence has been presented that these lesions progress to carcinoma. One study, however, has shown an association of tubal hyperplasia with malignant tumors in the upper genital tract (97).

Hyperplasia and atypia of tubal epithelium and mesothelium may occur in response to inflammation and may simulate an *in situ* or invasive adenocarcinoma (Fig. 15) (93,96). The hyperplastic epithelial changes include the formation of papillae and pseudoglands (Fig. 15) lined by cells with mild to moderate nuclear pleomorphism, hyperchromatism, and mitotic activity. The proliferation may involve the mucosa, muscularis, and serosa. When associated with pseudoglandular hyperplasia of the overlying mesothelial cells, which become incorporated within subserosal inflammatory and scar tissue, the combination of findings may lead to an erroneous interpretation of transmural carcinoma. These pseudocarcinomatous changes have long been recognized in tuberculous salpingitis (Fig. 5) but are also seen with other forms of bacterial salpingitis. A number of differences between carcinoma and pseudocarcinomatous inflammatory lesions facilitate the differential diagnosis. The great majority of carcinomas are grossly evident, are not associated with significant inflammation, and exhibit severe nuclear atypia. Pseudocarcinomatous changes simulating carcinoma, in contrast, are incidental microscopic findings associated with overt inflammatory manifestations. If atypical mesothelial proliferation is a component of the lesion, the mesothelial cells are typically cuboidal, often lined up in rows, and generally exhibit only mild nuclear atypia.

Heat artifact (prolonged intraoperative cautery or heating of the specimen inadvertently after surgical removal) may also simulate carcinoma by causing an appearance of marked cellular stratification and pseudoatypia (Fig. 16) (99).

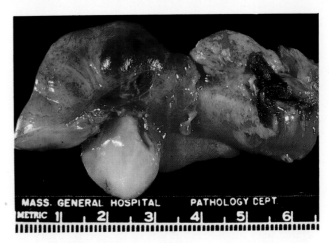

FIG. 17. Adenomatoid tumor. The tumor is well circumscribed and has a smooth, white, cut surface.

TUMORS

Adenomatoid Tumor

The adenomatoid tumor is the most common benign tumor of the fallopian tube (100–108). It is usually an incidental finding in the myosalpinx but may compress the tubal lumen or project from the serosa; it is typically 2.0 cm or less in diameter and is circumscribed, firm, and gray, white, or yellow (Fig. 17); rarely, it is bilateral

(104). The microscopic patterns include irregular gland-like spaces (Fig. 18), oval vacuoles, and small cords and clusters of cells. The neoplastic cells range from flattened cells sometimes confused with endothelium to large cells containing abundant eosinophilic cytoplasm. Nuclei are bland, and mitotic figures are rare. The glandular lumens and vacuoles may contain slightly basophilic fluid that is rich in hyaluronic acid. The stroma

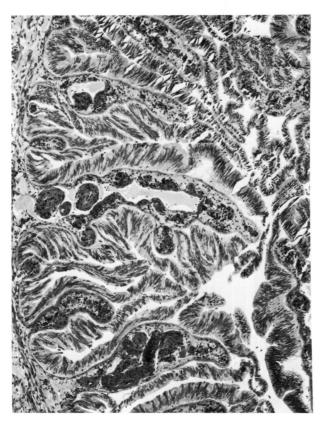

FIG. 16. Heat artifact due to cautery. The cells have a peculiar elongated appearance.

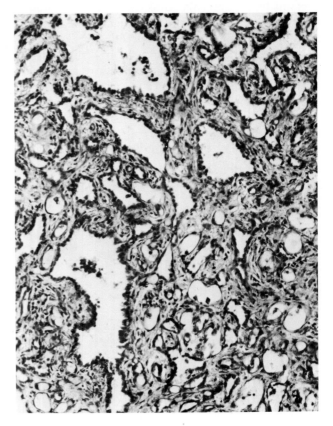

FIG. 18. Adenomatoid tumor. Small gland-like spaces and cysts are lined by cuboidal to flattened cells.

may be hyalinized and contain smooth muscle. Lymphocytes may form prominent follicles. An origin from mesothelium is now supported by most investigators, and continuity with the overlying mesothelium is occasionally seen (105). Adenomatoid tumor may be confused with other benign neoplasms, particularly lymphangiomas and leiomyomas. Careful examination of the tumor cells should permit their distinction from endothelium, and immunoperoxidase stains for cytokeratin and *Ulex europaeus* may aid in their recognition (108). Although smooth muscle may be present in tubal adenomatoid tumors, it is rarely as prominent as in analogous uterine tumors, and the characteristic spaces of an adenomatoid tumor are not seen in a leiomyoma. Adenomatoid tumors may also be confused with malignancy such as malignant mesothelioma and adenocarcinoma. The circumscribed gross appearance, bland cytologic findings, and mitotic inactivity characteristic of adenomatoid tumors allow distinction.

Benign Epithelial Tumors

Benign tumors of the types commonly encountered in the ovary are rare in the fallopian tube. Serous adenofibromas are similar to their ovarian counterparts (109–113). Rare adenomas, papillomas and adenomyomas have also been reported (109,114).

Benign Tumors of Soft Tissue Type

Benign tumors of soft tissue type may involve the fallopian tube or broad ligament. Leiomyomas are most common (115–120) and may undergo degenerative changes similar to those occurring in uterine smooth-muscle tumors. Most tubal leiomyomas are small; they may be submucosal, intramural, or subserosal. Rarer benign tumors in this category include neurilemoma (121), angiomyolipoma (122), lipoma (123), lymphangioma (124), ganglioneuroma (125), and hemangioma (126–129). Several tubal hemangiomas have resulted in hemoperitoneum.

Carcinoma of Fallopian Tube

Carcinoma of the fallopian tube is uncommon (130–156), accounting for only about 0.3% of gynecologic cancers (130). The distinctive presentation of intermittent, profuse, watery, clear to yellow (cholesterol-rich) vaginal discharge, accompanied by colicky abdominal pain and followed by a decrease in the size of an abdominal mass (hydrops tubae profluens) (130), is encountered in only a minority of cases and is not pathognomonic (132). The most common symptom of tubal carcinoma, seen in two-thirds of cases, is postmenopausal bleeding (133). The diagnosis is usually unsuspected preopera-

tively. Carcinoma cells in a cytologic smear from the lower genital tract, reported in approximately 10% of cases, is strongly suggestive if no other source of malignancy is identified (133,134,138,141,146). In some cases, fragments of tumor are discovered in an endocervical or endometrial curettage specimen (109,140,141). Most of the patients are postmenopausal with a mean age of 55 years (135,136,140–153); rare tumors occur in much younger patients (154–156).

Because primary tubal carcinoma is less common than secondary carcinoma of ovarian origin, gross as well as microscopic assessment is important in determining the primary site (140). When both tube and ovary are replaced by carcinoma compatible microscopically with an origin in either, the designation "tubo-ovarian carcinoma" has been applied (109). Occasionally a noninvasive, a superficially invasive, or, rarely, a borderline tubal carcinoma is associated with a similar serous tumor in the ovary. In such cases the tumors may reflect independent primary neoplasia, rather than spread from one organ to the other (150).

Carcinomas characteristically appear as fusiform swellings that may have the external appearance of a hydrosalpinx (Fig. 19) or hematosalpinx. Bilaterality has been reported in 10% to 20% of cases (130,132,146). On opening the tube, the tumor may be extensive (Fig. 19), or it may form a solitary, localized nodule (Fig. 20). In some cases it is predominantly or entirely endophytic (Fig. 19), and in others it is sessile with firm white tissue infiltrating the wall. Hemorrhage and necrosis are common, and cyst formation is occasionally seen.

Microscopically, tubal carcinoma is typically similar in appearance to serous ovarian carcinoma (Fig. 21). The tumors that grow primarily into the tubal lumen exhibit prominent papillarity (Fig. 21), whereas those that invade the wall usually have an alveolar pattern (Fig. 22). One reported tubal carcinoma had features of a serous papillary cystadenoma of borderline malignancy (157). Endometrioid adenocarcinoma (159,160),

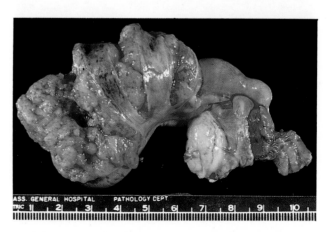

FIG. 19. Carcinoma of fallopian tube. A markedly expanded tube has been incised to disclose a friable, tan, papillary tumor.

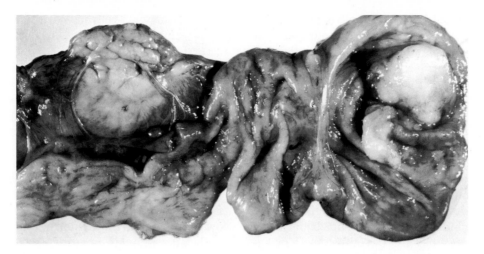

FIG. 20. Carcinoma of fallopian tube. The opened tube courses along the lower border of the left half of the specimen and occupies the entire right half, where an irregular nodule of carcinoma is seen on the mucosal surface. The ovary is visible at the upper left. (Reproduced with permission from ref. 108.)

adenoacanthoma (134,148), adenosquamous carcinoma (158,161,162), squamous-cell carcinoma (163), clear-cell carcinoma (164), and transitional-cell carcinoma (165,166) have also been encountered rarely. Squamous-cell carcinoma *in situ* secondary to upward spread from *in situ* or invasive cervical carcinoma has also been reported (167,168).

We have seen in consultation several examples of a peculiar tubal carcinoma characterized by a sieve-like pattern of small glands containing eosinophilic material,

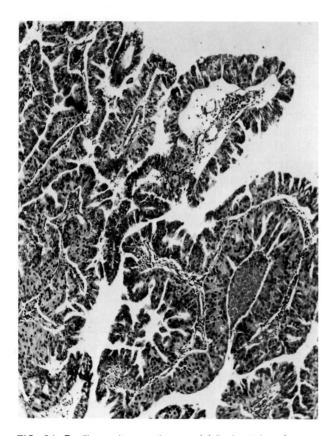

FIG. 21. Papillary adenocarcinoma of fallopian tube of serous type.

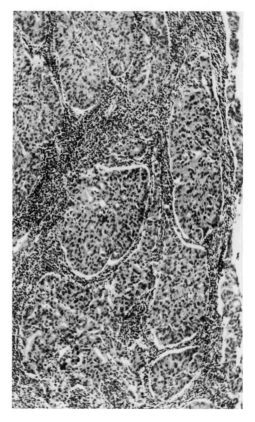

FIG. 22. Adenocarcinoma of the tube with a solid (alveolar) pattern.

suggesting the possibility of wolffian derivation. The intraluminal location of these tumors and the focal presence of endometrioid or serous type glands indicates, however, that these tumors are probably of müllerian origin.

Malignant Müllerian Mixed Tumor and Sarcomas

Approximately 35 malignant müllerian mixed tumors of the fallopian tube have been reported (169–172a). The age distribution and clinical presentation are similar to those of tubal carcinoma. The typical gross appearance is that of a large, sometimes polypoid mass protruding into the lumen (Fig. 23). The microscopic features and prognosis are similar to those of analogous tumors occurring elsewhere; both homologous and heterologous types have been encountered. Rare leiomyosarcomas of the tube and broad ligament have been reported (173–178).

Malignant Lymphoma and Leukemia

The female genital tract is involved in approximately 40% of women who die with disseminated lymphoma (179), and the fallopian tube is affected in many of these cases. In one large series of lymphoma presenting as an ovarian mass, 26% involved the tube (180). Tubal involvement is less common than ovarian involvement by lymphoma and is almost always less conspicuous on gross inspection. We are not aware of a reported case of lymphoma presenting in, and apparently confined to, the fallopian tube but have recently seen a case of this type. The tube may also be infiltrated in patients with leukemia (181).

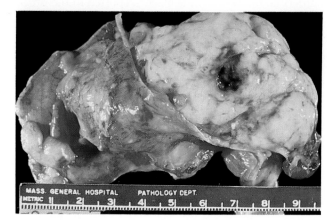

FIG. 23. Malignant müllerian mixed tumor. A markedly distended tube has been opened to disclose a large, soft, white tumor with focal hemorrhage.

Germ-Cell Tumors

Forty-eight teratomas of the tube have been reported (182–187). They are usually attached by a pedicle to the tubal mucosa and have ranged from 0.7 to 20 cm in diameter. Most of these tumors have been cystic and mature, but rare examples have been solid (187) or immature (186). One solid mature teratoma contained an area of insular carcinoid (187); another was composed entirely of thyroid tissue (188).

Trophoblastic Disease

Hydatidiform moles and choriocarcinomas occur rarely in the fallopian tube or mesosalpinx (189–193) and may mimic an ectopic pregnancy, both clinically and grossly.

Secondary Tumors of the Fallopian Tube

The tube may be involved secondarily by endometrial or cervical carcinoma (140,142) either by direct extension or by way of the tubal lumen. The tube is involved only occasionally by metastasis from an extragenital site. In a review of 149 cases of metastases to the genital tract from an extragenital site, there was only one tubal metastasis, in contrast to 113 ovarian metastases (194). In our experience, however, microscopic evidence of tubal metastasis is not as rare as the above figure indicates. In two other studies, 3% (140) and 7% (142) of metastases to the tube had their origin outside the genital tract.

Female Adnexal Tumor of Probable Wolffian Origin

This distinctive tumor has been interpreted as wolffian in origin because of its location and its microscopic patterns and cytologic features which are unlike those of müllerian tumors on both light and electron microscopic examination (195–200).

The patients have ranged from 18 to 72 (average 47) years of age. They typically have nonspecific clinical manifestations such as abdominal pain or swelling, or they have asymptomatic masses that are discovered incidentally. On gross examination, the tumors lie within the broad ligament (Fig. 24), or hang from it or from the fallopian tube by a pedicle. They average 8.0 cm in diameter and are typically rounded masses with bosselated external surfaces (Fig. 24). Cut surfaces are solid or solid and cystic (Fig. 25). The solid tissue varies from gray-white to tan or yellow and is usually firm or rubbery; hemorrhage and necrosis are rare. Microscopically, diffuse, tubular, cystic, and sieve-like patterns may be seen (Figs. 26 and 27). The tubules may be solid (Fig. 27) or may contain small lumens. They are lined by cuboidal

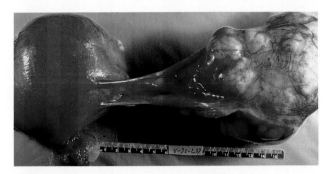

FIG. 24. Female adnexal tumor of probable wolffian origin. A bosselated solid mass is present within the leaves of the broad ligament. (From ref. 195.)

to columnar cells with scanty cytoplasm; occasional cells may contain abundant pale cytoplasm. The cysts are usually lined by flattened cells (Fig. 26). The nuclei are usually small, round to oval, and pale (Fig. 27). Some tumors have a focally prominent hyalinized stroma or fibrous bands that separate cellular foci into lobules. When the tumor cells grow in solid sheets, they may have a mesenchymal, spindle-shaped appearance; often vacuoles similar to those encountered in adenomatoid tumors are seen. Electron-microscopic examination of several tumors has shown a thick peritubular basal lamina, as well as an absence or paucity of cilia, Golgi complexes, secretory granules, and glycogen, features favoring a wolffian origin.

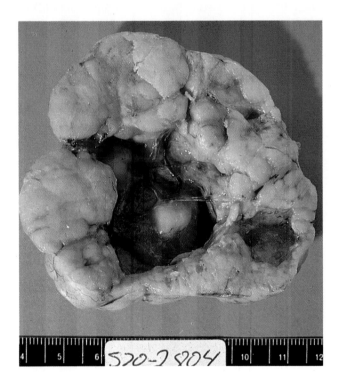

FIG. 25. Female adnexal tumor of probable wolffian origin. The sectioned surface of the tumor discloses lobulated, yellow-white tissue with cystic degeneration. (From ref. 195.)

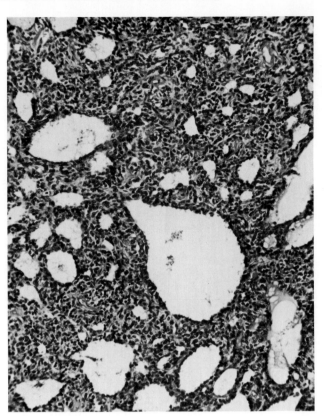

FIG. 26. Female adnexal tumor of probable wolffian origin with sieve-like pattern.

Most examples of this neoplasm occurring in the broad ligament have been benign, but two malignant tumors have been reported (196,200). Both recurred after 6 years, and one was fatal (200).

Serous and Other Müllerian Tumors of the Broad Ligament

Serous cystadenomas and serous cystadenomas of borderline malignancy have been reported in the broad ligament (201–206), typically in young women (mean age: 33 years). They have been unilateral, unilocular cysts ranging up to 13 cm in diameter. Typically they have an ovarian-like stroma but lack ova and follicular derivatives. Local excision has been curative. Rarely, carcinomas of müllerian-type arise in the broad ligament (207–210a).

Rare Tumors of the Broad Ligament

Three ependymomas of the broad ligament have been reported in patients 13, 45, and 47 years of age (211,212). They were 1.0, 9.5, and 13 cm in largest dimension and microscopically resembled ependymomas of the central nervous system. Immunoperoxidase stains for glial fibrillary acidic protein were positive in all cases.

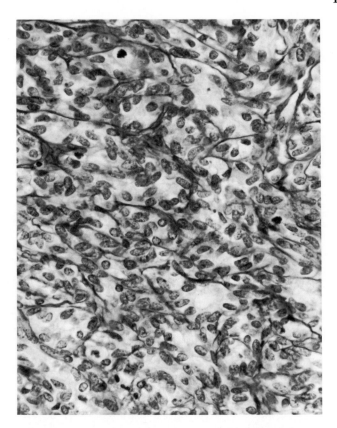

FIG. 27. Female adnexal tumor of probable wolffian origin. Closely packed solid tubules lined by cells with round to oval, uniform nuclei are present. Two mitotic figures are visible. (Periodic acid–Schiff stain.)

One tumor contained islands of cartilage. Intra-abdominal spread was present at presentation in one case and occurred 11 years later in a second (211). Rare examples of pheochromocytoma (213), extraskeletal Ewing's sarcoma (214), Brenner tumor (215), fibrothecoma (216), and papillary cystadenoma in a patient with von Hippel–Lindau disease (217) have also been reported in the broad ligament.

REFERENCES

1. Chow AW, Malkasian KL, Marshall JR, Guze LB. The bacteriology of acute pelvic inflammatory disease—value of cul-de-sac cultures and relative importance of gonococci and other aerobic or anaerobic bacteria. *Am J Obstet Gynecol* 1975;122:876–879.
2. Thadapalli H, Gorbach SL, Keith L. Anaerobic infections of the female genital tract: bacteriologic and therapeutic aspects. *Am J Obstet Gynecol* 1973;117:1034–1040.
3. Thompson SE, Hager WD, Wong K-H, Lopez B, Ramsey C, Allen SD, Stargel MD, Thornsberry C, Benigno BB, Thompson JD, Shulman JA. The microbiology and therapy of acute pelvic inflammatory disease in hospitalized patients. *Am J Obstet Gynecol* 1980;136:179–186.
4. Winkler B, Reumann W, Mitao M, Gallo L, Richart RM, Crum CP. Immunoperoxidase localization of chlamydial antigens in acute salpingitis. *Am J Obstet Gynecol* 1985;152:275–278.
5. Nassberg S, McKay DG, Hertig AT. Physiologic salpingitis. *Am J Obstet Gynecol* 1954;67:130–134.
6. Hellman LM. The morphology of the human fallopian tube in the early puerperium. *Am J Obstet Gynecol* 1949;57:154–163.
7. Smith HA, Greene RR. Physiologic salpingitis? *Am J Obstet Gynecol* 1956;72:174–179.
8. Schaefer G. Tuberculosis of the female genital tract. *Clin Obstet Gynecol* 1970;13:965–998.
9. Nogales-Ortiz F, Tarancón I, Nogales FF. The pathology of female genital tuberculosis. *Obstet Gynecol* 1979;53:422–428.
10. Lawrence WD, Scully RE. Pathology of the fallopian tube. In: Hunt RB, ed. *Atlas of female infertility surgery.* Chicago: Year Book Medical Publishers, 1986:11–24.
11. Bonar BE, Rabson AS. Gynecologic aspects of leprosy. *Obstet Gynecol* 1957;9:33–43.
12. Braby HH, Dougherty CM, Mickal A. Actinomycosis of the female genital tract. *Obstet Gynecol* 1964;23:580–583.
13. Paalman RJ, Dockerty MB, Mussey RD. Actinomycosis of ovaries and fallopian tubes. *Am J Obstet Gynecol* 1949;58:419–431.
14. Hamblen EC, Baker RD, Martin DS. Blastomycosis of the female reproductive tract with report of a case. *Am J Obstet Gynecol* 1935;30:345–356.
15. Murray JJ, Clark CA, Lands RH, Heim CR, Burnett LS. Reactivation blastomycosis presenting as a tuboovarian abscess. *Obstet Gynecol* 1984;64:828–830.
16. Bylund DJ, Nanfro JJ, Marsh WL Jr. Coccidioidomycosis of the female genital tract. *Arch Pathol Lab Med* 1986;110:232–235.
17. Saw EC, Smale LE, Einstein H, Huntington RW. Female genital coccidioidomycosis. *Obstet Gynecol* 1975;45:199–202.
18. Frost O. Bilharzia of the fallopian tube. *S Afr Med J* 1975;49:1201–1203.
19. Gelfand M, Ross MD, Blair DM, Weber MC. Distribution and extent of schistosomiasis in female pelvic organs with special reference to the genital tract, as determined at autopsy. *Am J Trop Med Hyg* 1971;20:846–849.
20. Arean VM. Manson's schistosomiasis of the female genital tract. *Am J Obstet Gynecol* 1956;72:1038–1053.
21. Symmers W St C. Pathology of oxyurasis. *Arch Pathol* 1950;50:475–516.
22. Abraham JL, Spore WW, Benirschke K. Cysticercosis of the fallopian tube: histology and microanalysis. *Hum Pathol* 1982;13:665.
23. Campbell JS, Nigam S, Hurtig A, Sahasrabudhe MR, Marino I. Mineral oil granulomas of the uterus and parametrium and granulomatous salpingitis with Schauman bodies and oxalate deposits. *Fertil Steril* 1964;15:278–289.
24. Elliott GB, Brody H, Elliott KA. Implications of "lipoid salpingitis". *Fertil Steril* 1965;16:541–548.
25. Rubin IC. Lipoidal granuloma in fallopian tubes localized by intra-uterine diodrast injection, with special reference to the value of follow-up x-ray films. *Radiology* 1939;33:350–353.
26. Brooks JJ, Wheeler JE. Granulomatous salpingitis secondary to Crohn's disease. *Obstet Gynecol* 1977;49:31s–33s.
27. Chalvardjian A. Sarcoidosis of the female genital tract. *Am J Obstet Gynecol* 1978;132:78–80.
28. Kay S. Sarcoidosis of the fallopian tubes. Report of a case. *J Obstet Gynaecol Br Emp* 1956;63:871–874.
29. Kunakemakorn P, Ontai G, Balin H. Pelvic inflammatory pseudotumor: a case report. *Am J Obstet Gynecol* 1976;126:286–287.
30. Shalev E, Zuckerman H, Rizescu I. Pelvic inflammatory pseudotumor (xanthogranuloma). *Acta Obstet Gynecol Scand* 1982;61:285–286.
31. McEntee GP, Coughlan M, Corrigan T, Dervan P. Pelvic inflammatory pseudotumor: problems in clinical and histological diagnosis. Case report. *Br J Obstet Gynaecol* 1985;92:1067–1069.
32. Chen KTK, Hendricks EJ. Malakoplakia of the female genital tract. *Obstet Gynecol* 1985;65:84s–87s.
33. Klempner LB, Giglio PG, Niebles A. Malacoplakia of the ovary. *Obstet Gynecol* 1987;69:537–540.
34. Czernobilsky B, Silverstein A. Salpingitis in ovarian endometriosis. *Fertil Steril* 1978;30:45–49.
35. Clement PB, Young RH, Scully RE. Necrotic pseudoxanthomatous nodules of ovary and peritoneum in endometriosis. *Am J Surg Pathol* 1988;12:390–397.
36. Herrera GA, Riemann BEF, Greenberg HL, Miles PA. Pigmentosis tubae, a new entity: light and electron microscopic study. *Obstet Gynecol* 1983;61:80s–83s.

37. Roberts JT, Roberts GT, Maudsley RF. Indolent granulomatous necrosis in patients with previous tubal diathermy. *Am J Obstet Gynecol* 1977;129:112–113.

38. Bell DA, Mondschein M, Scully RE. Giant cell arteritis of the female genital tract. A report of three cases. *Am J Surg Pathol* 1986;10:696–701.

39. Stock RJ. Histopathologic changes in fallopian tubes subsequent to sterilization procedures. *Int J Gynecol Pathol* 1983;2:13–27.

40. Copeland W, Hawlay PC, Teteris NJ. Gynecologic amyloidosis. *Am J Obstet Gynecol* 1985;153:555–556.

41. Schenken JR, Burns EL. A study and classification of nodular lesions of the fallopian tubes. "Salpingitis isthmica nodosa". *Am J Obstet Gynecol* 1943;45:624–636.

42. Benjamin CL, Beaver DC. Pathogenesis of salpingitis isthmica nodosa. *Am J Clin Pathol* 1951;21:212–222.

43. Majmudar B, Henderson PH III, Sample E. Salpingitis isthmica nodosa: a high-risk factor for tubal pregnancy. *Obstet Gynecol* 1983;62:73–78.

44. Wrork OH, Broders AC. Adenomyosis of the fallopian tubes. *Am J Obstet Gynecol* 1942;44:412–432.

45. Pauerstein CJ, Croxatto HB, Eddy CA, Ramzy I, Walters MD. Anatomy and pathology of tubal pregnancy. *Obstet Gynecol* 1986;67:301–308.

46. Budowick M, Johnson TRB, Genadry R, Parmley TH, Woodruff JD. The histopathology of the developing tubal ectopic pregnancy. *Fertil Steril* 1980;34:169–171.

47. Case Records of the Massachusetts General Hospital (Case 11-1976). *N Engl J Med* 1976;294:600–605.

48. Westerhout FC. Ruptured tubal hydatidiform mole. Report of a case. *Obstet Gynecol* 1964;23:138–139.

49. Filtenborg TA, Hertz JB. Torsion of the fallopian tube. *Eur J Obstet Gyn Reprod Biol* 1981;12:177–181.

50. Hibbard LT. Adnexal torsion. *Am J Obstet Gynecol* 1985;152:456–461.

51. Schultz LR, Newton WA, Clatworthy HW. Torsion of previously normal tube and ovary in children. *N Engl J Med* 1963;268:343–346.

52. Sebastian JA, Baker RL, Cordray D. Asymptomatic infarction and separation of ovary and distal uterine tube. *Obstet Gynecol* 1973;41:531–535.

53. Nissen ED, Kent DR, Nissen SE, Feldman BM. Unilateral tuboovarian autoamputation. *J Reprod Med* 1977;19:151–153.

54. Beyth Y, Bar-On E. Tuboovarian autoamputation and infertility. *Fertil Steril* 1984;42:932–933.

55. Sapan IP, Solberg NS. Prolapse of the uterine tube after abdominal hysterectomy. *Obstet Gynecol* 1973;42:26–32.

56. Ellsworth HS, Harris JW, McQuarrie HG, Stone RA, Anderson AE. Prolapse of the fallopian tube following vaginal hysterectomy. *JAMA* 1973;224:891–892.

57. Silverberg SG, Frable WJ. Prolapse of fallopian tube into vaginal vault after hysterectomy. *Arch Pathol* 1974;97:100–103.

58. Wheelock JB, Schneider V, Goplerud DR. Prolapsed fallopian tube masquerading as adenocarcinoma of the vagina in a postmenopausal woman. *Gynecol Oncol* 1985;21:369–375.

59. Anastasiades KD, Majmudar B. Prolapse of fallopian tube into urinary bladder, mimicking bladder carcinoma. *Arch Pathol Lab Med* 1983;107:613–614.

60. Sheldon RS, Wilson RB, Dockerty MB. Serosal endometriosis of fallopian tubes. *Am J Obstet Gynecol* 1967;99:882–884.

61. Lisa JR, Gioia JD, Rubin IC. Observations on the interstitial portion of the fallopian tube. *Surg Gynecol Obstet* 1954;99:159–169.

62. Rubin IC, Lisa JR, Trinidad S. Further observations on ectopic endometrium of the fallopian tube. *Surg Gynecol Obstet* 1956;103:469–474.

63. Donnez J, Casanas-Roux F, Ferin J, Thomas K. Tubal polyps, epithelial inclusions, and endometriosis after tubal sterilization. *Fertil Steril* 1984;41:564–568.

64. McLaughlin DS. Successful pregnancy outcome following removal of bilateral cornual polyps by microsurgical linear salpingotomy with the aid of the CO_2 laser. *Fertil Steril* 1984;42:939–941.

65. Fernstrom I, Lagerlof B. Polyps in the intramural part of the fallopian tubes. A radiographic and clinical study. *Br J Obstet Gynaecol* 1964;71:681–691.

66. David MP, Ben-Zwi D, Langer L. Tubal intramural polyps and their relationship to infertility. *Fertil Steril* 1981;35:526–531.

67. Cioltei A, Tasca L, Titiriga L, Maakaron G, Calciu V. Nodular salpingitis and tubal endometriosis. I. Comparative clinical study. *Acta Eur Fertil* 1979;10:135–141.

68. De Brux J. The contribution of pathological anatomy to the diagnosis and prognosis of different forms of tubal sterility. *Acta Eur Fertil* 1975;6:185–195.

69. Fortier KJ, Haney AF. The pathologic spectrum of uterotubal junction obstruction. *Obstet Gynecol* 1985;65:93–98.

70. Madelenat P, De Brux J, Palmer R. L'etiologie des obstructions tubaires proximales et son role dan le pronostic des implantations. *Gynecologie* 1977;28:47–53.

71. Sampson JA. Postsalpingectomy endometriosis (endosalpingiosis). *Am J Obstet Gynecol* 1930;20:443–480.

72. Sampson JA. Pathogenesis of postsalpingectomy endometriosis in laparotomy scars. *Am J Obstet Gynecol* 1945;50:597–620.

73. Stock RJ. Postsalpingectomy endometriosis: A reassessment. *Obstet Gynecol* 1982;60:560–570.

74. Rock JA, Parmley TH, King TM, Laufe LE, Su BC. Endometriosis and the development of tuboperitoneal fistulas after tubal ligation. *Fertil Steril* 1981;35:16–20.

75. Gardner GH, Greene RR, Peckham BM. Normal and cystic structures of the broad ligament. *Am J Obstet Gynecol* 1948;55:917–939.

76. Samaha M, Woodruff JD. Paratubal cysts: frequency, histogenesis, and associated clinical features. *Obstet Gynecol* 1985;65:691–694.

77. Gardner GH, Greene RR, Peckham B. Tumors of the broad ligament. *Am J Obstet Gynecol* 1957;73:536–555.

78. Samaha M, Woodruff JD. Paratubal cysts: frequency, histogenesis, and associated clinical features. *Obstet Gynecol* 1985;65:691–694.

79. Bransilver BR, Ferenczy A, Richart RM. Female genital tract remnants. An ultrastructural comparison of hydatid of Morgagni and mesonephric ducts and tubules. *Arch Pathol Lab Med* 1973;96:255–261.

80. Palomaki JF, Blair OM. Hilus cell rest of the fallopian tube. A case report. *Obstet Gynecol* 1971;37:60–62.

81. Lewis JD. Hilus-cell hyperplasia of ovaries and tubes. *Obstet Gynecol* 1964;24:728–731.

82. Honoré LH, O'Hara KE. Ovarian hilus cell heterotopia. *Obstet Gynecol* 1979;53:461–464.

83. Falls JL. Accessory adrenal cortex in the broad ligament. Incidence and functional significance. *Cancer* 1955;8:143–150.

84. Mason TE, Quagliarello JR. Ectopic pancreas in the fallopian tube. Report of a first case. *Obstet Gynecol* 1976;48:70s–73s.

85. Costa J. Peutz-Jeghers syndrome. Case presentation. *Obstet Gynecol* 1977;50:15s–17s.

86. Gloor E. Un cas de syndrome de Peutz-Jeghers associé a un carcinoma mammaire bilatéral, a un adénocarcinoma du col utérin et a des tumeurs des cordons sexuels a tubules annelés bilatérales dans les ovaires. *Schweiz Med Wochenschr* 1978;108:717–721.

87. Berger G, Frappart L, Berger F, Seffert P, Serain F, Lamerant P, Feroldi J. Tubules anneles de l'ovaire, metaplasie mucipare tubaire, hyperplasie glandulo-kystique et mucipare de l'endocol et syndrome de Peutz-Jeghers. *Arch Anat Cytol Pathol* 1981;29:353–357.

88. LiVolsi VA, Merino MJ, Schwartz PE. Coexistent endocervical adenocarcinoma and mucinous adenocarcinoma of ovary: a clinicopathologic study of four cases. *Int J Gynecol Pathol* 1983;1:391–402.

89. Young RH, Scully RE. Mucinous ovarian tumors associated with mucinous adenocarcinomas of the cervix. A clinicopathological analysis of 16 cases. *Int J Gynecol Pathol* 1988;7:99–111.

90. Fetissof F, Berger G, Dubois MP, Philippe A, Lansac J, Jobard P. Female genital tract and Peutz-Jeghers syndrome: an immunohistochemical study. *Int J Gynecol Pathol* 1985;4:219–229.

91. Saffos RO, Rhatigan RM, Scully RE. Metaplastic papillary tumor of the fallopian tube—a distinctive lesion of pregnancy. *Am J Clin Pathol* 1980;74:232–236.

92. Mills SE, Fechner RE. Stromal and epithelial changes in the fallopian tube following hormonal therapy. *Hum Pathol* 1980;11:583–585.

93. Dougherty CM, Cotten NM. Proliferative epithelial lesions of the uterine tube. I. Adenomatous hyperplasia. *Obstet Gynecol* 1964;24:849–854.

94. Pauerstein CJ, Woodruff JD. Cellular patterns in proliferative and anaplastic disease of the fallopian tube. *Am J Obstet Gynecol* 1966;96:486–492.

95. Moore SW, Enterline HT. Significance of proliferative epithelial lesions of the uterine tube. *Obstet Gynecol* 1975;45:385–390.

96. Mostoufizadeh M, Scully RE. Pseudocarcinomatous lesions of the fallopian tube. *Lab Invest* 1983;48:61a.

97. Stern J, Buscema J, Parmley T, Woodruff JD, Rosenshein NB. Atypical epithelial proliferations in the fallopian tube. *Am J Obstet Gynecol* 1981;140:309–312.

98. Ryan GM. Carcinoma *in situ* of the fallopian tube. *Am J Obstet Gynecol* 1962;84:198.

99. Cornog JL, Currie JL, Rubin A. Heat artifact simulating adenocarcinoma of fallopian tube. *JAMA* 1970;214:1118–1119.

100. Evans N. Mesotheliomas of the uterine and tubal serosa and the tunica vaginalis testis. *Am J Pathol* 1943;19:461–471.

101. Golden A, Ash JE. Adenomatoid tumors of the genital tract. *Am J Pathol* 1945;21:63–73.

102. Bolton RN, Hunter WC. Adenomatoid tumors of the uterus and adnexa. Report of eleven cases. *Am J Obstet Gynecol* 1958;76:647–652.

103. Jackson JR. The histogenesis of the "adenomatoid" tumor of the genital tract. *Cancer* 1958;11:337–350.

104. Youngs LA, Taylor HB. Adenomatoid tumors of the uterus and fallopian tube. *Am J Clin Pathol* 1967;48:537–545.

105. Pauerstein CJ, Woodruff JD, Quinton SW. Developmental patterns in "adenomatoid lesions" of the fallopian tube. *Am J Obstet Gynecol* 1968;100:1000–1007.

106. Salazar H, Kanbour A, Burgess F. Ultrastructure and observations on the histogenesis of mesotheliomas "adenomatoid tumors" of the female genital tract. *Cancer* 1972;29:141–152.

107. Taxy JB, Battifora H, Oyasu R. Adenomatoid tumors: a light microscopic, histochemical, and ultrastructural study. *Cancer* 1974;34:306–316.

108. Stephenson TJ, Mills PM. Adenomatoid tumors: an immunohistochemical and ultrastructural appraisal of their histogenesis. *J Pathol* 1986;148:327–335.

109. Green TH, Scully RE. Tumors of the fallopian tube. *Clin Obstet Gynecol* 1962;5:886–906.

110. Silverman AY, Artinian B, Sabin M. Serous cystadenofibroma of the fallopian tube: a case report. *Am J Obstet Gynecol* 1978;130:593–595.

111. Kanbour AI, Burgess F, Salazar H. Intramural adenofibroma of the fallopian tube. Light and electron microscopy. *Cancer* 1973;31:1433–1439.

112. De La Fuente AA. Benign mixed mullerian tumour—adenofibroma of the fallopian tube. *Histopathology* 1982;6:661–666.

113. Chen KTK. Bilateral papillary adenofibroma of the fallopian tube. *Am J Clin Pathol* 1981;75:229–231.

114. Gisser SD. Obstructing fallopian tube papilloma. *Int J Gynecol Pathol* 1986;5:179–182.

115. Crissman JD, Handwerker D. Leiomyoma of the uterine tube: report of a case. *Am J Obstet Gynecol* 1976;126:1046.

116. Klein HZ, Smith RL. Fibromyoma of the uterine tube. *Obstet Gynecol* 1965;26:515–517.

117. Roberts CL, Marshall HK. Fibromyoma of the fallopian tube. *Am J Obstet Gynecol* 1961;82:364–366.

118. Moore OA, Waxman M, Udoffia C. Leiomyoma of the fallopian tube: a cause of tubal pregnancy. *Am J Obstet Gynecol* 1979;134:101–102.

119. Talerman A. Leiomyoma of the fallopian tube. *Int J Gynaecol Obstet* 1974;12:145–147.

120. Honoré LH. Parauterine leiomyomas in women: a clinicopathologic study of 22 cases. *Europ J Obstet Gynecol Reprod Biol* 1981;11:273–279.

121. Okagaki T, Richart RM. Neurilemoma of the fallopian tube. *Am J Obstet Gynecol* 1970;106:929.

122. Katz DA, Thom D, Bogard P, Dermer MS. Angiomyolipoma of the fallopian tube. *Am J Obstet Gynecol* 1984;148:341–343.

123. Dede JA, Janovski NA. Lipoma of the uterine tube—a gynecologic rarity. *Obstet Gynecol* 1963;22:461–467.

124. Sanes S, Warner R. Primary lymphangioma of the fallopian tube. *Am J Obstet Gynecol* 1939;37:316–321.

125. Weber DL, Fazzini E. Ganglioneuroma of the fallopian tube: a hitherto unreported finding. *Acta Neuropathol (Berl)* 1970;16:173–175.

126. Ebrahimi T, Okagaki T. Hemangioma of the fallopian tube. *Am J Obstet Gynecol* 1973;115:864–865.

127. Patel DR, Kawalek R, Iger J. Cavernous hemangioma of the fallopian tube. *Int Surg* 1973;58:420–421.

128. Talerman A. Haemangioma of the fallopian tube. *J Obstet Gynaecol Br Commonwealth* 1969;76:559–560.

129. Joglekar VM. Haemangioma of the fallopian tube. Case report. *Br J Obstet Gynaecol* 1979;86:823–825.

130. Benedet JL, White GW. Malignant tumors of fallopian tube. In: Coppleson M, ed. *Gynecologic oncology: fundamental principles and clinical practice.* New York: Churchill Livingstone, 1981:621–629.

131. Goldman JA, Gans B, Eckerling B. Hydrops tubae profluens—a symptom in tubal carcinoma. *Obstet Gynecol* 1961;18:631–634.

132. Sedlis A. Primary carcinoma of the fallopian tube. *Obstet Gynecol Surv* 1961;16:209–226.

133. Amendola BE, LaRouere J, Amendola MA, McClatchey KD, Han IH, Morley GW. Adenocarcinoma of the fallopian tube. *Surg Gynecol Obstet* 1983;157:223–227.

134. Eddy GL, Copeland LJ, Gershenson DM, Atkinson EN, Wharton JT, Rutledge FN. Fallopian tube carcinoma. *Obstet Gynecol* 1984;64:546–552.

135. Roberts JA, Lifshitz S. Primary adenocarcinoma of the fallopian tube. *Gynecol Oncol* 1982;13:301–308.

136. Kinzel GE. Primary carcinoma of the fallopian tube. *Am J Obstet Gynecol* 1976;125:816–820.

137. Goldman JA, Eckerling B. Hydrops tubae profluens—a symptom in tubal carcinoma. *Obstet Gynecol* 1961;18:631–634.

138. Takashina T, Ito E, Kudo R. Cytologic diagnosis of primary tubal cancer. *Acta Cytol (Baltimore)* 1985;29:367–372.

139. Schiller HM, Silverberg SG. Staging and prognosis in primary carcinoma of the fallopian tube. *Cancer* 1971;28:389–395.

140. Finn WF, Javert CT. Primary and metastatic cancer of the fallopian tube. *Cancer* 1949;2:803–814.

141. Schenck SB, Mackles A. Primary carcinoma of fallopian tubes with positive smears. Case report. *Am J Obstet Gynecol* 1961;81:782–783.

142. Woodruff JD, Julian CG. Multiple malignancy in the upper genital cancer. *Am J Obstet Gynecol* 1969;103:810–819.

143. Hu CY, Taymor ML, Hertig AT. Primary carcinoma of the fallopian tube. *Am J Obstet Gynecol* 1950;59:58–67.

144. Momtazee S, Kempson RL. Primary adenocarcinoma of the fallopian tube. *Obstet Gynecol* 1968;32:649–656.

145. Benedet JL, White GW, Fairey RN, Boyes DA. Adenocarcinoma of the fallopian tube. Experience with 41 patients. *Obstet Gynecol* 1977;50:654–657.

146. Yoonessi M. Carcinoma of the fallopian tube. *Obstet Gynecol Surv* 1979;34:257–270.

147. Boutselis JG, Thompson JN. Clinical aspects of primary carcinoma of the fallopian tube. A clinical study of 14 cases. *Am J Obstet Gynecol* 1971;111:98–101.

148. Hershey DW, Fennell RH, Major FJ. Primary carcinoma of the fallopian tube. *Obstet Gynecol* 1981;57:367–370.

149. Raju KS, Barker GH, Wiltshaw E. Primary carcinoma of the fallopian tube. Report of 22 cases. *Br J Obstet Gynaecol* 1981;88:1124–1129.

150. Bannatyne P, Russell P. Early adenocarcinoma of the fallopian tubes. A case for multifocal tumorigenesis. *Diagn Gynecol Obstet* 1981;3:49–60.

151. Yeung HHY, Bannatyne P, Russell P. Adenocarcinoma of the fallopian tubes: a clinicopathological study of eight cases. *Pathology* 1983;15:279–286.

152. Amendola BE, LaRouere J, Amendola MA, McClatchey KD, Han IH, Morley GW. Adenocarcinoma of the fallopian tube. *Surg Gynecol Obstet* 1983;157:223–227.

153. Brown MD, Kohorn EI, Kapp DS, Schwartz PE, Merino M. Fallopian tube carcinoma. *Int J Radiat Oncol Biol Phys* 1985;11:583–590.

154. Johnston GA Jr. Primary malignancy of the fallopian tube: a clinical review of 13 cases. *J Surg Oncol* 1983;24:304–309.

155. Hanton EM, Malkasian GD Jr, Danlin DC, Pratt JH. Primary carcinoma of the fallopian tube. *Am J Obstet Gynecol* 1966;94:832–839.

156. Kahn ME, Norris S. Primary carcinoma of the fallopian tubes. *Am J Obstet Gynecol* 1934;28:393–402.

157. Gatto V, Selim MA, Lankerani M. Primary carcinoma of the fallopian tube in an adolescent. *J Surg Oncol* 1986;33:212–214.

158. Weiss PD, MacDougall MK, Reagan JW, Wentz WB. Primary adenosquamous carcinoma of the fallopian tube. *Obstet Gynecol* 1980;55:885–895.

159. Gaffney EF, Cornog J. Endometrioid carcinoma of the fallopian tube arising in endometriosis. *Obstet Gynecol* 1978;52:34s–36s.

160. Case Records of the Massachusetts General Hospital (Case 53-1967). *N Engl J Med* 1967;277:1415–1420.

161. Imm FC. Primary adenosquamous carcinoma of the fallopian tube. *South Med J* 1980;73:678–680.

162. Moore DH, Woosley JT, Reddick RL, Walton LA, Siegal GP. Adenosquamous carcinoma of the fallopian tube. A clinicopathologic case report with verification of the diagnosis by immunohistochemical and ultrastructural studies. *Am J Obstet Gynecol* 1987;157:903–905.

163. Malinak LR, Miller GV, Armstrong JT. Primary squamous cell carcinoma of the fallopian tube. *Am J Obstet Gynecol* 1966;95:1167–1168.

164. Voet RL, Lifshitz S. Primary clear cell adenocarcinoma of the fallopian tube: light microscopic and ultrastructural findings. *Int J Gynecol Pathol* 1982;1:292–298.

165. Hovadhanakul P, Nuerenberger SP, Ritter PJ, Taylor HB, Cavanagh D. Primary transitional cell carcinoma of the fallopian tube associated with primary carcinomas of the ovary and endometrium. *Gynecol Oncol* 1976;4:138–143.

166. Federman Q, Toker C. Primary transitional cell tumor of the uterine adnexa. *Am J Obstet Gynecol* 1973;115:863–864.

167. Kanbour AI, Stock RJ. Squamous cell carcinoma *in situ* of the endometrium and fallopian tube as superficial extension of invasive cervical carcinoma. *Cancer* 1978;42:570–580.

168. Qizilbash AH, DePetrillo AD. Endometrial and tubal involvement by squamous carcinoma of the cervix. *Am J Clin Pathol* 1975;64:668–671.

169. Manes JL, Taylor HB. Carcinosarcoma and mixed müllerian tumors of the fallopian tube. Report of four cases. *Cancer* 1976;38:1687–1693.

170. Hanjani P, Petersen RO, Bonnell SA. Malignant mixed müllerian tumor of the fallopian tube. Report of a case and review of the literature. *Gynecol Oncol* 1980;9:381–393.

171. Kahanpaa KV, Laine R, Saksela E. Malignant mixed müllerian tumor of the fallopian tube: report of a case with 5-year survival. *Gynecol Oncol* 1983;16:144–149.

172. Buchino JJ, Buchino JJ. Malignant mixed müllerian tumor of the fallopian tube. *Arch Pathol Lab Med* 1987;111:386–387.

172a. Muntz HG, Rutgers JL, Tarraza HM, Fuller AF. Carcinosarcomas and mixed Müllerian tumors of the fallopian tube. *Gynecol Oncol* 1989;34:109–115.

173. Sworn MJ, Hammond GT, Buchanan R. Mixed mesenchymal sarcoma of the broad ligament. Case report. *Br J Obstet Gynaecol* 1979;86:403–406.

174. Lowell DM, Karsh J. Leiomyosarcoma of the broad ligament. *Obstet Gynecol* 1968;32:107–110.

175. Ullmann AS, Roumell TL. Leiomyosarcoma of the broad ligament. *Mich Med* 1973;72:411–414.

176. Weed JC, Podger K. Leiomyosarcoma of the broad ligament coincident with ductal carcinoma of the breast. *South Med J* 1976;69:1379–1380.

177. DiDomenico A, Stangl F, Bennington J. Case report. Leiomyosarcoma of the broad ligament. *Gynecol Oncol* 1982;13:412–415.

178. Herbold DR, Fu YS, Silbert SW. Leiomyosarcoma of the broad ligament. A case report and literature review with follow-up. *Am J Surg Pathol* 1983;7:285–292.

179. Rosenberg SA, Diamond HD, Jaslowitz B, Craver LF. Lymphosarcoma—a review of 1269 cases. *Medicine* 1961;40:31–84.

180. Osborne BM, Robboy SJ. Lymphomas or leukemia presenting as ovarian tumors. An analysis of 42 cases. *Cancer* 1983;52:1933–1943.

181. Cecalupo AJ, Frankel LS, Sullivan MP. Pelvic and ovarian extramedullary leukemic relapse in young girls. A report of four cases and review of the literature. *Cancer* 1982;50:587–593.

182. Aaron JB. Dermoid cyst in the uterine tube: a case report with a review of the literature. *Am J Obstet Gynecol* 1941;42:1080–1086.

183. Grimes HG, Kornmesser JG. Benign cystic teratoma of the oviduct: report of a case and review of the literature. *Obstet Gynecol* 1960;16:85.

184. Mazzarella P, Okagaki T, Richart RM. Teratoma of the uterine tube. A case report and review of the literature. *Obstet Gynecol* 1972;39:381–388.

185. Horn T, Jao W, Keh PC. Benign cystic teratoma of the fallopian tube. *Arch Pathol Lab Med* 1983;107:48.

186. Sweet RL, Selinger HE, McKay DG. Malignant teratoma of the uterine tube. *Obstet Gynecol* 1975;45:553–556.

187. Scully RE. Germ cell tumors of the ovary and fallopian tube. In: *Progress in gynecology, vol. IV.* New York: Grune & Stratton, 1963:335–347.

188. Henricksen E. Struma salpingii. Report of a case. *Obstet Gynecol* 1955;5:833–835.

189. Westerhout FC Jr. Ruptured tubal hydatidiform mole. Report of a case. *Obstet Gynecol* 1964;23:138–139.

190. Govender NSK, Goldstein DP. Metastatic tubal mole and coexisting intrauterine pregnancy. *Obstet Gynecol* 1977;49:67s–69s.

191. Ober W, Maier RC. Gestational choriocarcinoma of the fallopian tube. *Diagn Gynecol Obstet* 1982;3:213–231.

192. Kay S, Schneider V, Litt J. Choriocarcinoma of the mesosalpinx masquerading as congestive heart failure: ultrastructural observations of the tumor. *Int J Gynecol Pathol* 1983;2:72–87.

193. Dekel A, van Iddekinge B, Isaacson C, Dicker D, Feldberg D, Goldman J. Primary choriocarcinoma of the fallopian tube. Report of a case with survival and postoperative delivery. Review of the literature. *Obstet Gynecol Surv* 1986;41:142–148.

194. Mazur MT, Hsueh S, Gersell DJ. Metastases to the female genital tract. Analysis of 325 cases. *Cancer* 1984;53:1978–1984.

195. Kariminejad MH, Scully RE. Female adnexal tumor of probable wolffian origin. A distinctive pathologic entity. *Cancer* 1973;31:671–677.

196. Taxy JB, Battifora H. Female adnexal tumor of probable wolffian origin. Evidence for a low grade malignancy. *Cancer* 1976;37:2349–2354.

197. Sivathondan Y, Salm R, Hughesdon PE, Faccini JM. Female adnexal tumour of probable wolffian origin. *J Clin Pathol* 1979;32:616–624.

198. Kao GF, Norris HJ. Juxtaovarian adnexal tumor—a clinical and pathologic study of 19 cases. *Lab Invest* 1978;38:350–351.

199. Demopoulos RI, Sitelman A, Flotte T, Bigelow B. Ultrastructural study of a female adnexal tumor of probable Wolffian origin. *Cancer* 1980;46:2273–2280.

200. Abbot RL, Barlogie B, Schmidt WA. Metastasizing malignant juxtaovarian tumor with terminal hypercalcemia: a case report. *Cancer* 1981;48:860–865.

201. Janovski NA, Bozzetti LP. Serous papillary cystadenoma arising in paramesonephric rest of the mesosalpinx. *Obstet Gynecol* 1963;22:684–687.

202. Honore LH, Nickerson KG. Papillary serous cystadenoma arising in a paramesonephric cyst of the parovarium. *Am J Obstet Gynecol* 1976;125:870–871.

203. d'Ablaing G, Klatt E, DiRocco G, Hibbard LT. Broad ligament serous tumor of low malignant potential. *Int J Gynecol Pathol* 1983;2:93–99.

204. Chandraratnam E, Leong AS. Papillary serous cystadenoma of borderline malignancy in a parovarian paramesonephric cyst. Light microscopic and ultrastructural observations. *Histopathology* 1983;7:601–611.

205. Duvall E, Survis JA. Borderline tumour of the broad ligament. Case report. *Br J Obstet Gynaecol* 1983;90:372–375.

206. Aslani M, Ahn G-H, Scully RE. Serous papillary cystadenoma of broad ligament: a report of 25 cases. *Int J Gynecol Pathol* 1988;7:131–138.

207. Clark JE, Wood H, Jaffurs WJ, Fabro S. Endometrioid-type cystadenocarcinoma arising in the mesosalpinx. *Obstet Gynecol* 1979;54:656–658.

208. Czernobilsky B, Lancet M. Broad ligament adenocarcinoma of müllerian origin. *Obstet Gynecol* 1972;40:238–242.

209. Stapleton JJ, Haber MH, Lindner LE. Paramesonephric papillary serous cystadenocarcinoma. A case report with scanning electron microscopy. *Acta Cytol (Baltimore)* 1981;25:310–316.

210. Rojansky N, Ophir E, Sharony A, Spira H, Suprun H. Broad ligament adenocarcinoma—its origin and clinical behavior. A literature review and report of a case. *Obstet Gynecol Surv* 1985;40:665–671.

210a.Aslani M, Sculls RE. Primary carcinoma of the broad ligament. Report of four cases and review of the literature. *Cancer* 1989;64:1540–1545.

211. Bell DA, Woodruff JM, Scully RE. Ependymoma of the broad ligament. A report of two cases. *Am J Surg Pathol* 1984;8:203–209.

212. Grody WW, Nieberg RK, Bhuta S. Ependymoma-like tumor of the mesovarium. *Arch Pathol Lab Med* 1985;109:291–293.

213. Al-Jafari MS, Panton HM, Gradwell E. Phaeochromocytoma of the broad ligament. Case report. *Br J Obstet Gynecol* 1985;92:649–651.

214. Longway SR, Lind HM, Haghighi P. Extraskeletal Ewing's sarcoma arising in the broad ligament. *Arch Pathol Lab Med* 1986;110:1058–1061.

215. Wagner I, Bettendorf U. Extraovarian Brenner tumor. Case report and review. *Arch Gynecol* 1980;229:191–196.

216. Merino MJ, LiVolsi VA, Trepeta RW. Fibrothecoma of the broad ligament. *Diagn Gynecol Obstet* 1980;2:51–54.

217. Gersell DJ, King TC. Papillary cystadenoma of the mesosalpinx in von Hippel–Lindau disease. *Am J Surg Pathol* 1988;12:145–149.

*Surgical Pathology of the Female
Reproductive System and Peritoneum,*
edited by Stephen S. Sternberg
and Stacey E. Mills. Raven Press, Ltd,
New York © 1991.

CHAPTER 8

Peritoneum

Philip B. Clement, Robert H. Young, and Robert E. Scully

INFLAMMATORY LESIONS

Acute Peritonitis

Acute diffuse peritonitis, characterized by a serosal fibrinopurulent exudate, is most commonly associated with a perforated viscus and is usually bacterial or chemical (bile or gastric or pancreatic juice) in origin. The lipases in pancreatic juice also typically produce fat necrosis. Spontaneous bacterial peritonitis occurs most often in children and in adults who are immunocompromised or have cirrhosis of the liver (1,2). Rare infectious causes of acute peritonitis include candida (3), actinomycetes (4), and amoebae (5). Recurrent attacks of acute peritonitis are an almost constant feature of familial Mediterranean fever (recurrent polyserositis; periodic disease) (6).

Granulomatous Peritonitis

A variety of infectious and noninfectious agents can cause granulomatous peritonitis. The peritoneum may be studded with nodules, which can mimic disseminated tumor at operation. The diagnosis rests on the histologic, and in some cases microbiologic, identification of the causative agent.

Infectious Causes

Tuberculous peritonitis may be secondary to spread from a focus within the abdominopelvic cavity or may be a manifestation of miliary spread (7,8). The granulomas are characterized by caseous necrosis and Langhans'-type giant cells; mycobacteria may be demonstrated by acid-fast stains or immunofluorescence methods. Rarely, granulomatous peritonitis is a complication of fungal infections, including histoplasmosis (9), coccidioidomycosis (10), and cryptococcosis (11), and

parasitic infestations, including schistosomiasis (12), oxyuriasis (13,14), echinococcosis (4), ascariasis (15), and strongyloidiasis (16).

Noninfectious Causes

Foreign material, typically recognizable on histologic examination, can elicit a granulomatous reaction on the peritoneum. Starch granules from surgical gloves (17–19), douche fluid (20), and lubricants (21) typically incite a granulomatous and fibrosing peritonitis; in occasional cases the inflammatory reaction may be of tuberculoid type with caseous necrosis (22). The periodic acid-Schiff (PAS)-positive starch granules exhibit a characteristic Maltese-cross configuration under polarized light. Talc was once an important cause of granulomatous and fibrosing peritonitis because of its use as a lubricant on surgical gloves (23,24), but talc-induced peritonitis has also been described more recently in drug abusers (25). Other iatrogenic causes of granulomatous peritonitis include: cellulose and cotton fibers from surgical pads and drapes (26–28); microcrystalline collagen hemostat (Avitene) (29); and oily materials (hysterosalpingographic contrast medium, mineral oil, paraffin) (30–32). The last three substances are associated with a lipogranulomatous reaction.

Escaped bowel contents, including vegetable matter, food-derived starch (33), and barium sulfate (34), can produce a peritoneal foreign-body reaction. Sebaceous material and keratin from ruptured dermoid cysts typically evoke an intense granulomatous, lipogranulomatous, and fibrosing peritoneal inflammatory reaction that may mimic a neoplasm at operation (35–37). Meconium, containing lanugo hair, squamous cells, keratin, bile, and pancreatic and intestinal secretions, produces a granulomatous peritonitis (Fig. 1); calcification may also be prominent (38–40). In boys, the process may involve the tunica vaginalis and may result in a

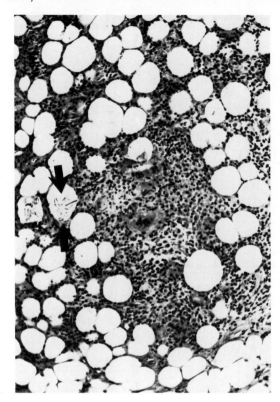

FIG. 1. Meconium peritonitis. The omentum is infiltrated with histiocytes, including foreign-body-type giant cells. Note keratin debris (*arrows*).

tumor-like scrotal mass (41). Keratin exfoliated from the surfaces of uterine and ovarian adenoacanthomas may incite a granulomatous response on the pelvic peritoneum; its presence is not considered to be evidence of implantation of carcinoma on the peritoneum (42). Chronic bile peritonitis may be associated with granulomatous inflammation and fibrosis; cholesterol crystals and bile pigment may be identifiable within giant cells (43). Granulomatous peritonitis has also been described secondary to Crohn's disease (44), sarcoidosis (45), and Whipple's disease (46).

Peritoneal Fibrosis

Reactive peritoneal fibrosis, often accompanied by fibrous adhesions, is a common sequela of prior peritoneal inflammation and is a frequent complication associated with surgical procedures (47). In occasional cases, it may be difficult to differentiate between markedly reactive peritoneal fibrosis and a desmoplastic mesothelioma, particularly in a small biopsy specimen (48). Features favoring a diagnosis of mesothelioma include nuclear atypia, necrosis, the presence of organized patterns of collagen deposition (fascicular, storiform), and infiltration of adjacent tissues (48).

Localized hyaline plaques are a common incidental

finding on the splenic capsule and are probably related to splenic congestion (49). Fibrous thickening of the peritoneum has been described in patients with hepatic cirrhosis and ascites (50).

Sclerosing peritonitis is a rare disorder characterized by a fibrous peritoneal thickening. Concato described pearly white thickening of the peritoneum, in the form of either discrete plaques or continuous sheets involving the hepatic, splenic, and diaphragmatic peritoneum (51). More recent reports have described a similar lesion that encases the small bowel ("abdominal cocoon"), causing bowel obstruction. It occurs in an idiopathic form, typically affecting adolescent girls (52,53), or it may be secondary to practolol therapy (54), chronic ambulatory peritoneal dialysis (55), or the use of a peritoneovenous (LeVeen) shunt (56). Sclerosing peritonitis should be distinguished from peritoneal encapsulation, a congenital malformation in which an accessory peritoneal membrane encases loops of small bowel in a sac-like structure (57,58).

Rare Types of Peritonitis

Eosinophilic peritonitis is seen rarely in cases of eosinophilic gastroenteritis and hypereosinophilic syndrome (59). Isolated cases of eosinophilic ascites have been associated with childhood atopy, peritoneal dialysis, vasculitis, lymphoma or metastatic carcinoma, and ruptured hydatid cysts (59). Rare cases of peritonitis may be secondary to peritoneal involvement by collagen-vascular diseases, including systemic lupus erythematosus (60) and Degos' disease (61).

TUMOR-LIKE LESIONS

Mesothelial Hyperplasia

Hyperplasia of mesothelial cells is a common response to inflammation and chronic effusions. Hyperplastic lesions may be noted at operation as solitary or multiple small nodules but more commonly are incidental findings on microscopic examination (48,62–64). Mesothelial hyperplasia may be confined to a hernia sac and in such cases may be due to trauma or incarceration (65). It often involves the adnexal areas in cases of chronic salpingitis and endometriosis and is occasionally encountered, particularly in the omentum, in association with ovarian tumors. In florid examples, solid, trabecular, or complex papillary or tubulopapillary patterns may be seen (Figs. 2 and 3), accompanied by limited degrees of extension of the mesothelial cells into the underlying tissues. In many cases the cells are arranged into more or less parallel thin layers, separated by fibrin or fibrous tissue. The mesothelial cells may contain intracellular vacuoles filled with acid mucin (predomi-

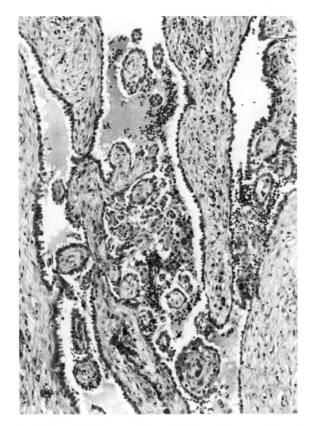

FIG. 2. Mesothelial hyperplasia of pelvic peritoneum. Reactive mesothelial cells line irregular spaces and form papillae. The stroma consists of inflamed fibrous tissue.

nantly hyaluronic acid) or, less commonly, may exhibit marked cytoplasmic clearing (48). Mild to moderate nuclear pleomorphism can be seen, along with mitotic figures and, occasionally, multinucleated cells (Fig. 3). Psammoma bodies are encountered in occasional cases, and rarely, eosinophilic strap-shaped cells resembling rhabdomyoblasts have been described (65). McCaughey and Al-Jabi (48) have pointed out that the presence of a grossly evident tumor mass, necrosis, severe nuclear pleomorphism, and deep infiltration favor malignant mesothelioma, although in occasional cases the distinction between a hyperplastic and malignant process may be difficult or impossible, particularly in a biopsy specimen. Immunohistochemical methods have not yet been of aid in the differential diagnosis. If the lesion in question is a malignant mesothelioma, follow-up usually reveals its nature within several months because of its typical rapid growth (48). Apparently benign, otherwise typical mesothelial proliferations, however, occasionally precede the appearance of malignant mesotheliomas (48).

Peritoneal Inclusion Cysts

Peritoneal inclusion cysts (PICs) typically occur in the peritoneal cavity of young women (66–73). Rarely, they

occur in males; similar lesions have been described in the pleural cavity (64,74–76). Some PICs are incidental findings at laparotomy in the form of single or multiple, small, thin-walled, translucent, unilocular cysts that may be attached or lie free in the peritoneal cavity. Occasionally they may involve the round ligament simulating an inguinal hernia (77). The cysts have a smooth lining, and their contents vary from a yellow watery fluid to a gelatinous fluid.

Other PICs, which have also been referred to as "benign cystic mesotheliomas," are large, fixed, multilocular cystic masses that may measure up to 20 cm in diameter (Fig. 4) (66,67). Unlike the smaller unilocular cysts, their septa and walls may contain considerable amounts of fibrous tissue. Their contents may resemble those of the unilocular cysts or may be serosanguinous or bloody. PICs of this type are usually associated with clinical manifestations—most commonly lower abdominal pain, a palpable mass, or both. A history of a prior abdominal operation, pelvic inflammatory disease, or endometriosis is present in at least one-third of the patients, suggesting a role for inflammation in the pathogenesis of the cysts in some cases (66,67,73,78–80). An inflammatory pathogenesis is also supported by the occurrence of cases in which the dividing line between a PIC and inflammation-associated florid adhesions may

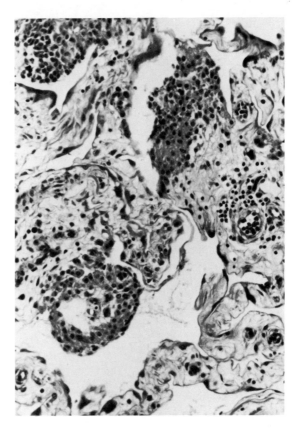

FIG. 3. Mesothelial hyperplasia of pelvic peritoneum. Some of the mesothelial cells form solid nests. Occasional mesothelial cells have hyperchromatic, pleomorphic nuclei.

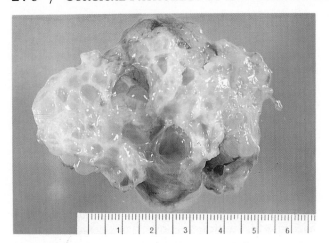

FIG. 4. Peritoneal inclusion cyst. The multilocular cystic mass consists of multiple cysts separated by fibrous tissue.

be difficult and arbitrary. With one exception (76), there has been no association with asbestos exposure. Follow-up examinations have not disclosed a malignant behavior, but in approximately 40% of the cases the lesions have recurred one or more times from months to many years postoperatively (71). It is possible, however, that at least some of these "recurrences" are the result of newly

formed postoperative adhesions. For these reasons, we prefer the designation "multilocular peritoneal inclusion cyst" to "benign cystic mesothelioma" until there is convincing evidence for their neoplastic nature (67).

On microscopic examination, PICs are typically lined by a single layer of flat to cuboidal mesothelial cells (Fig. 5); foci of squamous epithelium are seen in a minority of cases. The mesothelial cells typically lack significant atypia, stratification, or mitotic activity, but occasionally exhibit a hobnail appearance, as well as stratification, mild nuclear pleomorphism, and slight mitotic activity. The thin septa typically consist of a loose, fibrovascular connective tissue (Fig. 5) with a sparse inflammatory infiltrate. Less commonly (particularly in large multilocular cysts), marked acute and chronic inflammation, broad bands of proliferating fibrous tissue, and evidence of recent and remote hemorrhage may be seen in the cyst walls. In such cases, mural proliferations of atypical mesothelial cells arranged singly or as gland-like structures or nests may be encountered (Fig. 6), creating infiltrative patterns that should not be confused with a malignant tumor (73).

PICs should be distinguished from cysts of lymphatic origin, including unilocular lymphatic cysts and multilocular cystic lymphangiomas. The latter typically occur

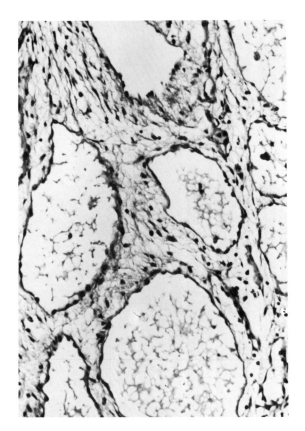

FIG. 5. Peritoneal inclusion cyst. Cystic spaces are lined by a single layer of flat to low cuboidal mesothelial cells. The stroma consists of loose fibrous tissue with a sparse chronic inflammatory-cell infiltrate.

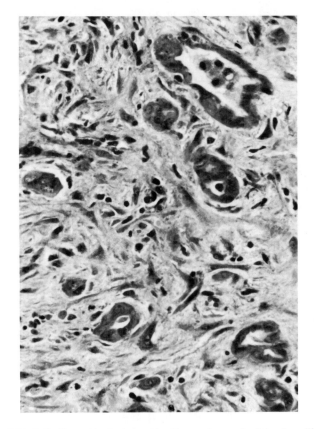

FIG. 6. Peritoneal inclusion cyst with mural mesothelial-cell proliferation. Atypical mesothelial cells form small nests and gland-like structures within a cellular inflamed fibrous stroma.

in children, more frequently in boys. In contrast to PICs, lymphatic cysts are typically located in the mesentery, frequently contain chylous fluid, and are characterized, at least focally, by a lining of flattened endothelial cells. Smooth muscle (in lymphangiomas) and a prominent lymphoid infiltrate are typically present within their walls. In problematic cases, immunohistochemical stains may be useful in distinguishing between endothelial cells (*Ulex europaeus* lectin reactivity) and mesothelial cells (vimentin and cytokeratin reactivity) lining lymphangiomas and PICs, respectively.

Splenosis

Splenosis, which results from implantation of splenic tissue, is typically an incidental finding at laparotomy months to years after splenectomy for traumatic rupture of the spleen (81–85). A few to innumerable red-blue peritoneal nodules, ranging from punctate to 7 cm in diameter, are scattered widely throughout the abdominal cavity but occur less commonly in the pelvic cavity. The intraoperative appearance may mimic endometriosis, hemangiomas, or metastatic tumor.

Melanosis

The three reported cases of melanosis, or melanotic pigmentation of the peritoneum, have all been associated with ovarian dermoid cysts; in two cases, the cysts had ruptured preoperatively (86–88). At laparotomy, focal or diffuse, tan to black, peritoneal staining or similarly pigmented, tumor-like nodules are encountered within the pelvis and in the omentum. Some of the cysts within the ovarian tumors exhibit pigmentation of their contents and lining. On histologic examination, the ovarian and peritoneal pigmentation consists of melanin-laden histiocytes within a fibrous stroma (Fig. 7). In

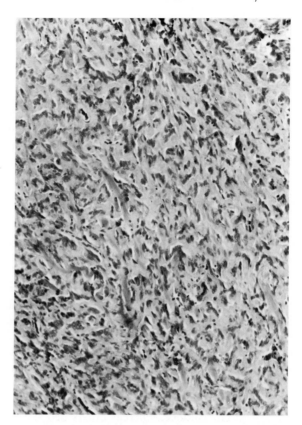

FIG. 8. Localized fibrous ''mesothelioma'' of the peritoneum.

at least two of the reported cases and in a third case we have encountered, gastric mucosa was prominent within an otherwise typical dermoid cyst. No obvious source for the pigment could be identified in any of the cases. These cases of benign peritoneal melanosis should obviously be distinguished from metastatic malignant melanoma.

MESOTHELIAL NEOPLASMS

Localized Fibrous "Mesothelioma"

Localized fibrous tumors of the type involving the pleura are extremely rare in the peritoneal cavity (Fig. 8) (89). They are now generally considered to originate from submesothelial fibroblasts (64).

Adenomatoid Tumor

This benign tumor of mesothelial origin rarely arises from extragenital peritoneum such as the omentum (90) or mesentery (91), but it is much more commonly encountered within the male and female genital tracts and is discussed in chapters dealing with these subjects.

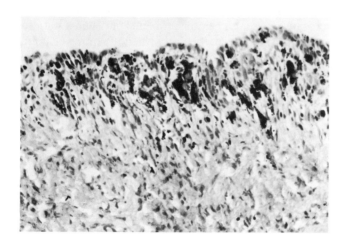

FIG. 7. Peritoneal melanosis. Melanin-laden histiocytes lie within the submesothelial connective tissue.

Well-Differentiated Papillary Mesothelioma

This rare lesion typically involves the peritoneum of females (62,69,92–94), but a few examples have been encountered in males (tunica vaginalis) and in extraperitoneal (pleura, epicardium) locations (64). The tumor is usually an incidental finding at operation but is occasionally associated with ascites or abdominal pain. None has been asbestos-related. All the patients with this type of tumor who have been followed have had a benign course, but only a few have had long-term follow-up; "well-differentiated" is therefore preferable to "benign" until knowledge of the natural history of this lesion is more complete.

On gross examination, the tumors appear as gray to white, firm, single or multiple, sometimes papillary lesions, several centimeters or less in diameter, typically involving the peritoneum of the omentum, mesentery, or stomach. Microscopic examination reveals a characteristic, uniform papillary pattern with fibrous papillae covered by single layers of well-differentiated, uniform, flattened to cuboidal mesothelial cells (Fig. 9). When multiple lesions are present, it is important that each be sampled histologically, because they may vary in appearance. We have seen one case in which a few lesions had a benign appearance, whereas others had the appearance of malignant mesothelioma.

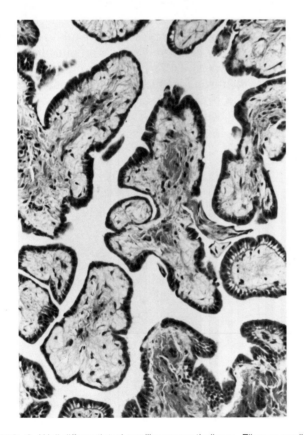

FIG. 9. Well-differentiated papillary mesothelioma. Fibrous papillae are lined by a single layer of uniform mesothelial cells.

Diffuse Malignant Mesothelioma

Diffuse malignant mesotheliomas (DMMs) of the peritoneal cavity are much less common than similar tumors in the pleural cavity. They are particularly rare in women, in whom the majority of malignant papillary neoplasms involving the peritoneum are examples of extraovarian papillary serous tumors of borderline malignancy or carcinomas (94,95).

The affected patients, who are typically middle-aged or elderly men, present with abdominal discomfort, distension, digestive disturbances, and weight loss (95). Over 80% of the patients in one large series had a history of asbestos exposure (95); occasional cases have followed abdominal irradiation. Rare examples have been preceded by recurrent peritonitis and atypical mesothelial hyperplasia (48,96). Most patients survive less than a year after diagnosis; more recently, however, intensive chemotherapy of patients with early tumors has resulted in improved survival (97).

At laparotomy, the visceral and parietal peritoneum appear diffusely thickened or extensively involved by nodules and plaques. The viscera are often encased by tumor and may be invaded, although local invasion and metastases to lymph nodes, liver, lungs, and pleura are less frequent than in association with carcinomas showing comparable degrees of peritoneal involvement (95). The histological features (Fig. 10) are identical to DMMs involving the pleura (see Chapter 24), except for an apparently lower frequency of purely sarcomatoid tumors (95). One unique case of peritoneal DMM was characterized by large numbers of foamy lipid-rich cells that were interpreted as histiocytes within the stroma of the tumor (98).

DMMs should be distinguished from diffuse peritoneal involvement by metastatic adenocarcinoma. Certain patterns of mesothelioma, such as the biphasic and the sarcomatoid, particularly when considered in conjunction with the gross characteristics of the tumor, are almost diagnostic. Tumors with a tubulopapillary pattern may present a greater problem, but such a pattern may be distinctive, particularly when the lining cells are characteristic of mesothelial cells. The presence of large numbers of psammoma bodies favors a diagnosis of papillary carcinoma of serous type. Special stains may be helpful in confirming the diagnosis. DMMs are characterized by an absence of neutral mucins and the presence of acid mucin (predominantly hyaluronic acid) within intracellular vacuoles or in an extracellular location, appreciable as alcian blue-positive, PAS-negative, hyaluronidase-sensitive material. Immunoreactivity for both cytokeratin and vimentin, in addition to negative staining for serous amylase, carcinoembryonic antigen (CEA), milk-fat globule protein, CA 125, beta$_1$ pregnancy-specific glycoprotein, and secretory component, favors a diagnosis of DMM over carcinoma (99–107).

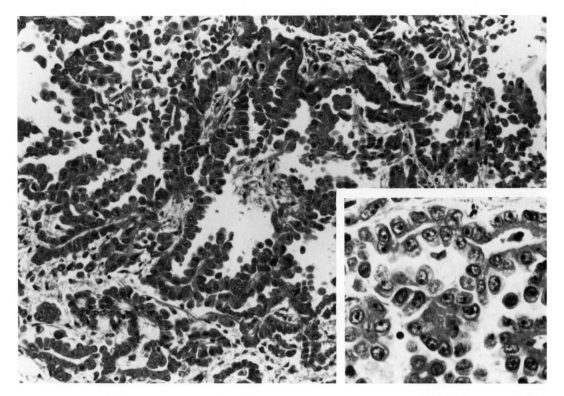

FIG. 10. Diffuse malignant mesothelioma with tubulopapillary pattern. Tumor cells have malignant features (**inset**).

METASTATIC TUMORS

Peritoneal involvement by metastatic tumor is typically a result of seeding from a primary tumor arising within the abdomen or pelvis, most commonly the ovary. Peritoneal serous tumors in which the ovaries are normal or only minimally involved may arise directly from the peritoneum (see next section) or rarely are metastatic from a serous papillary carcinoma of the endometrium. Other primary tumors that may be associated with peritoneal seeding include carcinomas of the breast (108) and gastrointestinal tract, especially the colon and stomach, and the pancreas. In such cases, the metastatic tumor may take the form of signet-ring cells widely scattered in a fibrous stroma (Fig. 11). Occasionally the signet-ring cells can have relatively bland nuclear features, resulting in a deceptively benign appearance (Fig. 11).

Peritoneal extension of a mucinous neoplasm may be accompanied by pseudomyxoma peritonei. Histologic examination discloses large pools of mucin surrounded by well-differentiated mucinous epithelium of intestinal type. The neoplastic epithelium may be inconspicuous, and if pseudomyxoma is suspected from the intraoperative appearance, extensive histologic sampling should be performed before the diagnosis is excluded. The collections of mucin typically elicit a proliferation of dense, often hyalinized, fibrous stroma. Pseudomyxoma peritonei is most commonly associated with a mucinous ovarian tumor, typically of borderline malignancy or, less commonly, benign or carcinomatous (see Chapter 49). An appendiceal lesion is also usually present in such cases, typically a low-grade adenocarcinoma similar in appearance to the ovarian tumor (109–112). It may be difficult or impossible to determine whether the appendiceal and ovarian tumors are independent lesions or whether the latter is metastatic from the former. Because primary ovarian carcinomas have no known association with primary intestinal carcinomas in general, most cases of combined appendiceal and ovarian mucinous tumors probably reflect metastatic spread from the appendix to the ovary. Careful microscopic examination of the appendix is important, therefore, in all cases of ovarian tumors associated with pseudomyxoma peritonei. Pseudomyxoma peritonei is rarely associated with other mucin-secreting tumors, including carcinomas of the stomach, colon, pancreas, gallbladder, uterine corpus, and urachus (113). Pseudomyxoma peritonei should be distinguished from localized collections of

These special stains may be less conclusive in distinguishing a DMM from a papillary peritoneal carcinoma of serous type. Occasional papillary peritoneal tumors that exhibit staining patterns intermediate between those of these two tumors are best classified on the basis of their appearance with routine stains.

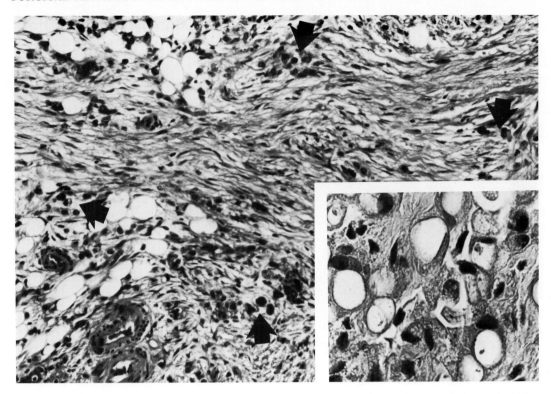

FIG. 11. Metastatic signet-ring carcinoma to the omentum. Note sparsely distributed tumor cells (*arrows*) within an abundant fibrous stroma. Typical signet-ring tumor cells are seen at higher power (**inset**).

acellular mucin surrounding a ruptured mucinous ovarian tumor or appendiceal mucocele. These mucin collections are associated with a self-limiting inflammatory reaction and fibrosis.

LESIONS OF THE SECONDARY MÜLLERIAN SYSTEM

These lesions share an origin from the so-called "secondary müllerian system," that is, the pelvic and lower abdominal mesothelium and the subjacent mesenchyme of females (114–116). The müllerian potential of this layer is consistent with its close embryonic relation to the primary müllerian system (the müllerian ducts), which arises by invagination of the coelomic epithelium. Lesions of the secondary müllerian system include those containing endometrioid, serous, and mucinous epithelium, simulating normal or neoplastic endometrial, tubal, and endocervical epithelium. The metaplastic potential of the pelvic peritoneum also includes differentiation toward cells of transitional (urothelial) type, exemplified most commonly by Walthard nests. Proliferation of the subjacent mesenchyme may accompany epithelial differentiation of the mesothelium or may give rise to a variety of pure mesenchymal lesions composed of endometrial stromal-type cells, decidua, or smooth muscle.

ENDOMETRIOSIS

Endometriosis is defined as the presence of endometrial tissue outside the endometrium or myometrium. Usually, both epithelium and stroma are seen, but occasionally the diagnosis of endometriosis can be made when only one component is present (116a). Etiologic, pathogenetic, and clinical aspects of endometriosis, which have been reviewed in detail elsewhere (116), are not considered here, as they do not have a significant bearing on histological interpretation. The occurrence of endometriosis in extraperitoneal sites is also discussed elsewhere (116,116b).

Macroscopic Features

Depending on their duration and their superficial or deep location in relation to the peritoneal surface, endometriotic foci may appear as punctate, red, blue, brown, or white spots or patches with either a slightly raised or puckered surface (Fig. 12) (117–119). Ecchymotic or brown areas have sometimes been described as "powder burns." The endometriotic foci are frequently associated with dense fibrous adhesions. The lesions may form nodules or cysts, or both. Rarely, pelvic peritoneal endometriosis may present as multiple, polypoid masses

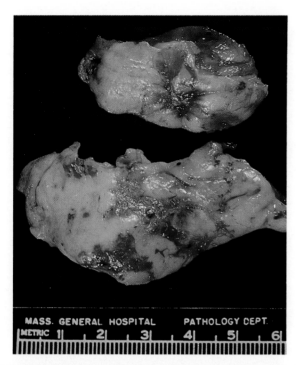

FIG. 12. Endometriosis of ovaries. Multiple hemorrhagic and pigmented foci involve the serosal surfaces. Some of the lesions have a puckered appearance.

of soft gray tissue that fill the pelvis, simulating a malignant tumor (120–122).

Endometriotic cysts (endometriomas) most commonly involve the ovaries, where they may partially or almost completely replace the normal tissue; bilateral involvement occurs in one-third to one-half of the cases (123,124). The cysts rarely exceed 15 cm in diameter; larger examples are more likely to harbor a neoplasm. Endometriotic cysts are commonly covered by dense fibrous adhesions, which may result in fixation to adjacent structures. The cyst walls are usually thick and fi-

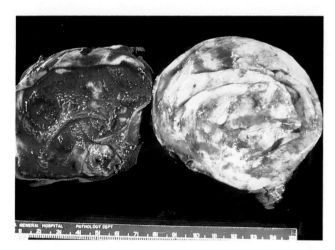

FIG. 13. Endometriotic cysts of ovaries. One of the cysts is filled with thick chocolate-colored material.

brotic, with a smooth or shaggy, brown to yellow lining (Fig. 13). The cyst contents typically consist of altered, semifluid or inspissated, chocolate-colored material (Fig. 13); rarely, the cyst is filled with watery fluid. Any solid areas in the cyst wall or intraluminal polypoid projections should be sampled histologically, because they may be malignant tumors arising from the epithelial or stromal component of the cyst. Rare complications of endometriosis, typically during pregnancy, include rupture (usually ovarian or intestinal) producing acute abdominal symptoms (125–127) or hemorrhage from endometriotic lesions that have undergone decidual transformation (128).

Histologic Features

The appearance of endometriotic tissue varies with the extent of its response to the normal hormonal fluctuations of the menstrual cycle and the duration of the process (Figs. 14 and 15). When the appearances of simultaneous samples of eutopic endometrium and endometriotic foci are compared, the latter exhibit cyclic changes in approximately 80% of the cases, although considerable variability in glandular morphology is observed (129). When more than one endometriotic focus is examined in the same patient, the appearances of the specimens do not differ significantly from one to an-

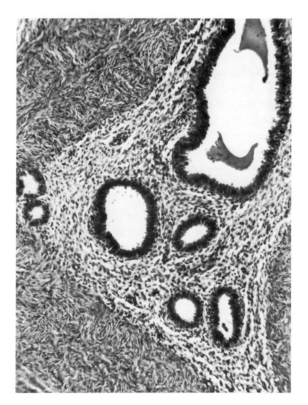

FIG. 14. Endometriosis of ovary. The endometriotic focus, composed of proliferative-type endometrial glands and stroma, is surrounded by ovarian stroma.

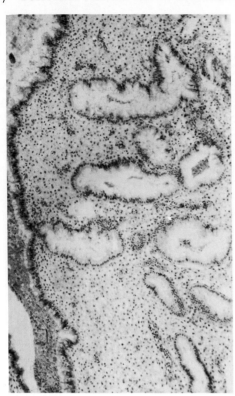

FIG. 15. Endometriosis of cul-de-sac showing a secretory appearance.

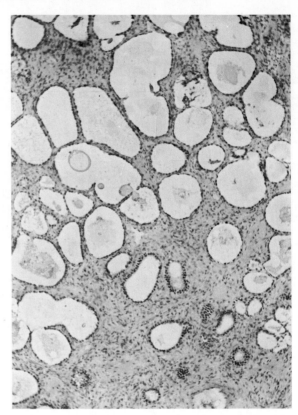

FIG. 16. Endometriosis in a postmenopausal woman. The cystic endometriotic glands are lined by flattened cells and are separated by a fibrous stroma.

other (129). In most postmenopausal patients with endometriosis, the endometriotic tissue is atrophic with glands that are occasionally cystic and lined by flattened epithelial cells surrounded by a dense fibrotic stroma (Fig. 16); the appearance is similar to that of simple or cystic atrophy of the endometrium (130). In a minority of cases, however, the endometriotic tissue has an active appearance, with or without the metaplastic and hyperplastic changes that are more commonly present in premenopausal women (see below).

Menstruation into endometriotic foci results in hemorrhage within the stroma and glandular lumens, as well as a secondary inflammatory response consisting predominantly of a diffuse infiltration of histiocytes. The latter typically convert the extravasated red blood cells into glycolipid and granular brown pigment, becoming so-called "pseudoxanthoma cells" (Figs. 18 and 19) (131–133). Most of the pigment appears to be hemofuscin, and hemosiderin is typically present to a much lesser extent (133). The amount of pigment in an endometriotic lesion appears to increase with its age, and early lesions are typically nonpigmented (118). Variable numbers of lymphocytes and smaller numbers of other inflammatory cells may be present. Large numbers of neutrophils with microabscess formation should raise the possibility of secondary bacterial infection (134).

In endometriotic cysts, the epithelial cells lining the cyst may be large and cuboidal with abundant eosinophilic cytoplasm and large atypical nuclei (Fig. 17) (135–138). The significance of such nuclear atypia is unclear. Although it may be reactive, we have seen cells with these feature merge with clear-cell adenocarcinomas and borderline mucinous neoplasms of müllerian type (137,138). The epithelial and stromal lining of

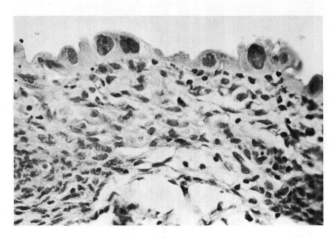

FIG. 17. Lining of endometriotic cyst. The lining epithelial cells have abundant cytoplasm and large atypical nuclei.

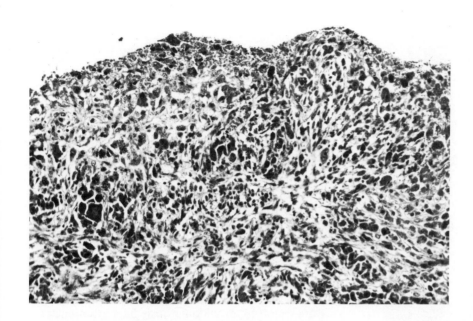

FIG. 18. Lining of endometriotic cyst. The lining consists of heavily pigmented histiocytes (pseudoxanthoma cells) and fibrous tissue.

an endometriotic cyst frequently becomes attenuated, and the former may be reduced to a single layer of cuboidal cells that may retain some endometrial characteristics but that are often devoid of specific features (117). In such circumstances, recognition of the cyst as endometriotic may only be possible if a rim of subjacent endometrial stroma persists. Commonly, the cyst lining of endometrial epithelium and stroma is totally lost and is replaced by granulation tissue, dense fibrous tissue, and variable numbers of pseudoxanthoma cells (Fig. 18). Occasionally, ovarian and extraovarian endometriosis is manifested by the presence of necrotic pseudoxanthomatous nodules characterized by a central zone of necrosis surrounded by pseudoxanthoma cells, often in a palisaded arrangement, hyalinized fibrous tissue, or both (Fig. 19); typical endometriotic glands and stroma may be few or absent (133). Rare examples of endometriosis are composed exclusively of endometriotic stroma ("stromal endometriosis") (116a).

Endometriosis that involves smooth muscle in the uterine ligaments or in the walls of hollow viscera is typically associated with striking proliferation of the smooth muscle, creating an appearance similar to that of adenomyosis (Fig. 20) (121). The endometriotic stroma itself may also undergo smooth-muscle metaplasia, which is most often encountered within the walls of ovarian endometriotic cysts but occasionally encountered elsewhere (139–142). Extensive amounts of smooth muscle within the endometriotic stroma can result in "endomyometriosis" (uterus-like masses), which has been described within an obturator lymph node (139), the ovary (140,143), broad ligament (144), and lumbosacral region (145), and, in males, in the scrotum (141). The appearance of a uterus-like mass in the region of the ovary has also been ascribed to a congenital malformation (146).

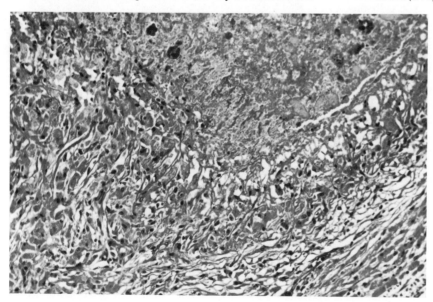

FIG. 19. Necrotic pseudoxanthomatous nodule of endometriosis. Pseudoxanthoma cells surround a central zone of necrotic tissue.

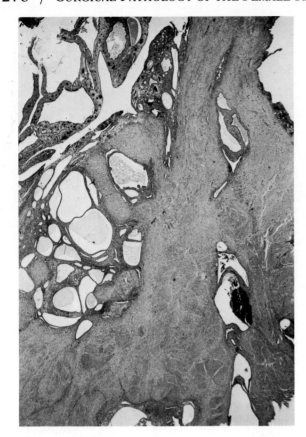

FIG. 20. Endometriosis of ureter. The wall of the ureter is thickened by hyperplastic smooth muscle that surrounds the foci of endometriosis containing cystic glands. Polypoid endometriosis projects into the lumen of the ureter (*top left corner*).

Metaplastic changes similar to those occurring in eutopic endometrial glands have been described in endometriotic glands. These include tubal (ciliated) (114,135,147), hobnail (135), and, rarely, squamous (148) and mucinous metaplasia; the latter may be characterized by the presence of endocervical-type cells or, less often, goblet cells (149,150). Rarely, endometriotic stroma may exhibit a myxoid appearance, or focal ossification and calcification (151,152). Perineural (153) and vascular invasion (154) have been reported rarely in otherwise typical, benign endometriotic lesions.

A variety of hyperplastic and atypically hyperplastic changes similar to those occurring in the endometrium have been described in endometriotic glands, sometimes related to an endogenous or exogenous estrogenic stimulus (Fig. 21) (135,155–158). It is logical to conclude that such atypical changes have a malignant potential similar to those in the endometrium, although there is little evidence on which to base such a conclusion. Rare cases of hyperplastic endometriosis, however, have preceded the development of an adenocarcinoma in the same area (156,158). Endometriotic tissue may also exhibit progestational changes, typically during pregnancy (Fig. 22) or progestin therapy (Fig. 23) (159). In such

cases, examination reveals a decidual reaction with atrophy of the endometrial glands, which are small and lined by cuboidal or flattened epithelial cells (Fig. 22). In pregnancy, the glands rarely exhibit an Arias-Stella reaction, optically clear nuclei, or both (160,161). Necrosis of the decidual cells, foci of marked stromal edema, and infiltration by lymphocytes are additional findings in patients receiving progestational agents (159). Atrophic changes similar to those that are seen typically in the endometriotic foci of postmenopausal patients may be present in premenopausal patients treated with oral contraceptives or danazol (162–164). In one study, one-third of the endometriotic foci disappeared or were replaced by fibrous tissue after danazol therapy (164).

Associated Lesions and Differential Diagnosis

Rare examples of endometriosis have been encountered in intimate association with foci of peritoneal leiomyomatosis (165–167), glial implants of ovarian teratomas (168,169), and nodules of splenosis (170). Endometriosis may also be accompanied by, and should be distinguished from, endosalpingiosis, which is characterized by glands lined by benign tubal-type epithelium, unassociated with endometrial stroma (see subse-

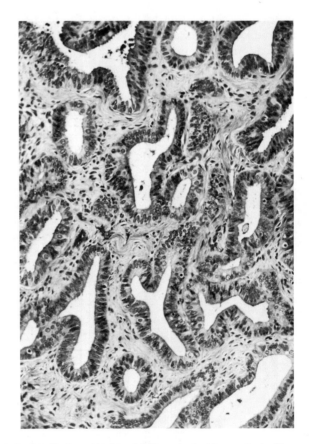

FIG. 21. Endometriosis exhibiting atypical hyperplasia. The endometriotic glands exhibit both architectural and cytologic atypia.

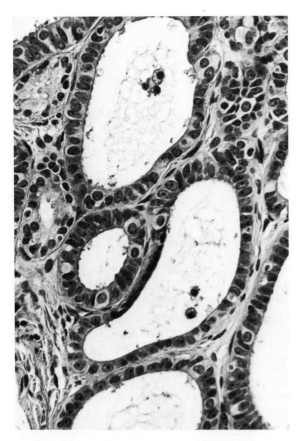

FIG. 24. Endosalpingiosis of omentum. The glands are lined by a single layer of uniform, cuboidal to columnar cells. Occasional cells have pale cytoplasm and are ciliated.

Extraovarian Serous Tumors

Occasional tumors resembling ovarian serous border-line tumors are characterized by (a) extraovarian peritoneal involvement and (b) absence of, or minimal, ovarian surface involvement. Patients with these tumors are typically under the age of 35 years, often present with infertility, and may have fibrous adhesions associated with the neoplastic foci (210,210a). Microscopic examination reveals superficial tumor that may be predominantly epithelial (Fig. 25) or may be associated with a marked desmoplastic response and numerous psammoma bodies (Fig. 26, 211). When the latter are present in very large numbers, the term "psammocarcinoma" has sometimes been used (Fig. 26). Myometrial lymphatic involvement has been described in two cases of "psammocarcinoma" (211a). The tumors may be associated with a very good long-term prognosis (210).

Occasionally, serous carcinomas with invasive properties also appear to arise from the pelvic peritoneum (212–216a–d). When there is more than minimal ovarian involvement in a patient with extensive peritoneal serous carcinoma, the tumor is better classified as an ovarian carcinoma, even though the possibility that it

arose multifocally on the peritoneum cannot be excluded.

Rare extraovarian serous tumors take the form of localized, typically cystic masses, usually within the broad ligament (see Chapter 50) and less commonly within the retroperitoneum. Serous papillary cystadenomas and adenofibromas, serous borderline tumors, and serous carcinomas have been described in these sites (217–225).

Extraovarian serous tumors are identical to their ovarian counterparts on histologic, immunohistochemical, and ultrastructural examination (62,94,225). The differential diagnosis of benign extraovarian serous tumors includes rare cysts of developmental origin with an endosalpingeal lining and a smooth-muscle wall (226).

PERITONEAL MUCINOUS LESIONS

Benign glands of endocervical type involving the peritoneum ("endocervicosis") are rare, but examples involving the posterior uterine serosa and cul-de-sac have been documented (114). Mucinous neoplasms, similar to those occurring within the ovary, have been described

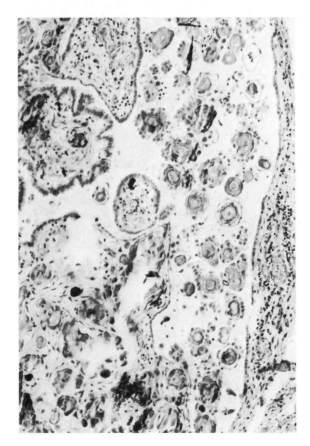

FIG. 25. Extraovarian borderline serous tumor involving the pelvic peritoneum. The ovaries were grossly unremarkable, but their serosal surfaces were involved microscopically by similar tumor.

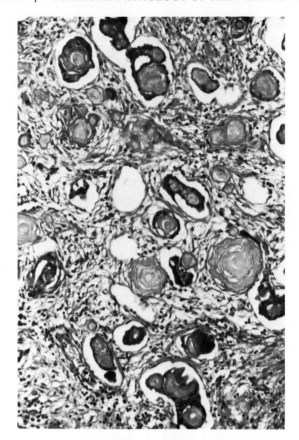

FIG. 26. Extraovarian borderline serous tumor ("psammocarcinoma") involving the omentum. The tumor consists almost entirely of psammoma bodies within a dense fibrous stroma. Some of the psammoma bodies are surrounded by a thin rim of neoplastic epithelial cells.

in extraovarian sites, typically in the retroperitoneum (114,227–230); a single case has been described in the inguinal region (231). These tumors form large cystic masses which, on histologic examination, have resembled ovarian mucinous cystadenomas, borderline tumors, or cystadenocarcinomas, typically containing stroma resembling ovarian stroma in their walls. Although it is possible that some of these tumors originate within a supernumerary ovary, the great rarity of the latter, the absence of follicles or their derivatives within the ovarian-like stroma, and the rare occurrence of similar tumors in males (230) strongly support a peritoneal origin.

PERITONEAL TRANSITIONAL CELL LESIONS

Nests of transitional (urothelial) epithelium, referred to as "Walthard nests," are commonly present on the pelvic peritoneum in women of all ages, typically involving the serosal surfaces of the fallopian tubes, mesosalpinx, and mesovarium (232–234). They are uncommon on the ovarian surface but may be seen in the hilus,

probably originating from the peritoneum of the mesovarium. Walthard nests, which are also seen in men, usually in the vicinity of the epididymis (235), are discussed in more detail in Chapter 50.

SUBPERITONEAL MESENCHYMAL LESIONS

Ectopic Decidua

Clinical and Operative Findings

An ectopic decidual reaction similar to that seen in the lamina propria of the fallopian tube, cervix, and vagina may also be seen within the submesothelial stroma of the peritoneal cavity (236–247). Frequent sites of ectopic decidua include the submesothelial stroma of the fallopian tubes, uterus and uterine ligaments, and appendix and omentum; ectopic decidua is also found within pelvic adhesions. Rare sites have included the serosal surfaces of the diaphragm, liver, and spleen (241,243) as well as the renal pelvis (242).

Submesothelial decidua is typically an incidental microscopic finding, but florid lesions may be visible at the time of cesarean section or postpartum tubal ligation as multiple, gray to white, focally hemorrhagic nodules or plaques studding the peritoneal surfaces and simulating a malignant tumor (243,244). Several cases have been associated with massive, occasionally fatal, intraperitoneal hemorrhage during the third trimester, labor, or the puerperium (244–247). Other rare clinical presentations include abdominal pain, which may simulate that of appendicitis, and hydronephrosis and hematuria secondary to renal pelvic involvement (242,245).

Histologic Appearance

Microscopic examination discloses submesothelial decidual cells disposed individually or arranged in nodules or plaques (Fig. 27). Smooth-muscle cells, probably derived from submesothelial myofibroblasts (237), may be admixed. The decidual foci are typically vascular and contain a sprinkling of lymphocytes. Focal hemorrhagic necrosis and varying degrees of nuclear pleomorphism and hyperchromasia of the decidual cells may suggest a tumor such as a malignant mesothelioma (248), but their generally bland appearance and mitotic inactivity militate against such a diagnosis. We have seen an unusual case of an omental decidual reaction in which most of the decidual cells exhibited striking vacuolation with basophilic mucin and an eccentric location of the nucleus; the appearance of the cells in that case raised the possibility of metastatic signet-ring-cell carcinoma.

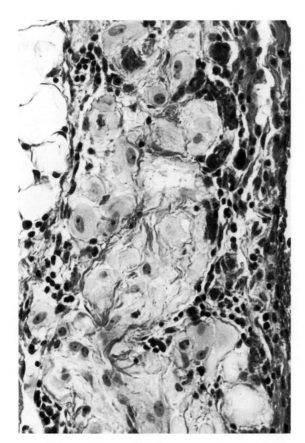

FIG. 27. Ectopic decidua within the omentum. The focus of decidua lies immediately beneath the surface mesothelium and is surrounded by chronic inflammatory cells.

Leiomyomatosis

Disseminated peritoneal leiomyomatosis is a rare disorder characterized by the presence of multiple submesothelial nodules of cytologically benign smooth muscle, frequently associated with uterine leiomyomas and, rarely, ovarian leiomyomas (165–167, 237, 249–252). The nodules are generally considered to arise from multipotential submesothelial mesenchymal cells. This disorder is discussed elsewhere (see Chapter 48).

RETROPERITONEAL LYMPH-NODE LESIONS

Benign Glands of Müllerian Type

Clinical Features

Benign glands of müllerian type are most commonly encountered within pelvic and para-aortic lymph nodes of females (203,205,253–257) and, less often, in inguinal and femoral lymph nodes (258,259). Because these glands are almost always incidental microscopic findings in lymph nodes removed in cases of pelvic carcinoma, their reported frequency has varied, depending on the number of lymph nodes removed and the extent of the histologic sampling. The frequency figures have ranged from 2% to 41%. Almost all of the patients have been adults, although rare occurrences have been reported in children (205). In males, the presence of similar glands have been recorded rarely within lymph nodes in the pelvis and abdomen (260,261) and mediastinum (262). Although typically without clinical or intraoperative manifestations, rare examples of lymph nodes containing müllerian-type glands have been associated with a false-positive lymphangiogram (263), ureteral obstruction secondary to lymph-node enlargement (264), or visible enlargement at the time of operation (265).

In a number of patients, intranodal glandular inclusions have been accompanied by endosalpingiosis of the peritoneum (203,205), salpingitis isthmica nodosa, or acute and chronic salpingitis (205,255,265). Other patients have had coexistent ovarian serous tumors, which have been benign, or borderline tumors, or carcinomas (253,259).

Pathologic Features

On gross examination, the glands are usually not apparent, although rarely they are recognizable as cysts measuring up to a few millimeters in diameter (264,266). The glands are typically located in the periphery of the node, most commonly within its capsule or between the lymphoid follicles in the superficial cortex (Fig. 28); rarely, they lie free within the subcapsular sinuses (255). In florid cases, they can be diffusely distributed throughout the lymph node (255,265). Intraglandular or periglandular psammoma bodies are commonly present. Intranodal glands may be surrounded by a thin rim of fibrous tissue or may abut directly on the surrounding lymphoid cells.

The glands may be round and cystically dilated or may exhibit an irregular contour due to infolding. They are most commonly lined by a single layer of cuboidal to columnar tubal-type epithelium, with an admixture of ciliated, secretory, and intercalated cell types (Fig. 28). With special stains, mucin can be demonstrated in the apical portion of the secretory cells and within the gland spaces (254,265). Acute and chronic inflammatory cells may be present within the lumina. The cells have a benign appearance with regular, basally oriented or pseudostratified, oval to round nuclei, fine nuclear chromatin, and occasional small nucleoli; mitotic figures are typically absent. In rare cases, the cells can exhibit varying degrees of atypia and stratification; the latter can produce an intraglandular cribriform pattern or luminal obliteration by sheets of cells (Fig. 28) (203,253,265).

Examples of intranodal glandular inclusions lined by benign endometrioid epithelium (114,256), mucinous epithelium of endocervical (256,266) or goblet-cell type (261), or metaplastic squamous epithelium (259,267)

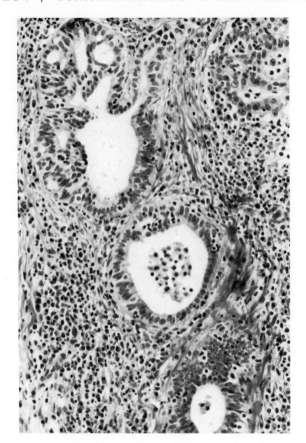

FIG. 28. Typical and atypical endosalpingiotic glands in subcapsular region of a pelvic lymph node. Two glands (*bottom*) are lined by a single layer of benign, ciliated columnar cells. In other glands, the lining cells are atypical and form cribriform arrangements and solid nests that obliterate their lumens.

have been reported. Rarely, endometriotic stroma is present around the glands, warranting a diagnosis of endometriosis.

Differential Diagnosis

In most cases the distinction between glandular inclusions and metastatic adenocarcinoma is not difficult unless a primary ovarian serous tumor of low malignant potential is present, in which case the distinction may be difficult or impossible. Features favoring a benign diagnosis include the following: a capsular or interfollicular location of the glands; lining cells of multiple types, including ciliated forms; a lack of significant cellular atypia and mitotic activity; periglandular basement membranes; and an absence of a desmoplastic stromal reaction (255). Complicating the differential diagnosis is the very rare development of borderline or frankly malignant change in müllerian glandular inclusions in lymph nodes (253, 268). Similarly, intranodal nests of benign squamous epithelium should not be mistaken for metastatic squamous-cell carcinoma (267). Features fa-

voring a benign diagnosis include bland cytological features, mitotic inactivity, and, in some cases, an origin within benign glands.

Ectopic Decidua

Ectopic decidua, unassociated with endometriosis, has been described as a rare, incidental microscopic finding in para-aortic and pelvic lymph nodes, usually removed as part of a radical hysterectomy for carcinoma of the cervix in pregnant patients (240,267,269–272). A subserosal ectopic decidual reaction may be present elsewhere in the pelvis (271). On careful macroscopic examination, the decidual tissue may be recognized as tiny, gray, subcapsular nodules (271). Microscopic examination reveals that the decidual nests typically occupy the subcapsular sinus and superficial cortex (Fig. 29), although more central parts of the lymph node may also be involved. The cells appear benign but may contain occasional bizarre, hyperchromatic nuclei, mimicking metastatic squamous-cell carcinoma (271). The absence of mitotic activity, keratinization, and stromal desmoplasia, should facilitate the diagnosis.

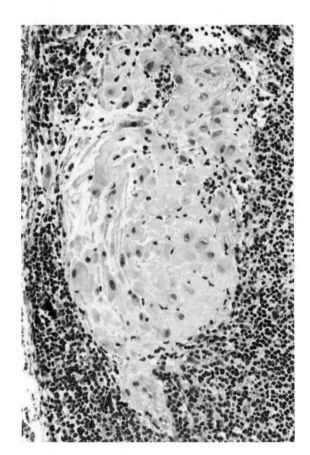

FIG. 29. Ectopic decidua in subcapsular region of a pelvic lymph node.

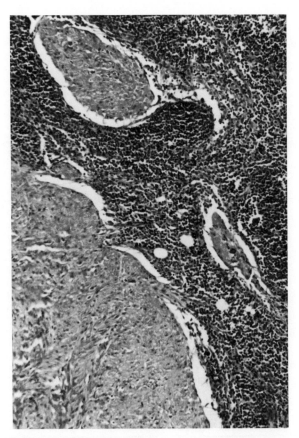

FIG. 30. Leiomyomatosis of pelvic lymph node. Islands of benign smooth muscle replace the normal nodal parenchyma.

Leiomyomatosis

Rare cases of lymph-node involvement by mitotically inactive, cytologically benign smooth muscle have been described (Fig. 30) (165,273–278). Most patients have had concurrent, typical uterine leiomyomas and, less commonly, disseminated peritoneal leiomyomatosis (276) or similar nodules within the lungs (273,275). In pregnant patients, the process may merge with an ectopic decidual reaction (276). The possible histogenesis of the lesion includes an origin from entrapped subcoelomic mesenchyme (278), myofibroblastic organization of intranodal decidua (276), and lymphatic spread from uterine leiomyomas (273,274,277). The presence of benign-appearing smooth muscle in a lymph node should also bring into consideration the diagnosis of lymphangioleiomyomatosis (279), in which there is usually, but not invariably, associated pulmonary involvement.

Benign intranodal smooth muscle should be distinguished from metastatic, well-differentiated leiomyosarcoma of uterine origin. Patients with the latter usually have a large uterine mass, and on histological examination the intranodal tumor is cellular and exhibits evidence of cellular atypicality and mitotic activity.

REFERENCES

1. Targan SR, Chow AW, Guze LB. Role of anaerobic bacteria in spontaneous peritonitis of cirrhosis. Report of two cases and review of the literature. *Am J Med* 1977;62:397–403.
2. Weinstein MP, Iannini PB, Stratton CW, et al. Spontaneous bacterial peritonitis. A review of 28 cases with emphasis on improved survival and factors influencing prognosis. *Am J Med* 1978;64:592–598.
3. Bayer AS, Blumenkrantz MJ, Montgomerie JZ, et al. Candida peritonitis. Report of 22 cases and review of the English literature. *Am J Med* 1976;61:832–840.
4. Williams GT. The peritoneum. In: Morson BC, ed. *Alimentary tract.* New York: Churchill Livingstone, 1987:417–450 (Symmers WSC, ed. Systemic pathology, vol. 3).
5. Kapoor OP, Nathwani BN, Joshi VR. Amoebic peritonitis. A study of 73 cases. *J Trop Med Hyg* 1972;75:11–15.
6. Sohar E, Gafni J, Pras M, et al. Familial Mediterranean fever. A survey of 470 cases and review of the literature. *Am J Med* 1967;43:227–253.
7. Bastani B, Shariatzadeh MR, Dehdashti F. Tuberculous peritonitis. Report of 30 cases and review of the literature. *Q J Med* 1985;56:549–557.
8. Haddad FS, Ghossain A, Sawaya E, et al. Abdominal tuberculosis. *Dis Colon Rectum* 1987;30:724–735.
9. Reddy P, Gorelick DF, Brasher CA, et al. Progressive disseminated histoplasmosis as seen in adults. *Am J Med* 1970;48:629–636.
10. Saw EC, Shields SJ, Comer TP, et al. Granulomatous peritonitis due to coccidioides immitis. *Arch Surg* 1974;108:369–371.
11. Watson NE Jr, Johnson AH. Cryptococcal peritonitis. *South Med J* 1973;66:387–388.
12. Blumberg H, Srinivasan K, Parnes IH. Peritoneal schistosomiasis simulating carcinoma. *NY State J Med* 1966;66:758–761.
13. Sjovall A, Akerman M. Peritoneal granulomas in women due to the presence of *Enterobius S. oxyuris vermicularis*. *Acta Obstet Gynecol Scand* 1968;47:361–372.
14. Dalrymple JC, Hunter JC, Ferrier A, et al. Disseminated intraperitoneal oxyuris granulomas. *Aust NZ J Obstet Gynaecol* 1986;26:90–91.
15. Reddy CRRM, Venkateswar Rao D, Sarma ENB, et al. Granulomatous peritonitis due to ascaris lumbricoides and its ova. *J Trop Med Hyg* 1975;78:146–149.
16. Lintermans JP. Fatal peritonitis, an unusual complication of strongyloides stercoralis infestation. *Clin Pediatr (Phila)* 1975;14:974–975.
17. Coder DM, Olander GA. Granulomatous peritonitis caused by starch glove powder. *Arch Surg* 1972;105:83–86.
18. Ignatius JA, Hartmann WH. The glove starch peritonitis syndrome. *Ann Surg* 1972;175:338–397.
19. Holmes EC, Eggleston JC. Starch granulomatous peritonitis. *Surgery* 1972;71:85–90.
20. Hidvegi D, Hidvegi I, Barrett J. Douche-induced pelvic peritoneal starch granuloma. *Obstet Gynecol* 1978;52:15S–18S.
21. Saxen L, Kassinen A, Saxen E. Peritoneal foreign-body reaction caused by condom emulsion. *Lancet* 1963;1:1295–1296.
22. Nissim F, Ashkenazy M, Borenstein R, et al. Tuberculoid cornstarch granulomas with caseous necrosis. *Arch Pathol Lab Med* 1981;105:86–88.
23. Eiseman B, Seelig MG, Womack NA. Talcum powder granuloma: a frequent and serious postoperative complication. *Ann Surg* 1947;126:820–832.
24. Postlethwait RW, Howard HL, Schanher PW, et al. Comparison of tissue reaction to talc and modified starch glove powder. *Surgery* 1949;25:22–29.
25. Castelli MJ, Armin A, Husain A, et al. Fibrosing peritonitis in a drug abuser. *Arch Pathol Lab Med* 1985;109:767–769.
26. Tinker MA, Burdman D, Deysine M, et al. Granulomatous peritonitis due to cellulose fibers from disposable surgical fabrics. *Ann Surg* 1974;180:831–835.
27. Godleski JJ, Gabriel KL. Peritoneal responses to implanted fabrics used in operating rooms. *Surgery* 1981;90:828–834.
28. Janoff K, Wayne R, Huntwork B, et al. Foreign body reactions secondary to cellulose lint fibers. *Am J Surg* 1984;147:598–600.

29. Park SA, Giannattasio C, Tancer ML. Foreign body reaction to the intraperitoneal use of avitene. *Obstet Gynecol* 1981;58:664–668.

30. Norris JC, Davison TC. Peritoneal reaction to liquid petrolatum. *JAMA* 1934;103:1846–1847.

31. Teilum G, Madsen V. Endometriosis ovarii et peritonaei caused by hysterosalpingography. *Br J Obstet Gynaecol* 1950;57:10–16.

32. Marshall SF, Forse RA. Peritoneal adhesions: report of a case of paraffinoma. *Surg Clin North Am* 1952;32:903–908.

33. Davies JD, Ansell ID. Food-starch granulomatous peritonitis. *J Clin Pathol* 1983;36:435–438.

34. Kay S. Tissue reaction to barium sulfate contrast medium. *Arch Pathol* 1954;57:279–284.

35. Waxman M, Boyce JG. Intraperitoneal rupture of benign cystic ovarian teratoma. *Obstet Gynecol* 1976;48:9S–13S.

36. Stuart GCE, Smith JP. Ruptured benign cystic teratomas mimicking gynecologic malignancy. *Gynecol Oncol* 1983;16:139–143.

37. Stern JL, Buscema J, Rosenshein NB, et al. Spontaneous rupture of benign cystic teratomas. *Obstet Gynecol* 1981;57:365–366.

38. Freedman SI, Ang EP, Herz MG, et al. Meconium granulomas in post-cesarean section patients. *Obstet Gynecol* 1982;59:383–385.

39. Herz MG, Stanley WD, Toot PJ, et al. Symptomatic maternal intraperitoneal meconium granulomata. Report of two cases. *Diagn Gynecol Obstet* 1982;4:147–149.

40. Tibboel D, Gaillard JLJ, Molenaar JC. The importance of mesenteric vascular insufficiency in meconium peritonitis. *Hum Pathol* 1986;17:411–416.

41. Forouhar F. Meconium peritonitis. Pathology, evolution, and diagnosis. *Am J Clin Pathol* 1982;78:208–213.

42. Chen KTK, Kostich ND, Rosai J. Peritoneal foreign body granulomas to keratin in uterine adenoacanthoma. *Arch Pathol Lab Med* 1978;102:174–177.

43. Sanner RF Jr. Chronic idiopathic bile peritonitis. *JAMA* 1965;194:238–240.

44. Daum F, Boley SJ, Cohen MI. Miliary Crohn's disease. *Gastroenterol* 1974;67:527–530.

45. Wong M, Rosen SW. Ascites in sarcoidosis due to peritoneal involvement. *Ann Intern Med* 1962;57:277–280.

46. Isenberg JI, Gilbert SB, Pitcher JL. Ascites with peritoneal involvement in Whipple's disease. *Gastroenterol* 1971;60:305–310.

47. Weibel MA, Majno G. Peritoneal adhesions and their relation to abdominal surgery. *Am J Surg* 1973;126:345–353.

48. McCaughey WTE, Al-Jabi M. Differentiation of serosal hyperplasia and neoplasia in biopsies. In: Sommers SC, Rosen PR, Fechner RE, eds. *Pathology annual, part 1.* New York: Appleton-Century-Crofts, 1986:271–292.

49. Wanless IR, Bernier V. Fibrous thickening of the splenic capsule. *Arch Pathol Lab Med* 1983;107:595–599.

50. Buhac I, Jarmolych J. Histology of the intestinal peritoneum in patients with cirrhosis of the liver and ascites. *Dig Dis Sci* 1978;23:417–422.

51. Concato L. Sulla poliomenorrhea scrofolosa o tisi delle sierose. *G Intern Sci Med* 1881;3:1037–1053.

52. Dehn TCB, Lucas MG, Wood RFM. Idiopathic sclerosing peritonitis. *Postgrad Med J* 1985;61:841–842.

53. Foo KT, Ng KC, Rauff A, et al. Unusual small intestinal obstruction in adolescent girls: the abdominal cocoon. *Br J Surg* 1978;65:427–430.

54. Marshall AJ, Baddeley H, Barritt DW, et al. Practolol peritonitis. A study of 16 cases and a survey of small bowel function in patients taking beta adrenergic blockers. *Q J Med* 1977;46:135–149.

55. Bradley JA, McWhinnie DL, Hamilton DNH. Sclerosing obstructive peritonitis after continuous ambulatory peritoneal dialysis. *Lancet* 1983;2:113–114.

56. Cambria RP, Shamberger RC. Small bowel obstruction caused by the abdominal cocoon syndrome: possible association with the LeVeen shunt. *Surgery* 1984;95:501–503.

57. Sayfan J, Adam YG, Reif R. Peritoneal encapsulation in childhood. Case report, embryologic analysis, and review of literature. *Am J Surg* 1979;138:725–727.

58. Sieck JO, Cowgill R, Larkworthy W. Peritoneal encapsulation and abdominal cocoon. Case report and review of the literature. *Gastroenterology* 1983;84:1597–1601.

59. Adams HW, Mainz DL. Eosinophilic ascites. A case report and review of the literature. *Dig Dis Sci* 1977;22:40–42.

60. Metzger AL, Coyne M, Lee S, et al. *In vivo* LE cell formation in peritonitis due to systemic lupus erythematosus. *J Rheumatol* 1974;1:130–133.

61. Lomholt G, Hjorth N, Fischermann K. Lethal peritonitis from Degos' disease (malign and atrophic papulosis). *Acta Chir Scand* 1968;134:495–501.

62. Foyle A, Al-Jabi M, McCaughey WTE. Papillary peritoneal tumors in women. *Am J Surg Pathol* 1981;5:241–249.

63. Hansen RM, Caya JG, Clowry LJ Jr, et al. Benign mesothelial proliferation with effusion. Clinicopathologic entity that may mimic malignancy. *Am J Med* 1984;77:887–892.

64. McCaughey WTE, Kannerstein M, Churg J. Tumors and pseudotumors of the serous membranes. In: *Atlas of Tumor Pathology,* series 2, fascicle 20. Washington, DC, Armed Forces Institute of Pathology, 1985.

65. Rosai J, Dehner LP. Nodular mesothelial hyperplasia in hernia sacs. A benign reactive condition stimulating a neoplastic process. *Cancer* 1975;35:165–175.

66. Weiss SW, Tavassoli FA. Multicystic mesothelioma. An analysis of pathologic findings and biologic behavior in 37 cases. *Am J Surg Pathol* 1988;12:737–746.

67. Ross MJ, Welch WR, Scully RE. Multilocular peritoneal inclusion cysts (so-called cystic mesotheliomas). *Cancer* 1989;64:1336–1346.

68. Katsube Y, Mukai K, Silverberg SG. Cystic mesothelioma of the peritoneum. A report of five cases and review of the literature. *Cancer* 1982;50:1615–1622.

69. Dumke K, Schnoy N, Specht G, et al. Comparative light and electron microscopic studies of cystic and papillary tumors of the peritoneum. *Virchows Arch [A]* 1983;399:25–39.

70. Mennemeyer R, Smith M. Multicystic, peritoneal mesothelioma. A report with electron microscopy of a case mimicking intra-abdominal cystic hygroma (lymphangioma). *Cancer* 1979;44:692–698.

71. Miles JM, Hart WR, McMahon JT. Cystic mesothelioma of the peritoneum. Report of a case with multiple recurrences and review of the literature. *Cleve Clin Q* 1986;53:109–114.

72. Moor JH Jr, Crum CP, Chandler JG, Feldman PS. Benign cystic mesothelioma. *Cancer* 1980;45:2395–2399.

73. McFadden DE, Clement PB. Peritoneal inclusion cysts with mural mesothelial proliferation. A clinicopathological analysis of six cases. *Am J Surg Pathol* 1986;10:844–854.

74. Blumberg NA, Murrary JF. Multicystic peritoneal mesothelioma. *SA Med J* 1981;59:85–86.

75. Sienkowski I, Russell AJ, Dilly SA, et al. Peritoneal cystic mesothelioma: an electron microscopic and immunohistochemical study of two male patients. *J Clin Pathol* 1986;39:440–445.

76. Kjellevold K, Nesland JM, Holm R, et al. Multicystic peritoneal mesothelioma. *Pathol Res Pract* 1986;181:767–771.

77. Harper GB Jr, Awbrey BJ, Thomas CG Jr, et al. Mesothelial cysts of the round ligament simulating inguinal hernia. Report of four cases and review of the literature. *Am J Surg* 1986;151:515–517.

78. Demopoulos RI, Kahn MA, Feiner HD. Epidemiology of cystic mesotheliomas. *Int J Gynecol Pathol* 1986;5:379–381.

79. Gussman D, Thickman D, Wheeler JE. Postoperative peritoneal cysts. *Obstet Gynecol* 1986;68:53S–55S.

80. Lees RF, Feldman PS, Brenbridge NAG, et al. Inflammatory cysts of the pelvic peritoneum. *AJR* 1978;131:633–636.

81. Auerbach RD, Kohorn EI, Cornelius EA, et al. Splenosis: a complicating factor in total abdominal hysterectomy. *Obstet Gynecol* 1985;65:65S–68S.

82. Brewster DC. Splenosis. *Am J Surg* 1973;126:14–19.

83. Fleming CR, Dickson ER, Harrison EG Jr. Splenosis: autotransplantation of splenic tissue. *Am J Med* 1976;61:414–419.

84. Overton TH. Splenosis: a cause of pelvic pain. *Am J Obstet Gynecol* 1982;143:969–970.

85. Watson WJ, Sundwall DA, Benson WL. Splenosis mimicking endometriosis. *Obstet Gynecol* 1982;59:51S–53S.

86. Afonso JF, Martin GM, Nisco FS, et al. Melanogenic ovarian tumors. *Am J Obstet Gynecol* 1962;84:667–676.

87. Fukushima M, Sharpe L, Okagaki T. Peritoneal melanosis sec-

ondary to a benign dermoid cyst of the ovary: a case report with ultrastructural study. *Int J Gynecol Pathol* 1984;2:403–409.

88. Lee D, Pontifex AH. Melanosis peritonei. *Am J Obstet Gynecol* 1975;122:526–527.

89. Young, RH, Clement PB, McCaughey WTE. Solitary fibrous tumors ("Fibrous mesotheliomas") of the peritoneum. A report of three cases and a review of one literature. *Arch Pathol Lab Med* 1990;114:493–495.

90. Hanrahan JB. A combined papillary mesothelioma and adenomatoid tumor of the omentum. Report of a case. *Cancer* 1963;16:1497–1500.

91. Craig JR, Hart WR. Extragenital adenomatoid tumor. Evidence for the mesothelial theory of origin. *Cancer* 1979;433:1678–1679.

92. Daya D, McCaughey WTE. Well-differentiated papillary mesothelioma of the peritoneum. A clinicopathologic study of 22 cases. *Cancer* 1990;65:292–296.

93. Goepel JR. Benign papillary mesothelioma of peritoneum: a histological, histochemical and ultrastructural study of six cases. *Histopathology* 1981;5:21–30.

94. McCaughey WTE. Papillary peritoneal neoplasms in females. In: Sommers SC, Rosen PR, Fechner RE, eds. *Pathology annual, part 2.* New York: Appleton-Century-Crofts, 1985:387–404.

95. Kannerstein M, Churg J. Peritoneal mesothelioma. *Hum Pathol* 1977;8:83–94.

96. Riddell RH, Goodman MJ, Moossa AR. Peritoneal malignant mesothelioma in a patient with recurrent peritonitis. *Cancer* 1981;48:134–139.

97. Antman KH, Klegar KL, Pomfret EA, et al. Early peritoneal mesothelioma: a treatable malignancy. *Lancet* 1985;2:977–981.

98. Kitazawa M, Kaneko H, Toshima M, et al. Malignant peritoneal mesothelioma with massive foamy cells. *Acta Pathol Jpn* 1984;34:687–692.

99. Churg A. Immunohistochemical staining for vimentin and keratin in malignant mesothelioma. *Am J Surg Pathol* 1985;9:360–365.

100. Loosli H, Hurlimann J. Immunohistological study of malignant diffuse mesotheliomas of the pleura. *Histopathology* 1984;8:793–803.

101. Gibbs AR, Harach R, Wagner JC, et al. Comparison of tumour markers in malignant mesothelioma and pulmonary adenocarcinoma. *Thorax* 1985;40:91–95.

102. Tron V, Wright JL, Churg A. Carcinoembryonic antigen and milk-fat globule protein staining of malignant mesothelioma and adenocarcinoma of the lung. *Arch Pathol Lab Med* 1987;111:291–293.

103. Silcocks PB, Herbert A, Wright DH. Evaluation of PAS-diastase and carcinoembryonic antigen staining in the differential diagnosis of malignant mesothelioma and papillary serous carcinoma of the ovary. *J Pathol* 1986;149:133–141.

104. Otis CN, Carter D, Cole S, et al. Immunohistochemical evaluation of pleural mesothelioma and pulmonary adenocarcinoma. A bi-institutional study of 47 cases. *Am J Surg Pathol* 1987;11:445–456.

105. Blobel GA, Moll R, Franke WW, et al. The intermediate filament cytoskeleton of mesotheliomas and its diagnostic significance. *Am J Pathol* 1985;121:235–247.

106. Kondi-Paphitis A, Addis BJ. Secretory component in pulmonary adenocarcinoma and mesothelioma. *Histopathology* 1986;10:1279–1287.

107. Mainguene C, Aillet G, Kremer M, et al. Immunohistochemical study of ovarian tumors using the OC 125 monoclonal antibody as a basis for potential *in vivo* and *in vitro* applications. *J Nucl Med Allied Sci* 1986;30:19–22.

108. Merino MJ, Livolsi VA. Signet ring carcinoma of the female breast: a clinicopathologic analysis of 24 cases. *Cancer* 1981;48:1830–1837.

109. Qizilbash AH. Mucoceles of the appendix. Their relationship to hyperplastic polyps, mucinous cystadenomas, and cystadenocarcinomas. *Arch Pathol* 1975;99:548–555.

110. Higa E, Rosai J, Pizzimbono CA, et al. Mucosal hyperplasia, mucinous cystadenoma, and mucinous cystadenocarcinoma of the appendix. A re-evaluation of appendiceal "mucocele". *Cancer* 1973;32:1525–1541.

111. Campbell JS, Lou P, Ferguson JP, et al. Pseudomyxoma peritonei et ovarii with occult neoplasms of appendix. *Obstet Gynecol* 1973;42:897–902.

112. Limber GK, King RE, Silverberg SG. Pseudomyxoma peritonaei: a report of ten cases. *Ann Surg* 1973;178:587–593.

113. Chejfec G, Rieker WJ, Jablokow VR, et al. Pseudomyxoma peritonei associated with colloid carcinoma of the pancreas. *Gastroenterology* 1986;90:202–205.

114. Lauchlan SC. The secondary mullerian system. *Obstet Gynecol Surv* 1972;27:133–146.

115. Ober WB, Black MB. Neoplasms of the subcoelomic mesenchyme. *Arch Pathol Lab Med* 1955;59:698–705.

116. Clement PB. Endometriosis, lesions of the secondary mullerian system, and pelvic mesothelial proliferations. In: Kurman RJ, ed. *Blaustein's pathology of the female genital tract.* New York: Springer-Verlag, 1987:516–559.

116a.Clement PB, Young RH, Scully RE. Stromal endometriosis of the uterine cervix. A variant of endometriosis that may simulate a sarcoma. *Am J Surg Pathol* 1990;14:449–455.

116b.Clement PB. Pathology of endometriosis. *Pathology Annual* 1990;25(1):245–295.

117. Fox H, Buckley CH. Current concepts of endometriosis. *Clin Obstet Gynaecol* 1984;11:279–287.

118. Jansen RPS, Russell P. Nonpigmented endometriosis: clinical, laparoscopic, and pathologic definition. *Am J Obstet Gynecol* 1986;155:1154–1159.

119. Dmowski WP. Pitfalls in clinical, laparoscopic and histologic diagnosis of endometriosis. *Acta Obstet Gynecol Scand [Suppl]* 1984;123:61–66.

120. Cantor JO, Fenoglio CM, Richart RM. A case of extensive abdominal endometriosis. *Am J Obstet Gynecol* 1979;134:846–847.

121. Scully RE, Richardson GS, Barlow JF. The development of malignancy in endometriosis. *Clin Obstet Gynecol* 1966;9:384–411.

122. Mostoufizadeh M, Scully RE. Malignant tumors arising in endometriosis. *Clin Obstet Gynecol* 1980;23:951–963.

123. Dmowski WP, Radwanska E. Current concepts on pathology, histogenesis and etiology of endometriosis. *Acta Obstet Gynecol Scand [Suppl]* 1984;123:29–33.

124. Egger H, Weigmann P. Clinical and surgical aspects of ovarian endometriotic cysts. *Arch Gynecol* 1982;233:37–45.

125. Floberg J, Backdahl M, Silfersward C, Thomassen PA. Postpartum perforation of the colon due to endometriosis. *Acta Obstet Gynecol Scand* 1984;63:183–184.

126. Anderson M, Edmond RM. Rupture of an endometriotic cyst in late pregnancy. *Br J Obstet Gynaecol* 1974;81:907–908.

127. Rossman F, D'Ablaing III G, Marrs RP. Pregnancy complicated by ruptured endometrioma. *Obstet Gynecol* 1983;62:519–521.

128. Rogers WS, Seckinger DL. Decidual tissue as a cause of intraabdominal hemorrhage during labor. *Obstet Gynecol* 1965;25:391–397.

129. Bergqvist A, Ljungberg O, Myhre E. Human endometrium and endometriotic tissue obtained simultaneously: a comparative histological study. *Int J Gynecol Pathol* 1984;3:135–145.

130. Kempers RD, Dockerty MB, Hunt AB, et al. Significant postmenopausal endometriosis. *Surg Gynecol Obstet* 1960;111:348–356.

131. Hamperl H. Uber fluorescierende Kornchensellen ("Fluorocyten"). *Virchows Arch* 1950;318:33–47.

132. Novak ER. Pathology of endometriosis. *Clin Obstet Gynecol* 1960;3:413–428.

133. Clement PB, Young RH, Scully RE. Necrotic pseudoxanthomatous nodules of the ovary and peritoneum in endometriosis. *Am J. Surg Pathol* 1988;12:390–397.

134. Schmidt CL, Demopoulos RI, Weiss G. Infected endometriotic cysts: clinical characterization and pathogenesis. *Fertil Steril* 1981;36:27–30.

135. Czernobilsky B, Morris WJ. A histologic study of ovarian endometriosis with emphasis on hyperplastic and atypical changes. *Obstet Gynecol* 1979;53:318–323.

136. Schuger L, Simon A, Okon E. Cytomegaly in benign ovarian cysts. *Arch Pathol Lab Med* 1986;110:928–929.

137. Rutgers JL, Scully RE. Ovarian müllerian mucinous papillary cystadenomas of borderline malignancy: a clinicopathological analysis. *Cancer* 1988;61:340–348.

138. Rutgers JL, Scully RE. Ovarian mixed-epithelial papillary cystadenomas of borderline malignancy of mullerian type: a clinicopathological analysis. *Cancer* 1988;61:546–554.

139. Rohlfing MB, Kao KJ, Woodard BH. Endomyometriosis: possible association with leiomyomatosis disseminata and endometriosis [Letter]. *Arch Pathol Lab Med* 1981;105:556–557.

140. Cozzutto C. Uterus-like mass replacing ovary. Report of a new entity. *Arch Pathol Lab Med* 1981;105:508–511.

141. Scully RE. Smooth-muscle differentiation in genital tract disorders [Editorial]. *Arch Pathol Lab Med* 1981;105:505–507.

142. McDougal RA, Roth LM. Ovarian adenomyoma associated with an endometriotic cyst. *South Med J* 1986;79:640–642.

143. Pueblitz-Peredo S, Luevano-Flores E, Rincon-Taracena R, Ochoa-Carrillo FJ. Uteruslike mass of the ovary: endomyometriosis or congenital malformation? A case with a discussion of histogenesis. *Arch Pathol Lab Med* 1985;109:361–364.

144. Chalmers JA. Mulleroma—a rare cause of dysmenorrhoea. *Br J Obstet Gynaecol* 1961;68:762–764.

145. Kurman RJ, Funk RL, Kirshenbaum AH. Spina bifida with associated choristoma of mullerian origin. *J Pathol* 1969;99:324–327.

146. Rosai J. Uteruslike mass replacing ovary [Letter]. *Arch Pathol Lab Med* 1982;106:364.

147. Lauchlan SC. The cytology of endometriosis. *Am J Obstet Gynecol* 1966;94:533–535.

148. von Numers C. Observations on metaplastic changes in the germinal epithelium of the ovary and on the aetiology of ovarian endometriosis. *Acta Obstet Gynecol Scand* 1965;44:107–116.

149. Leiman G, Naylor G. Mucinous metaplasia in scar endometriosis. Diagnosis by aspiration cytology. *Diagn Cytopathol* 1985;1:153–156.

150. Young RH, Prat J, Scully RE. Endometrioid stromal sarcomas of the ovary. A clinicopathologic analysis of 23 cases. *Cancer* 1984;53:1143–1155.

151. Gerbie AB, Greene RR, Reis RA. Heteroplastic bone and cartilage in the female genital tract. *Obstet Gynecol* 1958;11:573–578.

152. Shipton EA, Meares SD. Heterotopic bone formation in the ovary. *Aust NZ J Obstet Gynaecol* 1965;5:100–102.

153. Roth LM. Endometriosis with perineural involvement. *Am J Clin Pathol* 1973;59:807–809.

154. Abdel-Shahid RB, Beresford JM, Curry RH. Endometriosis of the ureter with vascular involvement. *Obstet Gynecol* 1974;43:113–117.

155. Kapadia SB, Russak RR, O'Donnell WF, Harris RN, Lecky JW. Postmenopausal ureteral endometriosis with atypical adenomatous hyperplasia following hysterectomy, bilateral oophorectomy, and long-term estrogen therapy. *Obstet Gynecol* 1984;64:60S–63S.

156. Granai CO, Walters MD, Safaii H, et al. Malignant transformation of vaginal endometriosis. *Obstet Gynecol* 1984;64:592–595.

157. Ray J, Conger M, Ireland K. Ureteral obstruction in postmenopausal woman with endometriosis. *Urology* 1985;26:577–578.

158. Young EE, Gamble CN. Primary adenocarcinoma of the rectovaginal septum arising from endometriosis. Report of a case. *Cancer* 1969;24:597–601.

159. Kistner RW. Current status of the hormonal treatment of endometriosis. *Clin Obstet Gynecol* 1966;9:271–292.

160. Moller NE. The Arias-Stella phenomenon in endometriosis. *Acta Obstet Gynecol Scand* 1959;38:271–274.

161. Sobel HJ, Marquet E, Schwarz R, et al. Optically clear endometrial nuclei. *Ultrast Pathol* 1984;6:229–231.

162. Fechner RE. The surgical pathology of the reproductive system and breast during oral contraceptive therapy. In: Sommers SC, Rosen PR, eds. *Pathology annual.* New York: Appleton-Century-Crofts, 1971:299–319.

163. Pedersen H, Rank F. Morphology of endometriosis before and during treatment with danazol. *Acta Obstet Gynecol Scand* [Suppl] 1984;123:13–14.

164. Schweppe KW, Wynn RM. Endocrine dependency of endometriosis: an ultrastructural study. *Eur J Obstet Gynecol Reprod Biol* 1984;17:193–208.

165. Horie A, Ishii N, Matsumoto M, et al. Leiomyomatosis in the pelvic lymph node and peritoneum. *Acta Pathol Jpn* 1984;34:813–819.

166. Kaplan C, Bernirschke K, Johnson KC. Leiomyomatosis peritonealis disseminata with endometrium. *Obstet Gynecol* 1980;55:119–122.

167. Kuo T, London SN, Dinh TV. Endometriosis occurring in leiomyomatosis peritonealis disseminata. Ultrastructural study and histogenetic consideration. *Am J Surg Pathol* 1980;4:197–204.

168. Albukerk JN, Berlin M, Palladino VC, et al. Endometriosis in peritoneal gliomatosis [Letter]. *Arch Pathol Lab Med* 1979;103:98–99.

169. Bassler R, Theele CH, Labach H. Nodular and tumorlike gliomatosis peritonei with endometriosis caused by a mature ovarian teratoma. *Pathol Res Pract* 1982;175:392–403.

170. Sinder C, Dochat GR, Wentsler NE. Splenoendometriosis. *Am J Obstet Gynecol* 1965;92:883–884.

171. Herbold DR, Frable WJ, Kraus FT. Isolated noninfectious granuloma of the ovary. *Int J Gynecol Pathol* 1984;2:380–391.

172. Brooks JJ, Wheeler JE. Malignancy arising in extragonadal endometriosis. A case report and summary of the world literature. *Cancer* 1977;40:3065–3073.

173. Russell P. The pathological assessment of ovarian neoplasms. II. The proliferating "epithelial" tumours. *Pathology* 1979;11:251–282.

174. Goldberg MI, Ng ABP, Belinson JL, et al. Clear cell adenocarcinoma arising in endometriosis of the rectovaginal septum. *Obstet Gynecol* 1978;51:38S–40S.

175. Gray LA, Barnes ML. Relation of endometriosis to ovarian carcinoma. *Am Surg* 1965;31:798–806.

176. Lele SB, Piver S, Barlow JJ, et al. Squamous cell carcinoma arising in ovarian endometriosis. *Gynecol Oncol* 1978;6:290–293.

177. Chen KTK, Weilert M. Squamous cell carcinoma arising in endometriosis. *Diagn Gynecol Obstet* 1982;4:343–346.

178. Berkowitz RS, Ehrmann RL, Knapp RC. Endometrial stromal sarcoma arising from vaginal endometriosis. *Obstet Gynecol* 1978;51:34S–37S.

179. Crum CP, Wible J, Frick HC, Fenoglio CM, Richart RM, Williamson S. A case of extensive pelvic endometriosis terminating in endometrial sarcoma. *Am J Obstet Gynecol* 1981;140:718–719.

180. Chumas JC, Thanning L, Mann WJ. Malignant mixed mullerian tumor arising in extragenital endometriosis: report of a case and review of the literature. *Gynecol Oncol* 1986;23:227–233.

181. Cooper P. Mixed mesodermal tumour and clear cell carcinoma arising in ovarian endometriosis. *Cancer* 1978;42:2827–2831.

182. Mahoney AD, Waisman J, Zeldis LJ. Adenomyoma. A precursor of extrauterine mullerian adenosarcoma? *Arch Pathol Lab Med* 1977;101:579–584.

183. Lankerani MR, Aubrey RW, Reid JD. Endometriosis of the colon with mixed "germ cell" tumor. *Am J Clin Pathol* 1982;78:555–559.

184. Rutgers JL, Young RH, Scully RE. Ovarian yolk sac tumor arising from an endometrioid carcinoma. *Hum Pathol* 1987;18:1296–1299.

185. Hafiz MA, Toker C. Multicentric ovarian and extraovarian cystadenofibroma. *Obstet Gynecol* 1986;68:94S–98S.

186. Ortega I, Nogales F, Gonzalez-Campora R, et al. Extragenital endometrioid cystadenofibroma. *Acta Obstet Gynecol Scand* 1982;61:283–284.

187. Clark JE, Wood H, Jaffurs WJ, et al. Endometrioid-type cystadenocarcinoma arising in the mesosalpinx. *Obstet Gynecol* 1979;54:656–658.

188. Ulbright TM, Kraus FT. Endometrial stromal tumors of extrauterine tissue. *Am J Clin Pathol* 1981;76:371–377.

189. Hasiuk AS, Petersen RO, Hanjani P, et al. Extragenital malignant mixed mullerian tumor. Case report and review of the literature. *Am J Clin Pathol* 1984;81:102–105.

190. Bard ES, Bard DS, Vargas-Cortes F. Extrauterine mullerian adenosarcoma; a clinicopathologic report of a case with distant metastases and review of the literature. *Gynecol Oncol* 1978;6:261–274.

191. Clement PB, Scully RE. Extrauterine mesodermal (mullerian) adenosarcoma. A clinicopathologic analysis of five cases. *Am J Clin Pathol* 1978;69:276–283.

192. Russell P, Slavutin L, Laverty CR, et al. Extrauterine mesodermal (mullerian) adenosarcoma. A case report. *Pathology* 1979;11:557–560.

193. Zinsser KR, Wheeler JE. Endosalpingiosis in the omentum. A study of autopsy and surgical material. *Am J Surg Pathol* 1982;6:109–117.

194. Tutschka BG, Lauchlan SC. Endosalpingiosis. *Obstet Gynecol* 1980;55:57S–60S.

195. Holmes MD, Levin HS, Ballard LA. Endosalpingiosis. *Cleve Clin Q* 1981;48:345–352.

196. Kern WH. Benign papillary structures with psammoma bodies in culdocentesis fluid. *Acta Cytol* 1969;13:178–180.

197. Chen KTK. Psammoma bodies in pelvic washings [Letter]. *Acta Cytol* 1983;27:377–379.

198. Sneige M, Fernandez T, Copeland LJ, et al. Mullerian inclusions in peritoneal washings. *Acta Cytol* 1986;30:271–276.

199. Picoff RC, Meeker CI. Psammoma bodies in the cervicovaginal smear in association with benign papillary structures of the ovary. *Acta Cytol* 1970;14:45–47.

200. McCaughey WTE, Kirk ME, Lester W, et al. Peritoneal epithelial lesions associated with proliferative serous tumours of the ovary. *Histopathology* 1984;8:195–208.

201. Burmeister RE, Fechner RE, Franklin RR. Endosalpingiosis of the peritoneum. *Obstet Gynecol* 1969;34:310–318.

202. Bryce RL, Barbatis C, Charnock M. Endosalpingiosis in pregnancy. Case report. *Br J Obstet Gynecol* 1982;89:166–168.

203. Chen KTK. Benign glandular inclusions of the peritoneum and periaortic lymph nodes. *Diagn Gynecol Obstet* 1981;3:265–268.

204. Dallenbach-Hellweg G. Atypical endosalpingiosis: a case report with consideration of the differential diagnosis of glandular subperitoneal inclusions. *Pathol Res Pract* 1987;182:180–182.

205. Shen SC, Bansal M, Purrazzella R, et al. Benign glandular inclusions in lymph nodes, endosalpingiosis, and salpingitis isthmica nodosa in a young girl with clear cell adenocarcinoma of the cervix. *Am J Surg Pathol* 1983;7:293–300.

206. Dore N, Landry M, Cadotte M, et al. Cutaneous endosalpingiosis. *Arch Dermatol* 1980;116:909–912.

207. Sinykin MB. Endosalpingiosis. *Minn Med* 1960;43:759–761.

208. Schuldenfrei R, Janovski NA. Disseminated endosalpingiosis associated with bilateral papillary serous cystadenocarcinoma of the ovaries. A case report. *Am J Obstet Gynecol* 1962;84:382–389.

209. Bransilver BR, Ferenczy A, Richart RM. Female genital tract remnants. An ultrastructural comparison of hydatid of Morgagni and mesonephric ducts and tubules. *Arch Pathol Lab Med* 1973;96:255–261.

210. Bell DA, Scully RE. Serous borderline tumors of the peritoneum. *Am J Surg Path* 1990;14:230–239.

210a. Bell DA, Scully RE. Benign and borderline serous lesions of the peritoneum in women. *Pathology Annual* 1989;24(2):1–21.

211. McCaughey WTE, Schryer MJP, Lin X, et al. Extraovarian pelvic serous tumor with marked calcification. *Arch Pathol Lab Med* 1986;110:78–80.

211a. Gilks CB, Bell DA, Scully RE. Serous psammomocarcinoma of the ovary and peritoneum. *Int J Gynecol Pathol* 1990;9:110–121.

212. Kannerstein M, Churg J, McCaughey WTE, et al. Papillary tumors of the peritoneum in women: mesothelioma or papillary carcinoma. *Am J Obstet Gynecol* 1977;127:306–314.

213. Mills SE, Anderson WA. Fechner RE, Austin MB. Serous surface papillary carcinoma. A clinicopathologic study of 10 cases and comparison with stage III-IV ovarian serous carcinoma. *Am J Surg Pathol* 1988;12:827–832.

214. August CZ, Murad TM, Newton M. Multiple focal extraovarian serous carcinoma. *Int J Gynecol Pathol* 1985;4:11–23.

215. Gooneratne S, Sassone M, Blaustein A, et al. Serous surface papillary carcinoma of the ovary: a clinicopathologic study of 16 cases. *Int J Gynecol Pathol* 1982;1:258–269.

216. White PF, Merino MJ, Barwick KW. Serous surface papillary carcinoma of the ovary: a clinical, pathologic, ultrastructural, and immunohistochemical study of 11 cases. In: Sommers SC, Rosen PR, Fechner RE, eds. *Pathology annual, part 1.* New York: Appleton-Century-Crofts, 1985:403–418.

216a. Fromm G, Gershenson DM, Silva EG. Papillary serous carcinoma of the peritoneum. *Obstet Gynecol* 1990;75:89–95.

216b. Truong LD, Maccata ML, Awalt H, Cagle PT, Schwartz MR, Kaplan AL. Serous surface carcinoma of the peritoneum: A clinicopathologic study of 22 cases. *Human Pathol* 1990;21:99–110.

216c. Raju U, Fine G, Greenwald KA, Ohorodnik JM. Primary papillary serous neoplasia of the peritoneum: A clinicopathologic and ultrastructural study of eight cases. *Hum Pathol* 1989;20:426–436.

216d. Dalrymple JC, Bannatyne P, Russell P, et al. Extraovarian peritoneal serous papillary carcinoma. A clinicopathologic study of 31 cases. *Cancer* 1989;64:110–115.

217. Genadry R, Parmley T, Woodruff JD. The origin and clinical behaviour of the parovarian tumor. *Am J Obstet Gynecol* 1977;129:873–879.

218. Honore LH, Nickerson KG. Papillary serous cystadenoma arising in a paramesonephric cyst of the parovarium. *Am J Obstet Gynecol* 1976;125:870–871.

219. Kanbour A, Salazar H, Stock R. Papillary cystadenoma originating in hydatid cyst of morgagni: clinicopathologic study and observations on histogenesis [Abstract]. *Lab Invest* 1978;38:350.

220. Steinberg L, Rothman D, Drey NW. Mullerian cyst of the retroperitoneum. *Am J Obstet Gynecol* 1970;107:963–964.

221. Czernobilsky B, Lancet M. Broad ligament adenocarcinoma of mullerian origin. *Obstet Gynecol* 1972;40:238–242.

222. Chandraratnam E, Leong AS-Y. Papillary serous cystadenoma of borderline malignancy arising in a parovarian paramesonephric cyst. Light microscopic and ultrastructural observations. *Histopathology* 1983;7:601–611.

223. D'Ablaing III G, Klatt EC, DiRocco G, et al. Broad ligament serous tumor of low malignant potential. *Int J Gynecol Pathol* 1983;2:93–99.

224. Stapleton JJ, Haber MH, Lindner LE. Paramesonephric papillary serous cystadenocarcinoma. A case report with scanning electron microscopy. *Acta Cytol* 1981;25:310–316.

225. Ulbright TM, Morley DJ, Roth LM, et al. Papillary serous carcinoma of the retroperitoneum. *Am J Clin Pathol* 1983;79:633–637.

226. Harpaz N, Gellman E. Urogenital mesenteric cyst with fallopian tubal features. *Arch Pathol Lab Med* 1987;111:78–80.

227. Williams PP, Gall SA, Prem KA. Ectopic mucinous cystadenoma. A case report. *Obstet Gynecol* 1971;38:831–837.

228. Douglas GW, Kastin AJ, Huntington RW Jr. Carcinoma arising in a retroperitoneal mullerian cyst, with widespread metastasis during pregnancy. *Am J Obstet Gynecol* 1965;91:210–216.

229. Fujii S, Konishi I, Okamura H, et al. Mucinous cystadenocarcinoma of the retroperitoneum: a light and electron microscopic study. *Gynecol Oncol* 1986;24:103–112.

230. Roth LM, Ehrlich CE. Mucinous cystadenocarcinoma of the retroperitoneum. *Obstet Gynecol* 1977;49:486–488.

231. Sun CJ, Toker C, Masi JD, et al. Primary low grade adenocarcinoma occurring in the inguinal region. *Cancer* 1979;44:340–345.

232. Bransilver BR, Ferenczy A, Richart RM. Brenner tumors and Walthard cell nests. *Arch Pathol Lab Med* 1974;98:76–86.

233. Roth LM. The Brenner tumor and the Walthard cell nest. An electron microscopic study. *Lab Invest* 1974;31:15–23.

234. Teoh TB. The structure and development of Walthard nests. *J Pathol* 1953;66:433–439.

235. Sundarasivarao D. The mullerian vestiges and benign epithelial tumours of the epididymis. *J Pathol Bacteriol* 1953;66:417–432.

236. Bersch W, Alexy E, Heuser HP, Staemmler HJ. Ectopic decidua formation in the ovary. *Virchows Arch [A]* 1973;360:173–177.

237. Herr JC, Platz CE, Heidger PM Jr, et al. Smooth muscle within ovarian decidual nodules: a link to leiomyomatosis peritonealis disseminata? *Obstet Gynecol* 1979;53:451–456.

238. Israel SL, Rubenstone A, Meranze DR. The ovary at term I. Decidua-like reaction and surface cell proliferation. *Obstet Gynecol* 1954;3:399–407.

239. Ober WB, Grady HG, Schoenbucher AK. Ectopic ovarian decidua without pregnancy. *Am J Pathol* 1957;33:199–214.

240. Zaytsev P, Taxy JB. Pregnancy-associated ectopic decidua. *Am J Surg Pathol* 1987;11:526–530.

241. Harbitz HF. Ectopic decidua. *Acta Pathol Microbiol Scand [Suppl]* 1936;26:16–20.

242. Bettinger HF. Ectopic decidua in renal pelvis. *J Pathol Bacteriol* 1947;5:686–687.

243. O'Sullivan D, Heffernan CK. Deciduosis peritonei in pregnancy. Report of two cases. *Br J Obstet Gynaecol* 1960;67:1013–1016.

244. Kwan D, Pang LSC. Deciduosis peritonei. *Br J Obstet Gynecol* 1964;71:804–806.

245. Hulme-Moir I, Ross MS. A case of early postpartum abdominal

pain due to hemorrhagic deciduosis peritonei. *Br J Obstet Gynaecol* 1969;76:746–749.

246. Sabatelle R, Winger E. Postpartum intraabdominal hemorrhage caused by ectopic deciduosis. *Obstet Gynecol* 1973;41:873–875.

247. Richter MA, Choudhry A, Barton JJ, et al. Bleeding ectopic decidua as a cause of intraabdominal hemorrhage. A case report. *J Reprod Med* 1983;28:430–432.

248. Talerman A, Montero JR, Chilcote RR, et al. Diffuse malignant peritoneal mesothelioma in a 13-year-old girl. Report of a case and review of the literature. *Am J Surg Pathol* 1985;9:73–80.

249. Parmley TH, Woodruff JD, Winn K, et al. Histogenesis of leiomyomatosis peritonealis disseminata (disseminated fibrosing deciduosis). *Obstet Gynecol* 1975;46:511–516.

250. Pieslor PC, Orenstein JM, Hogan DL, et al. Ultrastructure of myofibroblasts and decidualized cells in leiomyomatosis peritonealis disseminata. *Am J Clin Pathol* 1979;72:875–882.

251. Tavassoli FA, Norris HJ. Peritoneal leiomyomatosis (leiomyomatosis peritonealis disseminata): a clinicopathologic study of 20 cases with ultrastructural observations. *Int J Gynecol Pathol* 1982;1:59–74.

252. Valente PT. Leiomyomatosis peritonealis disseminata. A report of two cases and review of the literature. *Arch Pathol Lab Med* 1984;108:669–672.

253. Ehrmann RL, Federschneider JM, Knapp RC. Distinguishing lymph node metastases from benign glandular inclusions in low-grade ovarian carcinoma. *Am J Obstet Gynecol* 1980;136:737–746.

254. Karp LA, Czernobilsky B. Glandular inclusions in pelvic and abdominal para-aortic lymph nodes. *Am J Clin Pathol* 1969;52:212–218.

255. Kheir SM, Mann WJ, Wilkerson JA. Glandular inclusions in lymph nodes. The problem of extensive involvement and relationship to salpingitis. *Am J Surg Pathol* 1981;5:353–359.

256. Russell P, Laverty CR. Benign "müllerian" rests in pelvic lymph node. *Pathology* 1980;12:129–130.

257. Schnurr RC, Delgado G, Chun B. Benign glandular inclusions in para-aortic lymph nodes in women undergoing lymphadenectomies. *Am J Obstet Gynecol* 1978;130:813–816.

258. Silton RM. More glandular inclusions [Letter]. *Am J Surg Pathol* 1979;3:285–286.

259. Schneider V. Benign glandular lymph node inclusions. *Diagn Gynecol Obstet* 1980;2:313–320.

260. Huntrakoon M. Benign glandular inclusions in the abdominal lymph nodes of a man. *Hum Pathol* 1985;16:644–646.

261. Tazelaar HD, Vareska G. Benign glandular inclusions. *Hum Pathol* 1986;17:100–101.

262. Longo S. Benign lymph node inclusions. *Hum Pathol* 1976;7:349–354.

263. Schneider V, Walsh JW, Goplerud DR. Benign glandular inclusions in para-aortic lymph nodes: a cause for false positive lymphangiography. *Am J Obstet Gynecol* 1980;138:350–352.

264. Weir JH, Janovski NA. Paramesonephric lymph-node inclusions—a cause of obstructive uropathy. *Obstet Gynecol* 1963;21:363–367.

265. Kempson RL. Consultation Case. *Am J Surg Pathol* 1978;2:321–325.

266. Ferguson BR, Bennington JL, Haber SL. Histochemistry of mucosubstances and histology of mixed mullerian pelvic lymph node glandular inclusions. Evidence for histogenesis by mullerian metaplasia of coelomic epithelium. *Obstet Gynecol* 1969;33:617–625.

267. Mills SE. Decidua and squamous metaplasia in abdominopelvic lymph nodes. *Int J Gynecol Pathol* 1983;2:209–215.

268. Koss LG. Miniature adenoacanthoma arising in an obturator lymph node. Report of a case. *Cancer* 1963;16:1369–1372.

269. Ashraf M, Boyd CB, Beresford WA. Ectopic decidual reaction in para-aortic and pelvic lymph nodes in the presence of cervical squamous cell carcinoma during pregnancy. *J Surg Oncol* 1984;26:6–8.

270. Burnett RA, Millan D. Decidual change in pelvic lymph nodes: a source of possible diagnostic error. *Histopathology* 1986;1089–1092.

271. Covell LM, Disciullo AJ, Knapp RC. Decidual change in pelvic lymph nodes in the presence of cervical squamous cell carcinoma during pregnancy. *Am J Obstet Gynecol* 1977;127:674–676.

272. Yoonessi M, Satchindanand SK, Ortinez CG, et al. Benign glandular elements and decidual reaction in retroperitoneal lymph nodes. *J Surg Oncol* 1982;19:81–86.

273. Boyce CR, Buddhdev HN. Pregnancy complicated by metastasizing leiomyoma of the uterus. *Obstet Gynecol* 1973;42:252–258.

274. Abell MR, Littler ER. Benign metastasizing uterine leiomyoma. Multiple lymph nodal metastases. *Cancer* 1975;36:2206–2213.

275. Cramer SF, Meyer JS, Kraner JF, et al. Metastasizing leiomyoma of the uterus. S-phase fraction, estrogen receptor, and ultrastructure. *Cancer* 1980;45:932–937.

276. Hsu YK, Rosenshein NB, Parmley TH, et al. Leiomyomatosis in pelvic lymph nodes. *Obstet Gynecol* 1981;57:91S–93S.

277. Idelson MG, Davids AM. Metastasis of uterine fibroleiomyomata. *Obstet Gynecol* 1963;21:78–85.

278. Rigaud C, Bogomoletz WV. Leiomyomatosis in pelvic lymph node [Letter]. *Arch Pathol Lab Med* 1983;107:153–154.

279. Bhattacharyya AK, Balogh K. Retroperitoneal lymphangioleiomyomatosis. A 36-year benign course in a postmenopausal woman. *Cancer* 1985;56:1144–1146.

Subject Index